Essentials of Vascular Surgery for the General Surgeon

Vivian Gahtan • Michael J. Costanza
Editors

Essentials of Vascular Surgery for the General Surgeon

Springer

Editors
Vivian Gahtan, MD, FACS
Chief, Division of Vascular Surgery
and Endovascular Services
SUNY Upstate Medical University
Syracuse, NY, USA

Lead Physician, Vascular Surgery
Department of Veterans Affairs Healthcare
Network Upstate New York at Syracuse
Syracuse, NY, USA

Michael J. Costanza, MD, FACS
VA Health Care Network Upstate
New York at Syracuse
SUNY Upstate Medical University
Manlius, NY, USA

Vascular Surgeon
Department of Veterans Affairs Healthcare
Network Upstate New York at Syracuse
Syracuse, NY, USA

ISBN 978-1-4939-1325-1 ISBN 978-1-4939-1326-8 (eBook)
DOI 10.1007/978-1-4939-1326-8
Springer New York Heidelberg Dordrecht London

Library of Congress Control Number: 2014950048

Printed on acid-free paper

Springer is part of Springer Science+Business Media (www.springer.com)

Preface

Strictly defined, vascular surgery involves performing procedures on blood vessels outside the heart and brain. Although this definition is technically accurate, it only scratches the surface of vascular surgery in the twenty-first century. Vascular surgeons operate on arterial and venous disease, repair hemorrhagic injuries, perform endovascular interventions, create vascular access, and manage diabetic foot infections to name just a few areas of practice. Although vascular surgery emerged as a subspecialty in the 1980s, this field still plays an important role in general surgery training and practice. Since fewer than 3,000 board certified vascular surgeons practice in the USA, many general surgeons rely on their vascular surgery experience during residency to treat patients with vascular problems. In a recent review of operative logs from nearly 5,000 surgeons, the American Board of Surgery found that general surgeons performed 46 % of vascular surgery procedures [1]. Although efforts to increase the number of vascular surgeons have begun, general surgeons will continue to care for vascular patients given the rapidly increasing elderly population and the comparatively small number of residency and fellowship trained vascular surgeons entering the work force each year. Unfortunately, the training that general surgery residents receive in vascular surgery has become less consistent as vascular practice moves toward endovascular therapy. For many general surgery residents, the breadth of their case volume in vascular surgery experience has narrowed to dialysis access, amputation, and varicose vein management.

Therefore, finding an appropriate reference book for general surgeons who treat vascular patients can be challenging. Multi-volume textbooks of vascular surgery provide an extremely detailed and comprehensive approach to vascular conditions that may not readily translate into real-world practice. At the other extreme, general surgery textbooks condense vascular surgery into a few chapters that often lack the technical details and treatment guidelines valued by a practicing surgeon. This book directly addresses the needs of general surgeons who perform vascular surgery during residency training, clinical practice, or both. As a clinically oriented resource this book focuses on the diagnosis and clinical management of vascular conditions while describing the technical details and pitfalls to avoid when performing common vascular surgery procedures. Ideally this book will serve as a "one stop" information source that surgeons and trainees will turn to as a valuable reference, surgical atlas, and study guide.

The contributing authors have used clear illustrations and evidence based treatment recommendations to create clinically relevant chapters. The first chapter provides an organized approach to the vascular patient with an emphasis on history, physical exam, risk factors, and diagnostic options. Most vascular conditions require some form of physiologic study or imaging exam to clarify the diagnosis and assist with treatment planning. Chapter 2 lays the foundation for successful vascular surgery by illustrating common vascular exposures and describing fundamental technical principles unique to arterial surgery. The rest of the book is organized into parts on arterial disease, venous disease, vascular trauma, vascular access, and complex vascular conditions.

The chapters on acute arterial disease outline the management and surgical techniques for the treatment of acute limb ischemia, compartment syndrome, and diabetic foot infections. Restoring flow to an acutely ischemic limb is one of the defining interventions of vascular surgery. In many cases, an expeditious surgical thrombectomy as described in Chap. 3 can be the difference between limb salvage and major amputation. Likewise, compartment syndrome represents a limb threatening condition that may require immediate intervention by a general surgeon. Chapter 4 explains and illustrates the steps involved in a fasciotomy which can be a limb saving procedure. Diabetic foot infections are included in this part (Chap. 5) because of their tendency to require acute surgical intervention. Failure to recognize and adequately debride diabetic foot infections when indicated can have devastating local and systemic consequences.

Chronic arterial disease is addressed in chapters on the management of claudication, critical limb ischemia, and lower extremity amputation. Peripheral arterial disease (PAD) affects tens of millions of patients and can cause disabling symptoms. Chapter 6 discusses the diagnosis and risk factors associated with claudication while providing an overview of the medical, endovascular, and surgical treatment options. Chronic critical limb ischemia can manifest as ischemic rest pain, non-healing ulcers, or gangrene. Chapter 7 focuses on recognizing critical limb ischemia and preparing patients for limb salvage which may involve surgical, endovascular, and medical therapy. In some patients, complete limb preservation is not possible and an amputation is required. A well performed amputation of the toe, forefoot, or leg can have a significant impact on a patient's recovery potential and quality of life. Chapter 8 provides guidelines for choosing the appropriate level of amputation and gives a detailed description of several common amputations.

The part on venous disease includes chapters on deep and superficial venous thrombosis, chronic venous insufficiency, varicose veins, and inferior vena cava (IVC) filter placement. Acute deep venous thrombosis (DVT) poses an immediate life threatening problem if it becomes a pulmonary embolism (PE) and a long term disability risk if it causes venous dysfunction. Chapter 9 discusses the medical, endovascular, and surgical treatment modalities for acute DVT which are aimed at minimizing the short and long term clinical impact of venous thrombosis. Rarely, anti-coagulation failure or contraindication warrants placement of an IVC filter to reduce the risk of pulmonary embolism. Chapter 13 outlines the indications and risks associated with IVC filters and describes the technical aspects of placing and retrieving IVC filters. Superficial venous thrombosis (SVT) can complicate intravenous access and may become an important clinical problem with the increasing use of peripherally inserted central catheters (PICC lines). Chapter 10 provides practical guidelines for recognizing and managing SVT. Chronic venous disease encompasses a wide spectrum of clinical disorders ranging from spider veins to non-healing venous ulcers. Chapter 11 focuses on the pathophysiology and non-interventional treatment strategies for chronic venous insufficiency while Chap. 12 describes various techniques for treatment of varicose veins and superficial venous insufficiency.

The part on vascular trauma emphasizes surgical intervention for blood vessel injuries that occur in the neck, abdomen, and extremity. Modern management of vascular neck trauma incorporates the injury location, hemodynamic status of the patient, and imaging results. Chapter 14 describes the surgical approach and technical details involved in repairing arterial and venous injuries in each anatomic zone of the neck. Abdominal vascular injuries often prove to be fatal without prompt surgical exposure and effective vascular control. Chapter 15 illustrates and explains the maneuvers necessary to isolate, clamp, and repair the major abdominal vessels. Extremity vascular trauma poses an ischemic and hemorrhagic risk which may require immediate revascularization or temporary stabilization followed by delayed definitive repair. Chapter 16 reviews the management of extremity vascular injury including anatomic exposures, the use of tourniquets and shunts, and revascularization principles.

All surgeons regularly encounter patients with vascular access issues. Nearly half a million people receive hemodialysis in the USA, and most critically ill patients require some form of central venous access. Chapter 17 provides an overview of venous access options and describes insertion techniques aimed at maximizing safety and efficiency. Establishing and maintaining hemodialysis access can be a challenging undertaking that requires planning, persistence, and technical skill. Chapter 18 illustrates and explains the most common arteriovenous access procedures while Chap. 19 focuses on the recognition and management of vascular access complications.

The final part covers a wide range of vascular topics that are associated with more complicated clinical issues. These chapters provide a broad overview of the diagnosis and treatment principles for vascular conditions that usually warrant referral to a vascular specialist. Chapter 20 summarizes the most recent data and guidelines for managing patients with carotid, renal, and mesenteric stenosis. Chapter 21 describes the surgical and endovascular treatment options for aortic pathology including dissections, aneurysms, and traumatic transections. Non-atherosclerotic diseases often pose a diagnostic challenge because of their rarity and unusual clinical manifestations. Chapter 22 provides a well-organized and concise reference for evaluating patients with hypercoaguable disorders, vasculitis, and other uncommon conditions. All surgeons caring for vascular patients must be prepared to recognize and treat hemorrhagic and infectious complications. Chapter 23 uses clear treatment algorithms to explain the management of common complications associated with vascular surgery and endovascular interventions.

Approximately 75 % of general surgery residents plan to pursue fellowship training in one of a dozen or more clinical areas [2]. Despite this trend toward subspecialization, general surgeons still derive benefit from their training and experience in vascular surgery. The ability to control bleeding, restore perfusion, establish vascular access, and manage the increasing number of patients with atherosclerotic and venous disease remain valuable skills for general surgeons. Practicing surgeons and surgical trainees can now turn to this book as a concise and clinically oriented information source for vascular surgery.

Syracuse, NY, USA

Vivian Gahtan, MD, FACS
Michael J. Costanza, MD, FACS

References

1. Valentine JR, Jones A, Biester TW, Cogbill TH, Borman KR, Rhodes RS. General surgery workloads and practice patterns in the United States, 2007–2009: A 10 year update from the American Board of Surgery. Ann Surg. 2011;254:520–6.
2. Borman KR, Vick LR, Biester TW, Mitchell ME. Changing demographics of residents choosing fellowships: longterm data from the American Board of Surgery. J Am Coll Surg. 2008;206:782–8.

Contents

Contributors

Ahmed M. Abou-Zamzam, Jr., MD, FACS Division of Vascular Surgery, Loma Linda University School of Medicine, Loma Linda, CA, USA

Ali F. AbuRahma, MD Department of Surgery, Robert C. Byrd Health Sciences Center, West Virginia University, Charleston, WV, USA

Kwame S. Amankwah, MD, MSc, FACS Division of Vascular Surgery, Department of Surgery, SUNY Upstate Medical University, University Hospital, Syracuse, NY, USA

Department of Surgery and Radiology, Veterans Administration Hospital Upstate Healthcare Network, Syracuse, NY, USA

Enrico Ascher, MD Division of Vascular Surgery, Department of Surgery, Lutheran Medical Center, Brooklyn, NY, USA

Faisal Aziz, MD Department of Surgery/Vascular Surgery, Penn State Hershey College of Medicine, Heart and Vascular Institute, Hershey, PA, USA

Hussein Barayan, MD Jobst Vascular Institute, ProMedica Toledo Hospital, Toledo, OH, USA

Marshall E. Benjamin, MD Department of Vascular Surgery, University of Maryland Baltimore Washington Medical Center, Maryland Vascular Center, University of Maryland, Glen Burnie, MD, USA

Col (ret) Mark W. Bowyer, MD, FACS, DMCC The Norman M. Rich Department of Surgery, Uniformed Services University of the Health Sciences, Bethesda, MD, USA

Jeffrey P. Carpenter, MD Department of Surgery, Cooper Medical School, Camden, NJ, USA

Anjuli R. Cherukuri, MD Division of Vascular Surgery and Endovascular Services, Department of Surgery, SUNY Upstate Medical University, Syracuse, NY, USA

Jason T. Chiriano, DO, FACS Department of Cardiovascular and Thoracic Surgery, Loma Linda University Medical Center, Loma Linda, CA, USA

Anthony J. Comerota, MD, FACS, FACC Jobst Vascular Institute, ProMedica Toledo Hospital, Toledo, OH, USA

Section of Vascular Surgery, Cardiovascular Center, University of Michigan Medical Center, Ann Arbor, MI, USA

Michael J. Costanza, MD, FACS Division of Vascular Surgery and Endovascular Services, Department of Surgery, SUNY Upstate Medical University, Syracuse, NY, USA

Department of Veterans Affairs Healthcare Network Upstate New York at Syracuse, Syracuse, NY, USA

Mitchell W. Cox, MD Department of Surgery, Duke University School of Medicine, Duke University Medical Center, Durham, NC, USA

Mark G. Davies, MD, PhD, MBA Vascular and Endovascular Surgery, Houston Methodist DeBakey Heart &Vascular Center, Houston Methodist Hospital, Houston, TX, USA

Ellen D. Dillavou, MD, FACS, RPVI Department of Surgery/Vascular Surgery, University of Pittsburgh Medical Center, Pittsburgh, PA, USA

Hasan Haldun Dosluoglu, MD, FACS State University of New York at Buffalo, Buffalo, NY, USA

Department of Surgery, Division of Vascular Surgery, VA Western New York Healthcare System, Buffalo, NY, USA

Joseph J. DuBose, MD University of Maryland Health System, R Adams Cowley Shock Trauma Center, United States Air Force Baltimore Center for the Sustainment of Trauma and Readiness Skills (CSTARS), Baltimore, MD, USA

The Norman M. Rich Department of Surgery, The Uniformed Services University of the Health Sciences, Bethesda, MD, USA

Department of Cardiovascular Surgery, University of Texas Houston, Houston, TX, USA

William R. Flinn, MD Department of Vascular Surgery, University of Maryland Baltimore Washington Medical Center, Maryland Vascular Center, University of Maryland School of Medicine, Glen Burnie, MD, USA

Vivian Gahtan, MD, FACS Division of Vascular Surgery and Endovascular Services, SUNY Upstate Medical University, Syracuse, NY, USA

Department of Veterans Affairs Healthcare Network Upstate New York at Syracuse, Syracuse, NY, USA

Michael A. Golden, MD Division of Vascular Surgery and Endovascular Therapy, Department of Surgery, Penn Presbyterian Medical Center, Philadelphia, PA, USA

Linda M. Harris, MD Division of Vascular Surgery, Department of Surgery, Kaleida Health Buffalo General Medical Center, Buffalo, NY, USA

Jennifer A. Heller, MD, FACS Department of Surgery, John Hopkins Vein Centers, Johns Hopkins University, Baltimore, MD, USA

Anil Hingorani, MD Vascular Institute of New York, Lutheran Medical Center, Brooklyn, NY, USA

Division of Vascular Surgery, Department of Surgery, Lutheran Medical Center, Brooklyn, NY, USA

Shih Yau Grace Huang, MD Division of Vascular Surgery and Endovascular Therapy, University of Southern California, Los Angeles, CA USA

Chinenye O. Iwuchukwu, MD, MPH Department of General Surgery, SUNY Upstate University Hospital, Syracuse, NY, USA

Department of Surgery, SUNY Upstate Medical University, Syracuse, NY, USA

Department of Veterans Affairs Healthcare Network Upstate New York at Syracuse, Syracuse, NY, USA

Misaki M. Kiguchi, MD, MBA Department of Surgery/Vascular Surgery, University of Pittsburgh Medical Center, Pittsburgh, PA, USA

Purandath Lall, MBBS, FRCS(Ed), FACS Department of Surgery, Division of Vascular Surgery, South West Regional Health Authority, San Fernando, Trinidad and Tobago

James Lukan, MD Department of Surgery, Erie County Medical Center, University of Buffalo, Buffalo, NY, USA

Justin K. Nelms, MD Department of Vascular Surgery, University of Maryland Baltimore Washington Medical Center, Maryland Vascular Center, University of Maryland School of Medicine, Glen Burnie, MD, USA

David G. Neschis, MD Department of Surgery, Baltimore Washington Medical Center, Glen Burnie, MD, USA

Richard F. Neville, MD Division of Vascular Surgery, The George Washington University MFA, Washington, DC, USA

Patrick Joshua O'Brien, MD Department of Surgery, International Heart Institute of Montana, Missoula, MT, USA

Kathleen J. Ozsvath, MD The Vascular Group, Albany Medical College, Albany Medical Center Hospital, Albany, NY, USA

Todd E. Rasmussen, MD US Army Institute of Surgical Research, Joint Base Fort Sam Houston (San Antonio), San Antonio, TX, USA

US Combat Casualty Care Research Program, Fort Detrick, MD, USA

The Norman M. Rich Department of Surgery, The Uniformed Services University of the Health Sciences, Bethesda, MD, USA

Amy B. Reed, MD, FACS Department of Vascular Surgery, Penn State Hershey College of Medicine, Heart and Vascular Institute, Hershey, PA, USA

Afsoon D. Roberts, MD Division of Infectious Diseases, The George Washington University MFA, Washington, DC, USA

Vincent L. Rowe, MD, FACS Division of Vascular and Endovascular Surgery, Department of Surgery, Keck School of Medicine at University of Southern California, Los Angeles, CA, USA

Mathew Adam Schechter, MD Department of Surgery, Duke University School of Medicine, Duke University Medical Center, Durham, NC, USA

Gary L. Simon, MD, PhD Division of Infectious Diseases, The George Washington University MFA, Washington, DC, USA

Patrick A. Stone, MD Department of Surgery, Robert C. Byrd Health Sciences Center, West Virginia University, Charleston, WV, USA

Carlos H. Timaran, MD Division of Vascular and Endovascular Surgery, Department of Surgery, University of Texas Southwestern Medical Center, Dallas, TX, USA

Brant W. Ullery, MD Division of Vascular Surgery and Endovascular Therapy, Department of Surgery, University of Pennsylvania, Philadelphia, PA, USA

Sarah M. Wartman, MD Division of Vascular Surgery and Endovascular Therapy, University of Southern California, Los Angeles, CA, USA

Eanas S. Yassa, MD Department of Vascular Surgery, Frederik Meijer Heart and Vascular Institute, Spectrum Health, MI, USA

Part I

Basics of Vascular Surgery

1 Diagnosis and Imaging

Ali F. AbuRahma and Patrick A. Stone

The wide spectrum of vascular signs and symptoms requires an organized approach to the patient suspected of having arterial or venous disease. This chapter focuses on the essential information that a general surgeon needs to recognize and investigate patients with vascular disease. The basic concepts of noninvasive tests including ultrasound are also described because these exams play a central role in the diagnosis and confirmation of vascular disease. A brief description of the indications and limitations of other imaging options, e.g., magnetic resonance angiography, computed tomography, and catheter angiography, is also included.

Approach to the Patient with Vascular Disease

Key Points of History and Physical

The physical examination of the patient with vascular disease begins when he or she enters the office. Patients can be assessed for functional status: oxygen tank in hand, wheelchair, use of a cane, or normal ambulation and gait. With this initial assessment the surgeon can gauge the ability of the patient to tolerate a vascular reconstruction. Patients with limited functional status are unlikely to be ideal candidates for major surgery.

Carotid Artery Occlusive Disease

Approximately 80 % of strokes are ischemic and 20 % are hemorrhagic. Hemodynamically significant carotid stenosis is the most common cause of ischemic stroke accounting for 20–30 % of ischemic strokes. A directed history can help determine if a patient with carotid stenosis is symptomatic or asymptomatic. Ipsilateral monocular blindness or amaurosis fugax is usually described as a shade being pulled down over one eye. Vision loss lasts for a few minutes before returning to normal. Transient ischemic attacks (TIA) consist of contralateral episodic paresthesia and motor deficits, slurred speech, or aphasia. By definition, TIA symptoms resolve in less than 24 h; however, the typical TIA lasts only a few minutes. If a neurologic deficit persists for more than 24 h, it is considered a stroke. Brain imaging performed for atypical neurologic symptoms can confirm the presence of a stroke. In the landmark North American Symptomatic Carotid Endarterectomy Trial (NASCET), symptoms had to occur within the previous 120 days for patients to be classified as "symptomatic" [1].

Physical examination of the patient with suspected carotid stenosis should include an evaluation for conditions that could complicate surgical intervention including scars from previous surgery, soft tissue changes caused by neck radiation, and unfavorable body habitus (obesity, short neck). Voice quality should also be assessed to evaluate for a previous laryngeal nerve injury. Auscultation of the neck can detect carotid bruits which signify carotid stenosis in up to one third of patients.

Peripheral Artery Disease (PAD)

Clinical symptoms of PAD vary along a spectrum of severity ranging from mild intermittent claudication to limb-threatening trophic changes. Claudication involves lower extremity muscle pain precipitated by walking that resolves with rest. Pain localizes to the muscle groups one level distal to the arterial stenosis or occlusion. For example, disease involving the superficial femoral artery manifests as calf claudication while aortoiliac occlusive disease usually causes hip or thigh discomfort with walking. Patients with PAD and claudication have adequate blood flow at rest; pain

A.F. AbuRahma, MD (✉) • P.A. Stone, MD
Department of Surgery, Robert C. Byrd Health Sciences Center, West Virginia University, 3110 MacCorkle Ave., SE, Charleston, WV 25304, USA
e-mail: ali.aburahma@camc.org

V. Gahtan and M.J. Costanza (eds.), *Essentials of Vascular Surgery for the General Surgeon*, DOI 10.1007/978-1-4939-1326-8_1, © Springer Science+Business Media New York 2015

occurs only when the increased metabolic demand created by exercising muscle exceeds the available blood supply due to the degree of fixed arterial obstruction [2]. Aside from diminished distal pulses, physical findings are usually absent at this stage.

The differential diagnosis of intermittent claudication should include musculoskeletal and neurologic causes of lower extremity pain. Calf claudication symptoms can occur because of venous obstruction, chronic compartment syndrome, nerve root compression, or a Baker's cyst. Chronic compartment syndrome typically causes a tight bursting sensation in the calf while symptoms associated with venous obstruction often require leg elevation for relief. Hip or buttock claudication should be differentiated from pain related to spinal cord compression or hip arthritis. Patients with spinal cord compression often have a history of back pain and complain of leg symptoms that occur when standing and require a change in position as well as rest for relief. Arthritis causes pain in one or several joints that is triggered by variable amounts of exercise. Foot pain or in step claudication due to PAD rarely occurs and should be distinguished from other causes related to arthritis or inflammatory processes.

In patients with ischemic rest pain arterial occlusive disease is so severe that lower extremity perfusion fails to meet the basal metabolic demands of nerves in the foot. In this limb-threatening condition, burning pain in the forefoot typically increases when the patient is supine and is mitigated to some degree with the foot in a dependent position. Patients with ischemic rest pain occasionally present with chronic lower leg edema because of their tendency to keep the foot in a dependent position, often hanging the leg over the side of the bed at night. This physical finding can create a confusing clinical picture and trigger an evaluation for venous thrombosis unless the health care provider performs a careful history and physical to detect the presence of arterial disease. Physical findings in patients with advanced arterial disease include decreased skin temperature and delayed capillary refill, as well as Buerger's signs (dependent rubor and pallor on elevation). Trophic changes represent the most severe manifestations of chronically impaired lower extremity circulation. These changes range from subtle signs such as dependent rubor, cyanosis, loss of hair or nail substance, and atrophy of skin and muscle to frank ulceration and gangrene. The presence of trophic changes indicates impending limb loss and requires urgent intervention for limb salvage [3].

Many patients with PAD have disease in other vascular territories including the coronary, carotid, and renal arteries with consequences, i.e. renal impairment that may affect diagnostic strategies [4]. A thorough vascular evaluation should elicit symptoms of angina or transient ischemic attacks in addition to documenting a history of prior myocardial infarction or stroke. Men with PAD symptoms should be questioned about the presence of erectile dysfunction which frequently occurs in association with aortoiliac arterial occlusive disease.

Table 1.1 Classification of peripheral arterial disease (PAD): Rutherford categories

Grade	Category	Clinical description
0	0	Asymptomatic
I	1	Mild claudication
I	2	Moderate claudication
I	3	Severe claudication
II	4	Ischemic rest pain
III	5	Minor tissue loss
III	6	Major tissue loss

Reprinted from AbuRahma and Campbell [9], p. 269

Pulses should be palpated at all levels of the lower extremity: femoral, popliteal, dorsal pedal, and posterior tibial. Pulse strength can be quantified on a 3-point scale: +2 (normal), +1 (diminished), and 0 (no palpable pulse). If the pulse is not palpable, a handheld Doppler should be used to determine the presence or absence of flow in the vessel. If a Doppler signal is present, it should be described as monophasic, biphasic, or triphasic.

PAD Staging

After making the diagnosis of chronic lower extremity ischemia, efforts should focus on establishing the severity of disease. The stage of PAD and the natural history of each stage ultimately determine the most appropriate therapeutic modality. Most vascular surgeons use Rutherford's classification that defines claudication categories 0–3 as asymptomatic, mild, moderate, and severe, respectively (Table 1.1) [5]. Categories 4–6 encompass ischemic rest pain and minor and major tissue loss in patients with critical limb ischemia. Rutherford's classification provides a standardized method for describing the clinical situation and documenting improvement or deterioration over time [5]. The other classification that is used by our medical colleagues is the Fontaine classification. In this classification, the stages of the disease are categorized into class I through IV (class I corresponds to Rutherford category 0 and class IV corresponds to Rutherford's category 3).

Aneurysms

An aneurysm is defined as abnormal dilatation of a blood vessel greater than 1.5 times the size of the native vessel at that location. Most abdominal aortic aneurysms (AAA) are asymptomatic and are only detected by physical exam or as an incidental finding on an imaging study. Rare symptoms of an intact AAA include abdominal or back pain and compressive symptoms on the gastrointestinal tract or genitourinary system related to the size of the aneurysm. Although the classic triad of a ruptured AAA involves abdominal and/or back pain, hypotension, and a pulsatile abdominal mass, most patients do not have all three signs at their initial presentation.

Abdominal examination should include deep palpation of abdomen for the presence of a pulsatile mass. The width of the aortic pulsation provides some estimation of the size of the aneurysm. Rectal examination can be helpful to detect large aneurysms of the internal iliac arteries. The femoral and popliteal arteries should be examined in all patients with diagnosis of a AAA because of the association between abdominal and peripheral aneurysms. Widened pulses in the popliteal fossa are the most common finding in patients with popliteal aneurysms.

Venous Disease

Venous disease can present with a variety of symptoms. The spectrum of symptomatic venous reflux ranges from cosmetic concerns to leg swelling and lower extremity skin ulceration in severe cases. Physical examination should assess for edema, varicose veins, skin changes (stasis dermatitis or lipodermatosclerosis), and active or healing ulcerations which typically occur over the medial malleolus region.

Other Vascular Disorders

A directed history and physical exam plays an important role in planning vascular access in patients with chronic kidney disease. Patients should be questioned about previous central venous catheter, pacemaker, or defibrillator placement and a history of previous access surgery and/or radial artery harvest for coronary artery bypass should be elicited. The Kidney Disease Outcome Quality Initiative (K-DOQI) guideline recommends performing a preoperative venogram in patients with any of the above circumstances prior to proceeding with upper extremity vascular access creation. Physical examination in these patients should evaluate for signs of previous central venous access such as scars in neck or chest wall, as well as chest wall devices, i.e., ports, pacemakers, and automatic implantable cardioverter defibrillators. Prominent venous collaterals on the chest wall should also raise suspicion for chronic central venous stenosis or occlusion.

Cardiovascular Risk Factors

The probability that a patient has vascular disease depends in part on his or her demographics and underlying clinical conditions. These cardiovascular risk factors include hypertension, hypercholesterolemia, cigarette smoking, diabetes mellitus, obesity, stress, family history, and sedentary lifestyle.

Age

The incidence and prevalence of PAD significantly increase with age. Approximately 12 % of adult men aged between 55 and 74 years have PAD [6].

Gender

The prevalence of PAD is slightly higher in men than in women, particularly in the younger age group. The ratio of men to women in patients with intermittent claudication ranges between 1:1 and 2:1. Some studies involving patients with severe PAD report a male-to-female ratio exceeding 3:1 [6].

Smoking

Intermittent claudication is three times more common among smokers than nonsmokers. The association between smoking and PAD may be even stronger than that between smoking and coronary artery disease. People that smoke develop PAD a decade earlier than nonsmokers, and the severity of PAD increases with the number of cigarettes smoked. The incidence of claudication decreases with smoking cessation.

Diabetes Mellitus

Intermittent claudication is twice as common among diabetic patients as among nondiabetics. For every 1 % increase in hemoglobin A1c, there is a corresponding 26 % increased risk of PAD [7]. Major amputation is also five to ten times higher in diabetics than in nondiabetics.

Dyslipidemia

A fasting cholesterol level greater than 270 mg/dL doubles the incidence of intermittent claudication [8].

Hypertension

Although hypertension is associated with all forms of cardiovascular disorders, the relative risk of developing PAD is less for hypertension than for diabetes or smoking (Fig. 1.1).

Hyperhomocysteinemia

Hyperhomocysteinemia may be an independent risk factor for atherosclerosis as it is detected in about 30 % of young patients with PAD compared to 1 % in the general population [10].

Inflammatory Markers/C-Reactive Protein

Recent studies have shown that C-reactive protein (CRP) is higher in asymptomatic subjects who developed PAD in the subsequent 5 years, compared to an age-matched control group who remained asymptomatic [11].

Chronic Renal Insufficiency

PAD has been associated with chronic renal insufficiency.

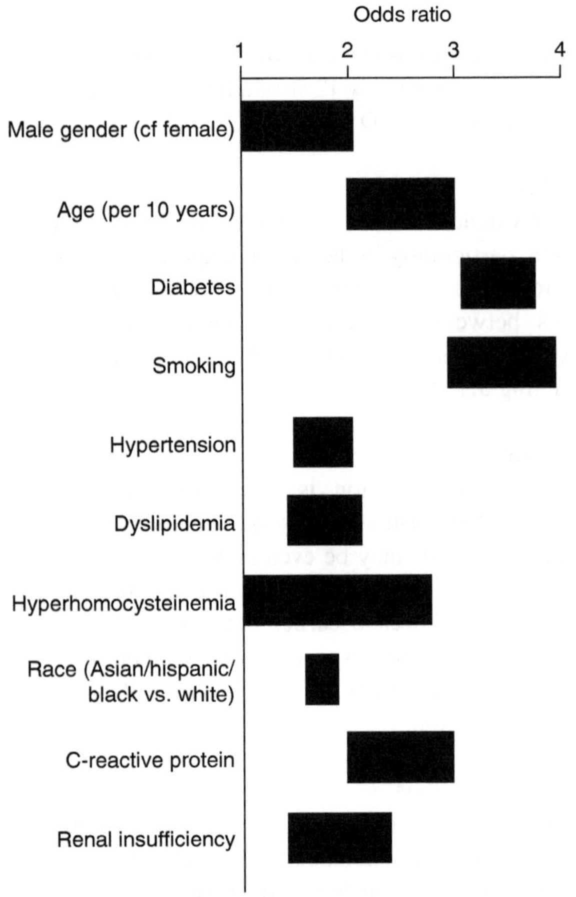

Fig. 1.1 Approximate range of odds ratios for risk factors for symptomatic peripheral arterial disease (Reprinted from Norgren et al. with permission from Elsevier [9]

Hypercoagulable States

Hyperviscosity and raised hematocrit have been detected in patients with PAD, which may be a consequence of smoking. Increased plasma fibrinogen levels have also been associated with PAD in some studies [6].

Ethnicity

PAD defined as an ABI of ≤0.9 was more common in non-Hispanic blacks (7.8 %) than in whites (4.4 %) [12].

Noninvasive Vascular Laboratory Exams

Cerebrovascular Noninvasive Vascular Testing

Carotid duplex ultrasound remains the initial exam of choice for evaluating patients with suspected cerebrovascular disease.

Indications

Common indications for carotid duplex sonography include a cervical bruit in an asymptomatic patient and the presence of symptoms suggesting a hemispheric or retinal TIA or stroke [13, 14]. Carotid duplex exams can provide a stroke risk assessment for patients with coronary disease and PAD as well as patients with multiple atherosclerotic risk factors. Other less common indications for carotid duplex sonography include intraoperative assessment during carotid surgery or stenting. Patients with posterior circulation symptoms which typically involve exertional lightheadedness or impaired vision associated with upper extremity exertion also warrant a carotid duplex exam.

Follow-Up After Carotid Intervention/ Surveillance

Patients with atherosclerotic risk factors and an initial duplex exam demonstrating less than 50 % stenosis of the internal carotid artery (ICA) can be reevaluated at 1–2-year intervals. Stenosis between 50 and 69 % should be followed at 6–12 month intervals whereas severe stenosis greater than 70 % should be considered for immediate intervention or surveillance every 6 months depending on the clinical scenario.

Limitations

The diagnostic accuracy of a carotid duplex exam depends on adequate sonographic visualization of the carotid arteries. Calcification creates acoustic shadows which impede ultrasound waves and prevent interrogation of blood flow velocities within the calcified arteries. Other conditions which prevent sonographic visualization include a cervical hematoma, soft tissue edema, the presence of sutures or skin staples, and exceptionally deep or tortuous vessels in patients with large necks.

A carotid duplex exam indirectly determines the severity of stenosis by measuring the blood flow velocity which is derived from the frequency shift using the Doppler equation. The accuracy of the exam therefore depends on measuring the true blood flow velocity with a known angle of insonation (usually 60°). Underestimating disease can occur in patients with long, smooth plaque formation which does not cause the accelerated, turbulent flow pattern usually associated with a focal, segmental stenosis. Failure to appreciate low-intensity echoes of soft plaque or using an inappropriate Doppler angle can also underestimate the degree of stenosis. Overestimating the severity of stenosis can occur when an artifact is mistaken for a carotid plaque and when physiologically accelerated flow is inappropriately attributed to stenosis. The presence of vessel kinking or tortuosity, significant contralateral stenosis or occlusion, and cardiac dysrhythmias makes it more difficult to evaluate the flow spectra. Large-caliber vessels generally have lower flow velocities compared to smaller-caliber vessels at the same flow intensity. Therefore, blood flow in a wide carotid sinus can be easily disturbed and this physiologic turbulence could be falsely attributed to arterial stenosis.

Table 1.2 Primary parameters for carotid duplex sonography

Duplex criteria	Interpretation
ICA PSV of <125 cm/s with no visible plaques	Normal carotid
ICA PSV of <125 cm/s with visible plaque of less than 50 % diameter reduction	Less than 50 % stenosis
ICA PSV range of 125–230 cm/s with a visible plaque estimate of greater than 50 % diameter reduction	50–69 % stenosis
ICA PSV of greater than 230 cm/s and a plaque estimate of greater than 50 % diameter reduction	Greater than 70 % stenosis but less than near occlusion
High, low, or undetectable PSV's with visible plaques, variable systolic ratio	Near occlusion
Undetectable flow with visible plaque, no detectable lumen	Total occlusion

Table 1.3 Other parameters recommended for use only in borderline data

Duplex criteria	Interpretation
ICA/CCA PSV ratio of less than 2 and an ICA EDV of less than 40 cm/s	Normal carotid
ICA/CCA PSV ratio of 2–4 and an ICA EDV of 40–100 cm/s	50–69 % stenosis
ICA/CCA ratio of greater than 4 and an ICA EDV greater than 100 cm/s	Greater than 70 % stenosis to near occlusion

Essentials of Examinations/Interpretation of Results

A duplex examination should provide detailed information of the extracranial carotid arteries. Grayscale (B-mode) imaging can characterize the plaque morphology within the common, internal, and external carotid arteries. Peak systolic and end diastolic velocities should be recorded at several points along the course of the common and internal carotid arteries as well as at least one point in the external carotid artery. The ratio of peak systolic velocity (PSV) in the internal carotid artery to the common carotid artery provides additional information to measure stenosis. Unfortunately many vascular laboratories do not meet the exam requirements and quality assurance guidelines required for accreditation by the Intersocietal Accreditation Commission (IAC). Exam reports from unaccredited labs often lack reliability and may limit the physician's ability to rely solely on this modality prior to carotid surgery. In 2003 Grant et al. reported consensus velocity criteria for duplex ultrasonography in an attempt to establish a more uniform method of classifying carotid stenosis (Tables 1.2 and 1.3) [15, 16]. Figures 1.2 and 1.3 show duplex ultrasound images of a normal carotid artery and severe stenosis of the ICA, respectively.

Abdominal Aortic Ultrasound

The infrarenal abdominal aorta is the most common site of aneurysmal degeneration of the aorta. An abdominal aortic ultrasound can function both as a screening exam for AAA and as a surveillance imaging modality for patients with small AAA's (Fig. 1.4).

Indications

An aortic ultrasound should be used to evaluate patients with a pulsatile abdominal mass. Patients with a history or presence of a popliteal artery aneurysm should also be evaluated for an AAA because of the strong association between peripheral and aortic aneurysms. Appropriate candidates to undergo a screening abdominal aortic ultrasound exam include men or women older than 60 who have a first-degree relative with an AAA and men older than 65 who have ever smoked cigarettes.

Limitations

Since ultrasound waves do not propagate well through air, the presence of excessive bowel gas prevents visualization of the aorta and renders the exam non-diagnostic. In morbidly obese patients, the depth of the abdominal aorta can exceed the penetration of even the lowest frequency ultrasound probe. Technically challenging ultrasound exams due to patient body habitus or previous abdominal surgery can compromise the spatial resolution of the sonographic images making it difficult to characterize aneurysm morphology. Ultrasound imaging may fail to identify saccular aneurysms which have an unpredictable natural history compared to the more commonly encountered fusiform aneurysms.

Surveillance

The Society for Vascular Surgery recommends the following schedule for abdominal aortic ultrasound examinations in patients with an AAA: every 6 months for aneurysms with maximum diameter of 4.5–5.4 cm, annually for aneurysms measuring 3.5–4.4 cm, every 3 years for 3–3.4 cm AAAs, and in 5 years if the aortic diameter is 2.6–2.9 cm. Aneurysms exceeding 5.5 cm in diameter should be evaluated with computed tomography to plan for surgical or endovascular repair.

Essentials of Evaluation/Interpretation

Grayscale images with a transverse view of the aorta allow for measurement of the maximal aneurysm diameter. Ultrasound measurements of the aorta have proven to be accurate and reproducible; the results usually come within 5 mm of measurements taken using computed tomography which is considered the gold standard [17]. It is important to clearly interpret the ultrasound exam report since some laboratories provide the length of the aneurismal segment in addition to its maximal diameter. The diameter and rate of

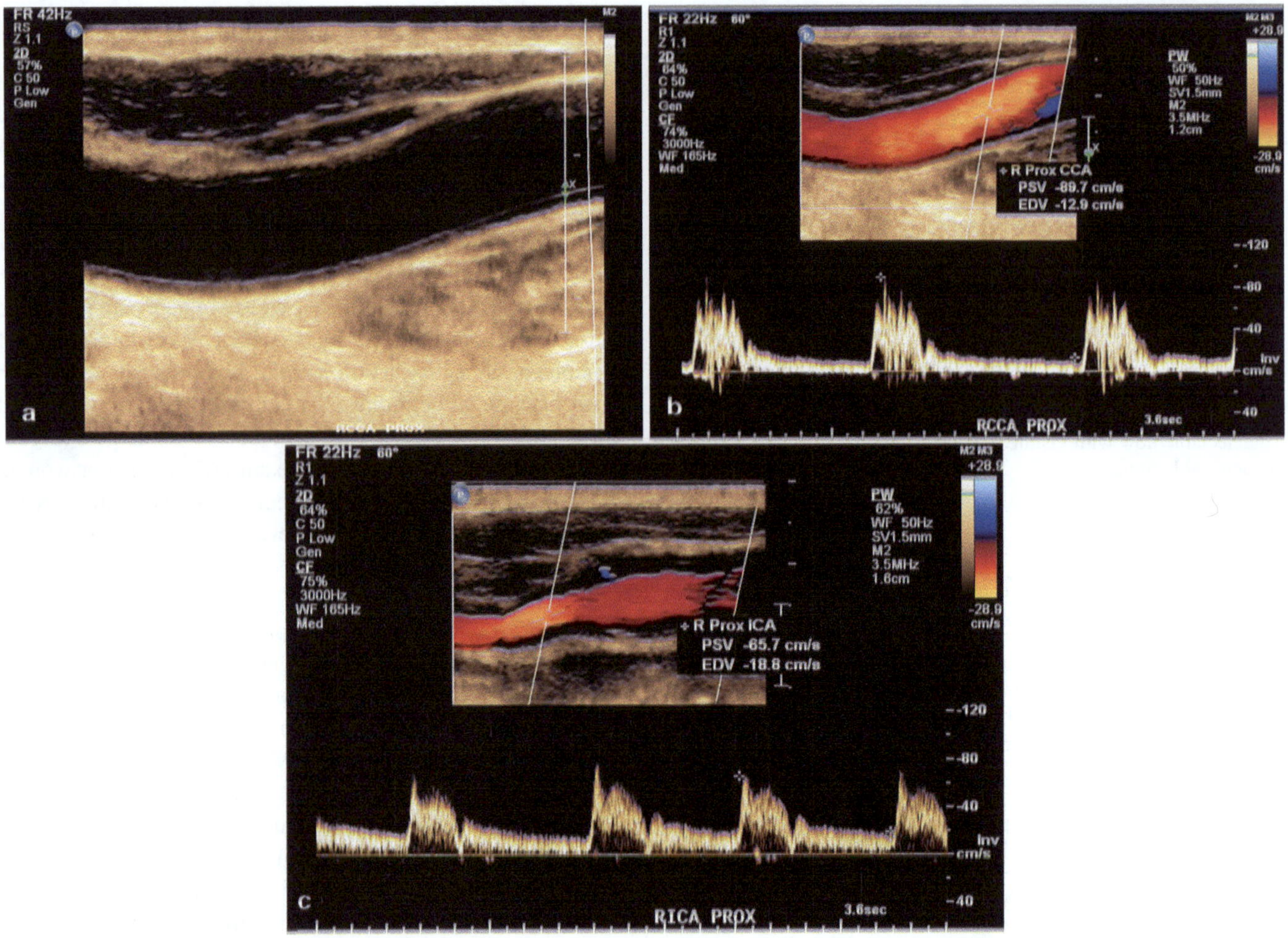

Fig. 1.2 (**a**) B-mode image of proximal common carotid artery. (**b**) Color flow of proximal common carotid artery. (**c**) Duplex image of normal proximal internal carotid artery: PSV of 66 cm/s and EDV of 19 cm/s, no plaquing

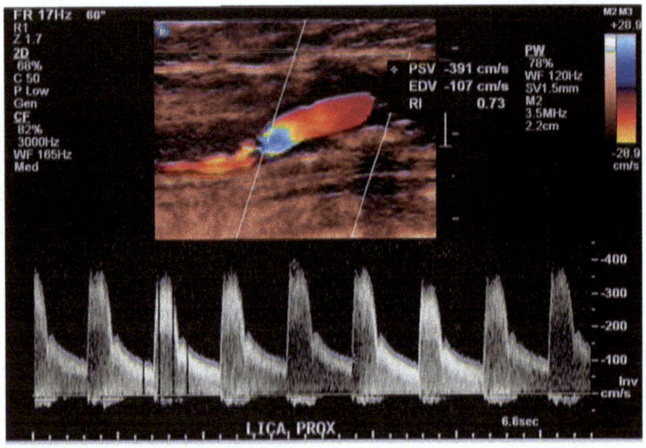

Fig. 1.3 Duplex ultrasound of severe internal carotid artery stenosis: PSV of 391 cm/s and EDV of 107 cm/s with significant carotid plaquing

growth are the clinically important data points in the assessment of infrarenal AAAs. Occasionally, urgent vascular surgery referrals are made for 8 cm aneurysms that turn out to be only 4 cm in diameter but 8 cm in length.

Ankle Brachial Index

The ankle brachial index (ABI) is the screening modality of choice for diagnosing patients with PAD. An ABI can be performed in virtually any clinical setting using a manual sphygmomanometer and a handheld continuous wave Doppler. The patient should be in the supine position. With the blood pressure cuff placed above the patient's ankle, the Doppler probe is used to locate the dorsal pedal or posterior tibial pulse. The blood pressure cuff is then inflated until the Doppler signal is no longer audible. The pressure at which the Doppler signal returns as the cuff slowly deflates is the systolic ankle pressure. The process is repeated for the remaining pedal pulse and then on the other leg. The brachial pressure in both arms should be measured using a similar technique with the blood pressure cuff around the upper arm and Doppler interrogation of the brachial, radial, or ulnar pulse. (The measured pressure is determined by cuff location, not the Doppler site.) The ABI is the ratio of the higher of the ankle pressures (posterior tibial or dorsal pedal) of the

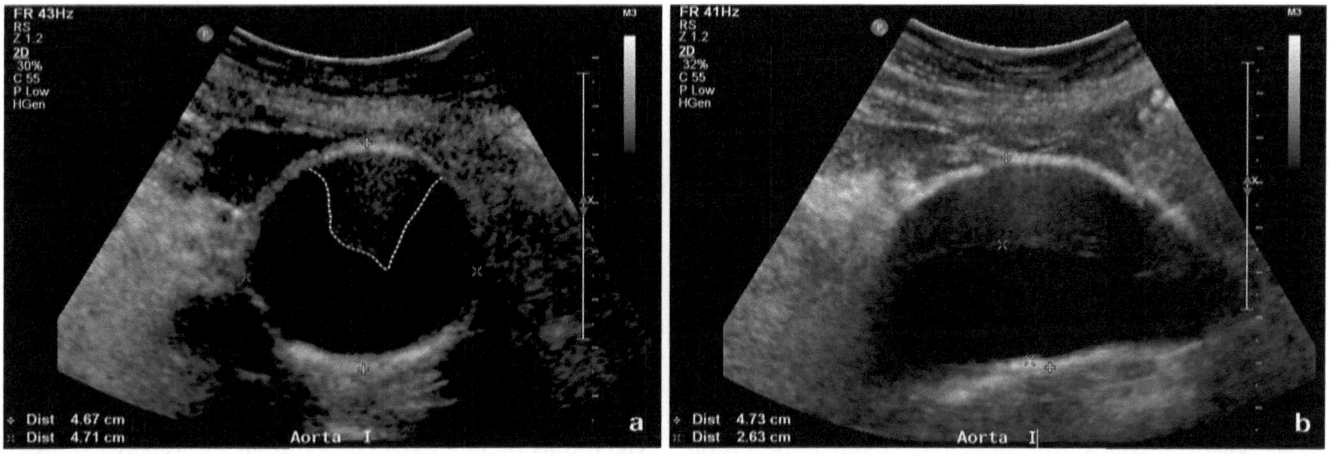

Fig. 1.4 Ultrasound of native aorta showing abdominal aortic aneurysm, (**a**) transverse view – notice intraluminal thrombus (*dotted line*), (**b**) sagittal view

ipsilateral lower extremity compared to the highest brachial pressure (either right or left arm). The ABI is a reliable predictor of long-term survival and future risk of limb loss. Men with an ABI of less than 0.9 had an 18 % cardiovascular-related mortality rate at 10-year follow-up compared to a 4 % mortality rate for men with a normal ABI [18, 19].

In addition to the ABI, segmental Doppler pressures of the lower extremity, including high thigh, low thigh (above knee), below knee, and ankle pressures can be measured using appropriately placed blood pressure cuffs (Fig. 1.5). These exams are usually performed in the noninvasive vascular lab and provide more precise localization of occlusive lesions in the lower limb [20]. Note that many vascular labs use a single wide cuff on the thigh instead of the two cuffs depicted in Fig. 1.5.

Indications

A screening ABI should be considered in patients with diminished or absent peripheral pulses and in patients with symptomatic PAD. Patients with diabetes and current or previous smokers over the age of 50 should also have a screening ABI.

Limitations

Calcified arteries can render the ABI inaccurate by falsely elevating the ankle pressure or making the tibial arteries noncompressible. These changes occur more frequently in patients with long-standing diabetes mellitus. In patients with noncompressible ABIs, the Doppler pressure in the toe accurately reflects arterial perfusion since calcification usually spares the small digital blood vessels. Toe pressures may also be a reasonable alternative in patients who cannot have an ABI because of the presence lower leg wounds which prevent application of a blood pressure cuff. Most noninvasive vascular laboratories have appropriately sized blood pressure cuffs to measure the toe pressure.

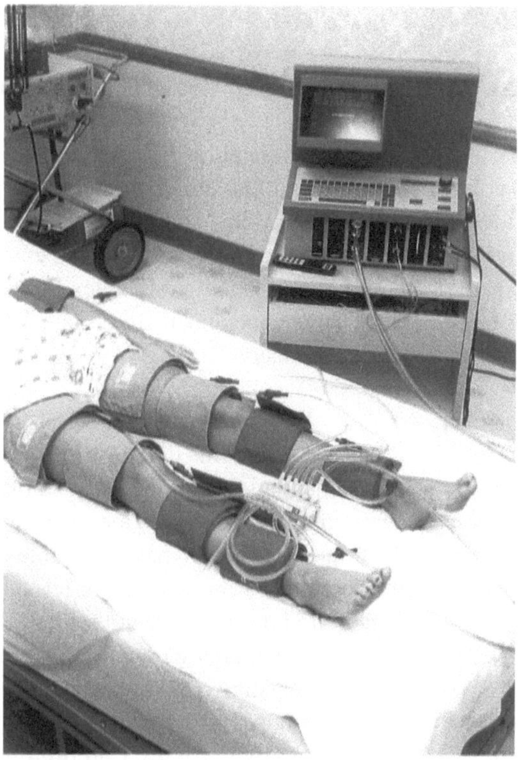

Fig. 1.5 Technique for measuring the segmental Doppler pressures using the four-cuff method

Interpretation of Results

Normally the systolic ankle pressure equals or slightly exceeds the systolic brachial pressure. Patients with normal lower extremity arterial pressure therefore have an ABI of 1.0–1.2. PAD is defined as an ABI of less than 0.9 and the severity of PAD increases as the ABI decreases (Table 1.4). Patients with significant medial calcinosis often have a falsely elevated ABI which can signify severe PAD and

Table 1.4 Ankle brachial index (ABI)

ABI	Interpretation
1.0–1.2	Normal
0.7–.09	Mild PAD
0.5–.07	Moderate PAD
0.3–0.5	Severe PAD
<0.3	Critical limb ischemia

predict poor long-term outcomes. Segmental blood pressure measurements indicate the presence of significant arterial disease if they demonstrate a pressure decrease of 30 mmHg or greater between adjacent segments, e.g., high thigh and above knee pressures (for superficial femoral occlusion, Fig. 1.6) or above knee and below knee pressures (for popliteal occlusion). Toe pressure and the calculated toe brachial index can predict wound healing following digital and foot amputations.

Duplex Ultrasound Exam of the Lower Extremity

An arterial duplex exam is a unique diagnostic tool that provides both anatomic and physiologic information. The exam involves grayscale imaging and blood flow velocity measurements along the entire course of the lower extremity. The level of detail provided by an arterial duplex can localize the diseased arterial segments and differentiate between stenosis and complete occlusion.

Indications

An arterial duplex exam is a valuable diagnostic tool to evaluate patients with symptomatic PAD including those with claudication, ischemic rest pain, or tissue loss. Patients with a leg or foot infection who do not have palpable pulses should also be considered for lower extremity arterial duplex evaluation. Since an arterial duplex does not require the use of intravascular contrast, this imaging modality is useful for evaluating patients with coexisting renal impairment. Arterial duplex exams also play an important role in the surveillance of patients with lower extremity bypasses. Careful follow-up using arterial duplex scans can improve the long-term patency of infrainguinal bypasses by detecting areas of progressive stenosis thereby allowing for therapeutic intervention before the bypass graft completely occludes.

Limitations

Arterial calcifications reflect ultrasound waves and may limit the ability to detect and measure the blood flow velocity. Patient factors such as severe lower extremity edema and obese body habitus increase the technical difficulty and decrease the accuracy of a lower extremity arterial duplex exam. Like other noninvasive ultrasound exams, the overall quality of an arterial duplex often depends on the skill and persistence of the sonographer.

Arterial duplex ultrasonography is an extremely sensitive and labor-intensive exam that should not be used to screen patients for the presence of PAD. The evaluation of patients suspected of having PAD should begin with the history and physical followed by an ABI. Arterial duplex should be reserved for patients with an unclear diagnosis or in patients in whom an intervention is being considered.

Duplex Ultrasound Interpretation in Patients with PAD

The results of an arterial duplex exam are usually expressed as peak-systolic velocity (PSV) and velocity ratio (VR) which is calculated by dividing the PSV at the stenosis by the PSV just proximal to the stenosis. Khan et al. defined greater than 70 % stenosis in the native femoropopliteal arteries as a PSV exceeding 200 cm/s and a VR greater than 2.5 [21]. Table 1.5 lists the velocity criteria proposed by Armstrong and Bandyk for de novo femoropopliteal arterial lesions [22].

The presence of a proximal stenotic or occlusive lesion can reduce downstream blood flow velocity. Preserving the accuracy and sensitivity of the arterial duplex exam may therefore require adjusting the velocity criteria for patients with multilevel occlusive disease. Figure 1.7 shows a duplex ultrasound of a hemodynamically significant stenosis in the superficial femoral artery.

Duplex Vein Mapping

Indication

The K-DOQI guidelines for arteriovenous access recommend preoperative duplex vein mapping for all patients who require hemodialysis access surgery. Duplex vein mapping increases the creation of native arteriovenous fistulas by detecting adequate caliber superficial veins in the upper extremity [23]. It is not uncommon to have a patient referred with a previous failed arteriovenous graft who still has suitable veins for autogenous fistula creation detected by duplex vein mapping. Preoperative duplex vein mapping of the saphenous veins (great and small) can be useful in patients who require lower extremity arterial bypass.

Limitations

The fluid status of the patient and the ambient room temperature can influence the diameter of superficial veins. Performing a duplex vein mapping on a dehydrated patient in a cool room can significantly underestimate the true caliber of the veins. In obese patients the large size of the arm can limit the ability to precisely measure vein diameter.

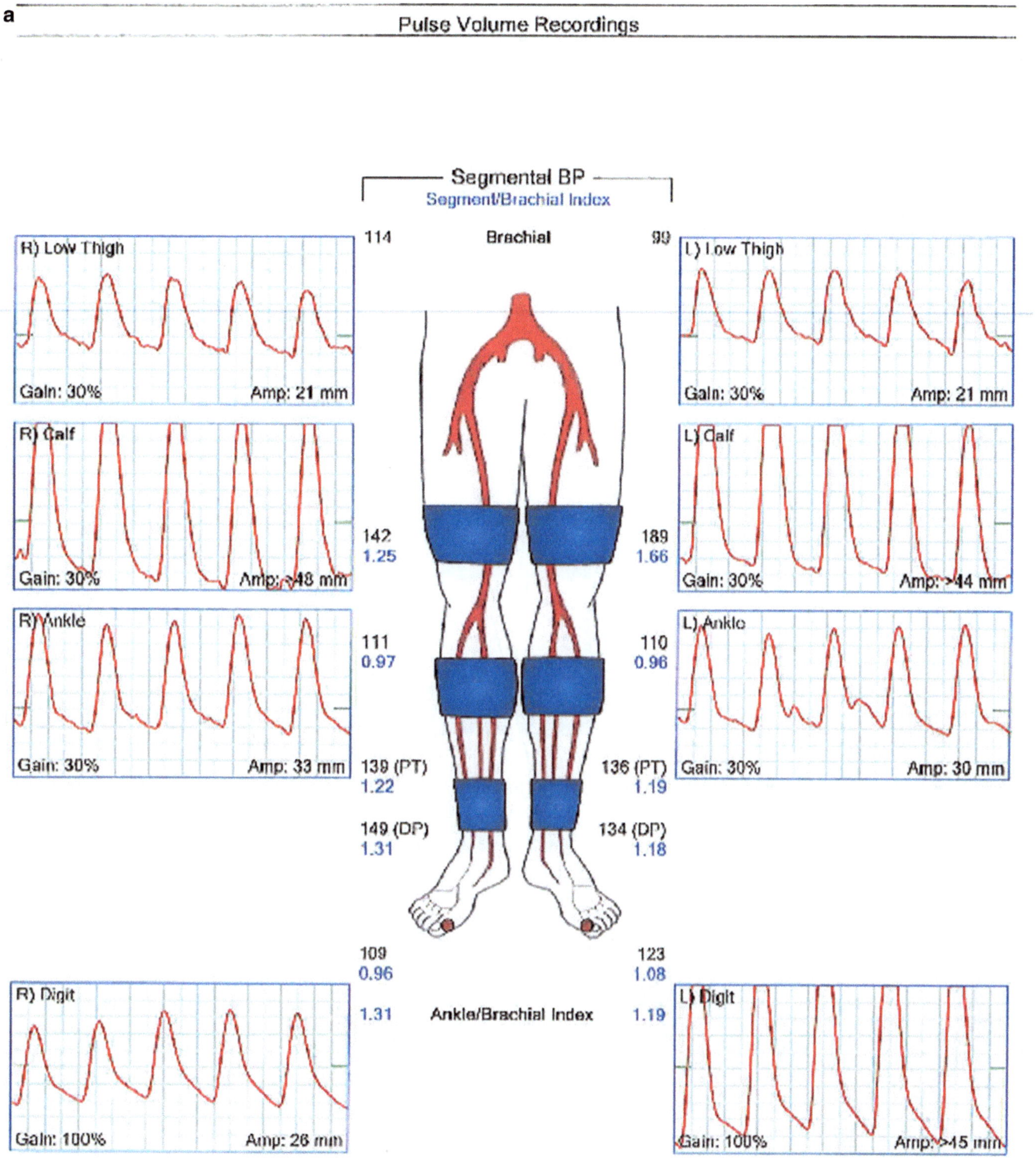

Fig. 1.6 Segmental systolic limb pressures and pressure volume recordings in a patient with normal lower extremity arterial perfusion (**a**) and in a patient with severe aortoiliac arterial occlusive disease (**b**)

b

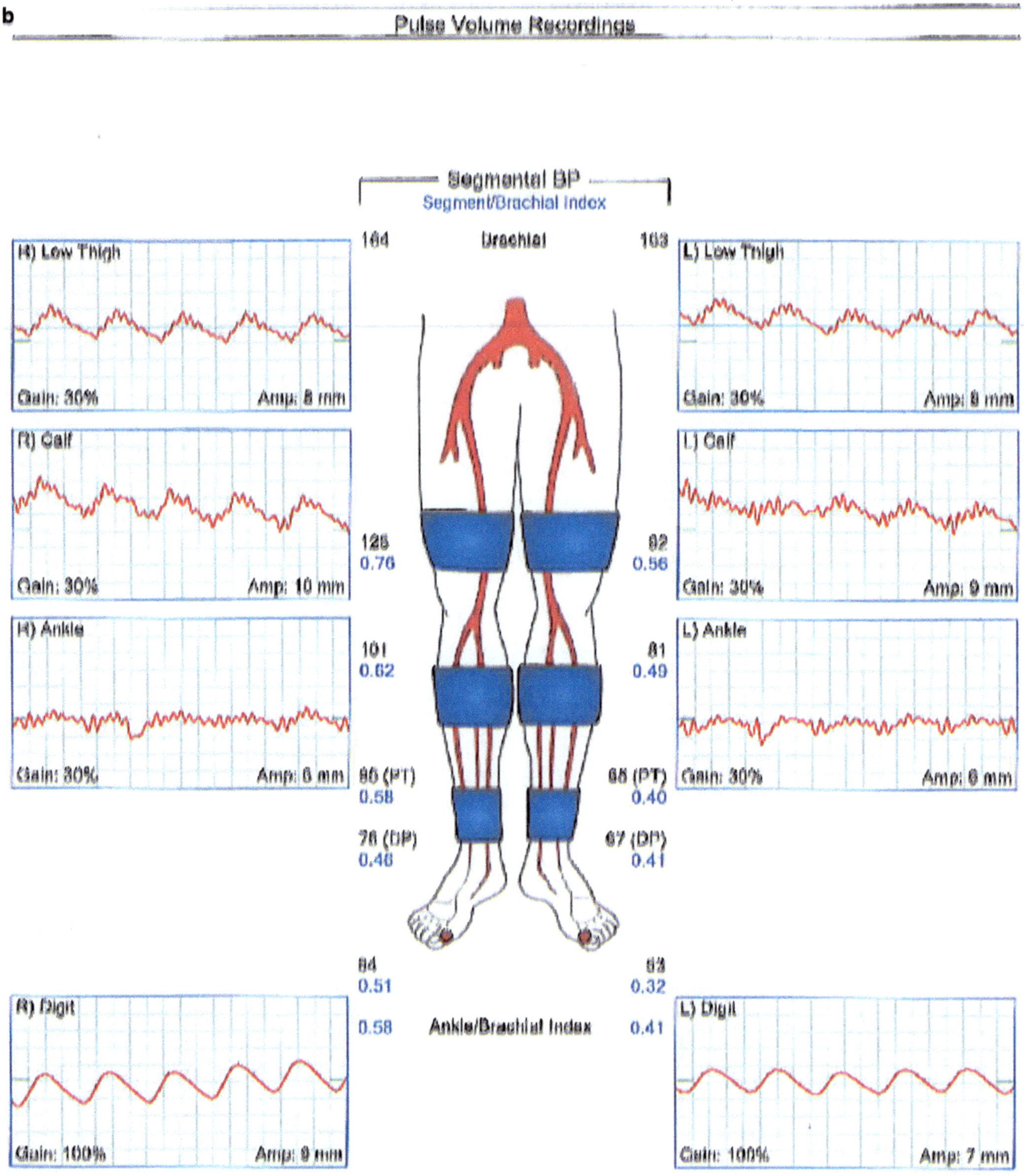

Fig. 1.6 (continued)

Table 1.5 Duplex-specific velocity criteria for femoropopliteal stenosis

PSV	VR	Degree of stenosis
<200 cm/s	≤2	Less than 50 %
200–300 cm/s	2–4	50–75 %
>300 cm/s	≥4	Greater than 75 %
No flow	–	Complete occlusion

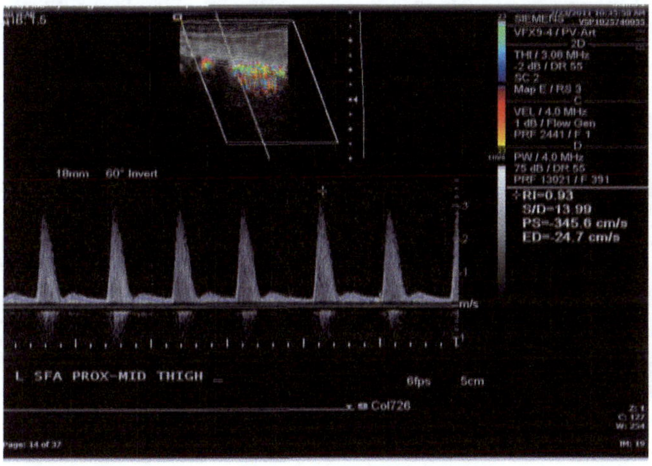

Fig. 1.7 Duplex scan of mid-thigh superficial femoral artery stenosis in a patient with calf claudication. At rest, a triphasic waveform was recorded proximal and at a focal stenosis with a PSV of 441 cm/s and VR of 8.4 (criteria indicating a >75 % diameter reducing stenosis [22])

Essentials of Evaluation/Interpretation of Results

Upper extremity vein mapping should be performed in a warm room on well-hydrated patients. The exam begins by evaluating the patency of the deep and superficial veins along their entire course in the upper arm and forearm. Patent veins demonstrate complete compressibility with gentle pressure from the ultrasound probe. Most vascular laboratories perform superficial vein diameter measurements with a tourniquet in place on the proximal upper arm. The anterior-posterior and transverse diameters of both the cephalic and basilic veins from the wrist to axilla should be recorded in chart form to enhance clarity. Superficial veins with a diameter of 3 mm or more have the best chance of maturing into a functional arteriovenous fistula. Evaluating vein diameters in the more proximal upper extremity in addition to recording the vein caliber at the proposed anastomotic site can identify sclerotic vein segments that could impede fistula maturation. The basilic vein in the upper arm always requires ultrasound evaluation since its location deep to the fascia prevents visual inspection.

A thorough preoperative exam for patients requiring hemodialysis access includes bilateral brachial blood pressure measurement and waveform analysis of the axillary, brachial, radial, and ulnar arteries. A greater than 20 mm Hg difference in upper extremity blood pressures warrants using the extremity with the higher pressure or performing preoperative angiography to assess for arterial occlusive lesions. Waveform analysis may indicate the presence of atherosclerotic disease in the upper extremity which can predispose the patient to develop hemodynamic steal symptoms after AV fistula creation. Patients with a history or physical exam findings which suggest central venous stenosis should be considered for preoperative venography to evaluate the central veins prior to access creation.

Venous Duplex Ultrasound for Endovascular Therapy

Endovenous ablation of the great saphenous vein has become one of the most common vascular procedures performed in the United States. Instead of surgically stripping an incompetent great saphenous vein, an endovenous ablation procedure uses percutaneous access to heat the inside of the vein. This intraluminal heat denatures the endothelium resulting in permanent occlusion of the vein. Duplex ultrasound plays a central role in both the preparation for and the performance of endovenous ablation procedures. Prior to an intervention, venous duplex sonography can evaluate for the presence of superficial venous reflux that is amenable to endovenous treatment. During the endovenous procedure, ultrasound provides imaging guidance for percutaneous access, placement of the ablation catheter, and infusion of tumescent anesthesia.

Indications

Patients with symptomatic varicose veins, chronic leg edema, lipodermatosclerosis, or venous ulcers should be considered for duplex ultrasound evaluation of both the superficial and deep venous systems. An endovenous ablation procedure may have therapeutic value for patients with duplex-proven reflux in the saphenous system and absence of occlusive thrombosis in the deep venous system. Varicose veins usually warrant intervention if the symptoms are refractory to leg elevation, prescription strength support hose, and minor analgesics.

Limitations

During the venous duplex exam, maneuvers designed to elicit venous reflux include having the patient stand up or perform the Valsalva maneuver. Patients with limited mobility or poor cooperation cannot participate in this part of the exam and therefore cannot be evaluated for venous reflux. Active ulcers and morbid obesity can also limit sonographic visualization especially during the evaluation for perforating veins and reflux segments.

Essentials of Evaluation

Duplex venous ultrasound exams should include the deep venous system, the superficial veins (great and small saphenous veins), and abnormal venous perforators when present.

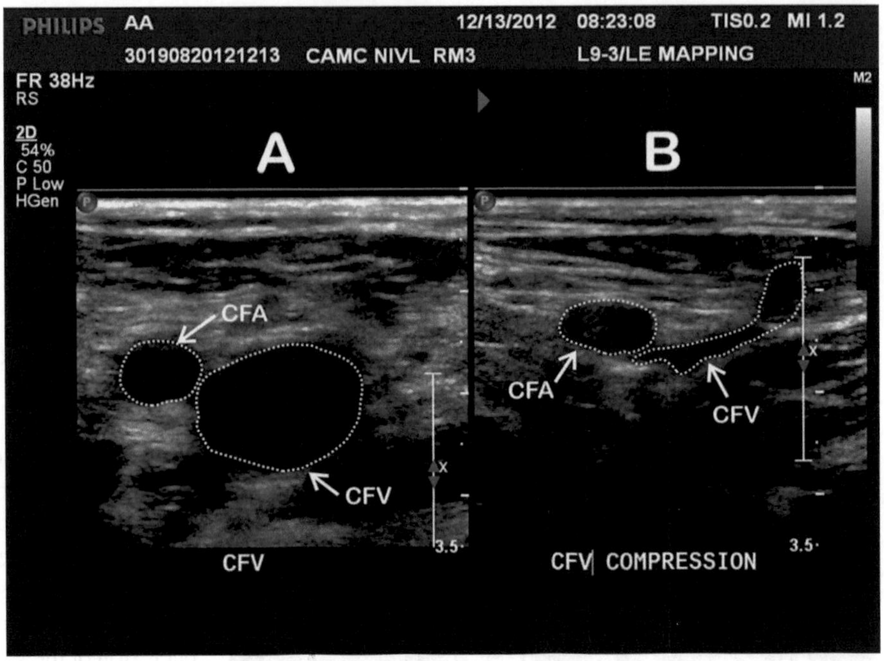

Fig. 1.8 Duplex ultrasound of a normal common femoral vein (*CFV*) with adjacent artery (*CFA*) (**a**) and compressibility of vein (**b**) (*arrow*)

The deep and superficial venous systems should be assessed for patency and the presence of venous reflux. Most vascular labs define abnormal reflux as retrograde venous flow that exceeds 1 s in the deep veins, 0.5 s in the superficial veins, and 0.3 s in the perforating veins. The diameter of the great and small saphenous veins should also be recorded from groin to ankle and popliteal fossa to ankle, respectively. The location of perforating veins which are usually present along the medial distal calf and thigh should be documented as well.

Venous Duplex for Deep Vein Thrombosis

Duplex ultrasonography to evaluate for deep venous thrombosis remains the most commonly performed noninvasive vascular exam. Patients with clinical findings suggestive of DVT and prothrombotic risk factors such as cancer, hypercoagulability, recent surgery or trauma, and immobility should be considered for duplex evaluation of the venous system.

Indications

Although many patients with a DVT have no symptoms, some patients experience new onset of pitting edema or symptomatic leg swelling with the entire limb or calf measuring more than 3 cm larger than contralateral extremity. Localized tenderness along the venous system and the presence of superficial collateral veins that are not varicose should also raise the suspicion of an underlying DVT. Patients recently diagnosed with a pulmonary embolism should undergo a lower extremity venous duplex exam to evaluate for the source of the embolic event.

Limitations

Any condition which prevents complete compression of the lower extremity veins including obesity, severe edema, and open wounds will decrease the diagnostic accuracy of duplex ultrasonography.

Essentials of Examination

Failure to completely compress a vein is the most sensitive sonographic sign of acute DVT [24]. Evaluating for compressibility involves obtaining a grayscale image of the vein in the transverse plane and exerting manual pressure with the ultrasound probe. This technique should be repeated along the entire course of the lower extremity deep veins from the groin to the ankle. A complete venous duplex exam also includes color flow assessment of the veins with and without augmentation and Doppler waveform evaluation. The Doppler signal in a normal vein varies with respiration and this is often described as a spontaneous phasic augmented signal (SPA) (Fig. 1.8). Waveform analysis can confirm augmentation of flow which is tested by compressing the leg distal to the vein segment being analyzed. Continuous, nonphasic venous flow signals which do not augment with distal compression suggest a proximal stenosis or obstruction.

In addition to assessing for compressibility, grayscale imaging should evaluate for venous dilation which often indicates acute deep venous thrombosis (Fig. 1.9). Differentiating an acute from a chronic DVT can be challenging since both conditions result in a noncompressible vein. Unlike veins with acute DVT, veins with chronic DVT are not dilated and may have hyperechoic signals within their lumen on grayscale imaging. Acute thrombus has the same

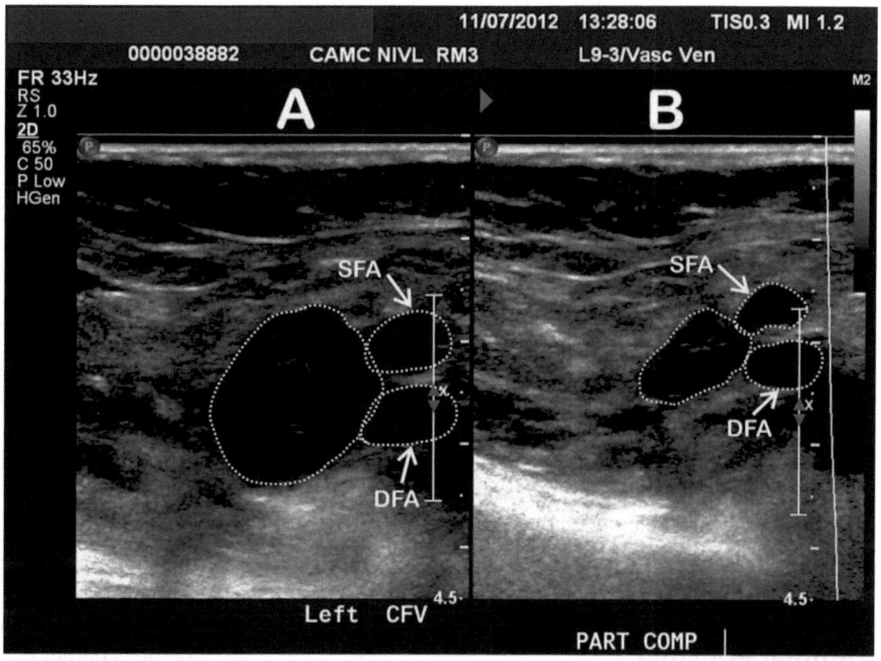

Fig. 1.9 Duplex ultrasound of acute deep vein thrombosis of the left common femoral vein (dilated, noncompressible with intraluminal echoes) with adjacent arteries (superficial femoral artery [*SFA*] and deep femoral artery [*DFA*]) (**a**); left common femoral vein (*CFV*) with partial compression (**b**)

density of blood and is therefore hypoechoic. In contrast, chronic thrombus becomes hyperechoic as it undergoes organization and fibrosis. Patients with chronic DVT may also have sonographically visible venous collaterals around the thrombosed vein.

Vascular Ultrasound General Principles

Since its introduction in 1959, vascular ultrasound has gained wide acceptance as an objective, accurate, and noninvasive diagnostic tool for evaluating patients with vascular disease [25]. Current applications of vascular ultrasound can identify and evaluate the morphology of blood vessels in addition to detecting and quantifying blood flow velocity. Blood flow velocity is derived from the Doppler effect, while tissue reflectance of transmitted ultrasound waves produces grayscale (B-mode) images of the blood vessels. Duplex ultrasound exams include a combination of both Doppler and grayscale imaging.

Although Satomura developed the first Doppler flow meter in 1959, Strandness et al. pioneered its clinical application in 1966 [25, 26]. Since then, vascular ultrasound has evolved through a series of technological advances and clinical applications. Working in obstetrics, Kossoff described grayscale ultrasound imaging techniques which ultimately paved the way for identifying blood vessels with ultrasound [27]. In 1969, Olinger reported on the use of ultrasound echo techniques to identify the carotid arteries launching efforts to develop high-resolution imaging technology [28]. These studies identified the walls of vessels as echodense parallel structures while the vessel lumen was an echo-free zone between the walls. Atherosclerotic lesions appeared as echodense structures projecting into the vessel lumen. Although it initially appeared that grayscale imaging alone would be able to detect and quantify the degree of atherosclerotic stenosis, vascular ultrasound proved to have several limitations. One drawback of sonographic imaging relates to the complex acoustic density of atherosclerotic plaques, particularly as the lesion severity progresses with areas of calcification and hemorrhage. Calcification serves as an acoustic barrier which obstructs the acoustic window and degrades the resolution of deeper structures [29]. In contrast, areas of hemorrhage are relatively echo-free and appear as defects within the plaque, rendering accurate delineation of the plaque surface more difficult. Although sonographic imaging alone can accurately characterize a homogeneous plaque, complex atherosclerotic plaques introduce a source of significant error. Finally, because flowing blood and acute thrombus have similar acoustic densities, differentiating between occluded and non-occluded arteries can be difficult using sonographic imaging alone.

To overcome these technical limitations, Barber et al. added a Doppler device to the ultrasound imaging component in 1974 [30]. It soon became apparent that the blood flow velocity detected by Doppler correlated closely with the severity of stenosis as measured by the gold standard of arteriography [31]. These findings gave rise to the first duplex scanning instruments which combined Doppler flow instrumentation with grayscale (B-mode) imaging to accurately evaluate arterial disease.

Duplex ultrasonography provides physiologic and anatomic information directly from the sites of vascular disease. Arterial occlusive lesions produce disturbances in blood flow patterns that can be detected and quantified by Doppler flow signal analyses. Although grayscale imaging detects arterial wall pathology including atherosclerotic plaque and calcifications, the classification of arterial disease severity is based primarily on the pulsed Doppler spectral waveform analysis. During a duplex ultrasound exam, grayscale imaging illustrates arterial anatomy and guides electronic placement of the pulsed Doppler sample volume within the artery of interest. The sample volume is the region in which flow is detected and evaluated by spectral wave analysis. Adjusting the size and position of the sample volume ensures that the center stream flow pattern can be evaluated without interference from flow disturbances near the arterial wall or in adjacent blood vessels.

Doppler Principle

Blood flow velocity measurements derive from observations made by the Austrian physicist Christian Doppler (1803–1853). He demonstrated that the frequency of light or sound increases as the source moves toward the observer and decreases as the source moves away from the observer. The magnitude of the change in frequency depends on the velocity of the moving source. A common example involves a whistle on a train which sounds higher in pitch (higher frequency, shorter wavelength) as the train approaches and lower in pitch (lower frequency, longer wave length) as the train moves away. Applying the Doppler effect to determine the velocity of blood flow yields the following equation:

$$\bar{V} = \frac{C\Delta f}{2f_o \cos\theta}$$

where $\bar{V}$ =average blood flow velocity, C=velocity of sound in tissue, Δf=Doppler frequency shift, f_o=transmitting frequency of ultrasound beam, and θ =angle of the incidence sound beam to the blood vessel being examined. Since transmitting frequency, angle of incidence, and sound velocity in tissue can remain constant, frequency shift (Δf) becomes proportional to the velocity of blood flow. In clinical practice, Doppler ultrasound detectors come in two varieties: continuous wave (CW) and pulsed Doppler ultrasound. Both types of instruments use the Doppler effect to detect blood flow.

Instrumentation

Commercially available Doppler instruments come in a variety of forms ranging from portable, pocket-sized models to more sophisticated instruments. CW Doppler detectors emit continuous ultrasound beams without interruption. These devices detect blood flow at any depth within the range of the instrument up to several centimeters, depending on the frequency of instrumentation. Figure 1.10 shows a commonly used portable CW Doppler unit (Dopplex D900, Huntleigh Diagnostics, Eatontown, NJ). In contrast, a pulsed Doppler detector transmits intermittent bursts of ultrasound waves and then receives the returning ultrasound echoes. Varying the time interval between transmission and reception allows for range resolution and the ability to detect flow at a specific distance from the transducer.

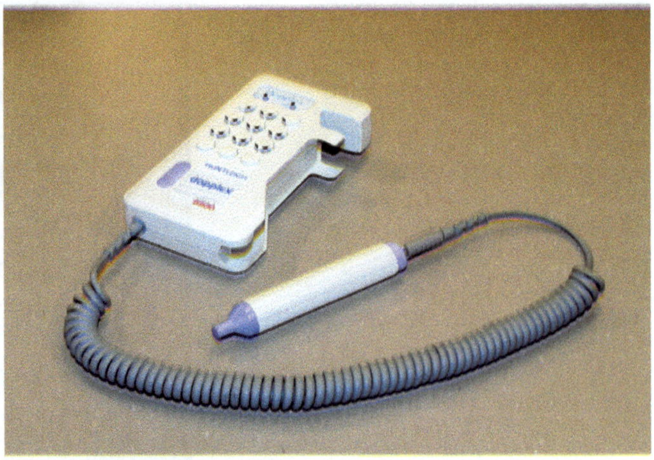

Fig. 1.10 Handheld Doppler ultrasound unit

Duplex Ultrasound Components

Real-Time Grayscale Imaging

Grayscale imaging was previously referred to as B-mode ultrasound with the "B" standing for brightness. The intensity or brightness of reflected ultrasound waves varies with the acoustic properties of different tissues. These variations in acoustic reflectance are represented visually by shades of gray on the image. The high reflectivity of the vessel wall usually makes it bright and easy to visualize sonographically.

Despite its ability to visualize soft tissue structures, grayscale imaging is often incapable of differentiating between flowing blood, thrombus, and non-calcified atherosclerotic plaques. With grayscale imaging alone, completely occluded vessels can appear patent and non-calcified plaques can be entirely missed or only partly visualized. Calcified atherosclerotic plaques also pose a technical challenge for grayscale imaging since calcium attenuates the penetration of ultrasound waves. A calcified plaque on the anterior wall of the vessel generates a very dense acoustic signal; however, there will be no information concerning the vessel lumen deep to the calcified segment. This imaging artifact is commonly

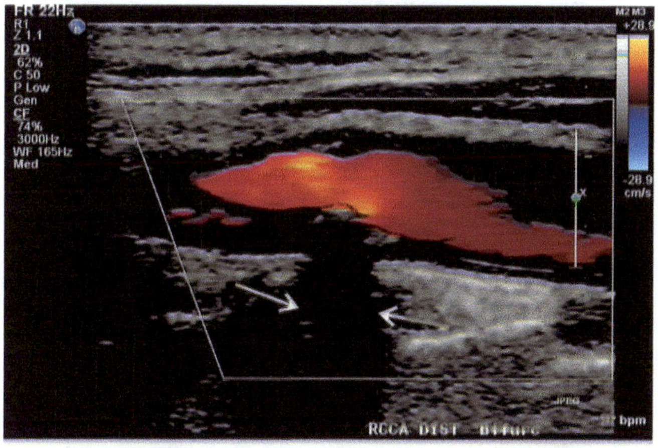

Fig. 1.11 Color duplex ultrasound image of an internal carotid artery showing calcified plaque where a very dense acoustic signal is registered with acoustic shadowing (*arrows*)

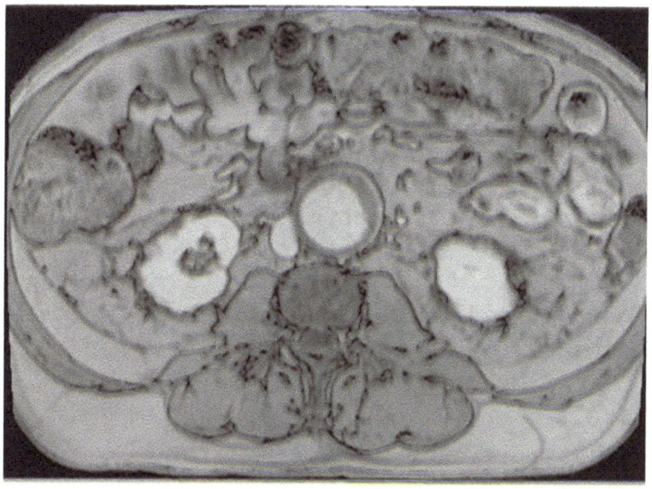

Fig. 1.12 MRA of abdomen with contrast. Axial imaging of mid-abdomen demonstrating an AAA with mural thrombus detected during workup of right kidney mass

referred to as acoustic shadowing (Fig. 1.11). These technical limitations can be overcome by combining grayscale imaging with Doppler-based blood flow detection techniques, such as spectral waveform analysis and color flow imaging.

Doppler Spectral Waveform Analysis

Understanding Doppler spectral waveform analysis requires a brief comparison of CW and pulsed Doppler techniques. A CW Doppler instrument sends out and receives signals that traverse the whole width of the insonated vessel as well as other vessels in close proximity. CW Dopplers therefore function as crude diagnostic tools that can only determine the mean velocity in the forward or reverse direction. In contrast, the pulsed Doppler technique can focus on the vessel of interest by providing velocity information from a known location. With pulsed Doppler the sonographer can interrogate a finite segment of the blood flow which is referred to as the "sample volume." Doppler spectral waveform analysis processes the Doppler signal that returns from this sample volume providing a more comprehensive evaluation of blood flow and detecting changes that would otherwise not be apparent with a CW device.

Doppler spectral waveform analysis processes the Doppler signal returning from the sample volume to generate a real-time display of the signal's frequency and amplitude. This spectral information is usually presented graphically with time on the horizontal axis and velocity (calculated from frequency shift) on the vertical axis. Each pixel on the spectral display theoretically represents the velocity of one blood cell as it travels through the sample volume at a single point in time. The amplitude of the Doppler signal is represented by the brightness of each pixel which is directly proportional to the number of blood cells traveling through the sample volume at that specific velocity and time point (see spectrum at bottom of figures 1.2B and C). Doppler spectral waveforms usually resemble an electrocardiogram (EKG) tracing since the velocity of blood cells varies with the time point of the cardiac cycle. The highest velocity occurs in systole (peak systolic velocity) while the lowest velocity is recorded during diastole (end diastolic velocity).

The width of the Doppler spectral waveform or spectral band can help gauge the arterial flow pattern. In a normal artery, the center stream flow pattern is uniform or laminar. Placing the pulsed Doppler sample volume in the center of the lumen generates a relatively narrow spectral band since most blood cells are traveling at the same velocity. Even relatively mild arterial stenosis disturbs laminar flow producing flow vortices and turbulence in the area distal to the stenosis. These flow disturbances are depicted as a wider spectral band which reflects the fact that blood cells are traveling at a variety of velocities at a given point in time. The magnitude of the flow disturbance and the decay in the laminar flow pattern correlates with the increase in spectral band width which is referred to as spectral broadening. In hemodynamically significant stenoses, not only is spectral broadening present, there is also a marked elevation in peak systolic velocity as a result of the high-speed jet of blood passing through and immediately beyond the stenosis. High-grade stenoses can therefore be recognized by the presence of both increased peak systolic velocity and diffuse spectral broadening [31]. The end-diastolic velocity also increases in areas of severe stenosis.

Color Duplex Ultrasound

Color duplex ultrasonography provides a qualitative display of the direction and magnitude of blood flow. Color flow imaging analyzes the Doppler flow information from a defined area which is superimposed on the grayscale image.

The size and location of this area or "color box" can be adjusted by the sonographer to evaluate the area of interest. Doppler flow signals within the color box are aggregated and assigned a color based on whether the overall direction of flow is toward or away from the transducer. The magnitude of flow velocity (calculated from the frequency shift) determines the hue or shade of the assigned color.

Overview of Imaging Options: MR, CT, Catheter Angiography – Advantages and Limitations

Magnetic Resonance Angiography

Magnetic resonance angiography (MRA) can provide accurate imaging of the peripheral vascular tree including the aorta, carotid arteries, and upper and lower extremities. MRA has the advantage of being a noninvasive test that does not require the use of conventional contrast or ionizing radiation. The limitations of MRA highlight the need for appropriate patient selection. First, achieving optimal images from an MRA requires that the patient remain completely still within a confined space for several minutes. Patients with claustrophobia may not tolerate this part of the exam. The presence of previously placed brain aneurysm clips or an implanted pacemaker or defibrillator may preclude the use of MRA due to the powerful magnetic forces generated. Finally, turbulent blood flow can result in loss of the MRA signal leading to an overestimation of the degree of stenosis [32].

MRA exams display arterial anatomy using one of two imaging protocols: time of flight (TOF) or contrast enhanced (CE MRA). TOF is a flow-dependent technique widely used to establish the diagnosis of carotid stenosis. This technique first establishes a "blank" background by minimizing the signal from stationary tissue within the imaging volume. Arteries then have relatively strong signals as blood flows into the imaging volume producing fresh magnetic spins superimposed on the "blank" stationary background [33]. TOF has two modes: two-dimensional which is more sensitive to slower flow and three-dimensional which depicts a wide range of flow velocities and has greater accuracy for defining internal and external carotid artery morphology [33]. As a flow-dependent technique, TOF can distort the carotid anatomy especially in lesions with high-grade stenosis or turbulent flow. In their review, Phillips and Bubash point out that TOF spins may remain in the imaging volume long enough to see numerous pulses and become saturated, thereby causing loss of signal within vessel lumen and inability to depict the vessel contiguous with the lesion [33]. This technical limitation can lead to overestimation of the degree of stenosis and a higher false-positive rate. The inherent sensitivity of TOF imaging results in a high negative predictive value. Carotid stenosis can be eliminated as a possible diagnosis in patients who have an MRA demonstrating minimal disease at the carotid bifurcation [34].

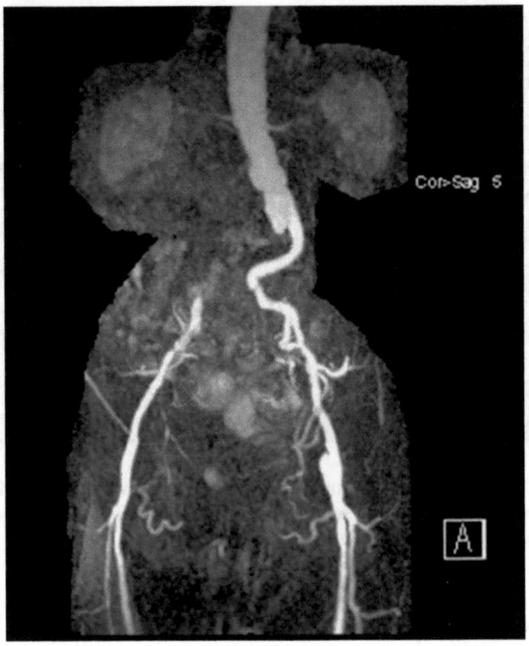

Fig. 1.13 MRA of abdomen/pelvis demonstrating right iliac occlusion

CE MRA generates images by detecting intravascular contrast on its first pass through the arteries within the imaging volume. The technique of CE MRA is somewhat similar to CTA and provides flow-independent anatomic information that can more accurately assess the degree of stenosis and visualize ulcerated plaques [33]. CE MRA requires timing the contrast bolus precisely to optimize the captured images. Once this technical challenge has been addressed, the shorter imaging time increases the accuracy of CE MRA by minimizing the risk of motion artifact. Figures 1.12, 1.13, 1.14, and 1.15 demonstrate MRA findings in patients with PAD and carotid disease. CE MRA using gadolinium as the contrast agent should be used with caution in patients with advanced renal disease. Gadolinium exposure can lead to nephrogenic systemic fibrosis in patients on dialysis and in patients with stage 5 chronic kidney disease or acute kidney injury [4].

Computed Tomographic Angiography

Computed tomography angiography (CTA) has gained prominence as a valuable imaging tool for evaluating patients with carotid, peripheral, and visceral artery stenosis. The technique of CTA involves timing a bolus of approximately 120 cc of intravenous contrast given through a 20-gauge intravenous catheter. Axial images are rapidly acquired while

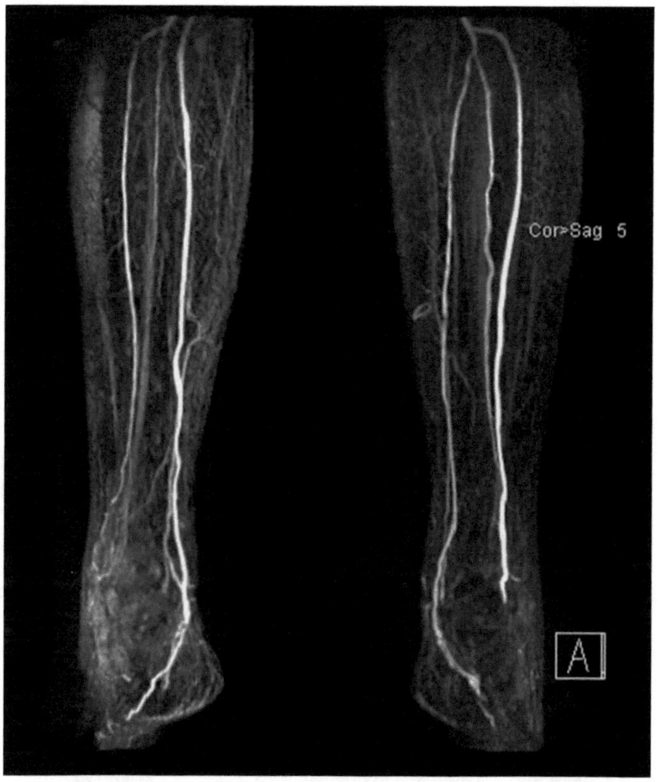

Fig. 1.14 MRA of tibial artery in same patient showing infrapopliteal runoff. Some artifacts appreciated with adjacent and superficial veins

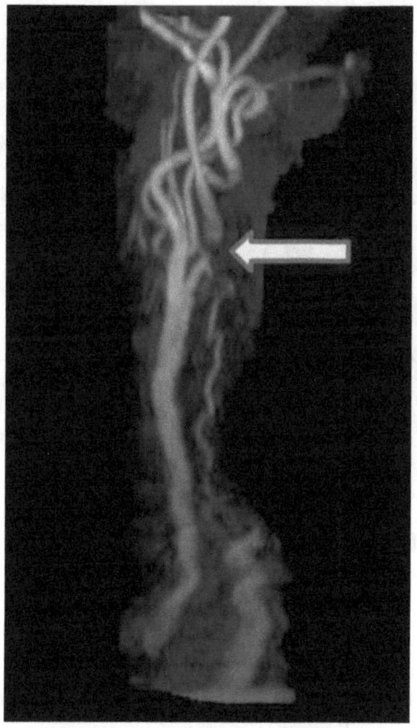

Fig. 1.15 MRA of carotid artery demonstrating flow gap (*arrow*) of left internal carotid artery significant stenosis

three-dimensional reconstructions require a specialized workstation and dedicated personnel for data processing.

Motion and interference artifacts are the primary source of error in data acquisition during a CTA exam. Since static images are generated, a CTA cannot evaluate flow dynamics nor can it diagnose subclavian steal and other flow-based lesions. Other limitations of CTA include higher cost (compared to duplex ultrasound), use of potentially nephrotoxic contrast, and radiation exposure. The presence of heavy arterial calcification can also limit the ability of CTA to distinguish intravascular contrast from calcium especially during post-processing imaging.

The advantages of CTA include its safety profile, ease of use, and quality images. Unlike digital subtraction angiography (DSA), a CTA does not require an arterial puncture. CTA images of the carotid arteries can be obtained without catheter manipulation thereby eliminating the stroke risk associated with carotid DSA. When performed on a high-quality helical scanner, CTA generates images that rival DSA in quality and detail. The ability to analyze axial and reformatted images also allows CTA to provide additional information about the morphology and composition of atherosclerotic occlusive lesions.

Compared to MRA, CTA is less likely to overestimate the severity of arterial stenosis. The rapid acquisition of spiral CT images can easily be synchronized with contrast administration minimizing the risk of signal loss or motion artifact. CTA is faster and less expensive than contrast-enhanced MRA and has the ability to simultaneously visualize soft tissue, bone, and blood vessels with better submillimeter spatial resolution (0.3 vs. 0.8 mm for contrast-enhanced MRA). CTA can also demonstrate vascular anomalies, quantify the extent of calcification, and interrogate the arterial tree from the aortic arch to the circle of Willis. Electronic microcalipers can be used on carotid CTA exams to measure stenoses based on NASCET or European Carotid Surgery Trial methods [35]. Given its accuracy, lower cost, and less invasive nature, computed tomography is increasingly being used as a surrogate for invasive angiography [36].

A meta-analysis of 28 studies analyzed the diagnostic accuracy of CTA compared to digital subtraction angiography. CTA had a pooled sensitivity of 85 % and specificity of 93 % for detecting severe (70–99 %) carotid stenosis and a sensitivity and specificity of 97 % and 99 % for detecting carotid occlusion [37]. CTA imaging did not perform as well in a study of patients who had a carotid endarterectomy. CTA had a lower diagnostic accuracy compared to MRA and duplex ultrasound when using the carotid plaque surgical specimen as the gold standard [38]. Previous studies with 4 and 16 multidetector computed tomographic (MDCT) angiography in the peripheral vasculature found adequate diagnostic accuracy versus digital subtraction angiography [39, 40].

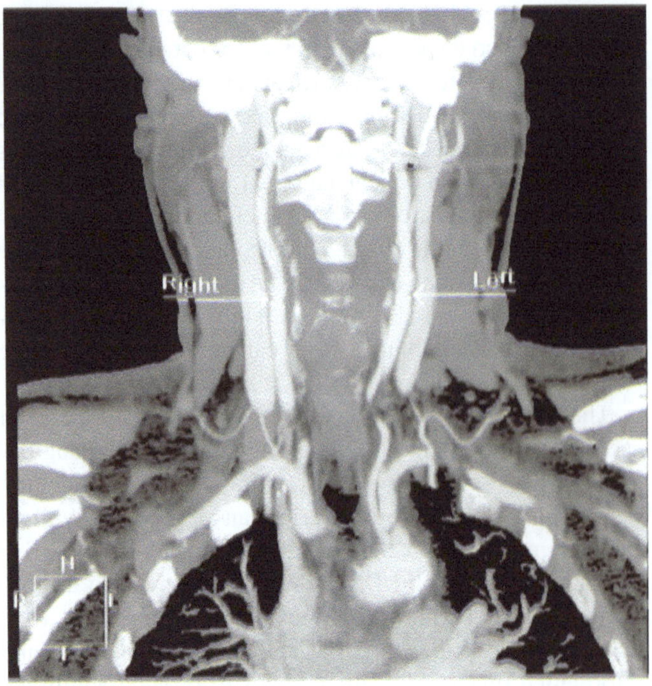

Fig. 1.16 CTA showing minimal carotid disease at right and left bifurcation (*arrow*)

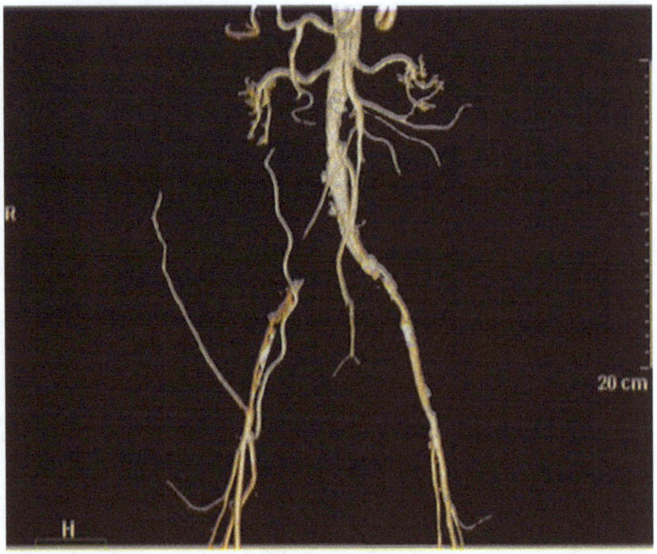

Fig. 1.18 CTA showing complete occlusion of right common iliac artery

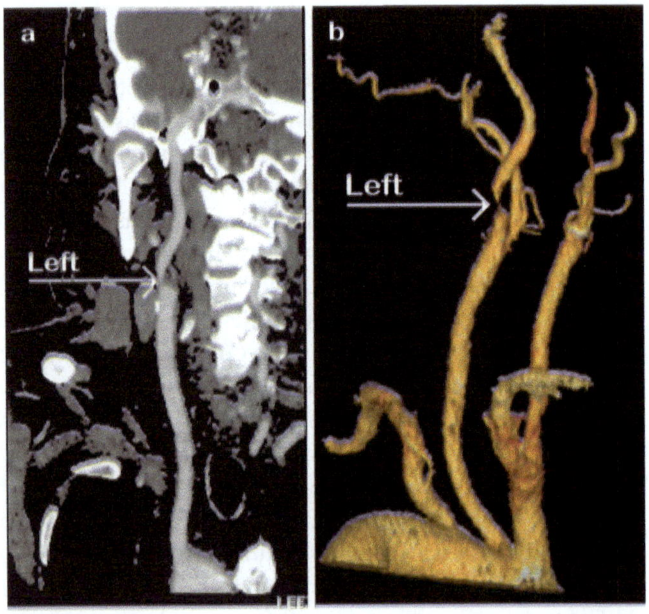

Fig. 1.17 CTA showing (**a**) severe left proximal internal carotid artery stenosis (*arrow*); (**b**) same patient showing aortic arch vessels (*arrow*)

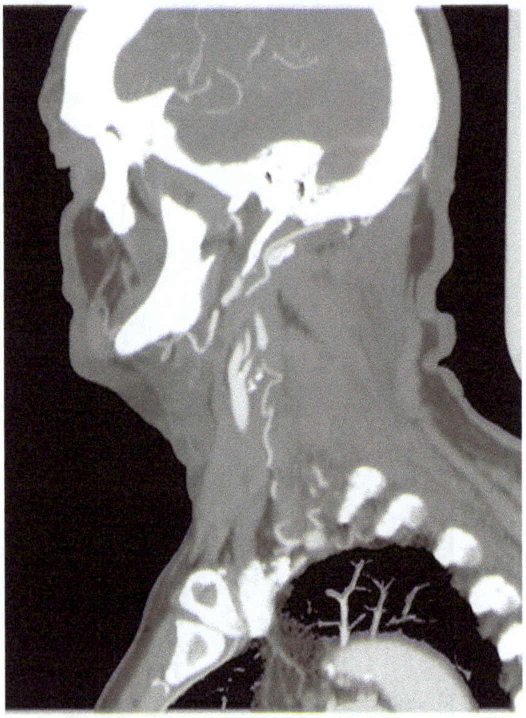

Fig. 1.19 CTA of left carotid artery demonstrating a "string sign" in a patient with acute left hemispheric deficit (sagittal view)

Figures 1.16, 1.17, 1.18, 1.19, 1.20, and 1.21 demonstrate CTA findings in patients with carotid artery disease and PAD.

The widespread use of diagnostic CT scans prompted Brenner and Hall to review the impact of radiation exposure associated with these exams [41]. CT involves larger radiation doses than conventional x-ray imaging and this increases the long-term risk of cancer in adults and especially children. Although the risks for any one person remain small, radiation exposure from diagnostic imaging exams may be a public health issue in the future [41]. Zhou made a similar observation in a study focused on patients with vascular disease [42].

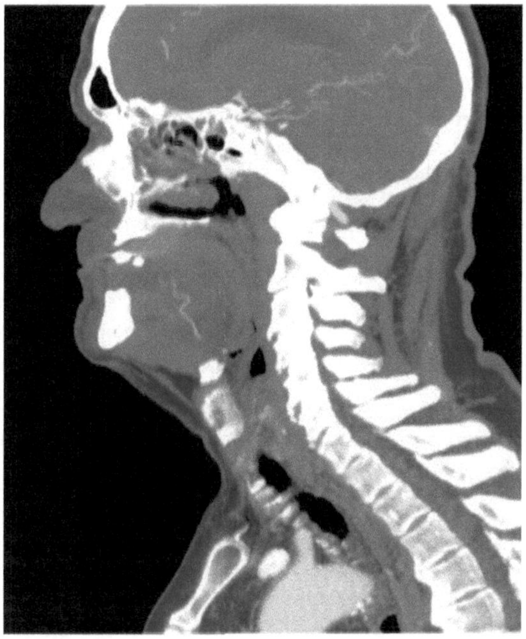

Fig. 1.20 During live scrolling the physician can locate the vertebral (bony landmark), i.e. level of the carotid lesion to aid in operative planning

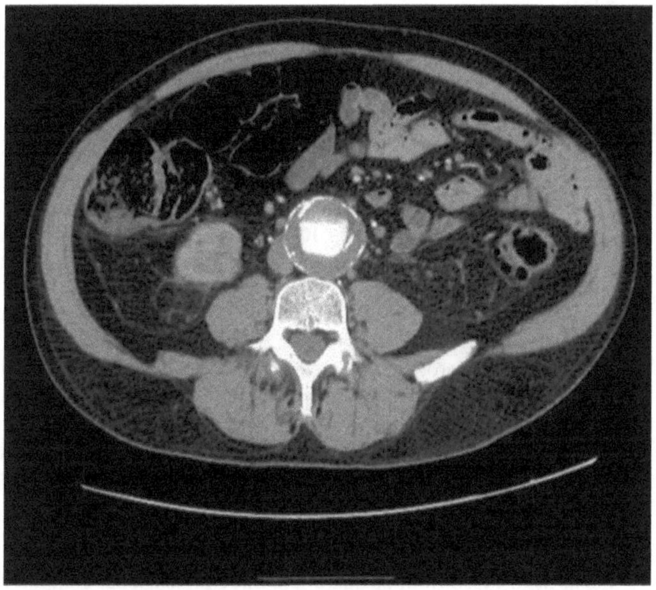

Fig. 1.21 CTA of abdomen/pelvis demonstrating AAA. Note the calcified rim of the aorta which is one of the short comings of CT imaging. Calcium artifacts are common (axial imaging)

Contrast Angiography (Digital Subtraction Angiography)

Catheter-directed angiography has a long track record as the gold standard for imaging the aorta and lower extremity vascular tree. The procedure involves arterial puncture followed by fluoroscopically guided advancement of a catheter into the area of interest. Contrast is then injected and fluoroscopic images are acquired in one or more planes.

Digital subtraction enhances the resolution of angiography by processing the video signal from a conventional signal image intensifier fluoroscopic system. Digital subtraction angiography (DSA) uses a time subtraction technique known as mask-mode radiography. With this technique, an initial fluoroscopic image is recorded and digitally processed. Contrast is then administered while additional images are recorded. The two sets of images are then digitally "subtracted" from each other to highlight the intravascular contrast. The resulting radiographs achieve a higher resolution using a smaller amount of contrast media than those obtained with conventional angiography [43].

Angiography carries the risk of an arterial puncture which can have thrombotic or hemorrhagic consequences. An arterial puncture can compromise the circulation due to thrombosis, embolism, or dissection. At the other end of the spectrum, inadequate hemostasis after arterial puncture can lead to bleeding complications in the form of hemorrhage, hematoma, or pseudoaneurysm formation. Intravascular contrast also has risks including allergic reactions, systemic vasodilatation, hypotension, convulsions, stroke, and renal insufficiency. Many of these risks can be minimized with adequate pre- and post-procedure hydration and the use of nonionic low-osmolarity contrast agents [44]. The overall complication rate for angiography may be as high as 7 %; however, more recent studies have reported lower major complication rates for peripheral arteriography (2.1 %) [45, 46]. The inherent risks associated with catheter-directed angiography preclude its use as a routine diagnostic exam, and angiography is now predominantly performed in conjunction with endovascular interventions. In selected patients with conflicting imaging studies, angiography may help clarify the decision to intervene or not.

AbuRahma et al. addressed the issue of surgeons performing angiographic procedures which had traditionally been the purview of interventional radiologists. They analyzed diagnostic arteriography performed by a vascular surgeon in a series of 558 patients and reported a complication rate of 3.8 % (1.3 % major) which was comparable to previous reports (1.9 and 2.9 %) but superior to what they published previously as performed by radiologists (7 %, $p<0.001$) [47]. A logistic regression analysis did not detect any variables that predicted a major complication. AbuRahma et al. concluded that diagnostic arteriography can be done safely by experienced vascular surgeons with low complication rates that compare favorably with what has been reported by interventional radiologists.

Endovascular Therapy

Most angiographic exams are now performed in conjunction with an endovascular intervention. Endovascular therapy is an evolving modality in which devices are introduced directly into the vessel lumen usually via percutaneous puncture. Stenotic or occluded arterial segments are then addressed using a variety of techniques:

1. Percutaneous transluminal angioplasty (PTA), in which a balloon is expanded across a stenotic area, thus fracturing the plaque and expanding the arterial lumen via a "controlled dissection"
2. Atherectomy, in which a specially designed catheter is used to shave a portion of the plaque from inside the vessel lumen
3. Stenting or stent grafting, which is an evolving technique involving the placement of an expandable metal stent across the stenotic area

The application of PTA for arterial occlusive disease of the lower extremities continues to increase and the long-term results of PTA are expected to improve with advances in technology. Overall, the initial technical success rates for open surgical procedures and PTA are similar; however, surgery results in superior long-term patency. On the other hand, angioplasty is often associated with lower mortality and morbidity rates, and late failure of PTA can often be treated successfully with a percutaneous reintervention [48].

Conclusion

All patients identified as having vascular disease should be counseled about lifestyle and medication adjustments to reduce their cardiovascular risk profile. Treatment decisions usually depend on the severity of vascular disease and its associated symptoms. An accurate diagnostic evaluation therefore plays a pivotal role in the management of a patient with vascular disease. The clinical history, physical exam, noninvasive tests, and imaging studies can detect, quantify, and monitor vascular disease. A firm understanding of the principles, advantages, and limitations of the various diagnostic modalities will help general surgeons deliver the highest level of care to patients with vascular disease.

References

1. North American Symptomatic Carotid Endarterectomy Trial Collaborators. Beneficial effect of carotid endarterectomy in symptomatic patients with high-grade carotid stenosis. N Engl J Med. 1991;325:445–53.
2. Imparato AM, Kim GE, Davidson T, Crowley JG. Intermittent claudication: its natural course. Surgery. 1975;78:795–9.
3. Boyd AM. The natural course of arteriosclerosis of lower extremities. Proc R Soc Med. 1962;55:591–3.
4. Perazella MA. Current status of gadolinium toxicity in patients with kidney disease. Clin J Am Soc Nephrol. 2009;4:461–9.
5. Rutherford RB, Baker JD, Ernst C, Johnston KW, Porter JM, Ahn S, et al. Recommended standards for reports dealing with lower extremity ischemia: revised version. J Vasc Surg. 1997;26:517–38.
6. Norgren L, Hiatt WR, Dormandy JA, Nehler MR, Harris KA, Fowkes FGR, on behalf of the TASC II Working Group. Inter-society consensus for the management of peripheral arterial disease (TASC II). J Vasc Surg. 2007;45(Suppl S):S5–67.
7. Selvin E, Marinopoulos S, Berkenblit G, Rami T, Brancati FI, Powe NR, et al. Meta-analysis: glycosylated hemoglobin and cardiovascular disease in diabetes mellitus. Ann Intern Med. 2004;141(6):421–31.
8. Kannel WB, Skinner Jr JJ, Schwartz MJ, Shurtleff D. Intermittent claudication: incidence in the Framingham Study. Circulation. 1970;41:875–83.
9. AbuRahma AF, Campbell JE. Overview of peripheral arterial disease of the lower extremity, Chapter 20. In: AbuRahma AF, Bandyk DF, editors. Noninvasive vascular diagnosis: a practical guide to therapy. 3rd ed. New York: Springer; 2012. p. 261–86.
10. van den Berg M, Stehouwer CDA, Bierdrager E, et al. Plasma homocysteine and severity of atherosclerosis in young patients with lower-limb atherosclerotic disease. Arterioscler Thromb Vasc Biol. 1996;16:165–71.
11. Ridker PM, Stampfer MJ, Rifai N. Novel risk factors for systemic atherosclerosis: a comparison of C-reactive protein, fibrinogen, homocysteine, lipoprotein(a), and standard cholesterol screening as predictors of peripheral arterial disease. JAMA. 2001;285(19):2481–5.
12. Kullo IJ, Bailey KR, Kardia SL, Mosley Jr TH, Boerwinkle E, Turner ST. Ethnic differences in peripheral arterial disease in the NHLBI Genetic Epidemiology Network of Arteriopathy (GENOA) study. Vasc Med. 2003;8(4):237–42.
13. AbuRahma AF. Duplex scanning of the extracranial carotid arteries, Chapter 7. In: AbuRahma AF, Bandyk DF, editors. Noninvasive vascular diagnosis: a practical guide to therapy. 3rd ed. New York: Springer; 2012. p. 79–110.
14. Culebras A, Kase CS, Masdeu JC, Fox AJ, Bryan RN, Grossman CB, et al. Practice guidelines for the use of imaging in transient ischemic attacks and acute stroke. A report of the Stroke Council, American Heart Association. Stroke. 1997;28:1480–97.
15. Grant EG, Benson CB, Moneta GL, Alexandrov AV, Baker JD, Bluth EI, et al. Carotid artery stenosis: gray-scale and Doppler US diagnosis – Society of Radiologists in Ultrasound Consensus Conference. Radiology. 2003;229:340–6.
16. AbuRahma AF, Srivastava M, Stone PA, Mousa AY, Jain A, Dean LS, et al. Critical appraisal of the carotid duplex consensus criteria in the diagnosis of carotid artery stenosis. J Vasc Surg. 2011;53:53–60.
17. Manning BJ, Kristmundsson T, Sonesson B, Resch T. Abdominal aortic aneurysm diameter: a comparison of ultrasound measurements with those from standard and three-dimensional computed tomography reconstruction. J Vasc Surg. 2009;50:263–8.
18. Ankle Brachial Index Collaboration. Ankle brachial index combined with Framingham Risk Score to predict cardiovascular events and mortality: a meta-analysis. JAMA. 2008;300:197–208.
19. ACCF/ACR/AIUM/ASE/ASN/ICAVL/SCAI/SCCT/SIR/SVM/SVS 2012 Appropriate use criteria for peripheral vascular ultrasound and physiological testing part 1: Arterial ultrasound and physiological testing. J Am Coll Cardiol. 2012;60:242–76.
20. Hass SM, AbuRahma AF. Segmental Doppler pressures and Doppler waveform analysis in peripheral vascular disease of the lower extremities, Chapter 21. In: AbuRahma AF, Bandyk DF, editors. Noninvasive vascular diagnosis: a practical guide to therapy. 3rd ed. New York: Springer; 2012. p. 287–302.

21. Khan SZ, Khan MA, Bradley B, Dayal R, McKinsey JF, Morrissey NJ. Utility of duplex ultrasound in detecting and grading de novo femoropopliteal lesions. J Vasc Surg. 2011;54:1067–73.
22. Armstrong PA, Parodi FE, Bandyk DF. Duplex scanning for lower extremity arterial disease, Chapter 23. In: AbuRahma AF, Bandyk DF, editors. Noninvasive vascular diagnosis: a practical guide to therapy. 3rd ed. New York: Springer; 2012. p. 311–20.
23. Silva MB, Hobson RW, Pappas PJ, Jamil Z, Araki CT, Goldberg MC, Gwertzman G, Padberg FT. A strategy for increasing use of autogenous hemodialysis access procedures: impact of preoperative noninvasive evaluation. J Vasc Surg. 1998;27:302–8.
24. Wells PS, Anderson DR, Bormanis J, Guy F, Mitchell M, Gray L, et al. Value of assessment of pretest probability of deep vein thrombosis in clinical management. Lancet. 1997;350:1795–8.
25. Satomura S, Kaneko Z. Ultrasonic blood rheograph. In: Proceedings of the third international conference on medical electronics. International Federation for Medical Electronics, London; 1960. p. 254.
26. Strandness Jr DE, McCutcheon EP, Rushmer RF. Application of transcutaneous Doppler flow meter in evaluation of occlusive arterial disease. Surg Gynecol Obstet. 1966;122:1039–45.
27. Kosoff G. Gray scale echography in obstetrics and gynecology. Report no. 60. Sydney: Commonwealth Acoustic Laboratories; 1973.
28. Olinger CP. Ultrasonic carotid echoarteriography. Am J Roentgenol. 1969;106:282–95.
29. Hartley DJ, Strandness Jr DE. The effects of atherosclerosis on the transmission of ultrasound. J Surg Res. 1969;9:575–82.
30. Barber FE, Baker DW, Nation AWC, et al. Ultrasonic duplex echo-Doppler scanner. IEEE Trans Biomed Eng. 1974;81:109–13.
31. Blackshear WM, Philips DJ, Chikos PM, Hartley JD, Thiele BL, Strandness Jr DE. Carotid artery velocity patterns in normal and stenotic vessels. Stroke. 1980;11:67–71.
32. Masaryk TJ, Modic MT, Ruggieri PM, Ross JS, Laub G, Lenz GW, et al. Three dimensional (volume) gradient-echo imaging of the carotid bifurcation: preliminary clinical experience. Radiology. 1989;171:801–6.
33. Phillips CD, Bubash LA. CT angiography and MR angiography in the evaluation of extracranial carotid vascular disease. Radiol Clin North Am. 2002;40:783–98.
34. Nederkoom PJ, Elgersma OE, Mali WP, Eikelboom BC, Kappelle LJ, van der Graaf Y. Overestimation of carotid artery stenosis with magnetic resonance angiography compared with digital subtraction angiography. J Vasc Surg. 2002;36:806–13.
35. Bartlet ES, Walters TD, Symons SP. Quantification of carotid stenosis on CT angiography. AJNR Am J Neuroradiol. 2006;27:13.
36. Lee SI, Miller JC, Abbara S, Achenbach S, Jang IK, Thrall JH, et al. Coronary CT angiography. J Am Coll Radiol. 2006;3:560–4.
37. Koelemay MJ, Nederkoom PJ, Reitsma JB, Majoie CB. Systematic review of computed tomographic angiography for assessment of carotid artery disease. Stroke. 2004;35:2306–12.
38. Gronholdt ML. B-mode ultrasound and spiral CT for the assessment of carotid atherosclerosis. Neuroimaging Clin N Am. 2002;12: 421–35.
39. Willmann JK, Baumert B, Schertler T, Wildermuth S, Pfammatter T, Verdun FR, et al. Aortoiliac and lower extremity arteries assessed with 16-detector row CT angiography: prospective comparison with digital subtraction angiography. Radiology. 2005; 236:1083–93.
40. Catalano C, Fraioli F, Laghi A, Napoli A, Bezzi M, Pediconi F, et al. Infrarenal aortic and lower extremity arterial disease: diagnostic performance of multi-detector row CT angiography. Radiology. 2004;231:555–63.
41. Brenner DJ, Hall EJ. Computed tomography – an increasing source of radiation exposure. N Engl J Med. 2007;357:2277–84.
42. Zhou W. Radiation exposure of vascular surgery patients beyond endovascular procedures. J Vasc Surg. 2011;53:39S–43.
43. Turnipseed WD. Diagnosis of carotid artery disease by digital subtraction angiography. In: AbuRahma AF, Diethrich EB, editors. Current noninvasive vascular diagnosis. Littleton: PSG Publishing; 1988. p. 337–55.
44. Katayama H, Yamaguchi K, Kozuka T, Takashima T, Seez P, Matsura K, et al. Adverse reactions to ionic and nonionic contrast media: a report from the Japanese Committee on the safety of contrast media. Radiology. 1990;175:621–8.
45. AbuRahma AF, Robinson PA, Boland JP, Umstot RK, Clubb EA, Grandia RA, et al. Complications of arteriography in a recent series of 707 cases: factors affecting outcome. Ann Vasc Surg. 1993;7: 122–9.
46. Balduf LM, Langsfeld M, Marek JM, Tullis MJ, Kasirajan K, Matteson B. Complication rates of diagnostic angiography performed by vascular surgeons. Vasc Endovascular Surg. 2002;36: 439–45.
47. AbuRahma AF, Elmore M, Deel J, Mullins B, Hayes J. Complication of diagnostic arteriography performed by a vascular surgeon in a recent series of 558 patients. Vascular. 2007;15:92–7.
48. Bates MC, AbuRahma AF. An update on endovascular therapy of the lower extremities. J Endovasc Ther. 2004;11:II-107–27.

Surgical and Endovascular Technique and Tools

2

Eanas S. Yassa and Jeffrey P. Carpenter

Introduction

There are few complications or traumatic injuries that elicit more distress in even the most seasoned surgeon than the possibility of uncontrolled hemorrhage from a major blood vessel. The vascular-trained surgeon has one key tool to manage this problem: the understanding of vascular exposures to obtain proximal and distal control. Herein, we discuss the basic exposures that any general surgeon would benefit to have at hand, the tools of the trade that can be foreign to those not familiar, and some basic steps in performing endovascular diagnostic studies. Although some of these exposures are common (e.g., femoral and brachial artery exposures), many are not relevant to an elective general surgical practice. The information may however be helpful in emergent/urgent situations for damage control or stabilization especially for surgeons practicing in rural settings.

Exposures

Aorta

Abdominal aortic exposure can be obtained through two primary approaches: transperitoneal and retroperitoneal. The benefits to each exposure listed in Table 2.1 have been discussed at length by many groups. The importance of the surgeon's comfort level with each exposure cannot be overstated in terms of minimizing injury to additional structures and optimizing the benefits of each approach.

E.S. Yassa, MD
Department of Vascular Surgery, Frederik Meijer Heart and Vascular Institute, Spectrum Health, 100 Michigan St NE, Grand Rapids, MI 49503, USA
e-mail: EANAS.YASSA@Spectrumhealth.org

J.P. Carpenter, MD (✉)
Department of Surgery, Cooper Medical School, 3 Cooper Plaza, Suite 411, Camden, NJ 08103, USA
e-mail: carpenter-jeffrey@cooperhealth.edu

Transperitoneal Abdominal Aortic Exposure

The abdomen is incised in the midline as for a standard laparotomy approach (Fig. 2.1). Adherence to the linea alba makes abdominal closure easier. To minimize the likelihood of bowel injury secondary to abdominal wall adhesions, select a site in the upper abdomen or away from any prior incision sites to enter the peritoneum sharply. Digital exploration ensures that no bowel is adherent to the abdominal wall prior to extending the laparotomy incision along the length of the abdomen from xiphoid to pubis. The falciform ligament should be divided between ties. Exposure of the infrarenal aorta begins with mobilization of the small bowel to the right of the midline (Fig. 2.2). When taking down the attachments at the ligament of Treitz and opening the retroperitoneum, care should be taken to incise slightly to the left of the midline. This technique leaves an adequate margin of tissue for suture closure of the retroperitoneum at the end of the case without risking inadvertent bowel injury.

Once the retroperitoneum has been opened, clamp sites for proximal and distal vascular control should be exposed as soon as possible. Distal control can be obtained at the level of the common iliac arteries or by isolating each external and internal iliac artery separately, if common iliac aneurysmal or occlusive disease is present. Circumferential control of the iliac arteries is not necessary and should be avoided to minimize the risk of iliac vein injury. Surgical dissection at the aortic bifurcation should also be avoided to prevent injury to the sympathetic nerve plexus at that location.

Proximal dissection in the retroperitoneum begins by exposing the left renal vein as it crosses anterior to the aorta. Failure to find the left renal vein indicates the presence of a retroaortic left renal vein which passes posterior to the abdominal aorta. This relatively common anomaly highlights the importance of avoiding unnecessary circumferential dissection of the abdominal aorta (Fig. 2.3). A slight cephalad retraction of the crossing renal vein usually exposes the bilateral renal arteries.

If suprarenal aortic clamping is required, exposure between the SMA and renal arteries is sometimes adequate.

V. Gahtan and M.J. Costanza (eds.), *Essentials of Vascular Surgery for the General Surgeon*,
DOI 10.1007/978-1-4939-1326-8_2, © Springer Science+Business Media New York 2015

Table 2.1 Comparative benefits of aortic approaches

Transperitoneal (supine patient)	Retroperitoneal
Easy access to upper extremities for line placement	Centripetal obesity and fatty abdominal viscera displaced
Bilateral groin access	Easy access to thoracic aorta and suprarenal aorta
Extension to median sternotomy	Abdominal viscera not in field
Access to abdominal viscera	Decreased post-op ileus
Ability to prep and drape prior to induction	Diminished risk of aortoenteric fistula secondary to decreased exposure of the suture lines

Adapted from Cronnenwett and Johnston [1]

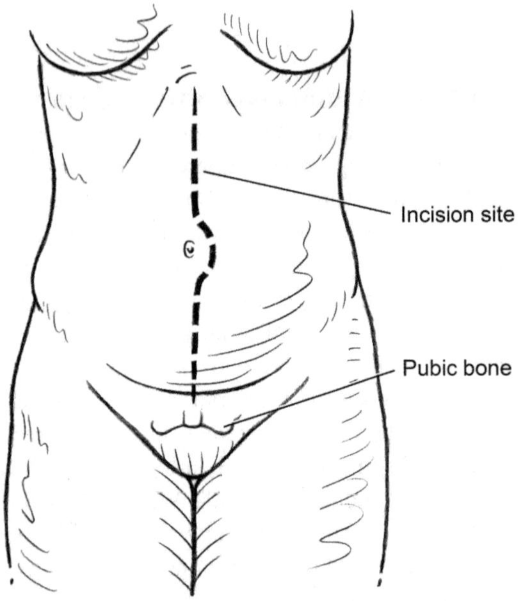

Fig. 2.1 Midline incision extending from the xiphoid to symphysis for transperitoneal approach to abdominal aortic exposure

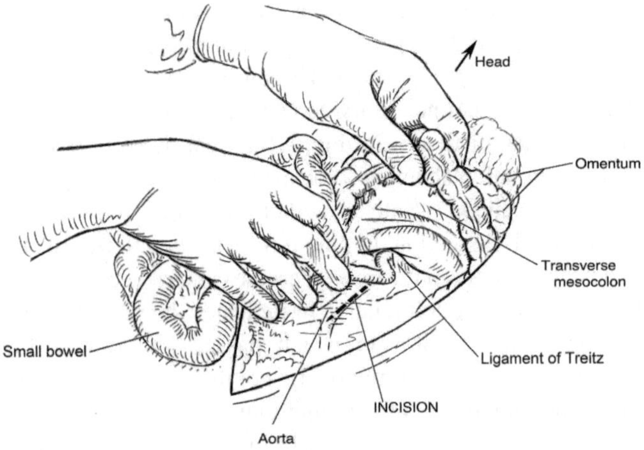

Fig. 2.2 The transverse colon and omentum are lifted cephalad and the small bowel retracted to the right to expose the retroperitoneum. Incision in the retroperitoneum is made slightly to left of the midline to allow closure of the retroperitoneum over the aorta after repair

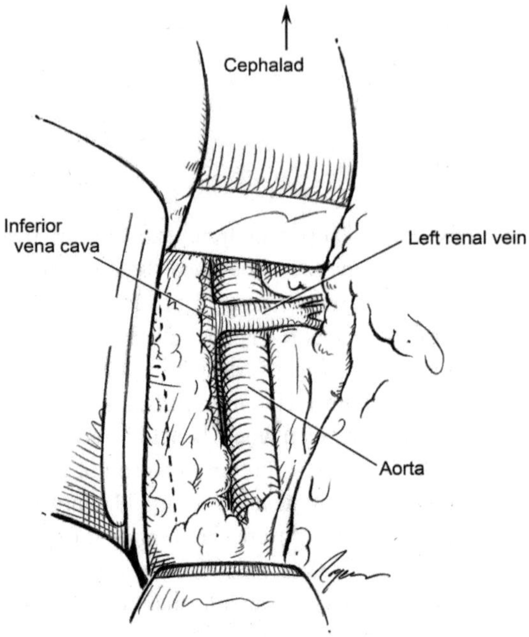

Fig. 2.3 The aorta with the crossing left renal vein. The crossing vein marks the approximate location of the renal arteries as well

Exposure between the SMA and celiac artery is rarely needed, and a clamp in this location leads to ongoing blood loss secondary to SMA backbleeding via collateral pathways fed by the celiac trunk. To avoid this problem, the next level of exposure obtained via a transperitoneal approach is the supraceliac aorta. Exposure in this location is facilitated by having a nasogastric or orogastric tube in place. In emergent situations, pulling the cardia of the stomach downward allows for manual palpation of the gastric tube. The aorta is then located where it crosses the diaphragmatic hiatus. The left anterior crus of the diaphragm should be sharply divided, and planes on each side of the aorta can be digitally developed enough to place a clamp in this location. Being able to palpate the spine on each side usually indicates that the aorta has been adequately cleared for clamping. Attempts to clamp the aorta before incising the periaortic tissues down to the spine will fail as the clamp slips off anteriorly. The most common error in this location is inadvertent clamping of the esophagus, typically caused by forgetting that the aorta is the

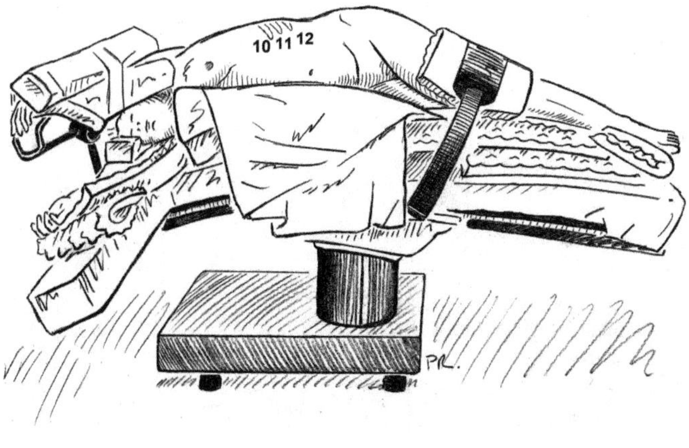

Fig. 2.4 Positioning patient in left lateral decubitus position for retroperitoneal aortic exposure

more posterior structure and the vertebral bodies are directly deep to it. Palpation of the gastric tube in the esophagus provides a constant reminder of its location and helps avoid esophageal injury and inadvertent clamping.

When exposure of the visceral segment of the aorta is needed, for example, in the setting of type IV thoracoabdominal aneurysm repair, we recommend a retroperitoneal approach to avoid obscuration by the overlying viscera.

Retroperitoneal Aortic Exposure

Retroperitoneal aortic exposure has the advantages discussed previously (Table 2.1). The key steps in positioning prior to this exposure are as follows:

1. Patient on a "sandbag" or "beanbag."
2. Ensuring that the flexion point or adjustable "kidney rest" of the operating table is at the level of the space between the iliac crest and the costal margin.
3. The patient is turned into a lateral decubitus position with the right side down. An axillary roll minimizes the possibility of right brachial plexus injury.
4. The left arm is extended upward and across the body and supported on either a Mayo stand or arm sling that can be secured to the operating table.
5. The lower extremities are carefully padded.
6. The "reflex" position of the bed obtained by raising the kidney rest opens the space between the costal margin and iliac crest and increases the intercostal spaces as well.
7. In patients with abdominal obesity, the pannus is allowed to fall forward while being supported with the beanbag. This position ensures that the benefits of retroperitoneal exposure are maximized (Fig. 2.4).

A curvilinear incision begins lateral to the rectus sheath, approximately 2 in. anterior to the anterior superior iliac spine (ASIS) and extends superiorly to the appropriate rib space as determined by the proximal extent of the aneurysm. For most abdominal aortic pathology, the incision is carried through the 10th interspace (the highest unattached rib) (Fig. 2.5).

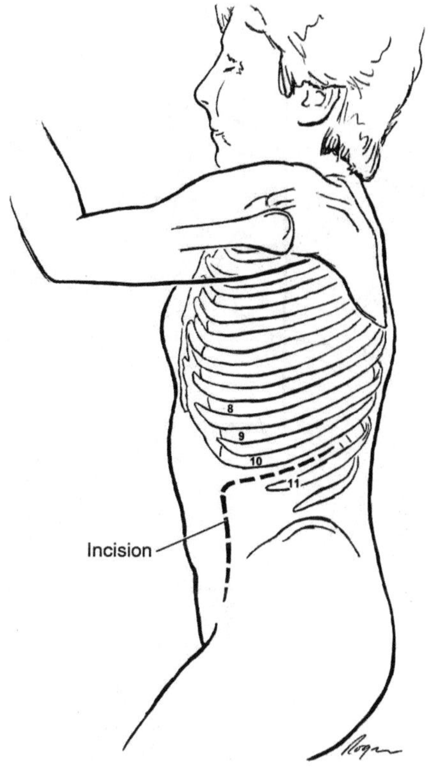

Fig. 2.5 Typical incision for juxtarenal aortic exposure is through the 10th interspace and then extends parallel to the rectus

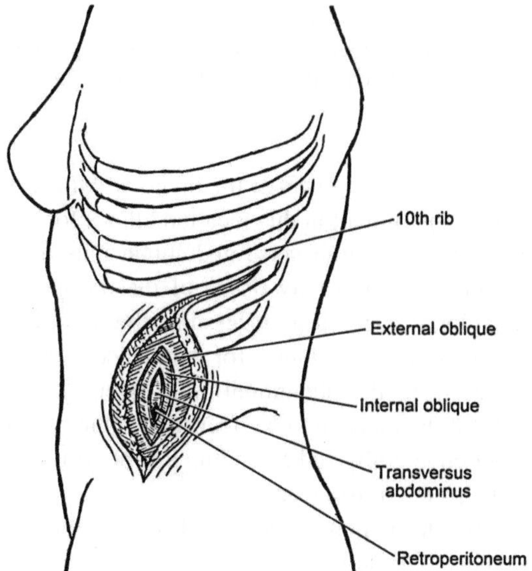

Fig. 2.6 Retroperitoneal aortic exposure demonstrates the muscle layers divided to expose the retroperitoneal space and avoid entry into the peritoneum

Careful attention to the layers of the abdominal wall in this location can help avoid inadvertent entrance into the peritoneum (Fig. 2.6). The first layer encountered is the external oblique aponeurosis. Incising this layer with elec-

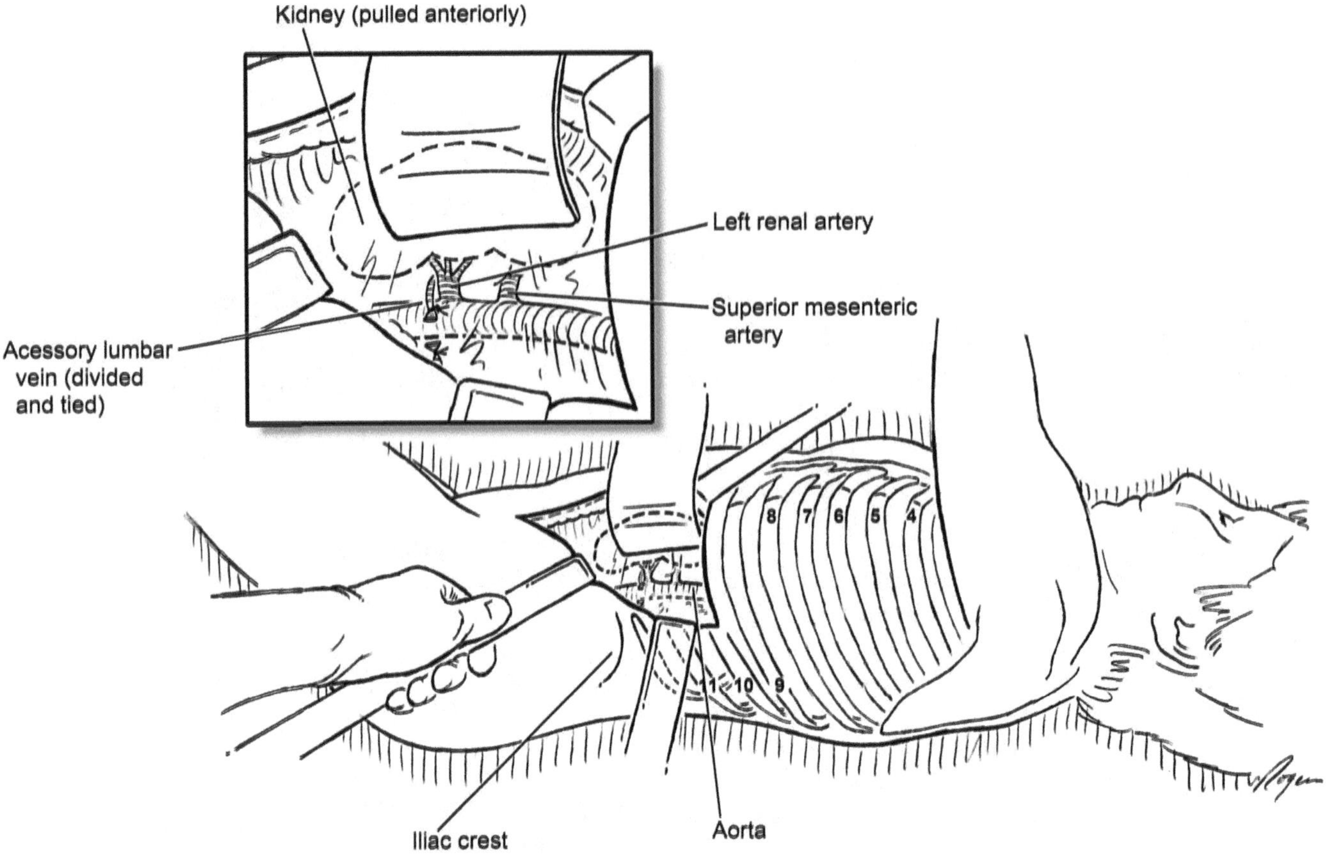

Fig. 2.7 Retroperitoneal aortic exposure with the left kidney reflected anteriorly. The left renal artery is traced back to its origin at the aorta, and the superior mesenteric artery can be felt slightly above. *Inset*: The accessory lumbar vein draining to the left renal vein is divided before the aorta is opened

trocautery exposes the fibers of the internal oblique. Using a blunt-tipped instrument in this location allows for spreading and exposure of the transverse abdominal muscular fibers, behind which lays the fatty tissue of the retroperitoneum. Digital exploration confirms access into the retroperitoneum not the peritoneum and allows for manual separation of the peritoneum from the abdominal wall layers to allow the remainder of the incision to be opened. Beginning this manual dissection laterally and extending it superiorly to the diaphragm helps maximize exposure.

Once the retroperitoneal space has been developed, manual displacement of the left kidney anteriorly allows for identification of the left renal artery and exposes the left diaphragmatic crus if needed. A self-retaining retractor assists with the exposure and can also be positioned to keep the left ureter out of the operative field. Exposure of the left renal artery and dissection proximally to its origin from the aorta takes the surgeon across an accessory lumbar vein that drains into the left renal vein. This vein should be preemptively divided to avoid avulsing it (Fig. 2.7). The aortic bifurcation can be located by palpation, and the bilateral common iliac arteries are usually bluntly exposed to minimize iliac vein injury while creating isolated clamp locations. If additional proximal exposure above the renal arteries is required, the right renal artery is usually lower than the left, and exposing above the left renal artery with a combination of blunt and sharp dissection allows the SMA pulsation to be appreciated. If space to clamp in this location is not adequate, the left crus can be divided which quickly exposes the supraceliac aorta. In emergent situations, the initial incision through the 10th intercostal space allows manual palpation of and clamp placement on the thoracic aorta until further exposure can be obtained. Thoracic aortic clamping is a temporary, salvage maneuver, and the clamp should be moved distally as soon as possible.

When planned intervention requires a supraceliac aortic clamp, the incision is often through the 9th interspace which requires division of the costochondral cartilage. If planned intervention is on the descending thoracic aorta primarily, or in addition to abdominal aorta, incision through the 6th rib space, with or without division of the diaphragmatic fibers, allows for proximal thoracic aortic clamping (Fig. 2.8). These procedures are typically performed with sequential clamp techniques and left heart bypass if the situation demands.

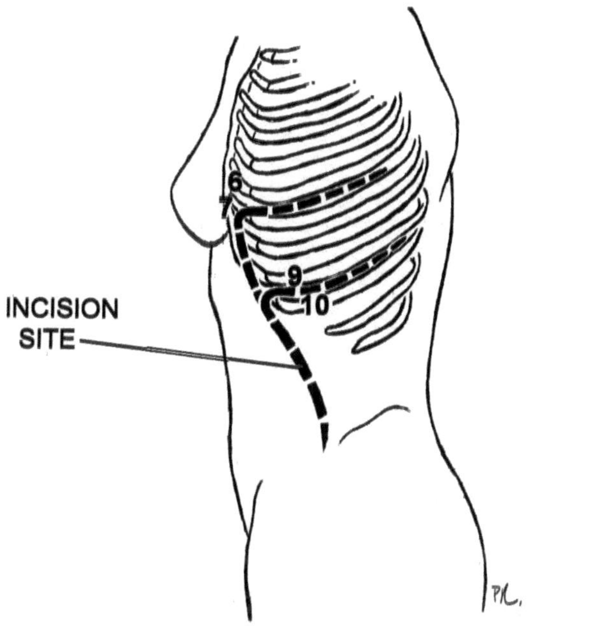

Fig. 2.8 Alternative incisions from retroperitoneal approach through the 9th interspace allows for improved exposure to the supraceliac aorta and through the 6th interspace allows for descending thoracic aortic exposure

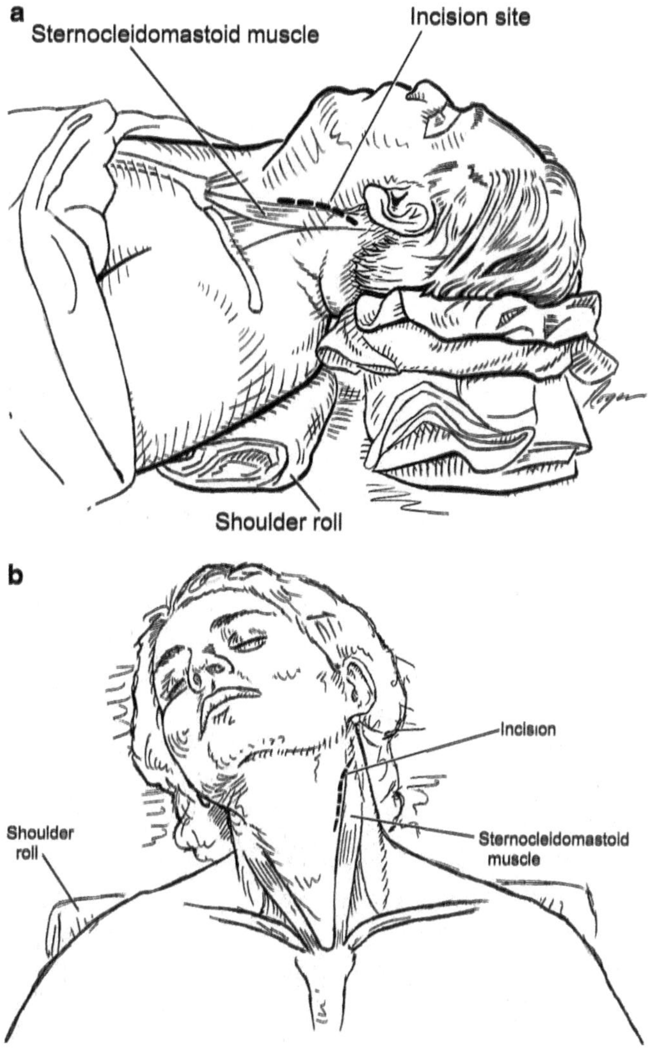

Fig. 2.9 (**a**, **b**) The lateral and anterior view of positioning for carotid exposure: the patient is positioned with the neck extended using a shoulder roll. Incision paralleling the anterior border of the sternocleidomastoid muscle and directing posteriorly before reaching the angle of the mandible

Descriptions of exposures to gain access to the aortic arch and the origin of the great vessels can be found in any cardiac or thoracic surgical atlas. Exposure of the ascending aorta, aortic arch, innominate artery, and left common carotid artery origin is obtained by way of a median sternotomy. To expose the origin of the left subclavian artery, a left anterior thoracotomy is performed through the fourth intercostal space.

Carotid, Subclavian, and Axillary Artery Exposures

Carotid Artery

The most common means of exposing the carotid artery, for both traumatic exploration and elective intervention, requires neck extension with the patient's head turned to the contralateral side whenever possible (Fig. 2.9a, b). The incision is placed along the anterior border of the sternocleidomastoid muscle. Care is taken to angle the incision posteriorly as it approaches to within 1–2 in. of the angle of the mandible as this minimizes the risk of injury to the marginal mandibular nerve. Injury to this nerve can manifest as unilateral downward drooping of the mouth and numbness.

After incising the skin, the platysma is divided in the same direction as the skin incision using the electrocautery. The external jugular vein is sometimes encountered and can be ligated and divided between ties. The anterior border of the sternocleidomastoid muscle should then be delineated and the muscle belly grasped and retracted posteriorly and laterally to allow for exposure of the internal jugular vein (Fig. 2.10a). Once the internal jugular vein is identified, mobilizing its anterior border leads to exposure of the facial vein. This crossing vein typically functions as a landmark for the level of the carotid bifurcation. The facial vein should be ligated and divided with care to avoid injury of the underlying hypoglossal nerve. The carotid artery is encased within its own sheath and lies deep and medial to the jugular vein. Before opening the carotid sheath, careful inspection sometimes reveals an anterior vagus nerve that should be protected. The vagus nerve is easily differentiated from the crossing branches of the ansa cervicalis by its larger size and its course which parallels the carotid artery. The inferior border of the dissection is typically the omohyoid muscle, while superiorly the dissection usually ends at the posterior belly of the digastric muscle (Fig. 2.10b).

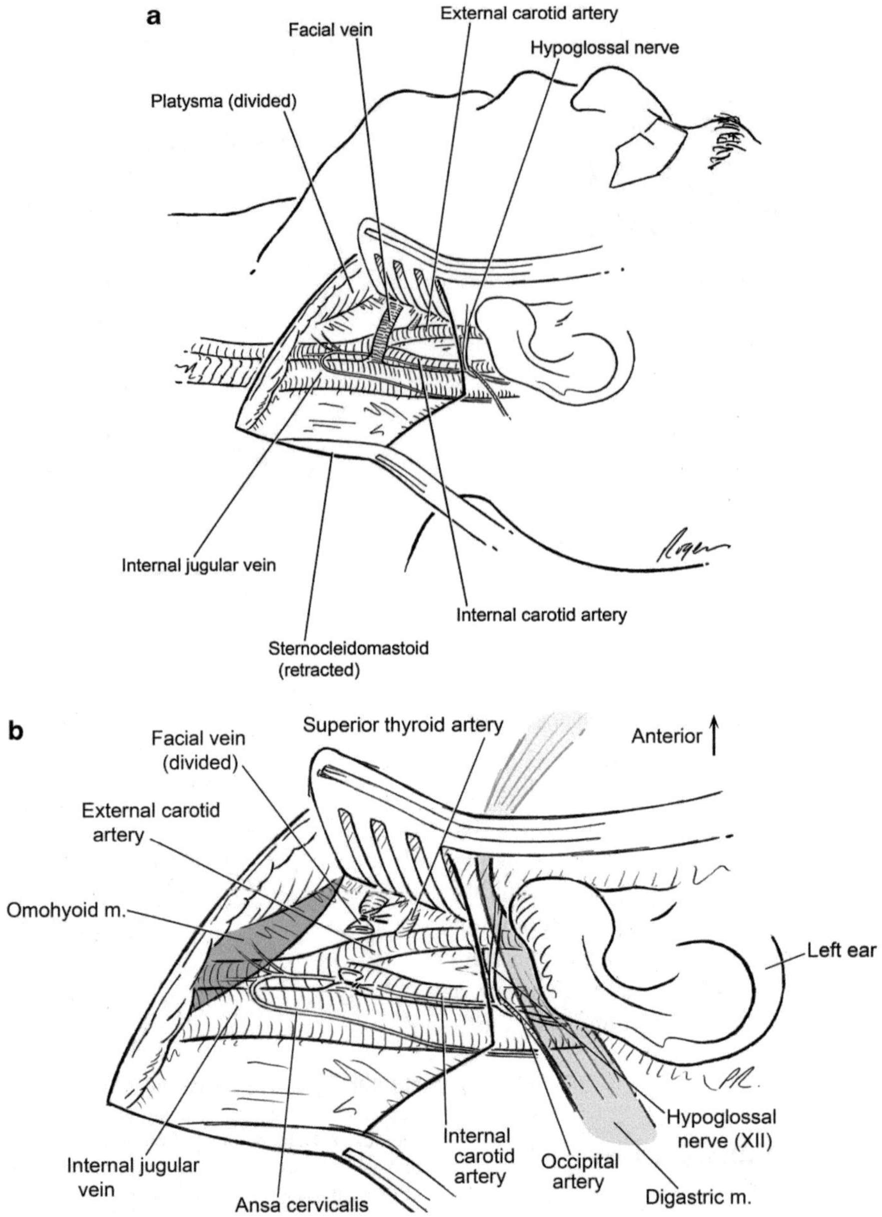

Fig. 2.10 (**a**) Carotid exposure: after division of the platysma and posterior retraction of the sternocleidomastoid muscle, the facial vein is noted to be crossing at the approximate level of the carotid bifurcation. (**b**) Once the facial vein is divided, the carotid bifurcation and superior thyroid artery can be exposed for further dissection and control. Note the omohyoid muscle at the inferior edge of the dissection and the posterior belly of the digastric muscle at the superior edge of the dissection. Can be either partially or completely divided for additional exposure if needed. Note the location of CN XII crossing the internal carotid artery

Division of either the omohyoid or digastric muscle belly allows for some additional exposure with minimal disability. Superior exposure of the internal carotid artery usually exposes the hypoglossal nerve which is held in place by an arterial branch to the sternocleidomastoid muscle. The division of this artery allows the hypoglossal nerve to be swung cephalad and protected from harm. Multiple small veins in this location also must be carefully dissected and preemptively divided to avoid unnecessary bleeding and blind placement of clips or cauterizing that can lead to nerve damage.

In the case of a planned carotid-subclavian bypass or transposition procedure, exposure of both the carotid and subclavian arteries can be obtained via a transverse supraclavicular incision centered over the medial third of the clavicle.

Supraclavicular Subclavian Artery Exposure

Supraclavicular exposure allows access to the subclavian artery as well as the origin of the vertebral artery if needed. The surgeon must remember that left-sided supraclavicular dissection risks injury to the thoracic duct, which arises deep

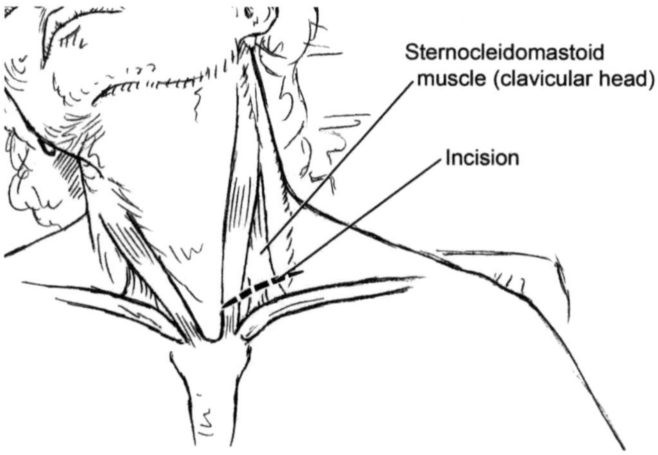

Fig. 2.11 Incision for supraclavicular exposure of the subclavian artery

and inferior in the wound to enter the posterior aspect of the internal jugular and subclavian vein confluence.

The patient is positioned with both arms tucked at the sides, the neck turned toward the contralateral side. A shoulder roll can be used when additional extension is needed to widen the space between the shoulder and neck. The incision is made approximately 1.5 cm above the clavicle and typically extends across the lateral head of the sternocleidomastoid (SCM) and 2 cm to either side (Fig. 2.11). The platysma muscle and the lateral head of the SCM are both divided. The authors recommend the scalene fat pad be mobilized inferomedially and then retracted superolaterally. Care is taken to not injure the phrenic nerve, which courses lateral to medial on the anterior surface of the anterior scalene muscle. Exposure of the subclavian artery typically requires the anterior scalene muscle to be divided. This is most safely done near its insertion onto the 1st rib. The muscle fibers can be elevated from the deeper brachial plexus using a right angle or straight dissector. Again, awareness of the trajectory and course of the phrenic nerve cannot be overstated.

Once the anterior scalene muscle is divided and reflected upward, the fascia overlying the subclavian artery can be sharply incised to mobilize the artery. The subclavian artery branches including the internal mammary, thyrocervical trunk, and vertebral artery can be individually encircled with vessel loops for control. Once mobilized, the subclavian artery easily elevates into the wound.

Infraclavicular Exposure of the Axillary Artery

Exposure of the axillary artery is most often used for axillofemoral bypass. The patient can be positioned supine with the arm tucked at the side or the arm abducted 90° on an arm board. The use of a shoulder roll to slightly elevate the side being exposed can also be helpful. Sterile skin preparation should include the neck and chest from the midline across to

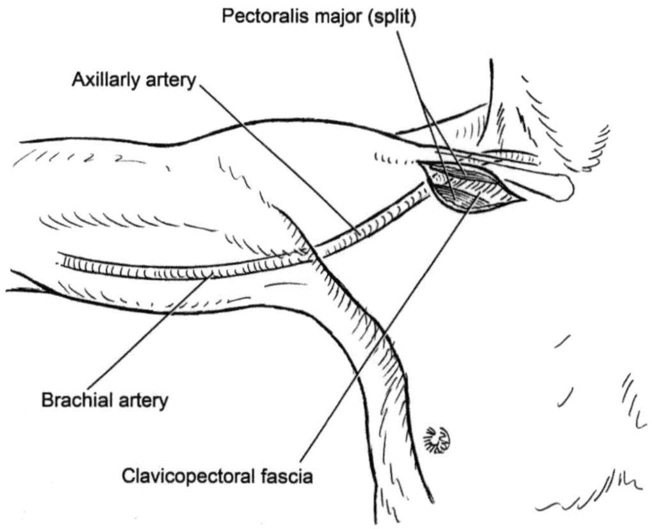

Fig. 2.12 Incision location and exposure of the infraclavicular axillary artery

the shoulder. An incision is made 2–4 cm below the clavicle extending from the deltopectoral groove to the lateral aspect of the clavicular head (Fig. 2.12). The fibers of the pectoralis major are then separated in the direction of their axis to expose the clavipectoral fascia beneath. The pectoralis minor lies laterally in the exposed space and should be divided in addition to the clavipectoral fascia to optimally expose the fibrofatty tissue surrounding the axillary artery and vein. The vein lies slightly anterior and inferior to the artery in this location, and care should be taken to avoid injury during circumferential dissection and control. In this location the thoracoacromial trunk should be divided to allow the artery to be pulled up into the wound, which is best done using atraumatic silastic vessel loops.

Exposure of the Lower Extremity Arteries

Femoral Artery

Understanding femoral vascular anatomy is critical to open, endovascular, and percutaneous procedures in vascular surgery. The inguinal ligament should be first delineated by the bony landmarks of the anterior superior iliac spine and the pubic tubercle. The femoral artery bisects the inguinal ligament with a slight medial to lateral trajectory.

For exposure of the femoral artery and its bifurcation, a vertical incision overlying and paralleling the expected course of the femoral artery is planned (Fig. 2.13) and is the preferred approach for occlusive disease. The overlying subcutaneous tissue is divided. The superficial epigastric vein is typically encountered and divided between ties or clips. Once the fibrofatty lymph tissue overlying the femoral artery is encountered, we recommend ligating and dividing this

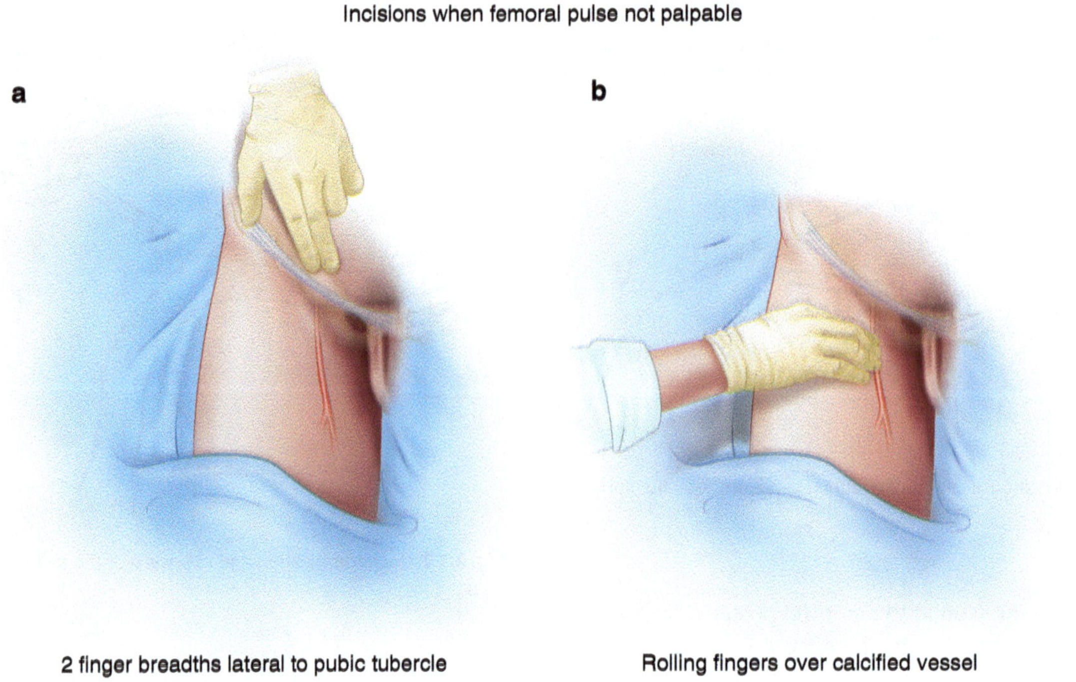

Fig. 2.13 Incision location and relevant bony landmarks of the anterior superior iliac spine and symphysis pubis for femoral artery exposure

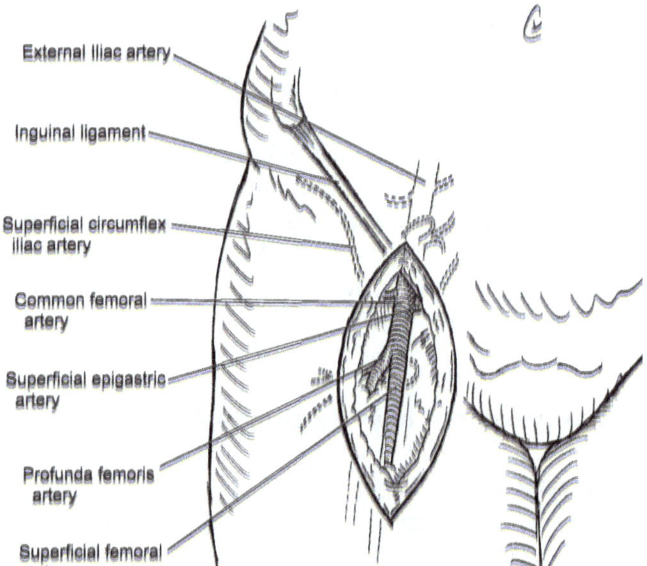

Fig. 2.14 With the fatty tissue divided and the femoral sheath open, the common femoral artery and its bifurcation is exposed

tissue between ties. This technique minimizes the risk of postoperative lymphatic leak, which is particularly troublesome when prosthetic graft material has been used in the groin.

The first step involves palpating for the femoral pulsation or the non-pulsatile but highly calcified femoral artery. Exposure of the inguinal ligament allows for proximal control as the common femoral artery passes beneath the ligament. The femoral circumflex and inferior epigastric arteries are small branches arising laterally and medially, respectively, from the proximal common femoral artery. These branches are usually located at the level of the inguinal ligament and mark the border of the distal external iliac artery from the proximal common femoral artery.

The common femoral artery bifurcates into the superficial femoral artery (SFA) and 1–2 profunda (or deep) femoral arteries. The SFA is a direct continuation of the common femoral artery which continues distally and passes deep to the sartorius muscle. The profunda femoral arteries follow a lateral course into the muscles of the thigh (Fig. 2.14).

Exposure for endovascular aortic procedures (which is generally an isolated common femoral artery dissection) can be via an oblique or transverse incision just below the expected location of the inguinal ligament. The incision is deepened until the inguinal ligament is seen, and then a vertically oriented dissection is performed on the fibrofatty tissue overlying the femoral artery. Again we recommend dividing this tissue between ties to decrease the risk of lymphatic leak.

Above-Knee Popliteal Artery

This may be one of the easiest exposures in vascular surgery once the basic anatomy is understood. The SFA becomes the popliteal artery when it exits the adductor canal, also known as "Hunter's canal." Hunter first described the pathology of popliteal aneurysms in stagecoach drivers, whom he postulated developed the aneurysms as a result of repeated trauma to the artery secondary to prolonged sitting. He also demonstrated that ligation of the artery above and below would not result in limb loss if time was allowed for the development of collateral pathways.

The lower extremity should be prepped circumferentially and positioned with external rotation and abduction at the hip and flexion at the knee. A "bump" of rolled towels or sheets is useful to maintain this position and is positioned under the calf (Fig. 2.15). An incision is made in the natural skin crease that is present between the sartorius and the quadriceps muscle group (Fig. 2.16). After retracting the sartorius muscle downward, the fascia between the adductor tendon and the semimembranous muscles is incised with electrocautery, and the adductor canal is entered. The adductor canal is identified by a space filled with fibrofatty tissue. The vastus medialis is then retracted superiorly (Fig. 2.17).

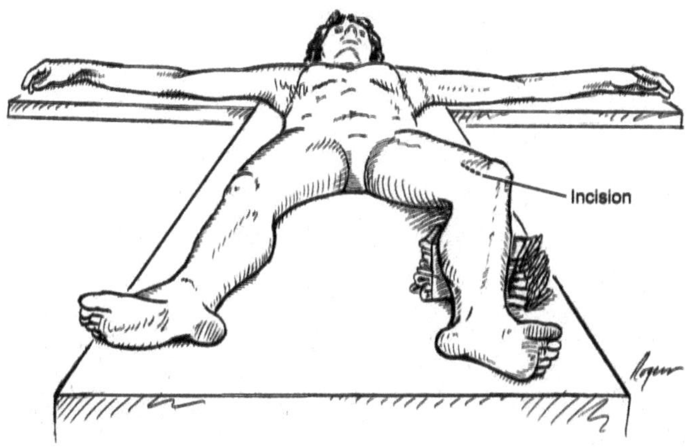

Fig. 2.15 Positioning for above-knee popliteal artery exposure. Note the operative leg slightly externally rotated and flexed at the knee with a bump below the gastrocnemius muscle

Blunt manual dissection spreads the fibrofatty tissue until the popliteal artery is easily felt by palpating along the posterior aspect of the femur. The popliteal artery is typically medial to the vein in this location (Fig. 2.18). The anterior tibial nerve, an in-line branch of the sciatic nerve, also courses posterior to the vascular structures in this location and should be protected from harm.

Behind-the-Knee Popliteal Artery

The prone position provides the best exposure of the popliteal artery directly behind the knee and may be useful for addressing selected popliteal artery aneurysms, popliteal entrapment syndrome, and adventitial cystic disease. The patient should be supported under the torso, waist, and ankles. A "lazy-S" incision decreases the risk of skin contracture and typically extends from the medial aspect of biceps femoris to the lateral head of the gastrocnemius at the calf (Fig. 2.19). The small saphenous vein is the first structure encountered and is at risk for an incidental injury. Depending on its caliber, the small saphenous vein can be mobilized and harvested for use as an interpositional bypass.

Running lateral to the small saphenous vein is the medial sural nerve, which can be traced back to the tibial nerve in the popliteal fossa. An incision in the fascia medial to the small saphenous vein allows access to the popliteal fossa. The apex of the fossa is formed by the semimembranous muscle medially and the biceps femoris laterally. The popliteal artery and vein typically lie deep and slightly medial to the tibial nerve in this location, so care is taken to protect the nerve injury during surgical exposure. A small silastic vessel loop can be used to gently retract the nerve laterally. The vein and artery take a parallel course at the apex of the popliteal fossa before the vein moves deep to the artery as the

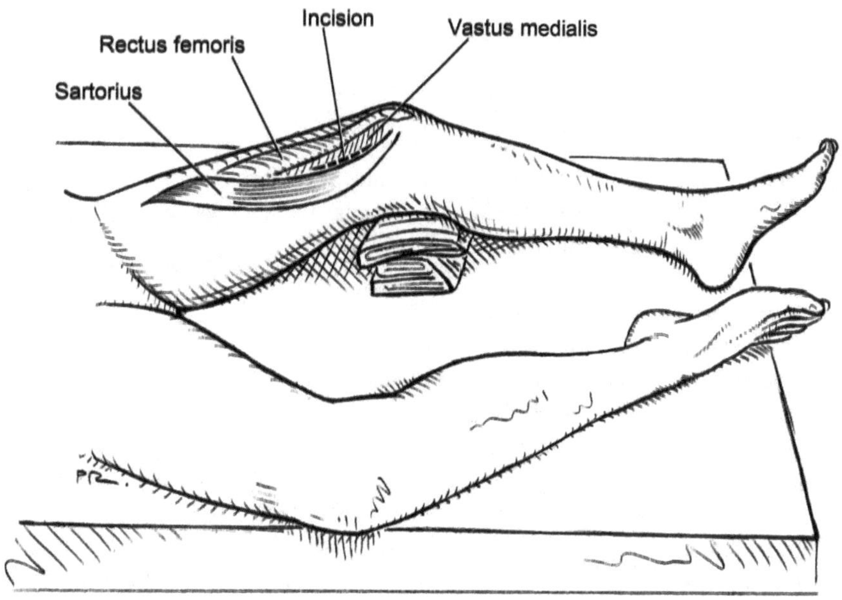

Fig. 2.16 The planned incision for above-knee popliteal artery exposure

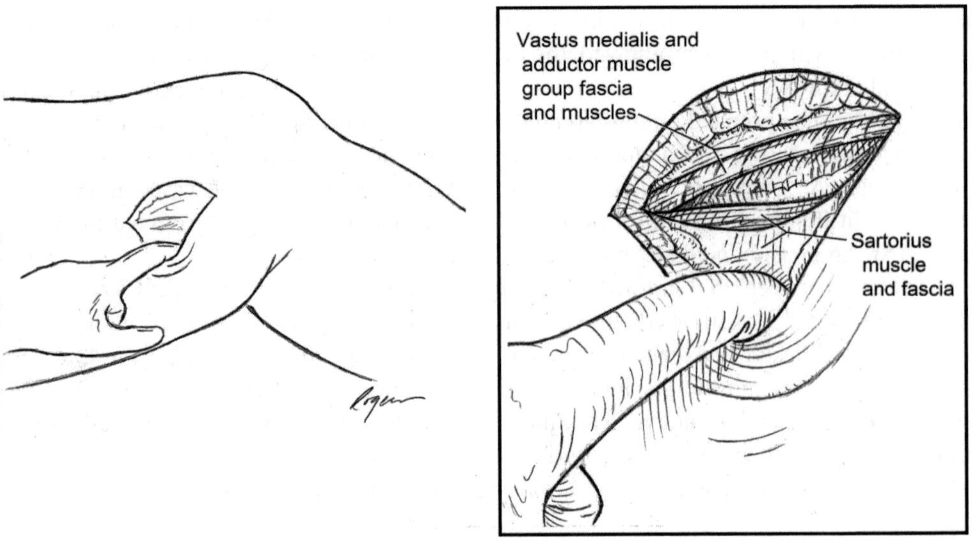

Fig. 2.17 Incision through the subcutaneous fat to the level of the fascia. *Inset:* the fascia is incised to allow entry to the space between the sartorius muscle, which will be retracted posteriorly, and the vastus medialis and adductor muscle group, which will be retracted anteriorly

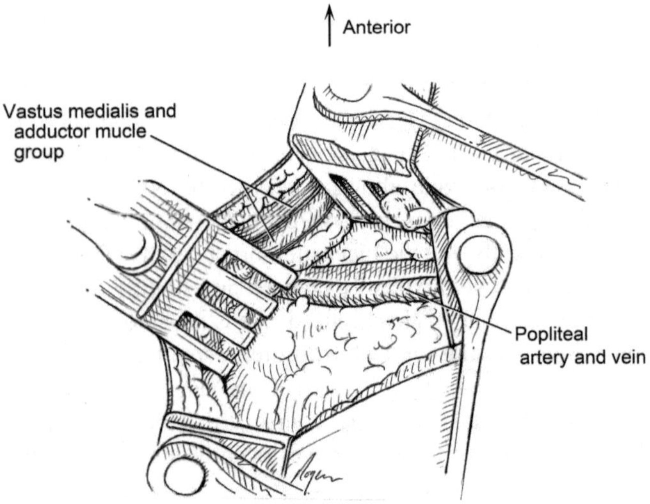

Fig. 2.18 After blunt digital dissection in the fibrofatty space. The popliteal artery and vein are exposed. Note that the artery is medial to the vein in this location and, thus, encountered first

dissection progresses distally. Proximal and distal arterial control in this location is obtained in the standard fashion as described elsewhere within this chapter.

Below-Knee Popliteal Artery and Proximal Anterior and Posterior Tibial Artery, Tibioperoneal Trunk, and Peroneal Arteries

Preparation is similar to the above-knee exposure with circumferential leg prep and external rotation/flexion/abduction positioning. For optimal exposure, a bump should be placed above the knee (Fig. 2.20a).

A medial calf begins at the level of the medial condyle approximately 2 in. posterior to and parallel to the tibial border. The fascia overlying the gastrocnemius medial head is incised and the muscle belly retracted inferiorly and posteriorly. We recommend dividing the tendinous insertions of the semitendinous, gracilis, and sartorius muscles to improve exposure and minimize extrinsic compression of anatomically tunneled grafts. This maneuver results in minimal, if any, morbidity.

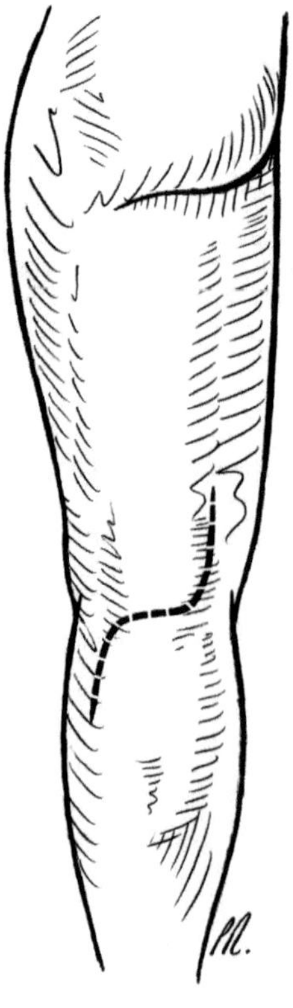

Fig. 2.19 "Lazy-s" incision for the posterior approach to the popliteal artery behind the knee

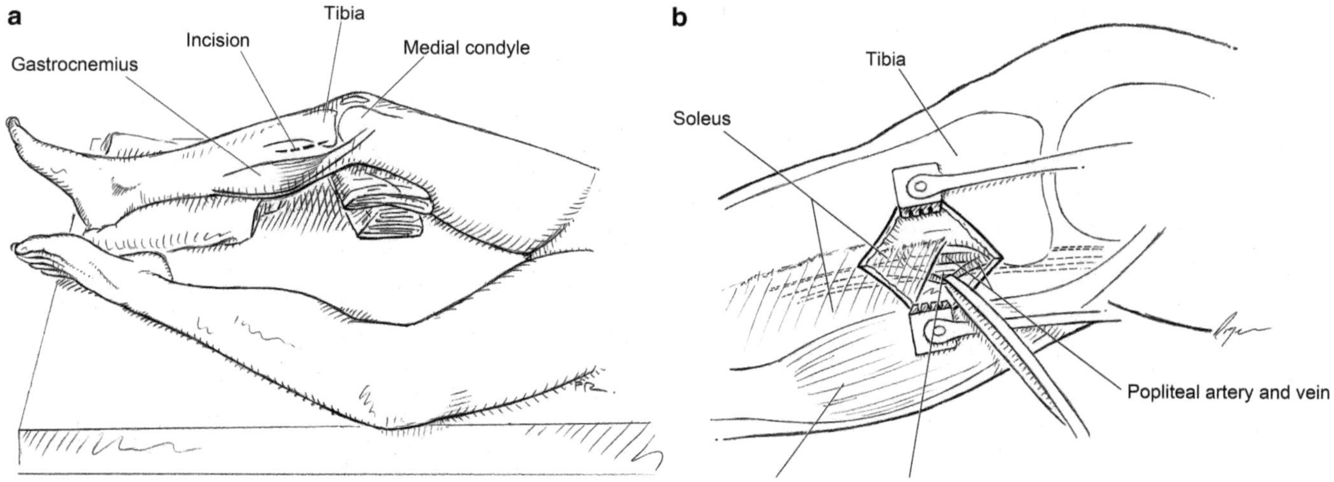

Fig. 2.20 (**a**) Positioning for below-knee popliteal artery exposure – note that the operative leg is slightly externally rotated at the hip and flexed at the knee. A bump positioned at the lower thigh allows the gastrocnemius muscle to fall away. (**b**) With the gastrocnemius muscle retracted posteriorly, the tibial nerve and popliteal artery and vein are exposed below the knee. The nerve and vein are medial to the artery and thus encountered first using this approach

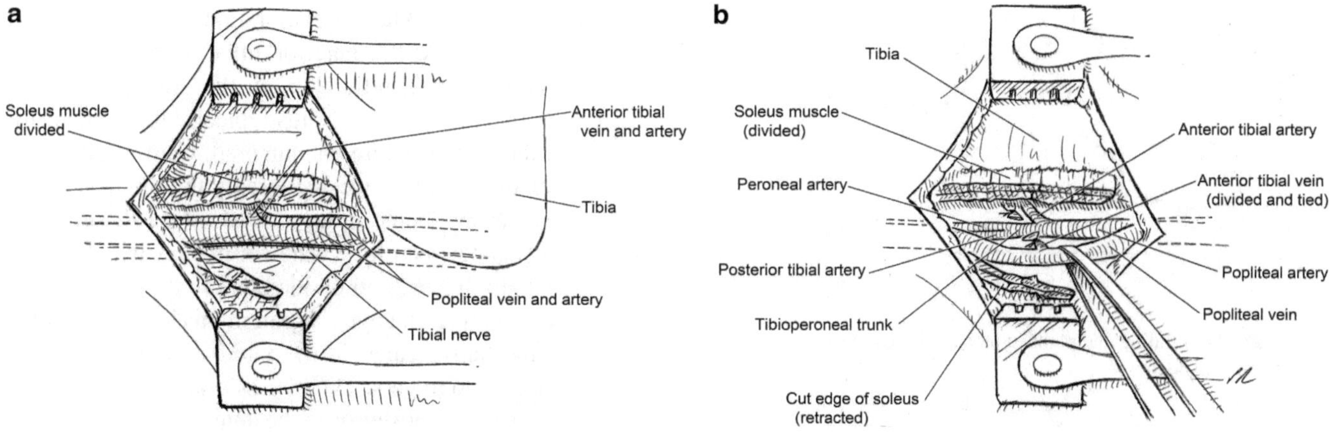

Fig. 2.21 (**a**) Takedown of the proximal soleus attachments to the tibia allows exposure of the anterior tibial vein. (**b**) Division of the anterior tibial vein exposes the popliteal bifurcation to the tibioperoneal trunk and anterior tibial artery

The below-knee popliteal artery is easily palpable by compressing the neurovascular bundle against the posterior aspect of the tibia. The nerve and popliteal vein are typically anterior to the artery so these structures need to be carefully dissected and retracted with the assistance of vessel loops and self-retaining retractors in order to expose the popliteal artery (Fig. 2.20b).

If exposure of the tibioperoneal trunk and anterior tibial artery origin is needed, these vessels can also be exposed through this approach. Taking down the soleus muscle from its insertion on the tibia exposes the remainder of the below-knee popliteal artery and the tibioperoneal trunk (Fig. 2.21a). The dissection can be carried as far distal as necessary to expose the bifurcation of the tibioperoneal trunk into the peroneal artery and posterior tibial artery origins (Fig. 2.21b). Crossing veins and the small, deep anatomic space mandate a careful and meticulous dissection.

The anterior tibial artery is identified as it originates laterally on the popliteal artery, deep to the crossing anterior tibial vein which is typically divided to facilitate exposure. From this exposure the artery travels "away" from the operating surgeon on its way to the anterior compartment. At this point, an anatomic tunnel can be created behind the knee. The index finger of each hand should be positioned just medial to the above- and below-knee neurovascular bundles (Fig. 2.22). Progressive sweeping maneuvers between the fingers will clear the minimal tissue that is in the popliteal fossa allowing for the fingers to touch. A large clamp, umbilical tape, or bypass graft can then be passed through the tunnel.

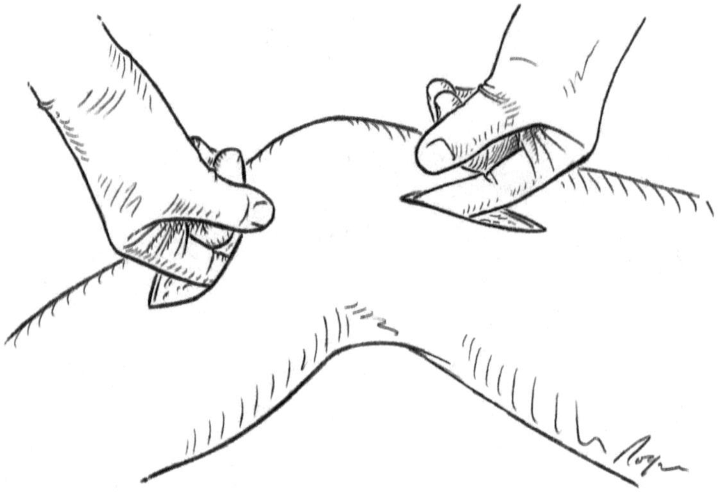

Fig. 2.22 To make an anatomic tunnel in the popliteal fossa for passage of graft, the index fingers of each hand are passed along the posterior surface of the above-knee and below-knee popliteal arteries

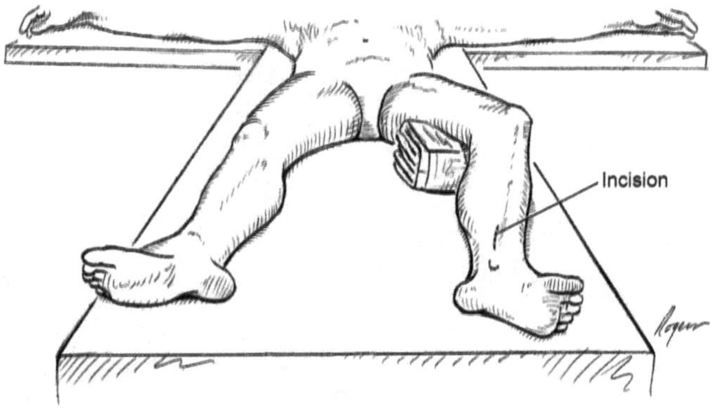

Fig. 2.23 Positioning and planned incision location for distal posterior tibial artery exposure

Distal Posterior Tibial Artery

The distal third of the posterior tibial artery, above the ankle, is best approached from a medial calf incision just posterior to the bony edge of the tibia (Fig. 2.23). The initial skin incision should expose the soleus fascia (Fig. 2.24a). The fascia is incised and muscle fibers spread in the direction of their travel. Just deep to the soleus muscle, the tendon of the flexor digitorum longus (Fig. 2.24b) is retracted anteriorly, and the posterior tibial neurovascular bundle lies immediately deep to it (Fig. 2.24c).

Mid to Distal Anterior Tibial Artery

As previously described, the origin of the anterior tibial artery is exposed as an extension of the below-knee popliteal artery exposure. Because the anterior tibial artery quickly passes through the interosseus membrane, more distal exposure is not pursued from the medial approach.

An anterolateral exposure begins with the hip and knee flexed approximately 30° and internally rotated. An incision is made midway between the tibia and the fibula at the desired exposure level. The fascia separating the tibialis anterior muscle and the extensor digitorum longus is incised using electrocautery. Manual exploration or a self-retaining retractor will expose the anterior tibial artery, veins, and peroneal nerve. The bundle rests on the interosseus membrane with one of the paired veins typically lying anteriorly making it the first structure encountered. Careful dissection will reveal the plane between the anterior tibial vein and artery. A constant theme of any tibial artery dissection is bridging veins between the venae comitantes which should be intentionally ligated and divided before they are avulsed. Anatomic tunneling of a bypass graft in this location requires enlarging the native canal in the interosseus membrane to accommodate two fingers. The bypass graft can then be tunneled from the deep posterior to the anterior compartment in a standard fashion.

Distal to the lower third of the tibia, the extensor hallucis longus (EHL) muscle originates from the medial tibia border. The anterior tibial neurovascular bundle follows a course between the EHL and the tibialis anterior muscle. The anterior tibial vein remains anterior, and the peroneal nerve remains posterior to the anterior tibial artery in this location as well.

Mid to Distal Peroneal Artery

Although the distal peroneal artery can be exposed via a medial approach, we prefer the lateral approach as described below. The lower extremity is circumferentially prepped and draped and positioned with the lower leg slightly flexed and internally rotated. An assistant is often needed to maintain this position for exposure. A longitudinal incision is made over the fibula extending above and below the level of planned peroneal artery exposure for a total length of approximately 15 cm. The common peroneal nerve should be protected as it wraps around the proximal fibular head. The

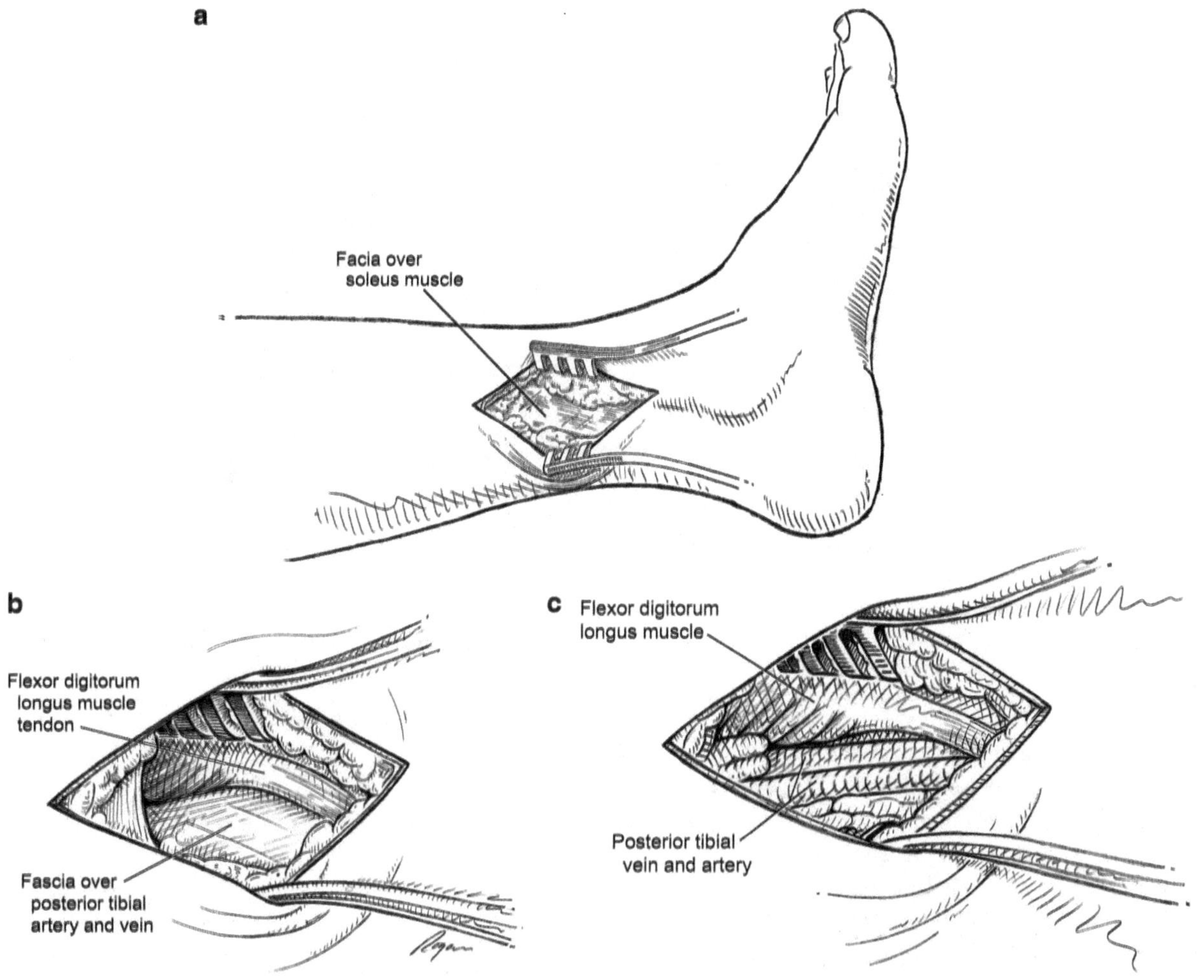

Fig. 2.24 Distal posterior tibial artery exposure. (**a**) Skin incision exposes underlying soleus fascia. (**b**) Incising the fascia exposes the flexor digitorum longus tendon anteriorly and the fascia overlying the neurovascular bundle. (**c**) Incising the fascia exposes the posterior tibial artery and its paired veins

peroneus longus and peroneus brevis muscles are stripped from their attachments to the fibula using a periosteal elevator. Confirm that the muscle has been stripped medially from the fibula before division to avoid inadvertent injury to the underlying peroneal vessels with fibular resection. The fibula is then resected using a bone cutter. Once this segment of fibula has been removed, the peroneal artery and paired veins can be seen in the underlying muscle bed.

For the medial approach to the peroneal artery, the patient is supine, the knee flexed, and the leg rotated laterally [2]. A medial vertical incision is made posterior to the tibia. The soleus muscle is detached from the tibia and retracted posteriorly. The fascia covering the flexor digitorum longus is incised and the plane entered to expose the vessels in the deep compartment. The posterior tibial vessels are encountered first, and the peroneal vessels are exposed by extending the dissection in this plane farther laterally (toward the fibula).

Upper Extremity Exposures

Brachial Artery

Exposure of the brachial artery can be achieved using a transverse incision a finger breadth above or below the antecubital fossa or a longitudinal upper arm incision directly over the brachial pulse. The "lazy-S" incision begins on the medial, distal upper arm and traverses the antecubital fossa before terminating on the proximal, lateral forearm [3]. The choice of incision depends on the reason for exposure. The transverse incision is typically used for arteriovenous access, while the "lazy-S" incision is used in the setting of upper extremity arterial thrombosis requiring an embolectomy or thrombectomy (Fig. 2.25).

Exposure of the brachial artery at above or below the antecubital fossa requires partial division of the biceps aponeurosis fibers that fan from the biceps tendon to the ulnar head. There are typically multiple superficial veins in this

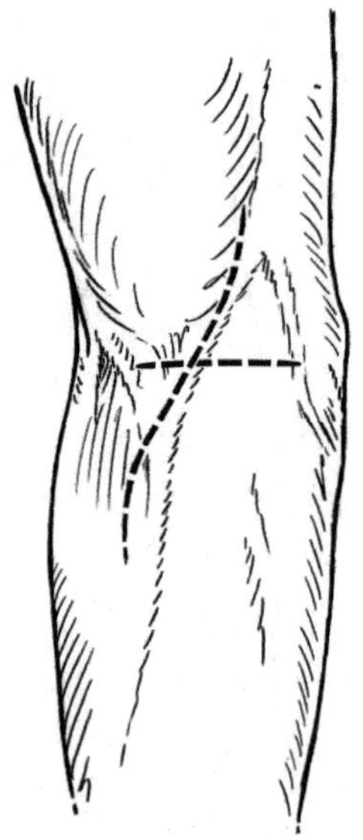

Fig. 2.25 Two incision choices for distal brachial artery exposure. The "lazy-s" incision allows for extension of exposure to the brachial bifurcation and is preferred in settings of thromboembolectomy

location, including the cephalic vein and medial antecubital vein which should be dissected free and protected from injury, particularly if the planned procedure is for creation of autogenous dialysis access (Fig. 2.26a, b).

The brachial artery typically runs between two venae comitantes, which must be sharply dissected free at the proximal and distal control sites. Crossing veins may be ligated between fine silk ties. The median nerve is medial to the brachial artery at this location and the proximal forearm, so careful sharp dissection also decreases the risk of nerve injury.

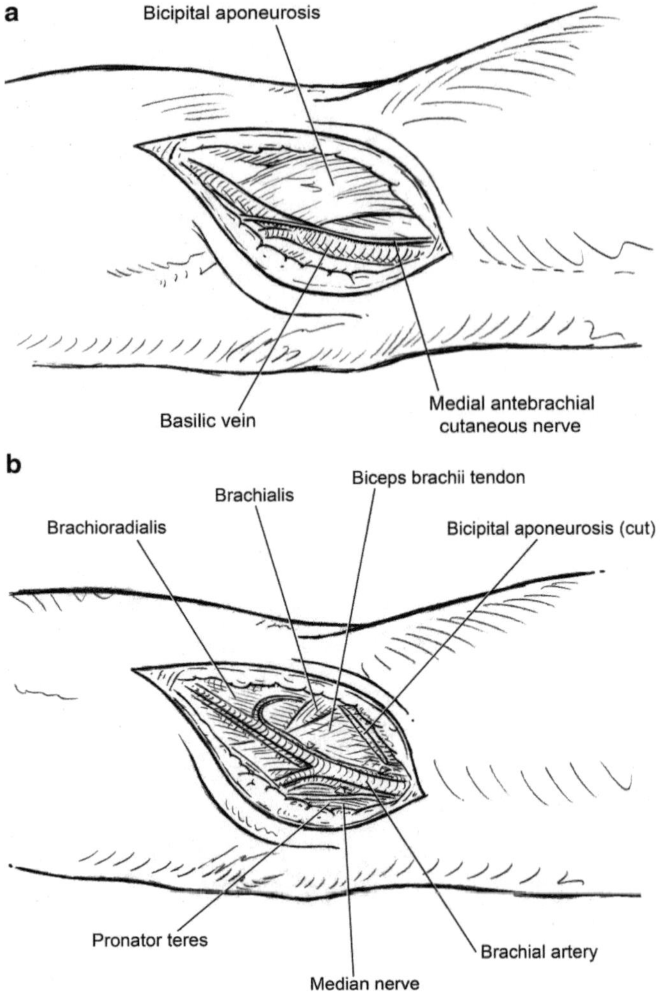

Fig. 2.26 Exposure of the distal brachial artery. (a) Initial skin incision exposes the bicipital aponeurosis and, medially, the forearm continuation of the basilica vein and the median antebrachial cutaneous nerve. (b) Incising the bicipital aponeurosis exposes the underlying brachial artery. The median nerve is medial and anterior to the artery

Proximal Radial Artery

Exposure of the proximal radial artery usually involves distal extension of the "lazy S" until the brachial artery bifurcation is encountered. This exposure is most often used during thrombectomy, when the ability to selectively guide a thrombectomy catheter down the radial and ulnar arteries is required. In the setting of trauma, proximal exposure for ligation of the radial artery can also be used to remotely decrease hemorrhage in the more distal and often traumatized surgical field.

Distal Radial Artery

Distal radial artery exposure is via a longitudinal forearm incision which parallels the course of the artery (Fig. 2.27). Care is taken to ensure the incision does not extend on to the mobile part of the wrist to minimize the risk of postoperative joint dysfunction. The fascia of the forearm is thin in this location and overlies the brachioradialis tendon. At the wrist, the radial artery becomes accessible by incising the fascia and retracting the brachioradialis tendon medially with a self-retaining retractor. The radial nerve does not accompany the artery at this location; however, the artery is surrounded by venae comitantes which can be easily injured. To reduce the risk of venous injury, sharp dissection to isolate the radial artery should be limited to the sites of planned proximal and distal control.

Distal Ulnar Artery

Like the distal radial artery, distal ulnar exposure is via a longitudinal forearm incision paralleling the course of the artery. Similarly, care is taken to ensure the incision does not extend onto the mobile part of the wrist to prevent contracture (Fig. 2.27).

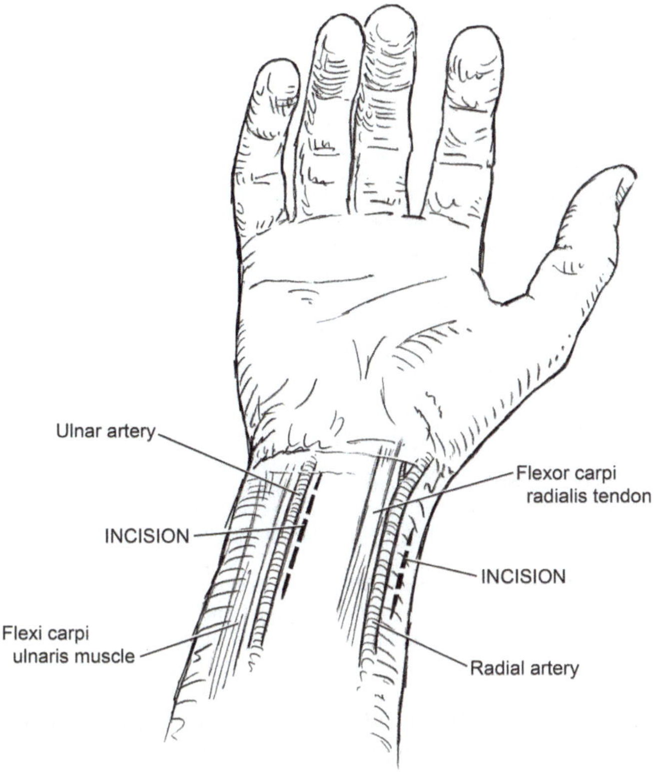

Fig. 2.27 Planned incision sites for exposure of either the distal radial artery or ulnar artery

Surgical Techniques

Methods of Obtaining Proximal and Distal Control

Adequate exposure is the prelude to the core principle of vascular surgery: proximal and distal vascular control. After anticoagulating the patient with heparin, one of the techniques described below can be used to gain vascular control.

Vessel Loop Control

Vessel loop control is ideal for thrombectomy or embolectomy procedures and when branch vessels need to be controlled. Silastic loops that come in varying thickness and strength can be passed around small- and medium-sized vessels. They are often single looped for venous control and double looped for arterial control. Tension can be placed on the loops to occlude the vessel lumen. Heavily calcified arteries often fail to occlude when a loop is tightened and may be difficult to control. Pulling on the loop for hemostasis can also distort the vessel wall. To avoid this situation, loops are often exchanged for clamps when an arteriotomy closure or anastomosis is required.

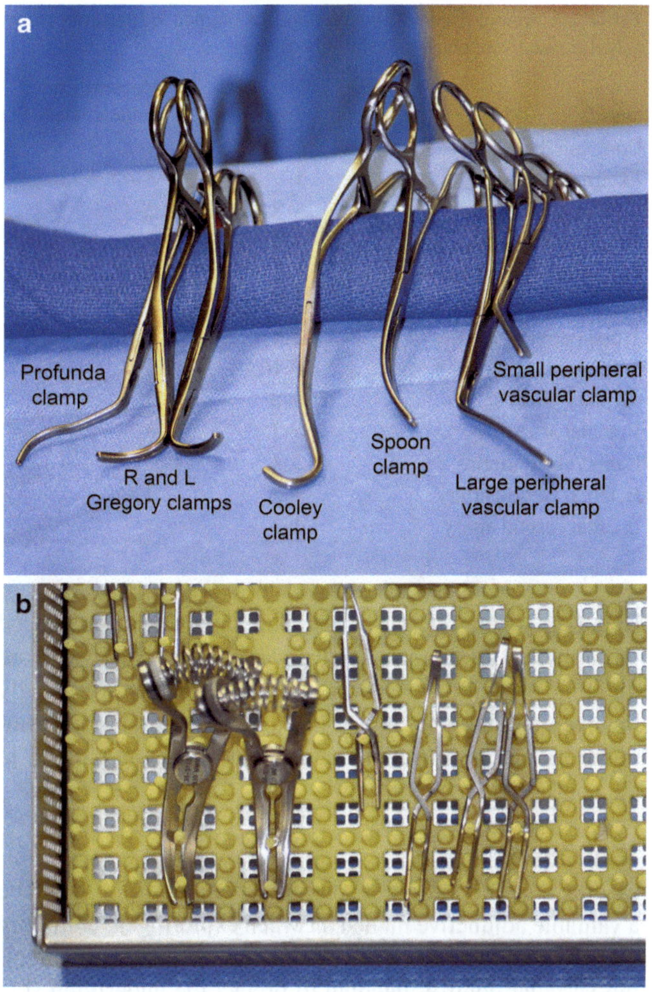

Fig. 2.28 (**a**) Optional clamps for peripheral vascular control. (**b**) Including peripheral "bulldog"-style clamps for smaller caliber vessels

Clamp Control

Although hundreds of vascular clamps are commercially available, each operating room's selection varies. We recommend a variety of large aortic clamps, side-biting clamps, small peripheral vascular clamps, and bulldog-style clamps that are relatively atraumatic for smaller arteries and veins (Fig. 2.28a, b).

Balloon Occlusion

Although balloon occlusion is often overlooked by the nonvascular surgeon, this technique can be lifesaving when dealing with highly diseased, calcified vessels or previously placed stents (see Table 2.2). An appropriately sized Fogarty balloon with a three-way stopcock can obtain intraluminal vascular control when vessels are too diseased to clamp without risking significant injury. Occlusion balloons specifically designed for this purpose come in a range of sizes.

Table 2.2 Vessel luminal diameter and recommended thrombectomy catheter size for occlusion or thrombectomy

Vessel	Size (mm)	Recommended catheter size (Fr)
Common iliac artery	6–12	4–5
External iliac artery	5–9	3–4
Common femoral artery	5–8	3–4
Superficial femoral artery	4–6	2–3
Profunda (deep) femoral artery	4–5	2–3
Popliteal artery	3–5	2–3
Tibial/peroneal arteries	2–4	2
Subclavian artery	6–10	3–4
Axillary artery	6–8	3–4
Brachial artery	5–7	3
Radial/ulnar arteries	2–4	2
External carotid artery	3–5	3
Internal carotid artery	4–7	3

Using an open approach, the balloon catheter is placed through the arteriotomy and advanced proximally before inflating the balloon. Endovascular balloon control usually involves percutaneous access through the contralateral femoral artery and fluoroscopic guidance to place the balloon in the appropriate location.

Tourniquet

Placing a sterile tourniquet on the upper arm or thigh can be a valuable adjunctive maneuver when exploring an extremity for possible vascular injury or anticipating difficulty obtaining vascular control. Padding to protect the underlying skin should be placed before the tourniquet is applied. To minimize backbleeding, the extremity is wrapped with an Esmarch bandage to empty the veins immediately before inflating the tourniquet to above systolic pressure.

Arteriotomies

Adequate exposure and proximal and distal control are the critical first steps that allow surgeons to operate safely on the vasculature. An arteriotomy is typically then made by using an 11-blade or 15-blade to make an initial entrance in to the vessel lumen. The arteriotomy is then extended using Potts or Metzenbaum scissors (Fig. 2.29a, b).

A transverse arteriotomy allows for primary closure of the artery without the risk of narrowing the vessel lumen. Embolectomy/thrombectomy procedures and arterial access for endograft delivery typically use a transverse arteriotomy. A longitudinal arteriotomy, paralleling the course of the vessel, is used for endarterectomy, proximal and distal bypass anastomoses, and AV fistulas and grafts or whenever extension of the arteriotomy is anticipated. In these circumstances, the vessel is generally not at risk for narrowing. In most cases, closing an endarterectomy with a patch angioplasty reduces the risk of restenosis.

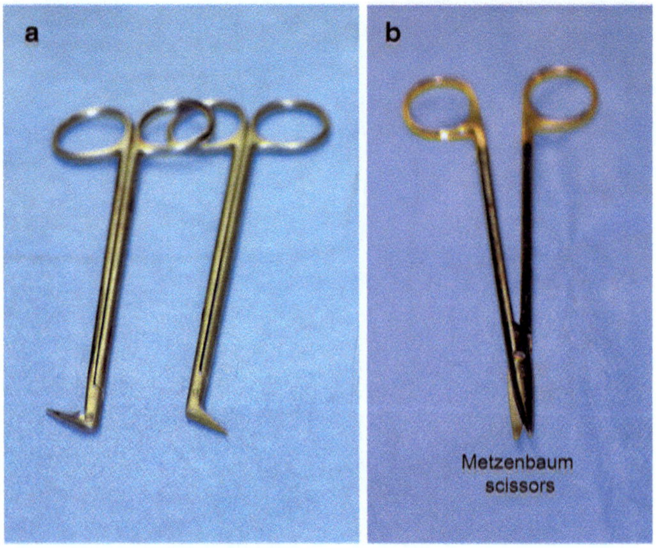

Fig. 2.29 (**a**) Scissors most often used during vascular exposure are the Metzenbaum scissors. (**b**) Potts scissors and reverse Potts scissors are often used to extend an initial arteriotomy made with a blade

Anastomotic Techniques

Instruments and Suture Material

Although each surgeon has a "preferred" anastomosis, a facility with several anastomotic techniques ensures flexibility to adjust to the exposure and vessel depth which can vary for each individual patient. Castroveijo needle drivers are ideal for most suture 5-0 or smaller in size, while Ryder or regular needle drivers can be used for larger sutures (Fig. 2.30). Several options for needle sizes and shapes exist depending on the site of the anastomosis. The following list describes the "rules of thumb" regarding suture size and material (Fig. 2.31):

- Aortic anastomosis: 3-0 nonabsorbable monofilament
  - Needle options: MH or SH (Ethicon)
- Iliac anastomosis: 4-0 nonabsorbable monofilament
  - Needle options: MH, SH, or BB
- Femoral and carotid anastomoses: 5-0 or 6-0 nonabsorbable monofilament
  - Needle options: C-1, BV1, or RB-2
- Popliteal, brachial, and radial: 6-0 nonabsorbable monofilament
  - Needle options: BV-1 or RB-2
- Tibial vessels: 6-0 versus 7-0 nonabsorbable monofilament
  - Needle options: BV-1 or CC

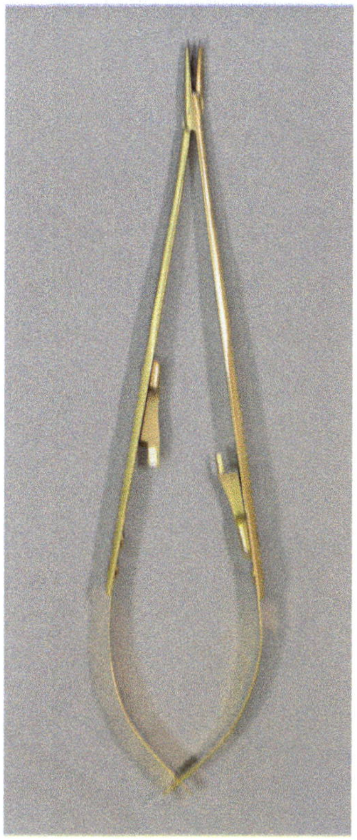

Fig. 2.30 Typical vascular needle drivers for handling fine suture and needles are called Castroveijo drivers

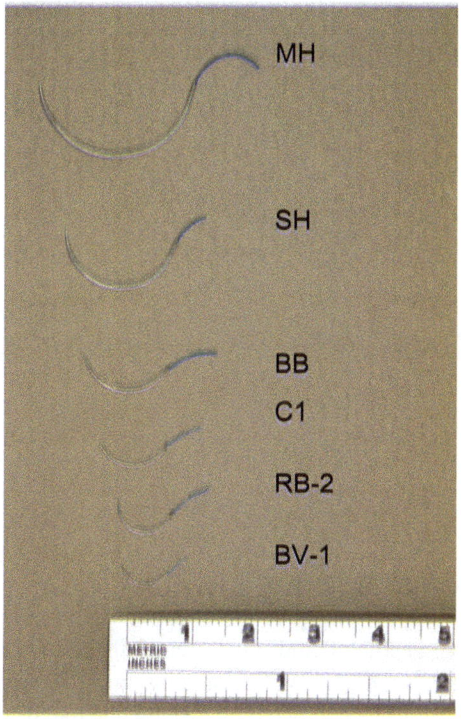

Fig. 2.31 Needles that are used often in vascular surgery

Techniques for Anastomosis

Parachute

This technique is ideally used when the site of the anastomosis is in a deep space. This style allows the back wall of the anastomosis to be visualized until the graft is pulled or "parachuted" into place. It is easiest to start on the side of the anastomosis farthest from the sewing surgeon (Fig. 2.32a–c).

End to End

This technique is used when the ends of two vessels are being brought together. To avoid narrowing, both vessel ends are cut at oblique angles or "spatulated" prior to beginning the anastomosis. Spatulation can correct size discrepancies between the vessels by creating an equal circumference for sewing and by spreading the distance of the sutures along the length of the vessels which prevents narrowing (Fig. 2.33).

End to Side

This common method involves suturing the cut and spatulated end of one vessel to a longitudinal arteriotomy in the sidewall of the second vessel (Fig. 2.34).

Thrombectomy

Choosing an appropriately sized thrombectomy catheter requires knowledge of the typical luminal size for various blood vessels. Table 2.2 provides a reference for the luminal size and corresponding recommended balloon catheter size. Thrombectomy catheters are used for clearing thromboembolism but can also provide "balloon control" of bleeding. To perform a thrombectomy, the catheter is passed beyond the level of the thrombus. While slowly pulling the catheter back, the balloon is inflated until the surgeon senses that the balloon has engaged the sidewalls of the vessel. The catheter is then withdrawn taking care to keep just enough inflation pressure on the balloon to engage the vessel sidewalls thereby dragging the thrombus out of the vessel through the arteriotomy. Overinflation of the thrombectomy balloon or inattention during catheter withdrawal can denude the arterial endothelium causing a significant injury.

Basics of Angiography

Like surgery, endovascular skills accumulate with time and experience. Percutaneous arterial punctures usually use ultrasound guidance to ensure that the suitability of the access vessel enhances safety. The choice of access vessel

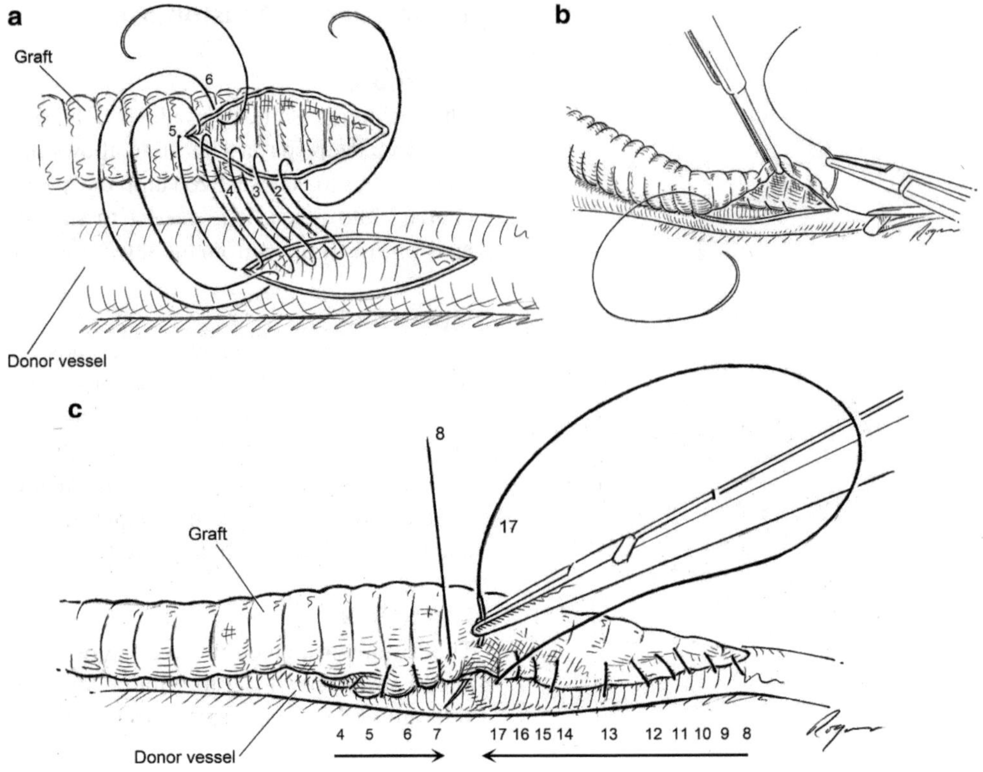

Fig. 2.32 Parachute anastomotic technique: (**a**) start throws from "out-to-in" on graft at about midpoint of the back wall. Carry around the "heel" to approximate the midpoint of the front wall before "parachuting" the graft into place. (**b**) The back wall suture is then carried around the toe in a standard running fashion. (**c**) The two suture ends come together at the midpoint of the front wall

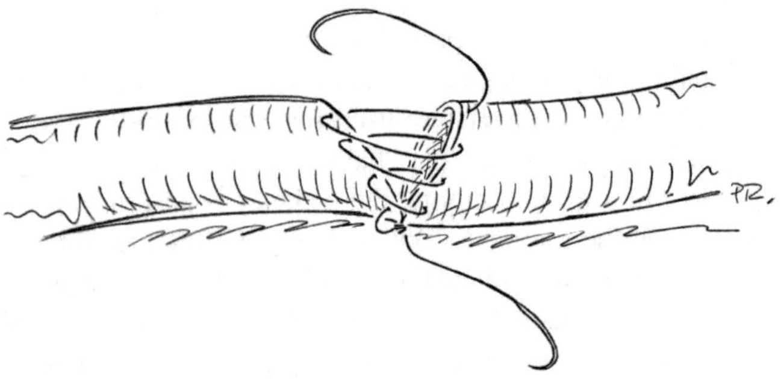

Fig. 2.33 End-to-end anastomosis. Both vessel ends are typically slightly spatulated in opposite directions to facilitate this anastomosis and accommodate any size mismatch

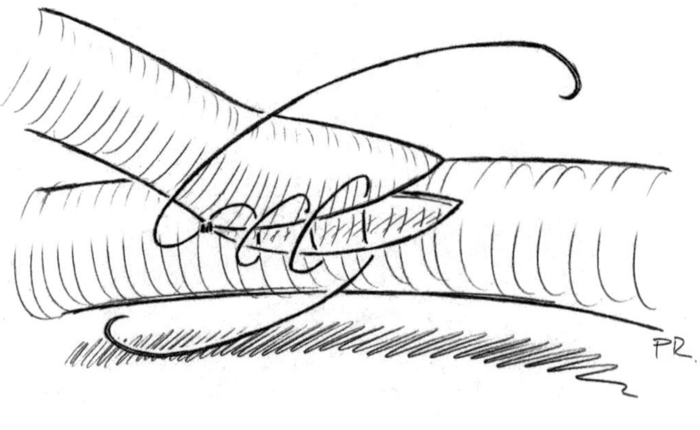

Fig. 2.34 End-to-side anastomosis. The initial bite is taken at the heel and a knot tied to the outside then run out of both corners to meet at the midpoint of the front or back wall

depends on the target for intervention. For most lower extremity interventions, contralateral femoral access is recommended; planned common iliac interventions are usually performed from ipsilateral femoral access. Renal and carotid interventions frequently use femoral access with the laterality determined by anatomy and surgeon handedness. Subclavian interventions can be performed with femoral or ipsilateral brachial access, and interventions for the celiac access or superior mesenteric artery can be performed through femoral or left brachial arterial access.

Femoral Access

The access needle should ideally enter the common femoral artery between the femoral bifurcation and the inguinal ligament. Punctures that stray too far distally into the SFA or too far proximally into the external iliac artery can result in bleeding complications. The SFA is too distal to be compressed against the head of the femur when holding pressure for hemostasis. In

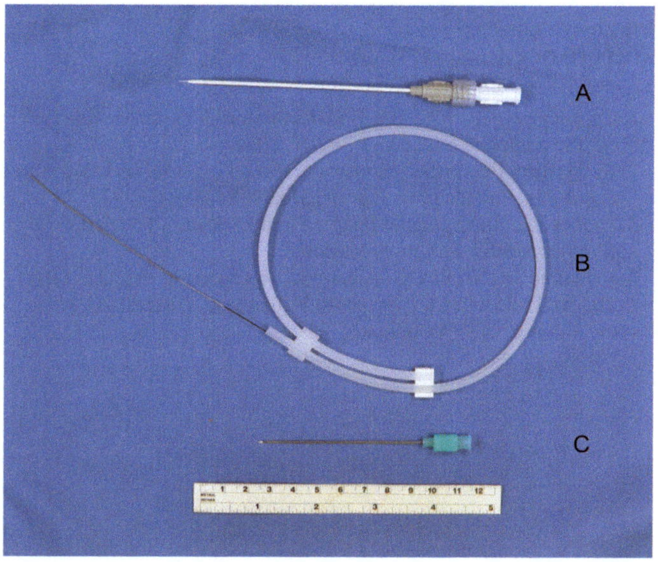

Fig. 2.35 Example of a micropuncture access kit (Angiodynamics™, Latham NY)

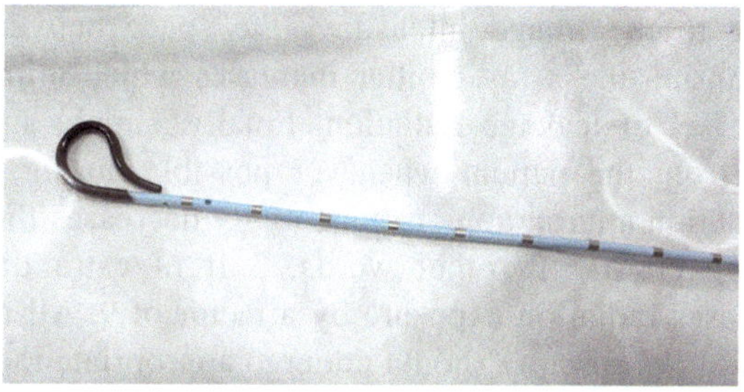

Fig. 2.36 Example of a flush catheter used for initial aortogram (Angiodynamics™, Latham NY)

the case of accidental percutaneous iliac access ("high stick"), manual pressure is usually held distal to the actual needle hole allowing unabated bleeding into the potential space of the retroperitoneum. It is difficult if not impossible to manually apply hemostatic pressure to a puncture site above the inguinal ligament. Use of a closure device is recommended in the event of a high puncture. Ultrasound guidance for percutaneous needle punctures helps to confirm vessel patency, identify the bifurcation, and assess the extent of calcification.

The femoral artery is best accessed using a micropuncture kit of some variety. This typically contains a 21Ga needle and a mandrel or micropuncture wire of 0.018 in. diameter (Fig. 2.35). After puncturing the artery, the wire should pass without resistance through the femoral and iliac arteries to the abdominal aorta. The position of the wire should be confirmed by fluoroscopy.

We recommend making a small skin nick using an 11-blade with the micropuncture needle still in place as a guide. The needle is then exchanged for the micropuncture sheath, using the standard Seldinger technique. The inner cannula of the microsheath as well as the .018″ guidewire is removed and the .035″ wire of the surgeon's choosing is then advanced, again under fluoroscopic guidance. Passing the larger caliber wire allows the micropuncture sheath to be exchanged for a working sheath of the required diameter, typically 4 Fr or 5 Fr for initial diagnostic angiography.

Any type of flush (side-hole containing) catheter (Fig. 2.36) can then be advanced into position for digital subtraction angiography. While vascular interventions are beyond the scope of this text, they can be found in textbooks of endovascular surgery or angiography.

Radiation Safety

All angiographic procedures involve radiation exposure, and the interventionist must make a concerted effort to ensure the safety of the patient and health care team. When performing fluoroscopy there are three potential sources of radiation exposure [4]:

1. Primary radiation comes directly from the x-ray tube to the patient. The proceduralist is only exposed to this when a hand, or other body parts, comes between the patient and the primary beam.
2. Scatter radiation is the primary exposure source of radiation for the proceduralist and is emitted in all directions from the patient after the imaging beam comes into contact with him or her.
3. Leakage radiation is emitted from the imaging system and accounts for minimal exposure when using modern imaging equipment.

Radiation safety begins with education and the use of appropriate personal protective equipment. A lead attire including a thyroid shield and lead safety glasses ensures maximum operator protection. Lead aprons should be checked for cracks and flaws biannually by the hospital's radiation safety officer. Appropriate lead aprons block more than 90 % of potential leakage radiation and 95–99 % of scatter radiation.

Some basic intra-procedural maneuvers to decrease radiation exposure include minimizing time spent on continuous fluoroscopy in favor of intermittent spot or pulse fluoroscopy. Collimating the imaging field also focuses the radiation beam so that the patient receives less radiation thereby decreasing the amount of scatter radiation that can reach the proceduralist. Minimizing the use of magnification also decreases the total radiation dose to the patient and the amount of radiation available for scatter. Decreasing the space between the patient and the image intensifier decreases the amount of scatter radiation, widens the imaging field, and improves image quality. With the patient closer to the image intensifier, the space between the patient and the x-ray emitter increases which minimizes the effect of leakage radiation. Finally, simply stepping back from the patient whenever possible during digital subtraction angiography exponentially decreases the radiation exposure. In other words, 3 ft of extra distance decreases radiation exposure by a factor of 9. All regular users of fluoroscopy should undergo appropriate radiation safety training and exposure monitoring.

References

1. Cronnenwett JL, Johnston KW. Rutherford's vascular surgery. 7th ed. Philadelphia: Saunders Elsevier; 2010.
2. Rutherford RB. Atlas of vascular surgery, basic techniques and exposures. Philadelphia: Elsevier Health Sciences; 1993.
3. Fauber TL. Radiographic Imaging and Exposure, Fourth Ed. 2013. Elsevier Mosby. St. Louis, Missouri.
4. Valentine JR, Wind GG. Anatomic exposures in vascular surgery. 2nd ed. Philadelphia: Lippincott, Williams & Wilkins; 2003.

Part II

Acute Arterial Disease

Peripheral Arterial Thrombosis/ Emboli

3

Amy B. Reed and Faisal Aziz

Etiology and Pathophysiology

The earliest epidemiologic data on acute limb ischemia came from a Swedish study which estimated the incidence to be 9 per 100,000 of the general population [1]. The Swedish vascular registry reported the incidence of acute limb ischemia to be 13 per 100,000 population [2]. Similarly, the Gloucestershire study from the United Kingdom estimated the incidence to be 14 per 100,000 of general population [3].

When evaluating a patient for acute limb ischemia, underlying peripheral artery disease (PAD) must be considered as this diagnosis may alter the treatment plan. Risk factors associated with PAD include advanced age, male gender, diabetes mellitus, smoking, hyperhomocysteinemia, dyslipidemia, end-stage renal disease, elevated C-reactive protein, and hypertension [4–6]. The clinician should inquire about a history of claudication or ischemic rest pain prior to the current ischemic event.

Acute limb ischemia occurs when the oxygen supply to the limb is suddenly stopped. The most common reasons for developing acute limb ischemia are embolism, thrombosis, and trauma. A thorough history and physical examination helps the clinician determine the underlying etiology, which has implications for treatment and long-term prognosis. Patients who present with thrombosis tend to be younger and have a higher risk of amputation, while patients who present with embolic events are usually older and have higher perioperative mortality rates [7, 8].

Embolus (from the Greek word *embolus* meaning plug) is any solid material which travels in the blood vessels. Most commonly, the source of embolism is the heart, where a mural thrombus is formed and ejected into the arterial system. Another potential source is atherosclerotic plaque in the aorta which can dislodge and travel downstream as emboli. The embolus keeps traveling in the arteries until it becomes trapped in an artery having the same diameter as the embolus, thus occluding blood flow at this level. Usually, the embolus lodges at arterial branch points. A large embolus can settle at the aortic bifurcation as a saddle embolus. An embolus that has passed beyond the aortic bifurcation usually gets lodged in the common femoral artery at its bifurcation into the superficial and profunda femoris arteries or in the popliteal artery at its bifurcation into the anterior tibial artery and tibioperoneal trunk. Patients who have no baseline PAD lack collaterals and sudden occlusion usually leads to acute severe pain. On physical examination, the leg appears pale or white and usually has a marked neurosensory deficit. Once direct blood flow is stopped at the site of embolic occlusion, distal stasis can lead to formation of secondary thrombus.

Usually at the time of embolectomy, a clear distinction can be made between the embolus and secondary thrombus. Embolus from a cardiac source is usually large, solid, and white in color (organized, platelet rich), while the secondary thrombus is generally plum-colored. With continued stasis, secondary thrombus propagates and starts extending into smaller blood vessels and capillaries. If not treated by intervention, the thrombus adheres to the endothelial lining making it difficult to remove with embolectomy catheters and resistant to dissolution by intra-arterial thrombolytic therapy.

Thrombosis of native arteries can result from several conditions including chronic progressive atherosclerosis, hypercoagulability, and arterial dissection. Atherosclerosis causes gradual narrowing of the arteries which can progress to a hemodynamically significant stenosis. If the narrowing gets worse and becomes a critical stenosis, blood flow through the artery slows down allowing for platelet aggregation, thrombus formation, and possible occlusion. Accumulated evidence shows that plaque disruption in carotid and coronary arteries can result in acute stroke and myocardial infarction,

A.B. Reed, MD, FACS (✉)
Department of Vascular Surgery, Penn State Hershey College of Medicine, Heart and Vascular Institute, 500 University Drive, Hershey, PA 17033-0850, USA
e-mail: abreed@psu.edu

F. Aziz, MD
Department of Surgery/Vascular Surgery, Penn State Hershey College of Medicine, Heart and Vascular Institute, Hershey, PA USA

V. Gahtan and M.J. Costanza (eds.), *Essentials of Vascular Surgery for the General Surgeon*,
DOI 10.1007/978-1-4939-1326-8_3, © Springer Science+Business Media New York 2015

respectively [9]. Although plaque disruption has not been shown to directly cause acute thrombosis in peripheral arteries, the composition of atherosclerotic plaques is similar regardless of the artery involved. Therefore, it is likely that plaque disruption plays a role in acute peripheral artery thrombosis. The slow progression of atherosclerosis allows most peripheral arterial beds to develop robust collaterals. The blood flow provided by these collaterals can minimize the impact of an acute thrombotic occlusion which explains why patients with acute thrombosis typically have less severe ischemic symptoms compared to patients with an embolic obstruction.

Diagnosis

Clinical presentation of acute limb ischemia depends on the adequacy of collateral blood vessels and the diameter of the occluded artery. For example, a saddle embolus at the aortic bifurcation occludes arterial inflow to the lower extremities leading to acute ischemic symptoms in both legs. Likewise, an embolic occlusion or traumatic arterial injury to the lower extremity in a person with normal arteries can lead to profound limb ischemia. In contrast, patients with chronic atherosclerotic disease of the superficial femoral artery (SFA) and well-developed collaterals may not develop ischemic symptoms even if the SFA acutely occludes.

Acute onset of limb pain is the most common symptom. Usually, the sensory nerves are affected first making sensory loss one of the earliest signs of acute ischemia. Motor nerves are affected next leading to muscle weakness. Skin is involved next, presenting as pallor and mottling in some cases. Muscles are affected later, and, therefore, calf muscle tenderness in patients with an acute arterial occlusion indicates more advanced ischemia.

The classic five Ps of acute limb ischemia remain useful in guiding the physical exam: pallor, pain, paresthesia, paralysis, and pulse deficit (with poikilothermia being a 6th). Standard vascular examination demonstrates absent pulses below the level of occlusion. Careful examination can distinguish a normal pulse from the prominent "water hammer pulse" at the site of obstruction. Skin color, capillary refill, and sensory and motor examination in the involved extremity should be performed to assess the severity of ischemia. The exact level of loss of pulse should be determined, as it helps identify the level of occlusion and guides therapy. For example, loss of the femoral pulses with mottling of both lower extremities suggests occlusion at the aortic level, whereas loss of one femoral pulse suggests ipsilateral iliac occlusion. Similarly, presence of a femoral pulse with loss of the distal pulses suggests SFA/popliteal artery occlusion, while presence of a popliteal pulse with loss of distal pulses suggests infrapopliteal arterial occlusion. The examiner should also assess heartbeat for arrhythmias and palpate for aneurysms in the abdominal aorta and femoral and popliteal arteries as possible sources of embolism or thrombosis.

The scoring system for assessing the severity of acute ischemia has been developed by the Society for Vascular Surgery and the International Society for Cardiovascular Surgery, which was later modified by TASC in 2007 (Table 3.1) [4, 10, 11]. The classification system ranges from patients with class I ischemia who have viable limbs to patients with class III ischemia who have unsalvageable extremities. There is no role for revascularization in class III ischemia and the major decision options are amputation versus comfort care. Patients with class II ischemia require revascularization, and it is crucial to accurately classify these patients into marginally threatened (IIa) and immediately threatened (IIb) categories. This classification determines the timing and type of therapy offered as will be discussed later in this chapter.

Imaging

The importance of a good clinical examination cannot be overstated. In a patient with imminent risk of limb loss, a well-performed clinical examination may provide enough diagnostic information to bring the patient directly to the operating room without wasting time on unnecessary imaging studies.

Table 3.1 Acute limb ischemia classifications

		Findings		Doppler signals	
Category	Description/prognosis	Sensory loss	Motor loss	Arterial	Venous
I. Viable	Not immediately threatened	None	None	Audible	Audible
II. Threatened					
(a) Marginally	Salvageable if promptly treated	Minimal (toes) or none	None	Inaudible	Audible
(b) Immediately	Salvageable with immediate revascularization	More than toes, associated with rest pain	Mild, moderate	Inaudible	Audible
III. Irreversible	Major tissue loss or permanent nerve damage inevitable	Profound, anesthetic	Profound, paralysis (rigor)	Inaudible	Inaudible

Adapted from Rutherford et al. [10]

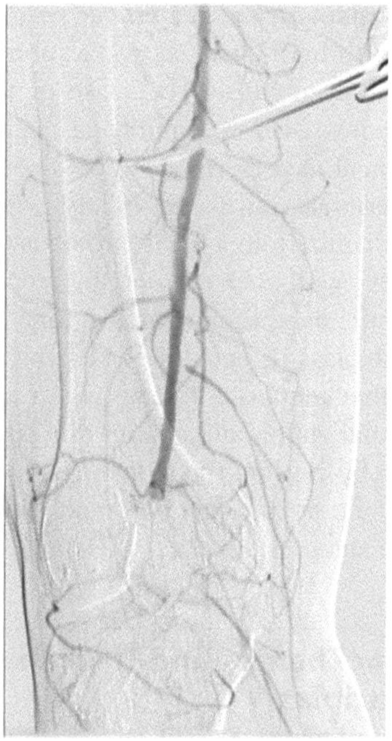

Fig. 3.1 Digital subtraction arteriogram showing embolic occlusion of the popliteal artery. Note the distinct cutoff of the popliteal and absence of collateral vessels

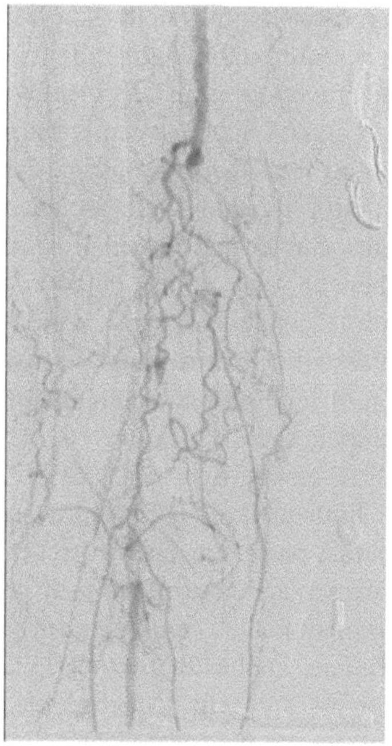

Fig. 3.2 Digital subtraction arteriogram showing arterial thrombosis with well-developed collaterals around the area of occlusion

Duplex Ultrasound

Duplex ultrasound can accurately determine the level of obstruction and the status of other blood vessels in the limb. More importantly, in cases of aortic dissections extending into one extremity, duplex ultrasound can identify the true and false lumens.

Computed Tomography Angiography (CTA)

Computed tomography angiography (CTA) is widely available in most emergency departments, and the imaging quality is similar to intra-arterial angiography. As a noninvasive imaging modality, CTA has an advantage in the evaluation of aortoiliac occlusions, dissections, traumatic limb injuries, and patients with significant underlying occlusive disease.

Digital Subtraction Angiography (DSA)

Digital subtraction angiography (DSA) is the mainstay diagnostic study, especially when thrombolytic therapy is anticipated. An angiogram can show the level of occlusion, the patency of distal blood vessels. In some cases, the angiographic images suggest the etiology of ischemia. For example, embolic occlusions will have a sharp cutoff sign with no collateral vessels (Fig. 3.1), while thrombotic occlusions will show collateral blood vessels around the occluded artery (Fig. 3.2). For collaterals to develop, the affected artery must have been stenosis over a long period of time implying that the ischemic event represents acute thrombosis of an already diseased artery. Hybrid operating rooms allow for a seamless transition between diagnostic angiography, endovascular therapy, and surgical intervention.

Treatment Decision Making

Treatment decisions concerning an acutely threatened limb can be challenging for even the most experienced surgeons. Making the best treatment choice requires a basic understanding of the etiology, pathophysiology, and consequences of limb ischemia. Younger patients with acute limb ischemia are at risk for limb loss, whereas older patients have a high risk of mortality in addition to the threat of limb loss. Patients with acute myocardial infarction and poor cardiac output have substantially higher postoperative mortality, regardless of the type of operation performed [12, 13]. Therefore, performing a thorough history and physical examination and accurately placing the patient in the appropriate category of limb ischemia are crucial.

Anticoagulation should be initiated on all patients with acute limb ischemia. Blaisdell introduced the role of heparin in preventing proximal and distal propagation of thrombus in patients with acute limb ischemia [14]. Although heparin does not have thrombolytic properties, it stabilizes and prevents extension of the already formed thrombus while preserving the patency of the microcirculation. An initial heparin bolus of 80 units/kg should be followed by a continuous infusion of 18 units/kg/h. Most patients are dehydrated and benefit from large bore intravenous access and hydration. Contrast which is required for angiographic imaging may be harmful to kidney function, especially in dehydrated patients.

Patients with class I limb ischemia have viable limbs which allows more time to get investigational studies that will guide definitive treatment. Revascularization for this group of patients can be performed less emergently, and patients may benefit from anticoagulation in the interim period. In addition, high surgical risk patients occasionally are not revascularized if their residual perfusion is adequate and the addition of long-term anticoagulation is felt to prevent further ischemic events.

Patients with reversible ischemia (class II) require revascularization for limb salvage. The majority of patients with acute limb ischemia present as class II ischemia and benefit the most from revascularization efforts. Any sensory or motor deficit in this group of patients must be identified, as the presence of these deficits implies that the peripheral nerve cells are getting ischemic and will soon become anoxic. Nerve death is followed by muscle necrosis and limb loss. Patients with class IIa ischemia have marginally threatened limbs allowing the surgeon more time to decide on definitive treatment. All of these patients should be immediately anticoagulated and undergo an imaging study. Revascularization can involve endovascular or open surgical techniques, depending on the surgeon's familiarity and comfort with the use of modern endovascular technology. The duration of symptoms can help guide treatment decisions. Patients who have less than 2 weeks duration of signs and symptoms benefit the most from endovascular treatment, while patients whose duration of symptoms is more than 2 weeks usually benefit more from open surgical procedures [15]. Intra-arterial thrombolytic therapy requires close clinical monitoring and interval angiography. If the patient cannot tolerate thrombolysis or develops worsening ischemia with motor loss, the treating surgeon must be prepared to perform an emergent open surgical revascularization to save the leg.

Patients with class IIb ischemia have acute critical ischemia and are at an extremely high risk for limb loss if emergent revascularization is not performed. Institutions with limited resources should consider transferring these patients to vascular centers of excellence which offer a full range of vascular and endovascular services. Evidence suggests that this strategy improves surgical outcomes in patients with acutely threatened limbs [3]. Historically, these patients had extremely high rates of limb loss. The advent of the embolectomy catheter by Fogarty in 1963 revolutionized the treatment of acutely threatened limbs [16]. Balloon catheter embolectomy became the gold standard surgical therapy for acute limb ischemia. Although low-dose intra-arterial thrombolytic treatment is effective for subcritical ischemia, the long treatment time required makes thrombolysis ill suited for threatened limbs requiring immediate reperfusion. Well-equipped endovascular centers can perform accelerated thrombolysis with high-dose, short-duration infusions [17] or pulse spray thrombolysis [18]. Use of these advanced techniques requires 24-h availability of angiography suites and a commitment to perform emergent open surgery if the limb status deteriorates during thrombolytic therapy. Patients with severe ischemia from a focal thrombus or embolus in a proximal vessel usually benefit more by proceeding directly to a definitive surgical thromboembolectomy.

Patients with class III acute limb ischemia have irreversible ischemia that cannot be treated with revascularization. In fact, revascularization attempts in this group of patients can be harmful by causing rhabdomyolysis and myoglobinuria. These patients are better served with limb amputation at the appropriate anatomic level.

Endovascular Therapy and Thrombolysis: General Principles

The use of thrombolytic therapy for acute limb ischemia has evolved over the last several decades with many reports in the literature describing its benefit. Systemic infusion of thrombolytic therapy has given way to catheter-directed thrombolysis (i.e., percutaneous placement of a catheter directly into the intra-arterial thrombus). Tissue plasminogen activator (TPA) has largely replaced streptokinase and urokinase and is infused in a variety of doses and infusion times. Although randomized trials have been performed, they failed to provide a clear-cut answer to the treatment dilemma of thrombolysis versus surgical revascularization. Meta-analyses have found similar mortality and amputation rates for both percutaneous thrombolysis and open surgery. Thrombolysis reduces the need for open major surgery at a cost of causing more bleeding and distal embolization [19, 20].

Patients who present with limb ischemia less than 14 days duration with intact motor and sensory function may benefit from intra-arterial catheter-directed thrombolysis followed by correction of the causative lesion. Treatment options for patients with an acutely occluded bypass graft include surgical graft thrombectomy, thrombolysis with correction of the causative lesion, or creation of a new bypass. Consideration needs to be given to the age of the graft, conduit availability, the duration and degree of ischemia, and the overall condition and comorbidities of the patient.

Absolute contraindications to thrombolysis are recent intracranial or retinal surgeries. The practitioner must be ready to abort thrombolysis in favor of open surgical revascularization if at any point thrombolysis is causing an unacceptable delay in revascularization. The decision to perform thrombolysis versus open surgical revascularization should be made by a surgeon familiar with both techniques in a center equipped to perform either procedure.

Femoral and Brachial Embolectomy Techniques

Femoral Artery Embolectomy

The majority of patients presenting with acute lower extremity ischemia have an embolism lodged at the common femoral artery bifurcation that can be surgically treated with a femoral embolectomy. All patients should receive full systemic heparinization while being prepared for emergent surgery. The operation can be performed under general anesthesia; however, local anesthesia with moderate sedation may be more appropriate for patients with significant pulmonary comorbidities. The sterile prep should extend from the umbilicus to the entire limb circumferentially down to the toes. A longitudinal or oblique incision can be made for femoral artery exposure. An oblique incision, while sometimes limiting exposure, is preferred by many surgeons for its superior healing especially in morbidly obese patients. Although oblique incisions can be associated with lymphatic issues such as lymphocele or lymphedema, these complications can be avoided by dissecting in a vertical plane once the superficial fascia has been opened.

For the standard vertical incision, the femoral artery lies approximately two fingerbreadths lateral to the pubic tubercle (Chap. 2, Fig. 2.13). In the patient with a pulseless femoral artery, the firm tubular structure of the clotted or atherosclerotic artery can be palpated by rolling one's fingers back and forth over the groin. A vertical incision should begin well above the inguinal crease, incising the lowermost fibers of the external oblique aponeurosis in order to gain full exposure to the proximal common femoral artery. Once the superficial fascia is opened, tributaries of the great saphenous vein will be encountered and require ligation as necessary to facilitate arterial exposure. Contrary to the popular mnemonic NAVEL (nerve, artery, vein, empty space, lymphatics) for structures organized lateral to medial, lymphatics can be present on both the medial and lateral sides of the vein. Carefully ligating and dividing this tissue helps avoid lymphatic complications.

The deep fascia should then be incised longitudinally. Encountering muscle indicates that the dissection is too far lateral, while visualization of venous structures suggests the approach is too medial. Repeat palpation or Doppler examination will keep the dissection on track and in the appropriate trajectory. Upon opening the deep fascia, the "bloodshot eye" appearance of the common femoral artery will be noted due to the unique appearance of the vasa vasorum on the surface of acutely occluded peripheral arteries. Sharp dissection should continue in close proximity to the artery in order to gain control of the vessel by encircling it with an umbilical tape. Gentle upward traction on the umbilical tape will elevate the artery facilitating further dissection proximally as necessary to ensure one has the common femoral artery isolated. As dissection continues distally, an abrupt change in caliber of the vessel indicates the femoral bifurcation. At the bifurcation, the profunda femoris artery usually travels posterolaterally while the SFA continues distally in the same plane as the common femoral artery (Chap. 2, Fig. 2.14). Both vessels should be encircled with atraumatic Silastic vessel loops, taking care to protect a sensory branch of the femoral nerve, which courses anteriorly from lateral to medial just distal to the femoral bifurcation.

Once arterial structures are dissected free from the surrounding tissues, the patient is bolused with heparin if a therapeutic heparin infusion is not already running. After 3 min, an angled soft-jaw clamp is applied to the proximal common femoral artery and the previously looped branches are secured. The arteriotomy can be performed in a transverse or longitudinal fashion. If the artery feels soft and free of atherosclerotic plaque and acute embolism is felt for certain to be the cause, a simple transverse arteriotomy should be used. This orientation will allow thrombus retrieval proximally and distally and can be closed with interrupted polypropylene suture (5.0 or 6.0) without concern for future stenosis at the arteriotomy site. If a significant amount of atherosclerotic plaque is appreciated and an acute-on-chronic etiology for acute limb ischemia is suspected, a longitudinal arteriotomy should be used. This type of arteriotomy usually requires closure with a patch angioplasty to prevent future stenosis.

The Fogarty embolectomy catheter is a thin-walled balloon attached to a hollow catheter with a hub at the end to which a syringe is attached (Fig. 3.3). Arterial embolectomy catheters range in size from 1F to 6F. The catheters are marked at 5–10 cm intervals. Before beginning the thromboembolectomy, placing the catheter on the patient will help gauge how far one will need to advance the catheter in order to reach the aortic bifurcation or the popliteal artery. Typically, a 4F or 5F catheter is repeatedly passed proximally until thrombus is no longer retrieved. Heparinized saline is instilled proximally and the artery reclamped. A similar process proceeds distally with initially a 4F catheter followed by a smaller 3F as necessary. When using the catheter, it is important that the individual pulling on the catheter is the one controlling the inflation of the balloon so that the drag and pull on the artery can be appreciated in order to avoid vascular injury to the intimal surface. The goal is to coapt the balloon against the arterial sidewall without excessive force. Fluoroscopy and an over-the-wire embolectomy catheter may be required to retrieve clot that extends into the tibial vessels,

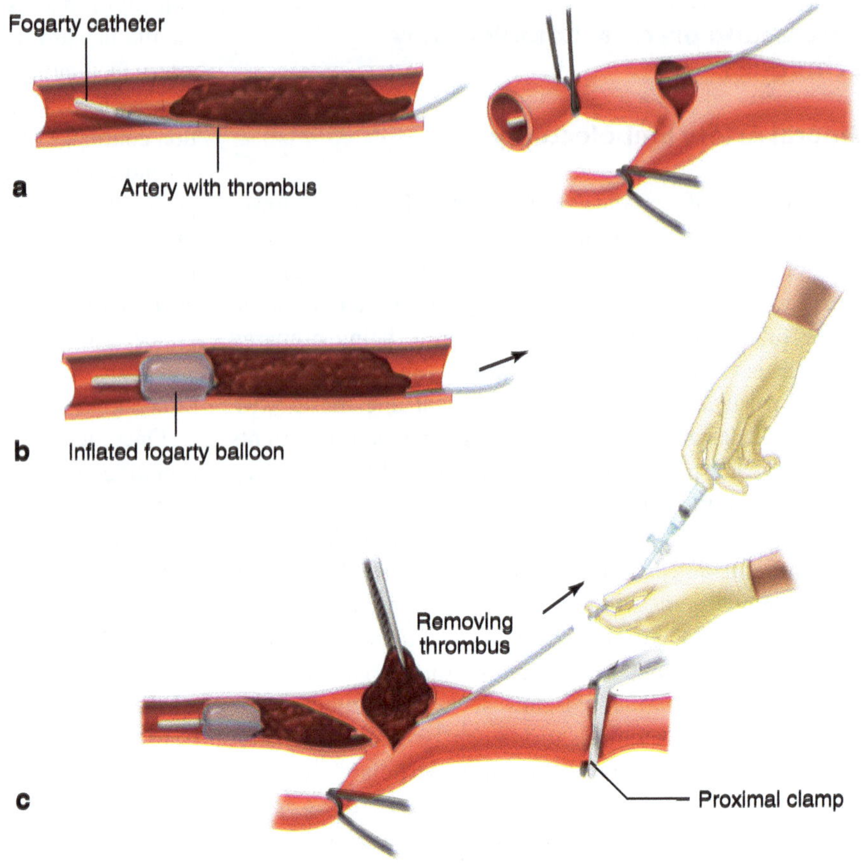

Fig. 3.3 Demonstration of performing an arterial thrombectomy/embolectomy. (**a**) Placement of the catheter tip just beyond the thrombus. (**b**) Inflation of the embolectomy balloon. (**c**) Removal of the thrombus through the arteriotomy using the embolectomy catheter

Once the thrombus has been cleared, a completion imaging study, such as intraoperative arteriography, should be used to assess the technical success of the procedure. In simple cases, a completion angiogram may not be necessary; however, unsuspected technical flaws can be detected in up to 10 % of cases [8]. The completion angiogram can be performed either before or after closure of the arteriotomy. If before, an angiocatheter is inserted through the arteriotomy and the vessel is snugged around it with a vessel loop. A short length of pressure tubing with a three-way stopcock on the end can make it easier to inject contrast and flush the artery with heparinized saline. Multiple digital subtraction runs may be necessary to image the entire extremity. A transverse arteriotomy can then be closed primarily with interrupted simple 5-0 polypropylene sutures. Longitudinal arteriotomies require closure with a small elliptical-shaped patch of nearby vein or synthetic material which is sutured into position in a running fashion. Arteriograms performed after closure of the arteriotomy require a needle puncture to introduce a cannula. The arterial inflow should be occluded while injecting contrast to optimize the image quality. If the arteriogram is satisfactory, a purse-string suture can be used to close the cannulation site. The groin incision is then closed in layers after achieving hemostasis.

Brachial Artery Embolectomy

The approach to acute upper extremity ischemia follows the same overall principles used for the lower extremity. The most common presentation involves an embolus from a cardiac source that lodges at the brachial bifurcation. After systemic anticoagulation, patients proceed to the operating room with similar anesthetic management as described above.

The most common exposure of the brachial artery centers over its bifurcation (please refer to Chap. 2, Figs. 2.25 and 2.26a, b). An "S"-shaped incision around the antecubital fossa decreases the chance of skin contractures during healing. The incision starts longitudinally on the medial upper arm proximal to the antecubital crease. It then takes a transverse course across the antecubital crease and terminates longitudinally on the lateral proximal forearm. The extent of the incision depends on the location of the brachial bifurcation and the severity of disease. After the incision is deepened, the aponeurosis of the biceps tendon can be partially divided to expose the brachial artery. Care should be exercised to avoid undue retraction on the median nerve, which is posteromedial to the brachial artery. Once the brachial artery is looped, gentle upward traction will facilitate isolating the radial and ulnar arteries with Silastic loops.

As with the femoral embolectomy, systemic heparinization is followed by proximal and distal clamping of the brachial artery and its branches. Chronic atherosclerotic occlusive disease is rare at the brachial artery; thus, a transverse arteriotomy can almost always be used. Exceptions to this rule include patients with a traumatic injury or multiple prior upper extremity surgeries for dialysis access. In these cases, chronic anastomotic stenosis may be present requiring a longitudinal arteriotomy. Generally 3F to 4F Fogarty balloon thrombectomy catheters are used for the upper extremity. The technique for thrombectomy/embolectomy is illustrated in Fig. 3.3.

Technical Tips/Pitfalls

1. Ensure that the incision is of adequate length in order to avoid struggling with the exposure.
2. Use self-retaining retractors with appropriate depth and grasp, readjusting at each level of dissection.
3. Beware of nerve injury from poorly placed retractors and use of electrosurgery near nerves.
4. Be wary of nearby lymphatics whether using an oblique or longitudinal incision for femoral exposure in the groin. Ligate or cauterize all lymphatics before transecting them.
5. Locate pulseless arteries by palpation as a firm tubular structure or by Doppler signal detected beyond the area of obstruction.
6. As soon as possible, dissect close to and around the artery. Encircling the artery with an umbilical tape and then applying traction facilitates its elevation and allows branches to be more readily dissected. This technique is safer than trying to dig the artery out that is lying in its bed at the depth of the wound.

Postoperative Management

The introduction of the Fogarty embolectomy catheter nearly 50 years ago has dramatically decreased mortality and limb loss from arterial embolism. Despite this advance, the comorbidities of patients presenting with acute limb ischemia portend a worse prognosis compared to patients with chronic atherosclerosis who present with less severe ischemia. Cardiac dysrhythmias, coronary artery disease, hypertension, hyperlipidemia, and diabetes are common comorbid states and bring their own set of complications to the postoperative setting despite an expeditious embolectomy through a small incision or needle puncture. Common complications related to surgical thrombectomy/embolectomy include hypotension, myocardial infarction, stroke, acute renal failure, infection, bleeding, compartment syndrome, and even death.

Therapeutic anticoagulation with heparin should continue postoperatively with conversion to long-term oral anticoagulation with warfarin. In general, therapeutic intravenous unfractionated heparin is used for the first 1–2 postoperative days due to the relatively short half-life and ability to discontinue it if there are bleeding complications. The author's preference is to convert from unfractionated heparin to low molecular weight heparin on the second postoperative day, if no additional procedures are being planned and the patient is recovering as expected. A course of anticoagulation with warfarin follows.

Compartment syndrome can develop postoperatively, particularly if there is a prolonged delay in achieving reperfusion. Patients who are not revascularized in an adequate time period – ischemia lasting more than 6 h – need to be considered for fasciotomy of the lower leg. In general, the upper extremity is more forgiving compared to the lower extremity due to its smaller muscle mass. Even if revascularization occurs within the 6-h time frame, patients should still be closely monitored for compartment syndrome postoperatively. Creatinine kinase levels may be followed along with physical examination of the compartments. Decreased first web space sensation on the foot and calf pain with passive stretch or dorsiflexion of the foot are early signs of compartment syndrome that should prompt urgent compartment pressure measurement and a low threshold for return to the operating room for fasciotomy.

The source of embolism is frequently cardiac in nature with atrial fibrillation being the most common etiology. In patients without cardiac dysrhythmia, transthoracic or transesophageal echocardiography is warranted to rule out ventricular thrombus or aneurysm. Computerized tomography (CT) of the chest, abdomen, and pelvis will provide imaging of the aorta and iliac arteries to identify aneurysms or extensive atherosclerotic disease, which can serve as sources of arterial embolization. Hypercoagulable workup should be performed for this patient population and may help guide long-term anticoagulation.

Patients are followed in the office after discharge to ensure complete healing of wounds and to monitor the arterial perfusion of the extremity. Arterial duplex and ankle brachial indices in the noninvasive vascular lab are useful and objective tools for surveillance.

Limb Salvage Predictors and Survival Implications

In general, patients with acute arterial embolism are more likely to die, while those with arterial thrombosis are more likely to require amputation. Limb salvage tends to be higher after embolization than thrombosis due to the ease of performing balloon embolectomy versus a distal tibial bypass [8]. In population studies, the 5-year survival rate for patients with acute arterial embolization was 17 % which is significantly lower than the expected survival of 62 % [21].

More patients with acute arterial thrombosis are alive at 5 years; however, the 44 % survival rate is still less than the expected 74 % for population-matched controls. This lower survival rate is likely due to the older age of those with embolic disease and the greater prevalence of cardiac disease.

Predictors of successful limb salvage include the absence of underlying lower extremity atherosclerotic disease, normal cardiac function, and younger age (less than 80 years). Clearly, those patients who seek treatment earlier in their acute ischemic process and undergo revascularization expeditiously stand a better chance of successful limb salvage.

Conclusion

This chapter emphasized the key concepts in the diagnosis, classification, and treatment of acute limb ischemia. Physical exam serves as the foundation for the diagnosis of acute limb ischemia while imaging studies provide confirmation and guidance for treatment decisions. Classifying the severity of ischemia determines the feasibility and urgency of revascularization. Treatment strategies for acute limb ischemia include endovascular therapy in the form of thrombolysis and surgical intervention involving thromboembolectomy. Surgeons treating acute limb ischemia should be familiar with the advantages, drawbacks, and technical details of the various options for revascularization. Achieving a successful outcome in patients with an acutely ischemic limb requires sound clinical judgment and technical expertise.

References

1. Dryjski M, Swedenborg J. Acute ischemia of the extremities in a metropolitan area during one year. J Cardiovasc Surg (Torino). 1984;25:518–22.
2. Bergqvist D, Troeng T, Elfstrom J, et al. Auditing surgical outcome: ten years with the Swedish Vascular Registry–Swedvasc. The Steering Committee of Swedvasc. Eur J Surg Suppl. 1998;581:3–8.
3. Clason AE, Stonebridge PA, Duncan AJ, Nolan B, Jenkins AM, Ruckley CV. Acute ischaemia of the lower limb: the effect of centralizing vascular surgical services on morbidity and mortality. Br J Surg. 1989;76:592–3.
4. Norgren L, Hiatt WR, Dormandy JA, Nehler MR, Harris KA, Fowkes FG. Inter-society consensus for the management of peripheral arterial disease (TASC II). J Vasc Surg. 2007;45 Suppl S:S5–67.
5. Fowkes FG, Housley E, Riemersma RA, et al. Smoking, lipids, glucose intolerance, and blood pressure as risk factors for peripheral atherosclerosis compared with ischemic heart disease in the Edinburgh Artery Study. Am J Epidemiol. 1992;135:331–40.
6. Powell JT, Edwards RJ, Worrell PC, Franks PJ, Greenhalgh RM, Poulter NR. Risk factors associated with the development of peripheral arterial disease in smokers: a case-control study. Atherosclerosis. 1997;129:41–8.
7. Dale WA. Differential management of acute peripheral arterial ischemia. J Vasc Surg. 1984;1:269–78.
8. Cambria RP, Abbott WM. Acute arterial thrombosis of the lower extremity. Its natural history contrasted with arterial embolism. Arch Surg. 1984;119:784–7.
9. Mackman N. Triggers, targets and treatments for thrombosis. Nature. 2008;451:914–18.
10. Rutherford RB, Baker JD, Ernst C, et al. Recommended standards for reports dealing with lower extremity ischemia: revised version. J Vasc Surg. 1997;26:517–38.
11. Suggested standards for reports dealing with lower extremity ischemia. Prepared by the Ad Hoc Committee on Reporting Standards, Society for Vascular Surgery/North American Chapter, International Society for Cardiovascular Surgery. J Vasc Surg. 1986;4:80–94.
12. Jivegard L, Arfvidsson B, Frid I, Haljamae H, Holm J. Cardiac output in patients with acute lower limb ischaemia of presumed embolic origin – a predictor of severity and outcome? Eur J Vasc Surg. 1990;4:401–7.
13. Ljungman C, Adami HO, Bergqvist D, Sparen P, Bergstrom R. Risk factors for early lower limb loss after embolectomy for acute arterial occlusion: a population-based case-control study. Br J Surg. 1991;78:1482–5.
14. Blaisdell FW, Steele M, Allen RE. Management of acute lower extremity arterial ischemia due to embolism and thrombosis. Surgery. 1978;84:822–34.
15. Ouriel K, Shortell CK, DeWeese JA, et al. A comparison of thrombolytic therapy with operative revascularization in the initial treatment of acute peripheral arterial ischemia. J Vasc Surg. 1994;19:1021–30.
16. Fogarty TJ, Cranley JJ, Krause RJ, Strasser ES, Hafner CD. A method for extraction of arterial emboli and thrombi. Surg Gynecol Obstet. 1963;116:241–4.
17. Braithwaite BD, Birch PA, Poskitt KR, Heather BP, Earnshaw JJ. Accelerated thrombolysis with high dose bolus t-PA extends the role of peripheral thrombolysis but may increase the risks. Clin Radiol. 1995;50:747–50.
18. Armon MP, Yusuf SW, Whitaker SC, Gregson RH, Wenham PW, Hopkinson BR. Results of 100 cases of pulse-spray thrombolysis for acute and subacute leg ischaemia. Br J Surg. 1997;84:47–50.
19. Palfrayman SJ, Booth A, Michaels JA. A systematic review of intra-arterial thrombolytic therapy for lower-limb ischaemia. Eur J Vasc Endovasc Surg. 2000;19:143–57.
20. Berridge DC, Kessel D, Robertson I. Surgery versus thrombolysis for acute limb ischaemia: initial management. Cochrane Database Syst Rev. 2002;(6):CD002784.
21. Aune S, Trippestad A. Operative mortality and long-term survival of patients operated on for acute lower limb ischaemia. Eur J Vasc Endovasc Surg. 1998;15(2):143–6.

4 Compartment Syndrome

Col (ret) Mark W. Bowyer

Introduction

Compartment syndrome (CS) is a condition in which increased pressure within a limited space compromises the circulation and function of affected tissues [1–6]. Arising from a wide variety of circumstances (Table 4.1), this condition is a limb and potentially life-threatening condition with which every surgeon should have intimate knowledge. Current knowledge unequivocally reflects that failure to identify and treat CS properly leads to tissue necrosis, permanent functional impairment, possible amputation, and potential renal failure and death [2, 7, 34–39]. In a 9-year review of extremity trauma, Feliciano et al. [40] found that 75 % of amputations in the lower extremity were related to a delay in performing fasciotomy or an incomplete fasciotomy.

Not only is disability resulting from CS of great consequence to the patient [41–43], but failure to diagnose or properly treat a CS is one of the most common causes of medical litigation, with significant malpractice liability [4]. Bhattacharyya and Vrahas [44] reported an average indemnity payment of $426,000 in nine cases settled between 1980 and 2003 in Massachusetts, and awards as high as $14.9 million have been made in cases of missed CS.

The average number of fasciotomies reported in case logs submitted to the American Board of Surgery for 2011 graduates of US surgical residencies was 1.2 [45], and the average number of fasciotomies reported by graduates of US vascular fellowships in the last decade has been between 0.8 and 1.4 per year [46]. As such, otherwise well-trained surgeons are ill-prepared to recognize and manage CS and to perform complete and adequate fasciotomies. Optimal outcomes result from early recognition of CS and aggressive, properly performed fasciotomy. Proper fasciotomy requires extensive knowledge of the anatomical landmarks and anatomy of the muscle compartments of the extremities.

The goal of this chapter is to review the pathophysiology, epidemiology, diagnosis, relevant anatomy, and treatment of CS with an emphasis on the proper performance of fasciotomy of the lower leg and complications associated with this vital limb and potentially life-saving procedure.

Pathophysiology

The pathophysiology of CS is relatively straightforward. Groups of muscles and their associated nerves and vessels are surrounded by thick fascial layers that define the various compartments of the extremities which are of relatively fixed volume. Compartment syndrome occurs either when compartment size is restricted or compartment volume is increased [7]. Several conditions have been implicated in causing CS [1, 7–33] and are detailed in Table 4.1.

As pressures increase because of internal or external forces, venous flow decreases and narrows the arteriovenous perfusion gradient, resulting in diminished tissue blood flow. This condition is self-perpetuating, leading to a continuous loop that must be broken with the timely initiation of definitive care [7]. Hippocrates may have been the first to describe the dangers of elevated intracompartmental pressures in 400 BC [47]. When untreated, permanent deformity of the distal extremity results, a phenomenon first described by Richard von Volkmann in the late nineteenth century [48]. In 1926, Jepson [49] was able to experimentally create CS in the extremities of dogs using external pressure (Esmarch's bandage), and he suggested drainage of the compartments would be of value in preventing deformity.

Cellular anoxia is the final common pathway of all compartment syndromes. However, the interrelation between

Disclaimer The views expressed herein are those of the author and are not to be construed as official or reflecting the views of the Department of Defense. The author has nothing to disclose.

M.W. Bowyer, MD, FACS, DMCC (✉)
The Norman M. Rich Department of Surgery,
Uniformed Services University of the Health Sciences,
4301 Jones Bridge Road, Bethesda, MD 20814, USA
e-mail: mark.bowyer@usuhs.edu

V. Gahtan and M.J. Costanza (eds.), *Essentials of Vascular Surgery for the General Surgeon*,
DOI 10.1007/978-1-4939-1326-8_4, © Springer Science+Business Media New York 2015

Table 4.1 Factors implicated with the development of acute limb compartment syndrome [1, 7–33]

Restriction of compartment size	Increased compartment volume
	From hemorrhage
	Fractures
Casts	Vascular injury
Splints	Drugs (anticoagulants)
Burn eschar	Hemophilia; sickle cell
Tourniquets	*From muscle edema/swelling*
Tight dressings	Crush – trauma, drugs, or alcohol
Fracture reduction	Rhabdomyolysis/blast injury
Closure of fascial defects	Sepsis
Incomplete skin release	Exercise induced
Military antishock trousers	Envenomation or bee sting
Prolonged extrication trapped limb	Massive resuscitation
Localized external pressure	Intracompartmental fluid infusion
Long leg brace	Phlegmasia cerulea dolens
Automated BP monitoring	Electrical burns
Malpositioning on OR table	Reperfusion injury
	Postpartum eclampsia

increased compartment pressure, blood pressure, and loss of tissue perfusion leading to cell death are incompletely understood. This incomplete understanding leads to diagnostic and treatment challenges. As ischemia continues, irreparable damage to tissue ensues and myoneural necrosis occurs. Development of CS depends on many factors, including the duration of the pressure elevation, the metabolic rate of the tissues, vascular tone, associated soft tissue damage, and local blood pressure [6]. Nerves demonstrate functional abnormalities (paresthesias and hypoesthesia) within 30 min of ischemic onset. Irreversible functional loss will occur after 12–24 h of total ischemia [1]. The muscle shows functional changes after 2–4 h of ischemia with irreversible loss of function beginning at 4–12 h.

A dynamic relationship exists among the blood pressure, the level of intracompartmental pressure (ICP), and the duration of time for which a raised pressure is maintained. It is known that the higher the pressure, the faster and greater is the damage, but a lower pressure maintained for a longer period of time may also cause similar tissue damage [38]. Many authors [50, 51] have concluded that catastrophic clinical results were inevitable if fasciotomies were delayed for over 12 h, whereas a full recovery was achieved if decompression was performed within 6 h of making the diagnosis. Compartment syndromes lasting longer than 8–12 h are likely to produce chronic functional deficits, such as contractures, sensory aberrations, and motor weakness. Clinically, a precise pressure threshold and duration do not exist above which significant damage is irreversible and below which recovery is assured.

Tissue that has been previously subjected to intervals of ischemia is especially sensitive to increased pressure. Bernot and colleagues [52] showed that tissue previously compromised by ischemia prior to elevated ICP has a lower threshold for metabolic deterioration and irreversible damage. It must be kept in mind that polytrauma patients with low blood pressures can sustain irreversible injury at lower compartment pressures than patients with normal blood pressures, and a very high index of suspicion should be maintained in this group.

Epidemiology/Risk Factors

Given the consequences of missing a CS, it is important to identify the population at risk, as well as factors which predict the occurrence of this condition. In a 10-year retrospective review of over 10,000 trauma patients sustaining extremity injury, Branco et al. described a fasciotomy rate of 2.8 % [35]. During this period, 315 fasciotomies were performed on 237 patients with 68.4 % done below the knee, 14.4 % on the forearm, and 8.9 % on the thigh (see Fig. 4.1). In a review of 294 combat-injured soldiers undergoing 494 fasciotomies, Ritenour et al. reported the calf as the most common site (51 %) followed by the forearm (22.3 %), the thigh (8.3 %), the upper arm (7.3 %), the hand (5.7 %), and the foot (4.8 %) [53].

Certain injury patterns have been associated with higher likelihood of needing fasciotomy. Blick et al. found a close association between grade of fracture, degree of comminution, and risk of development of CS in a retrospective review of 198 open tibia fractures [54]. Abouezzi et al. found a 28 % incidence of fasciotomy in patients with peripheral vascular injuries treated at a level I trauma center. They determined that injury to popliteal vessels was more likely (62 % cases) to result in fasciotomy than above the knee vascular injury (19 % cases) [55]. This finding was echoed by Gonzalez et al. [56] who reported that CS of the lower extremity was more likely to be associated with penetrating injuries below the knee (94 %) than above the knee. Another study evaluated femoral vascular injuries in particular and found that the rates of fasciotomy depended on whether there was isolated arterial (13 % fasciotomy) or venous injury (3 % fasciotomy) or a combination (38 % fasciotomy) [57].

Branco et al. [35] found that the incidence of fasciotomy varied widely by mechanism of injury (0.9 % after motor vehicle collision to 8.6 % after a gunshot wound). Additionally the need for fasciotomy was related to the type of injury ranging from 2.2 % incidence for patients with closed fractures up to 41.8 % in patients with combined venous and arterial injuries (see Fig. 4.2). The study by Branco identified the risk factors associated with the need for fasciotomy after extremity trauma: young males with penetrating or multisystem

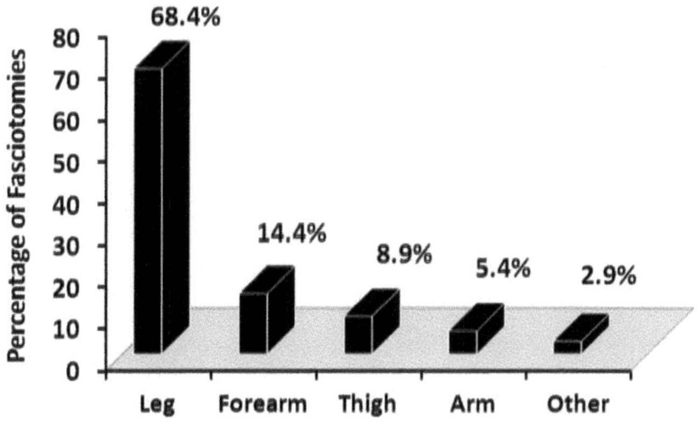

Fig. 4.1 Anatomic distribution of 315 fasciotomies done for extremity trauma. Other includes the foot and hand (Adapted, with permission from Elsevier, from Branco et al. [35])

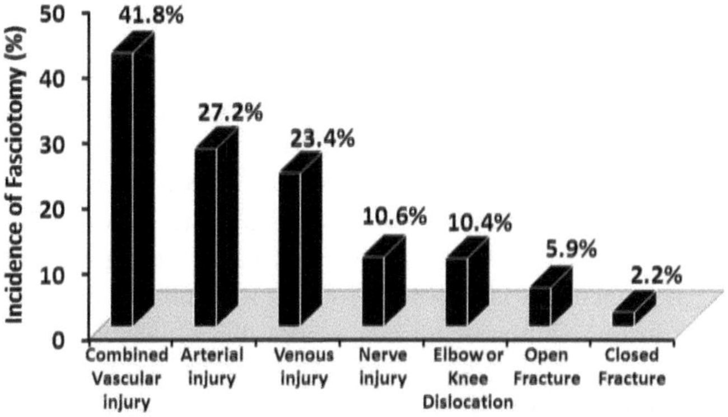

Fig. 4.2 Incidence of fasciotomy as a result of the injury type in 315 fasciotomies done for extremity trauma (Adapted, with permission from Elsevier, from Branco et al. [35])

trauma, requiring blood transfusion, and with open fractures, elbow or knee dislocations, or vascular injury (arterial, venous, or combined) are at the highest risk of requiring a fasciotomy after extremity trauma [35]. Taylor et al. [39] reiterate that age is a major prognostic factor with patients less than 35 more likely than older patients to develop CS following the same type of injury. These orthopedic authors list tibial shaft fractures as the most common antecedent cause (36 %) followed by soft tissue injury (23 %), distal radial fracture (9.8 %), crush syndrome (7.9 %), diaphyseal fracture of the radius/ulna (7.9 %), femoral fracture (3.0 %), and tibial plateau fracture (3.0 %) [39].

Diagnosis

Diagnosis depends on a high clinical suspicion and an understanding of risk factors, pathophysiology, and subtle physical exam findings. The diagnosis of CS is often based on subtle changes in symptoms and vague clinical exam findings. The physician must have a high degree of suspicion when treating these patients. Time to diagnosis is the most important prognostic factor for these patients. Insufficient understanding of the natural history and limited evaluation of signs and symptoms primarily account for delays in diagnosis [39]. It is important to realize that the aim is to recognize and treat raised intracompartmental pressure before irreversible cell damage occurs [47].

Numerous authors have stated that the diagnosis of CS is a clinical diagnosis [4, 6, 7, 33, 34, 39, 47, 58–62]. The classically described five "Ps" – pain, pallor, paresthesias, paralysis, and pulselessness – are said to be pathognomonic of CS. However, *these are usually late signs and extensive and irreversible injuries may have taken place by the time they are manifested.* In the earliest stages of CS, patients may report some tingling and an uncomfortable feeling in their extremity followed closely by pain with passive stretching of the muscles of the affected compartment. The most important symptom of CS is *pain greater than expected due to the injury alone.*

Nerve tissue is affected first by the subsequent end-tissue hypoxia causing pain on passive motion seen early in the development of CS, sparing distal pulses until late in the course [33]. The loss of pulse is a late finding, and the presence of pulses and normal capillary refill do not rule out CS! *The presence of open wounds does not exclude CS.* In fact, the worst open fractures are actually more likely to have a CS.

All clinical signs have inherent drawbacks in making the diagnosis. Pain is an unreliable and variable predictor. It can range from being very mild to severe and is already present in patients who have suffered acute trauma [63]. The pain of the obvious injury can mask that of an impending CS and cannot alone be depended upon to make the diagnosis [60]. Mubarak and colleagues [64] found that pain in response to passive stretching of the affected muscle compartment was also an unreliable sign and suggested that the presence of hypoesthesia was more dependable. However, Rorabeck and Macnab [65] found hypoesthesia to be the last clinical finding to develop as the syndrome progressed.

Although all have a role in the diagnosis of CS, the constellation of signs and symptoms and overall clinical picture are more important than the presence or absence of any particular finding [39]. Ulmer [41] undertook a review of over 1,900 articles on CS published in the English literature between 1966 and 2001 to assess whether published studies support basing the diagnosis of CS of the lower leg on clinical findings. This exhaustive review produced only four studies in which sensitivity, specificity, and positive and negative predictive values could be calculated [66–69]. Data from these studies suggest that the sensitivity of clinical findings for diagnosing CS is low (13–19 %). The positive predictive value of clinical findings was 11–15 %, and the specificity and negative predictive value were each 97–98 %. These findings suggest that the clinical features of CS are more useful by their absence in excluding the diagnosis than when they are present in confirming the diagnosis. When one clinical finding was present, the probability of a CS was 25 and 93 % when three clinical findings were present [41].

Given the findings of Ulmer's review and the fact that clinical findings may be absent in patients with altered sensorium, under the influence of drugs or alcohol, distracting injuries, or paralysis, many authors advise using tissue pressure measurements as an adjunct to clinical findings [36, 60, 64, 70]. Others advocate the use of compartment pressure measurement as a principle criterion for the diagnosis of CS [68, 71].

In actual practice, tissue pressure (compartment pressure) measurements have a limited role in making the diagnosis of CS. However, in polytrauma patients with associated head injury, drug and alcohol intoxication, intubation, spinal injuries, use of paralyzing drugs, extremes of age, unconsciousness, or low diastolic pressures, measuring compartment pressures may be of use in determining the need for fasciotomy.

The pressure threshold for making the diagnosis of CS is controversial. A number of authors recommend 30 mmHg [64], and others cite pressures as high as 45 mmHg. Ouellete [72] recommended that an ICP of 15–25 mmHg should be used in patients with clinical signs and greater than 25 mmHg for those without. Many surgeons use the "Delta-P" system. The compartment pressure is subtracted from the patient's diastolic blood pressure to obtain the Delta-P. Whitesides as early as 1975 proposed that the muscle was at risk when the ICP was within 10–30 mmHg of the diastolic pressure [73]. If the Delta-P is less than 30, the surgeon should be concerned that a CS may be present. For instance, if the diastolic blood pressure was 60 mmHg and the measured compartment pressure was 42 mmHg, the "Delta-P" would be 18 (60 − 42 = 18) and the patient is likely to have CS. Other factors to consider when considering fasciotomy are the length of time of transport to definitive care and ability to do serial exams.

One of the earliest champions of measuring compartment pressures was Whitesides [74], who used an 18-gauge needle inserted into the compartment connected to a mercury manometer to obtain pressure measurements. This and other methods to include the wick catheter technique developed by Mubarek [2], and the slit catheter technique developed by Rorabeck [75] have been widely used in the past, but suffer from the cumbersome nature of setting them up and user variability. A commercially available portable handheld, self-contained, electronic pressure monitor with a digital display is available (Stryker® intracompartmental pressure monitor system, Stryker® Surgical, Kalamazoo, Michigan) has replaced most of these less reproducible devices as the current standard (Fig. 4.3). Another commercially available device, Twin Star ECS® that was initially developed to remove fluid from compartments by tissue ultrafiltration [76] has recently received clearance to be used a continuous pressure monitor as well (Fig. 4.4). An alternative approach is to

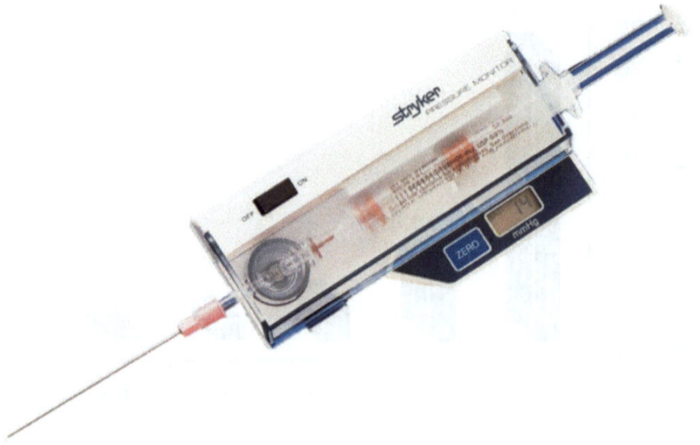

Fig. 4.3 Intracompartmental pressure monitor system manufactured by Stryker® Surgical, Kalamazoo, Michigan (Courtesy of Stryker® Instruments. Kalamazoo, Michigan)

use an 18-gauge needle attached to a side-port arterial line setup inserted into the compartment.

The use of pressure measurements to decide if fasciotomy is necessary can be very useful if significantly elevated, but there are several potential pitfalls when interpreting pressure measurements. It is important to keep in mind that the pressure in one compartment can be normal while that in the compartment immediately adjacent can be elevated. It is therefore essential to have thorough understanding of the anatomy of the compartments and the confidence that the pressure of all of the compartments of the suspicious extremity have been measured prior to making any conclusions about a normal pressure. Additionally, there may be variations of pressure within a compartment at different levels. Seiler et al. [77] demonstrated that there is significant intracompartmental variability within normal compartments, and Heckman et al. [70] showed that ICP measurements also show variability within an injured compartment.

There have been a variety of other noninvasive techniques proposed for making the diagnosis of CS to include near-infrared spectroscopy [78–80], laser Doppler flowmetry [81], pulsed phase-locked loop ultrasound [82–84], magnetic resonance imaging [85, 86], skin quantitative hardness measurement [87, 88], vibratory sensation [89, 90], and scintigraphy using 99Tcm-methoxyisobutyl isonitril (MIBI) [91]. Though some of these techniques have shown early promise, none have reached clinical use outside of protocols [92].

At the end of the day, CS remains primarily a clinical diagnosis fueled by a high index of suspicion and supported by objective examination findings. The reliance on clinical examination with a low threshold for fascial release may result in unwarranted fasciotomies, but it avoids the grave consequences of a missed diagnosis.

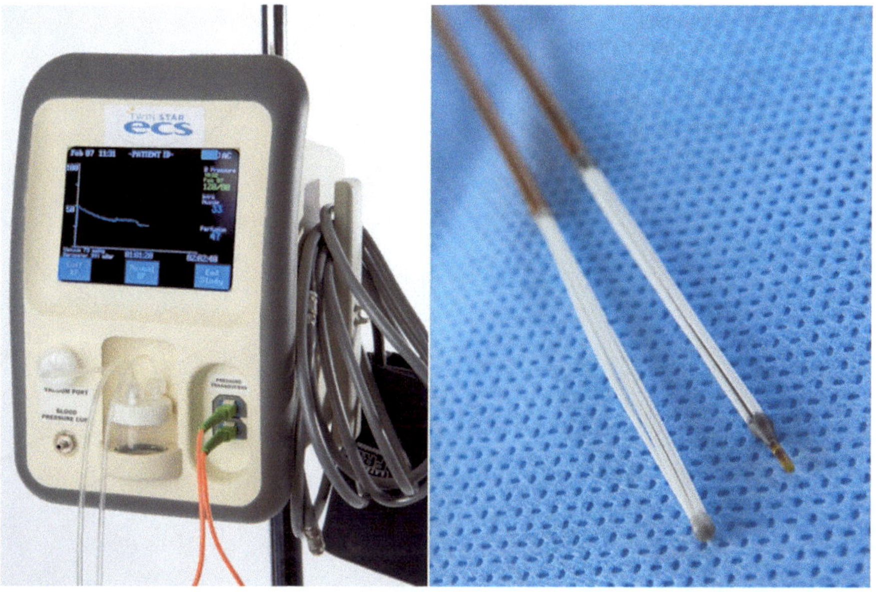

Fig. 4.4 Intracompartmental pressure monitor system and catheter tip manufactured by Twin Star Medical (Twin Star ECS®), Minneapolis, MN

Treatment

The definitive treatment of CS is *early and aggressive fasciotomy.* In patients with vascular injury in whom a fasciotomy in conjunction with a vascular repair is planned, it makes great sense to perform the fasciotomy *before* doing the repair. The rationale for this is that the ischemic compartment is likely to already be tight and thus will create inflow resistance to your vascular repair, making it susceptible to early thrombosis.

It is imperative that surgeons caring for traumatically injured patients fully understand the anatomy of the extremity compartments and the technique of fasciotomy for each. It is extremely embarrassing for the surgeon and life altering for the patient if an adequate or timely fasciotomy is not done and the patient loses the limb as a result. As previously mentioned in the series reported by Feliciano et al., 75 % of amputations of the lower extremity were related to a delay in performing, or performing an incomplete fasciotomy [41]. In a recent large review of combat patients, Ritenour et al. reported that patients who had incomplete or delayed fasciotomy had twice the rate of major amputation and three times the rate of mortality [53]. In spite of these alarming numbers, many otherwise well-trained surgeons continue to make these mistakes. The following section will focus on the recommended technique for performing fasciotomy of the lower extremity emphasizing the landmarks, relevant anatomy, and pitfalls.

Fasciotomy of the Lower Leg

As previously discussed, the lower leg (calf) is the most common site for CS requiring fasciotomy. The preferred technique for fasciotomy of the below the knee CS is the two-incision four-compartment fasciotomy. This technique was widely used in WWII and was the standard treatment for decompression in a syndrome involving more than one compartment [93]. An alternative single-incision approach in which the fibula is resected has been championed by some [94], but has been condemned by others as being unnecessarily mutilating, more likely to result in injury to the peroneal nerve, and likely to result in incomplete release of the compartments [3, 4]. Because it uses a lateral approach, the one-incision technique protects the great saphenous vein from injury during the fasciotomy.

In 2014, the standard approach to treating CS of the lower extremity in traumatically injured patients is the two-incision, four-compartment fasciotomy as popularized by Mubarak and Owen in 1977 [3]. As previously discussed, this procedure is not performed frequently by the majority of general or even vascular surgeons [45, 46], and the rate of delayed, incomplete, or improperly performed fasciotomy is alarmingly high with preventable morbidity and mortality as a result [53]. The most commonly missed compartments are the anterior followed closely by the deep posterior [53], and this likely occurs as a result of incomplete knowledge of the anatomy of the lower extremity. Successful fasciotomy of the lower extremity requires a thorough understanding of the anatomy and the relevant landmarks. The lower leg has four major tissue compartments bounded by investing the muscle fascia (Fig. 4.5). It is important to understand the anatomical arrangement of these compartments as well as some key structures within each compartment in order to perform a proper four-compartment fasciotomy (Fig. 4.6).

It is not necessary to remember the names of all the muscles (Fig. 4.6) in each compartment, but it is useful to remember the following: the anterior compartment contains the anterior tibial artery and vein and the deep peroneal nerve;

Fig. 4.5 Cross-sectional anatomy of the midportion of the left lower leg depicting the four compartments that must be released when performing a lower leg fasciotomy

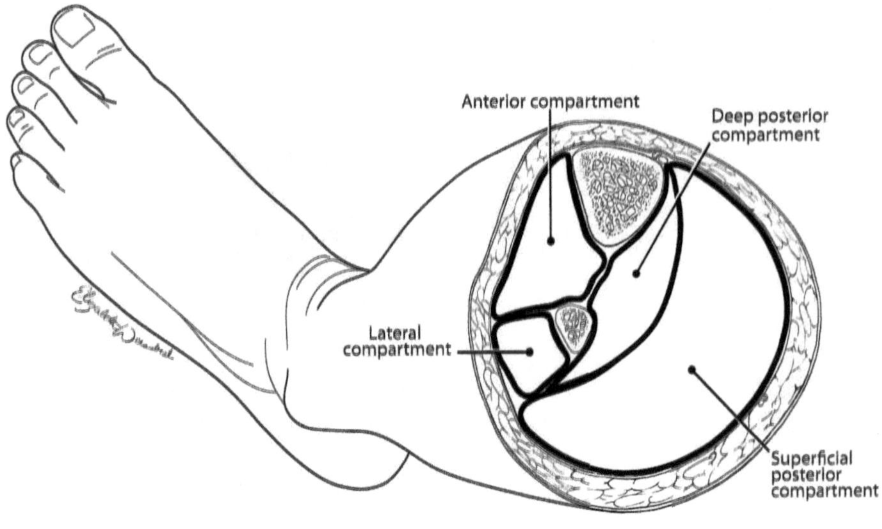

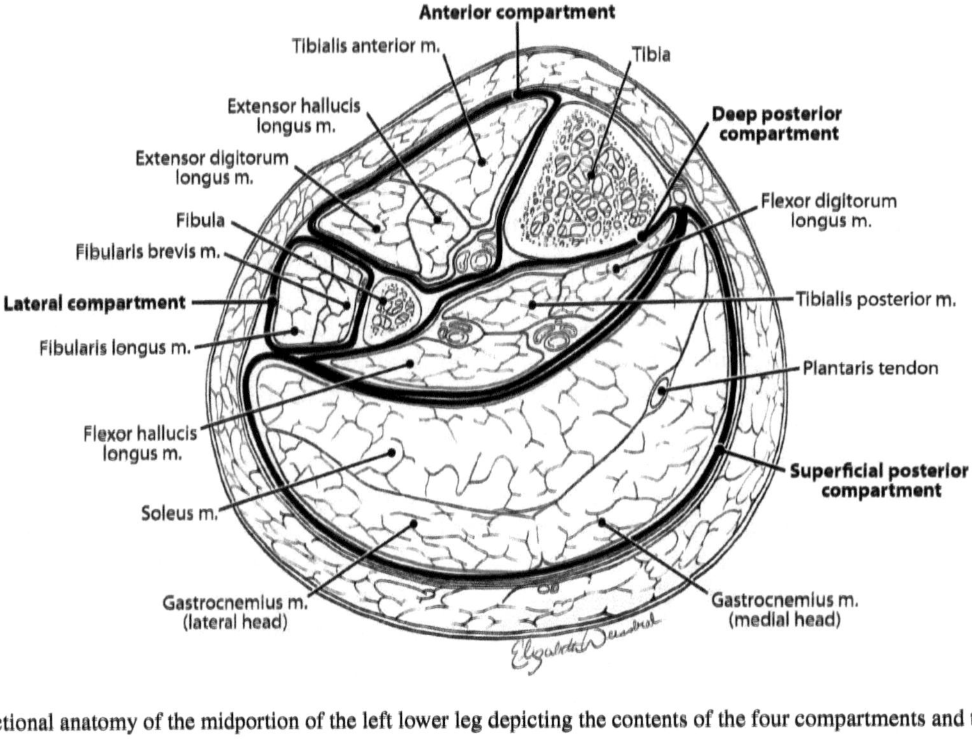

Fig. 4.6 Cross-sectional anatomy of the midportion of the left lower leg depicting the contents of the four compartments and their relationship to the tibia and fibula

the lateral compartment, the superficial peroneal nerve (which must not be injured); the superficial posterior compartment, the soleus and gastrocnemius muscles; and the deep posterior compartment, the posterior tibial and peroneal vessels and the tibial nerve (Fig. 4.7).

There are several key features that will enable performance of a successful two-incision four-compartment fasciotomy. Proper placement of the incisions is essential. As extremities needing fasciotomy are often grossly swollen or deformed, marking the key landmarks will aid in placement of the incisions. The tibial spine serves as a reliable midpoint between the incisions. The lateral malleolus and fibular head are used to identify the course of the fibula on the lateral portion of the leg (Fig. 4.8). The lateral incision is usually made just anterior (~1 fingerbreadth) to the line of the fibula, or *a finger in front of the fibula*. It is important to stay anterior to the fibula as this minimizes the chance of damaging the superficial peroneal nerve. The medial incision is made one thumb breadth below the palpable medial edge of the tibia, or *a thumb below the tibia* (Fig. 4.9). The extent of the skin

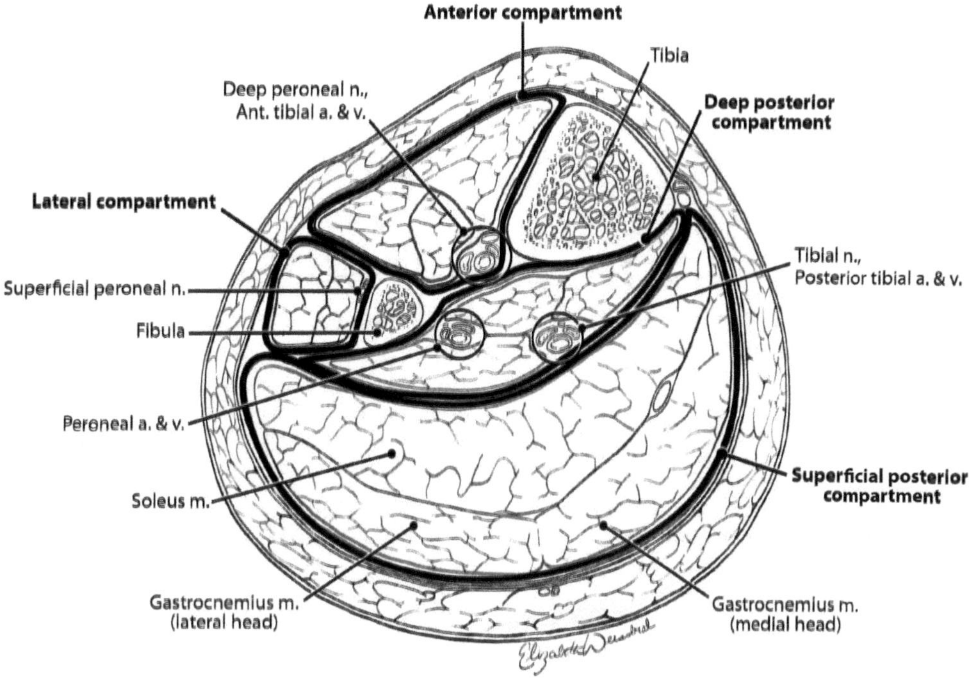

Fig. 4.7 Cross-sectional anatomy of the midportion of the left lower leg depicting the key structures and relationships that must be kept in mind when performing a two-incision four-compartment fasciotomy

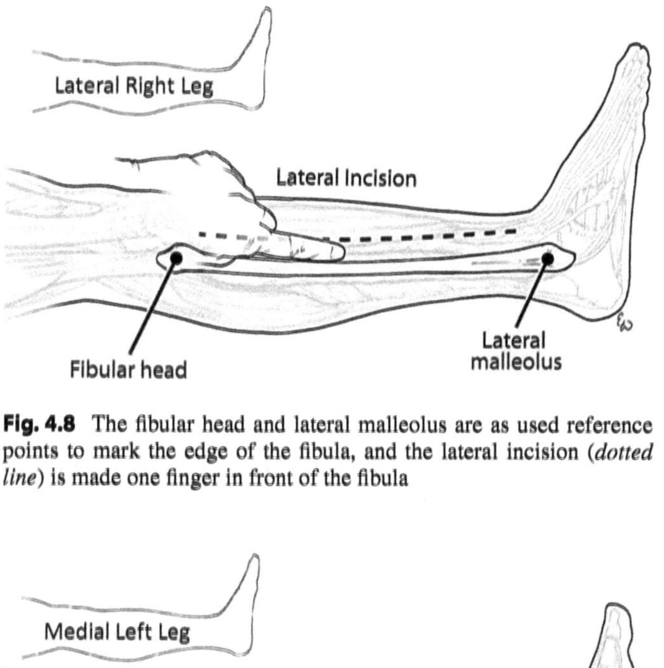

Fig. 4.8 The fibular head and lateral malleolus are as used reference points to mark the edge of the fibula, and the lateral incision (*dotted line*) is made one finger in front of the fibula

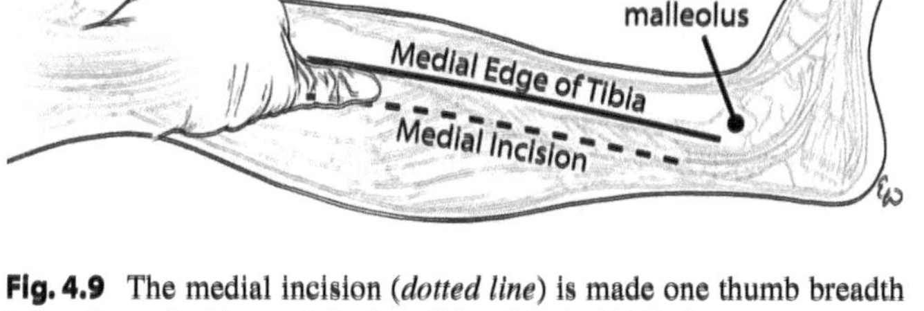

Fig. 4.9 The medial incision (*dotted line*) is made one thumb breadth below the palpable medial edge of the tibia (*solid line*)

incision should be approximately two fingerbreadths below the tibial tuberosity and above the malleolus on either side.

It is very important to mark the incisions on both sides prior to opening them, as the landmarks of the swollen extremity will become distorted once the incision is made.

The Lateral Incision of the Lower Leg

The lateral incision (Fig. 4.8) is made *one finger in front of the fibula* and should in general extend from two fingerbreadths below the head of the fibula down to two fingerbreadths above the lateral malleolus. The exact length of the skin incision will depend on the clinical setting, and care must be taken to make sure that it is long enough such that the skin does not serve as a constricting band. The skin and subcutaneous tissue are incised to expose the fascia encasing the lateral and anterior compartments. Care should be taken to avoid the lesser saphenous vein and peroneal nerve when making these skin incisions.

Once the skin flap is raised, the intermuscular septum is sought and identified. This is the structure which divides the anterior and lateral compartments. In the swollen or injured extremity, it may be difficult to find the intermuscular septum. In these circumstances, the septum can often be found by following the perforating vessels down to it (Fig. 4.10). Classically the fascia of the lower leg is opened using an "H"-shaped incision (Fig. 4.11). This will be accomplished by making the crosspiece of the "H" using a scalpel which

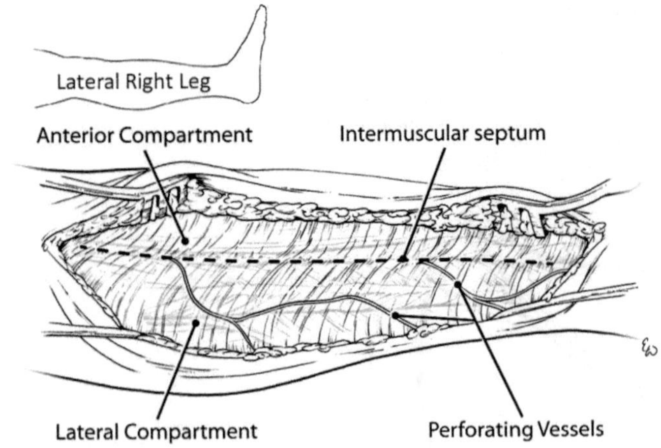

Fig. 4.10 The intermuscular septum separates the anterior and lateral compartments and is where the perforating vessels traverse. This is a representation of the lateral incision of the right lower leg

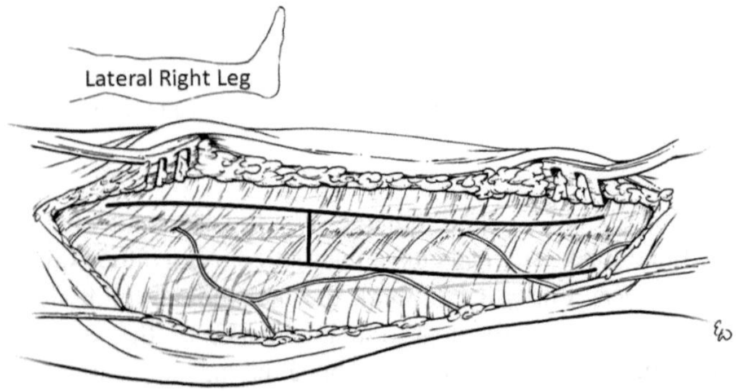

Fig. 4.11 The fascia overlying the anterior and lateral compartments is opened in an "H"-shaped fashion

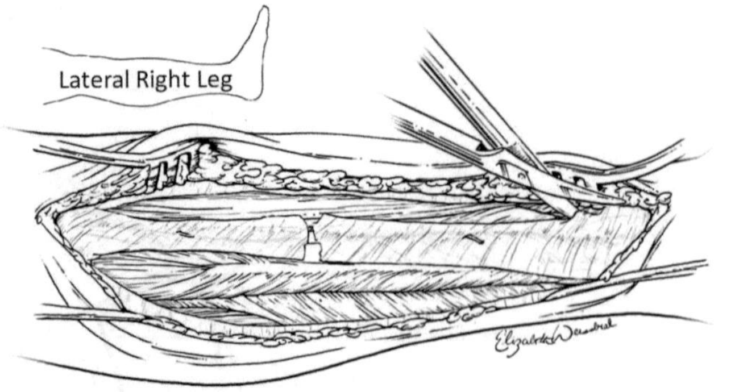

Fig. 4.12 The fascia overlying the anterior and lateral compartments is opened in an "H"-shaped fashion using scissors with the tips turned away from the septum

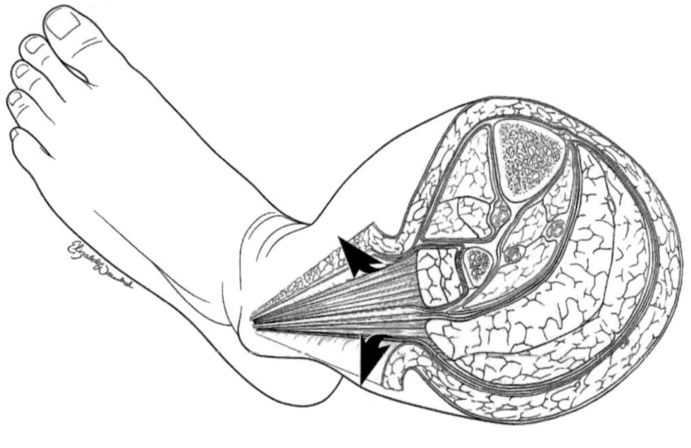

Fig. 4.13 When the lateral incision is made too far posterior, the septum between the lateral and superficial posterior compartments may be mistaken for that between the anterior and lateral leading to the anterior compartment not being opened

will expose both compartments and the septum. The legs of the "H" are made with curved scissors using just the tips which are turned away from the septum to avoid injury to the peroneal nerve (Figs. 4.11 and 4.12). It is important to identify the intermuscular septum and open the fascia at least one centimeter from it on either side, because the terminal branch of the deep peroneal nerve perforates the septum in the distal one third of the lower leg and this could be cut if care is not taken. The anterior and lateral compartments are then fasciotomized 1 cm in front and behind the intermuscular septum.

The fascia should be opened by pushing the partially opened scissor tips in both directions on either side of the septum opening the fascia from the head of the fibula down to the lateral malleolus in a line that is 1–2 cm from the septum. Inspection of the septum and identification of the deep peroneal nerve and/or the anterior tibial vessels confirm entry into the anterior compartment. The skin incision should be closely inspected and extended as needed to ensure that the ends do not serve as a point of constriction.

As previously stated, the anterior compartment is the one most commonly missed during lower-extremity fasciotomy. One of the reasons for missing the anterior compartment stems from making the incision too far posteriorly, either directly over or behind the fibula. When the incision is made in this manner, the septum between the lateral and the superficial compartment may be directly below the incision and is erroneously identified as the septum between the anterior and lateral compartments (Fig. 4.13). When the lateral incision is made *one finger in front of the fibula*, the intramuscular septum between the anterior and lateral compartments is found directly below the incision making successful decompression likely (Fig. 4.14).

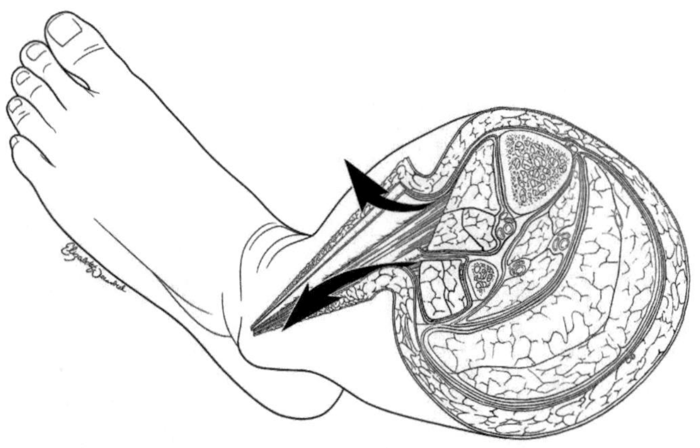

Fig. 4.14 When the lateral incision is made one fingerbreadth in front of the fibula, the septum between the anterior and lateral compartments is more readily identified allowing for adequate decompression of both the anterior and lateral compartments

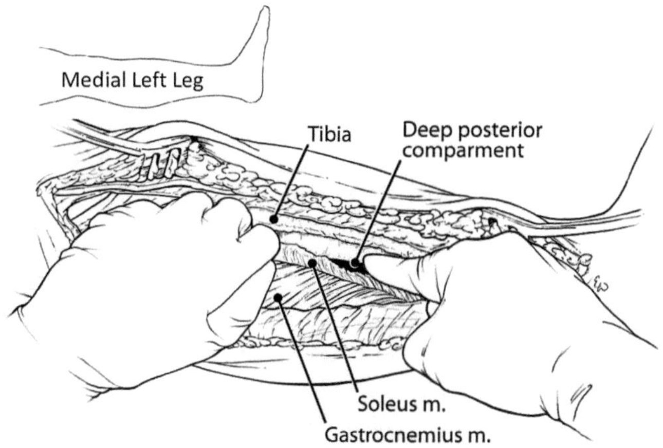

Fig. 4.16 The deep posterior compartment is entered by taking the soleus fibers down off the underside of the tibia

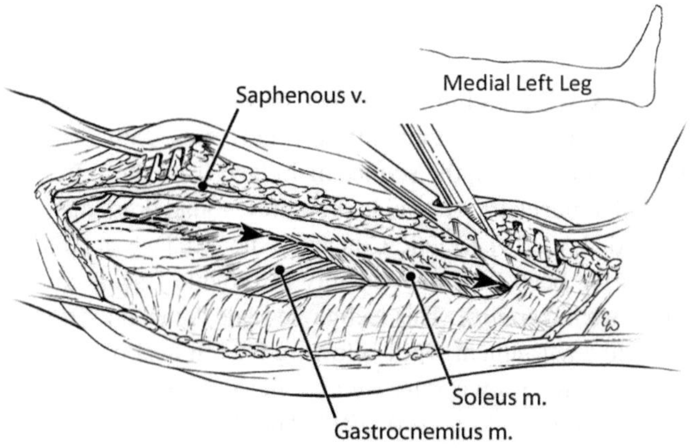

Fig. 4.15 The fascia overlying the superficial posterior compartment is opened with partially closed scissors from the tibial tuberosity to the medial malleolus

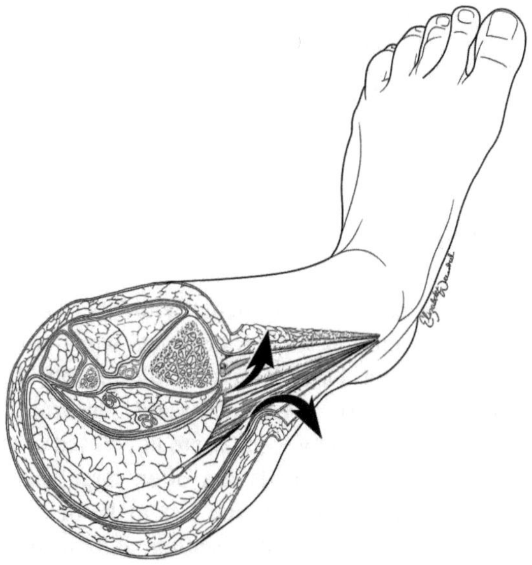

Fig. 4.17 A potential pitfall when doing the medial incision is to develop a plane between the gastrocnemius and soleus muscles and believing that this represents the plane between the superficial and deep posterior compartment

The Medial Incision of the Lower Leg

The medial incision is made one thumb breadth below the palpable medial edge of the tibia (Fig. 4.9). When making this incision, it is important to both identify and preserve the great saphenous vein and ligate any perforators to it, as these can bleed profusely. After dividing the skin and subcutaneous tissues, the fascia overlying the superficial posterior compartment which contains the soleus and gastrocnemius muscle is exposed. The fascia should be opened with partially opened scissors from the tibial tuberosity to the medial malleolus to effectively decompress this compartment (Fig. 4.15). The key to entering the deep posterior compartment is the soleus muscle. The soleus muscle attaches to the medial edge of the tibia, and dissecting these fibers (the "soleus bridge") completely free from and exposing the underside of the tibia ensures entry into the deep posterior compartment (Fig. 4.16). Identification of the posterior tibial neurovascular bundle confirms that the compartment has been entered.

As previously discussed, the deep posterior compartment can also be missed, and thorough understanding of the anatomy is key to ensuring that this does not happen. One potential way to miss the deep posterior compartment is to get into the plane between the gastrocnemius and soleus muscle and believe that the compartment has been released (Fig. 4.17). Proper decompression of the deep posterior compartment requires that the soleus fibers be separated from their attachment on the underside of the tibia (Figs. 4.16 and 4.18).

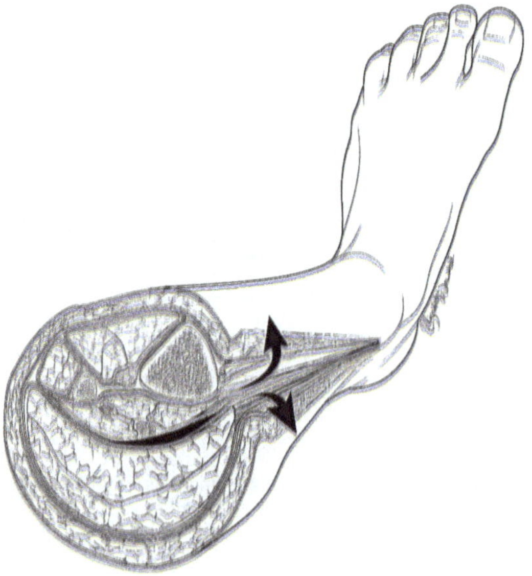

Fig. 4.18 Entry into and release of the deep posterior compartment requires separating both the gastrocnemius and soleus from the underside of the tibia. Identification of the neurovascular bundle confirms that the deep posterior compartment has been entered

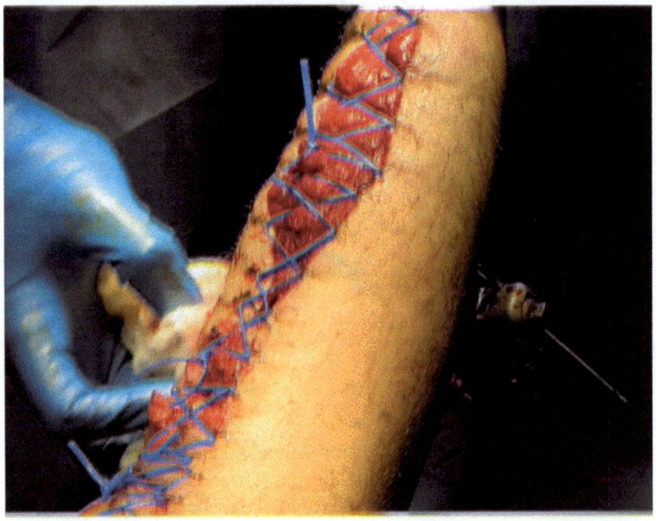

Fig. 4.19 The shoelace technique using vessel loops interlaced over the wound through staples placed at the skin edges is used to minimize skin retraction (Photo courtesy of Dr. John Kragh)

Wound Care

The muscle in each compartment should be assessed for viability. Viable muscle is pink, contracts when stimulated, and bleeds when cut. Dead muscle should be debrided back to healthy viable tissue when necessary. Generally in the trauma setting, fasciotomy wounds are not closed at the time of fasciotomy. These wounds are often large, and tissue swelling, skin retraction, or tissue loss make these wounds impossible to close at the initial setting, and closure would also defeat pressure decreases obtained by fasciotomy.

From the time of fasciotomy, wound management focuses on swelling control, allowing recovery of injured tissues and minimizing skin retraction, if possible. Patients are generally returned to the operating room every 24–72 h for dressing changes, reevaluation of muscle viability, and gradual closure of the wound. If the wounds cannot be primarily closed within 7–10 days, split-thickness skin grafts (STSG) may be required when both the patient and the wound are stable. Several techniques have been described to minimize skin retraction, possibly obviating the need for STSG [6, 95–100].

The vessel-loop or shoelace technique is commonly performed [96]. It involves using vessel loops interlaced over the wound through staples placed at the skin edges (Fig. 4.19). Although it uses equipment readily available, it suffers from several drawbacks. The thin vessel loops frequently do not have adequate tensile forces to allow minimal skin retraction in severe injuries because of the significant soft tissue swelling. It is common for such swelling to cause the vessel loops to break, eliminating any effect they may exert. Dressing changes are made more difficult and carry with them the potential of having the staples dislodged from the skin.

Subatmospheric (negative pressure) wound dressings (e.g., wound V.A.C.™, Kinetic Concepts, Inc (KCI), San Antonio, TX) have been used successfully to provide fasciotomy and open-wound control. This technique seals the wound from the outside environment while allowing for removal of exudates. Studies have shown improved capillary circulation with the use of these devices [100, 101]. The downside of this technique is that it requires a machine to provide suction and may be difficult to apply around external fixators. Janzing and Broos [98] reported on a comparison of three different techniques for closure of civilian fasciotomy wounds in 15 subjects. The mean time to wound closure for all groups was 9 days. They found that skin traction with vessel loops or prepositioned intracutaneous sutures provided good skin apposition without the necessity of skin grafting. The major advantage was that the material required was readily available in most operating rooms. However, they pointed out the potential risk for high compartment pressures during a prolonged time in the postoperative period requiring close monitoring of limb perfusion.

Singh and colleagues [95] described their experience caring for war casualties in Iraq using a dynamic wound-closure device (dynamic wound closure device – ABRA® Surgical Skin Closure, Canica, Almonte, ON, Canada) for closure of fasciotomy incisions. Eleven consecutive subjects who had undergone two-incision fasciotomies for CS were studied. Ten of the 11 subjects (91 %) had their wounds closed in a delayed primary fashion after application of the wound-closure device. They found that the subjects benefited from the use of the device and avoided the need to create additional wounds in multiple-injury patients. However, long-term follow-up of this small group was limited because of the rapid evacuation of soldiers to the United States and the expedient discharge from the hospital of host-nation soldiers.

Complications

In spite of numerous articles in the literature regarding fasciotomy, there is surprisingly little published about the complications of this procedure. Patients with open fasciotomy wounds are at risk for infection, and incomplete or delayed fasciotomies can lead to permanent nerve damage, loss of limb, multisystem organ failure, rhabdomyolysis, and death. If muscle injury is extensive, either from prolonged ischemia or from direct crush, significant amounts of myoglobin may be released as the muscle is reperfused after fasciotomy. Early recognition and aggressive fasciotomy will help to minimize these adverse outcomes. Some surgeons have questioned the practice of performing delayed fasciotomies because of the increased morbidity in the face of little to no functional benefit [101, 102]. Finkelstein and coauthors [102] reviewed the cases of five subjects who underwent a delayed fasciotomy for extremity CS at least 35 h after the injury, when ideally the fasciotomy would have been performed earlier. Of the five subjects, one subject died of septicemia and multiorgan failure, and the remaining four required lower-extremity amputation. They concluded that fasciotomies were consistently associated with severe infection and possible death when the recognition of the CS was delayed for more than 8–10 h.

Williams and colleagues [103] demonstrated in a retrospective study of 88 subjects that fasciotomy performed after 12 h was associated with a fourfold increase in infection compared with those performed before 12 h. The rates of limb salvage and neurologic sequelae were similar. They advocated that fasciotomy performed early was most effective, but that the similar rates of limb salvage, even with the increased risk for infection, justify the aggressive use of fasciotomy in extremity trauma regardless of the time of diagnosis.

Rush and colleagues [104] reported on a retrospective series of 127 lower-extremity fasciotomies performed for CS after acute ischemia and revascularization in subjects with either vascular trauma or arterial occlusive disease. Superficial infections occurred in five subjects and all resolved with local wound care. In their series, no limb loss was attributed to primary open fasciotomy. They concluded that the morbidity and mortality of fasciotomy were the result of refractory ischemia caused by associated injuries or underlying medical problems, but not from open fasciotomy wound complications.

In a retrospective study of 36 patients undergoing lower-extremity fasciotomy [59], complications were common (only seven were done as two-incision four-compartment fasciotomy, and the range of time from diagnosis to intervention was up to 9 days). Nerve damage occurred in 6 cases (15 %); bleeding was seen in 13 cases (35 %). Wound infection occurred in 10 cases (25 %). Functional outcome after fasciotomy was not always good. In this series, 18 legs (45 %) healed with good functional result, but in 11 cases (27.5 %) the final outcome was more or less a disabled leg. In 5 cases, the fasciotomy could not prevent amputation of the affected limb, and 6 patients died during the course of their hospitalization. None of the patients who underwent double-sided fasciotomy died, nor did they undergo amputation [59]. The cause of the CS appeared to be an important predictive factor for outcome. Posttraumatic CSs had a better outcome after fasciotomy than vascular injuries. At the time of discharge in this study, 45 % of patients had good limb function, 27.5 % had kept their leg with diminished function, 12.5 % underwent amputation, and 15 % died. These results are comparable with reported earlier studies by Rush et al. [104] and Jensen [105] showing 11–15 % mortality and 11–21 % amputation.

Fitzgerald and colleagues [106] found in a study of 60 requiring open fasciotomy of a traumatized limb a marked morbidity in terms of continued pain, altered sensation, and poor cosmetic result as perceived by the patients as well as ongoing wound morbidity. The majority of patients (95 %) in this study suffered continued altered sensation within the affected limb postoperatively. However, this altered sensation was restricted to within the limits of the fasciotomy wound in 77 % of patients. Furthermore, altered sensation was more marked in those whose wounds were split skin grafted rather than those where the wound was directly closed. Continuing pain existed in 55 % of patients in the affected limbs. However, only 10 % of patients had pain that could be solely attributed to their fasciotomy wounds. Much of the perceived pain was attributable to stiff joints on either side of either the underlying fracture or the fasciotomy wound that were relatively immobile for long periods of time. No patient in this study developed subsequent contracture or required amputation. The fasciotomy wounds were a considerable source of continuing morbidity in that eczematous changes (40 %), pruritus (33 %), discoloration (30 %), and recurrent ulceration (13 %) were all found to be present [106].

Fasciotomy of Other Compartments

As previously discussed in both civilian and combat trauma [35, 53], the lower leg is by far and away the most likely location of CS requiring fasciotomy (68.5 and 51 %, respectively), followed by the forearm (14 and 22 %) and the thigh (~8.5 %). A detailed description of CS and the technique for fasciotomy of the forearm and thigh is beyond the scope of this chapter, but the highlights will be briefly covered.

Compartment Syndrome and Fasciotomy of the Forearm and Hand

Compartment syndrome of the forearm may be associated with fractures, crush or blast injury, burns, or vascular injury [107–110]. CS of the hand can occur from trauma but is more commonly associated with infiltration of intravenous fluids. As there are no sensory nerves in the hand compartments, physical findings do not include sensory abnormalities, and the pressure threshold is much less than in the legs (15–20 mmHg is indication for release). The classic fasciotomy of the forearm is performed though a curvilinear incision on the volar surface (to release the anterior or volar and the lateral compartments) which is extended to the hand to release the carpal tunnel (Fig. 4.20). The dorsal or posterior compartment of the forearm is released through a linear dorsal incision, with two additional incisions on the dorsum of the hand to release the hand (Fig. 4.20).

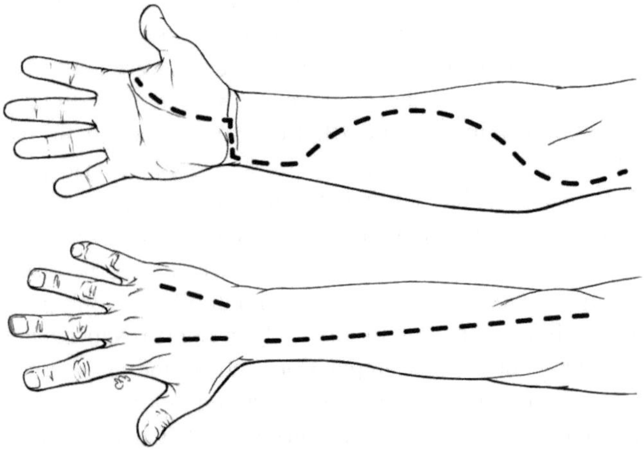

Fig. 4.20 The volar incision enables decompression of the anterior compartment of the forearm and is carried down onto the hand to release the carpal tunnel. The dorsal incision allows for decompression of the posterior compartment, and the two dorsal hand incisions enable release of the intraosseous compartments

Compartment Syndrome and Fasciotomy of the Thigh

Compartment syndrome is uncommon in the thigh because of the large volume that the thigh requires to cause an increase in interstitial pressure. In addition the compartments of the thigh blend anatomically with the hip allowing for extravasation of blood or fluid outside the compartment. Risk factors for thigh CS include: severe femoral fractures, severe blunt trauma/crush or blast injury to thigh, vascular injury, iliofemoral deep venous thrombosis, and the use of military antishock trousers or other external compression of the thigh [111–113]. The thigh contains three compartments – anterior, posterior, and medial. If CS of the thigh exists, a lateral incision with decompression of both the anterior and posterior compartments is often all that is needed, though on occasion with a severely swollen extremity a medial incision will be needed as well.

Compartment syndromes of the hand and foot are much less frequently encountered, and optimal outcomes are achieved with appropriate subspecialty input.

Summary

Compartment syndrome must be suspected in all polytrauma patients with extremity injury. It is essential that surgeons caring for these patients have an intimate knowledge of the pathophysiology, etiology, diagnostic evaluation, relevant anatomy, and the techniques for performing a proper fasciotomy. A high index of suspicion must be maintained (especially in patients with altered levels of consciousness), and early and aggressive fasciotomy will minimize the morbidity and mortality associated with failure to adequately treat compartment syndromes.

Acknowledgment The author is grateful to Ms. Elizabeth Weissbrod, MA, CFI, for her expert illustrations contained in this chapter.

References

1. Matsen FA. Compartment syndrome: a unified concept. Clin Orthop. 1975;113:8–14.
2. Mubarak SJ, Hargens AR, Owen CA, Garetto LP, Akeson WH. The wick catheter technique for the measurement of intramuscular pressure: a new research and clinical tool. J Bone Joint Surg. 1976;58A:1016–20.
3. Mubarak SJ, Owen CA. Double-incision fasciotomy of the leg for decompression in compartment syndromes. J Bone Joint Surg Am. 1977;59:184–7.
4. Bourne RB, Rorabeck CH. Compartment syndromes of the lower leg. Clin Orthop Relat Res. 1989;240:97–104.
5. Frink M, Klaus A-K, Kuther G, Probst C, Gosling T, Kobbe P, et al. Long term results of compartment syndrome of the lower limb in polytraumatised patients. Injury. 2007;38:607–13.

6. Kirk KL, Hayda R. Compartment syndrome and lower-limb fasciotomies in the combat environment. Foot Ankle Clin. 2010;15(1):41–61.
7. McGee DL, Dalsey WC. Compartment syndrome and amputations. Emerg Med Clin North Am. 1992;10:783–800.
8. Schreiber SN, Liebowitz MR, Berstein LH. Limb compression and renal impairment (crush syndrome) following narcotic overdose. J Bone Joint Surg. 1972;54A:1683.
9. Bowden REM, Gutman E. The fate of voluntary muscle after vascular injury in man. J Bone Joint Surg. 1949;31B:356–8.
10. Ashton H. Effect of inflatable plastic splints on blood flow. Br Med J. 1966;2:1427–30.
11. Kirby NG. Exercise ischemia in the fascial compartment of the soleus. J Bone Joint Surg. 1970;52B:738–40.
12. Cywes S, Louw JH. Phlegmasia cerulean dolens: successful treatment by relieving fasciotomy. Surgery. 1962;51:169–76.
13. Manson JW. Post-partum eclampsia complicated by the anterior tibial syndrome. Br Med J. 1964;2:1117–18.
14. Owen R, Tsimboukis B. Ischaemia complicating closed tibial and fibular shaft fractures. J Bone Joint Surg. 1967;49:268–75.
15. Sweeney HE, O'Brien GF. Bilateral anterior tibial syndrome in association with the nephrotic syndrome; report of a case. Arch Intern Med. 1965;116:487–90.
16. Weitz EM, Carson G. The anterior tibial compartment syndrome in a twenty month old infant: a complication of the use of a bow leg brace. Bull Hosp Joint Dis. 1969;30:16–20.
17. Beall S, Garner J, Oxley O. Anterolateral compartment syndrome related to drug induced bleeding. Am J Sports Med. 1983;11: 454–5.
18. Aerts P, DeBoeck H, Casteleyn PP, Opdecam P. Deep volar compartment syndrome of the forearm following minor crush injury. J Pediatr Orthop. 1989;9:69–71.
19. Aprahamian C, Gessert G, Bandyk OF, Sell L, Stiehl J, Olson DW. MAST associated compartment syndrome (MACS): a review. J Trauma. 1989;29:549–55.
20. Bass RR, Allison EJ, Reines HD, Yeager JC, Pryor Jr WH. Thigh compartment syndrome without lower extremity trauma following application of pneumatic antishock trouser. Ann Emerg Med. 1983;12:382–4.
21. Black KP, Schultz TK, Cheung NL. Compartment syndromes in athletes. Clin Sports Med. 1990;9:471–87.
22. Bogaerts Y, Lameire N, Ringoir S. The compartment syndrome: a serious complication of acute rhabdomyolysis. Clin Nephrol. 1982;17:206–11.
23. DeLee JC, Stiehl JB. Open tibia fracture with compartment syndrome. Clin Orthop. 1981;160:175–84.
24. Egan TO, Joyce SM. Acute compartment syndrome following a minor athletic injury. J Emerg Med. 1989;7:353–7.
25. Garfin SR, Mubarak SJ, Evans KL, Hargens AR, Akeson WH. Quantification of intracompartmental pressure and volume under plaster casts. J Bone Joint Surg. 1981;63:449–53.
26. Halpern AA, Nagel DA. Bilateral compartment syndrome associated with androgen therapy. Clin Orthop. 1977;128:243–6.
27. Hieb LD, Alexander H. Bilateral anterior and lateral compartment syndromes in a patient with sickle cell trait. J Bone Joint Surg. 1988;228:190–3.
28. Moscati R, Moore GP. Compartment syndrome with resultant amputation following interosseous infusion. Am J Emerg Med. 1990;8:470–1.
29. Peek RD, Haynes DW. Compartment syndrome as a complication of arthroscopy. Am J Sports Med. 1984;12:464–8.
30. Reedy PK, Kaye KW. Deep posterior compartmental syndrome: a serious complication of the lithotomy position. J Urol. 1984;132: 144–5.
31. Royle SG. Compartment syndrome following forearm fracture in children. Injury. 1990;21:73–6.
32. Stockley I, Harvey lA, Getty CJM. Acute volar compartment syndrome of the forearm secondary to fractures of the distal radius. Injury. 1986;19:101–4.
33. Rush RJ, Arrington E, Hsu J. Management of complex extremity injuries: tourniquets, compartment syndrome detection, fasciotomy, and amputation care. Surg Clin North Am. 2012;92:987–1007.
34. Matsen III FA, Krugmire Jr RB. Compartmental syndrome. Surg Gynecol Obstet. 1978;147:943–9.
35. Branco BC, Inaba K, Barmparas G, Schnüriger B, Lustenberger T, Talving P, et al. Incidence and predictors for the need for fasciotomy after extremity trauma: a 10-year review in a mature level I trauma centre. Injury. 2011;42:1157–63.
36. Rorabeck CH. The treatment of compartment syndromes of the leg. J Bone Joint Surg Br. 1984;66:93–7.
37. Janzing H, Broos P. Fasciotomies of the limbs: how to do it? Acta Chir Belg. 1998;98:187–91.
38. Gourgiotis S, Villias C, Germanos S, Foukas A, Ridolfini MP. Acute limb compartment syndrome: a review. J Surg Educ. 2007;64:178–86.
39. Taylor RM, Sullivan MP, Mehta S. Acute compartment syndrome: obtaining diagnosis, providing treatment, and minimizing medicolegal risk. Curr Rev Musculoskelet Med. 2012;5:206–13.
40. Feliciano D, Cruse P, Spjut-Patrinely V, Burch J, Mattox K. Fasciotomy after trauma to the extremities. Am J Surg. 1988;156: 533–6.
41. Ulmer T. The clinical diagnosis of compartment syndrome of the lower leg: are clinical findings predictive of the disorder? J Orthop Trauma. 2002;16:572–7.
42. Ellis H. Disabilities after tibial shaft fractures with special reference to Volkmann's ischemic contracture. J Bone Joint Surg. 1958;40B:190–7.
43. Horwitz T. Ischemic contracture of the lower extremity. Arch Surg. 1940;41:945–59.
44. Bhattacharyya T, Vrahas MS. The medical-legal aspects of compartment syndrome. J Bone Joint Surg. 2004;86-A:864–8.
45. Accreditation Council for Graduate Medical Education. http://www.acgme.org/acgmeweb/Portals/0/PDFs/GSNatData1011.pdf. Accessed 15 Dec 2012.
46. Accreditation Council for Graduate Medical Education. http://www.acgme.org/acgmeweb/Portals/0/PDFs/VSNatData1011.pdf. Accessed 15 Dec 2012.
47. Mars M, Hadley GP. Raised intracompartmental pressure and compartment syndromes. Injury. 1998;29:403–11.
48. von Volkmann R. Die ischamischen Muskellahmungen und-Kontrakturen. Zentralbl Chir. 1881;8:801–3.
49. Jepson PN. Ischemic contracture. Experimental study. Ann Surg. 1926;84:785–95.
50. McQueen MM, Christie J, Court-Brown CM. Acute compartment syndrome in tibial diaphyseal fractures. J Bone Joint Surg Br. 1996;78:95–8.
51. Mullet H, Al Abed K, Prasad CV, O'Sullivan M. Outcome of compartment syndrome following intramedullary nailing of tibial diaphyseal fractures. Injury. 2001;32:411–13.
52. Bernot M, Gupta R, Dobrasz J, Chance B, Heppenstall RB, Sapega A. The effect of antecedent ischemia on the tolerance of skeletal muscle to increased interstitial pressure. J Orthop Trauma. 1996;10:555–9.
53. Ritenour AE, Dorlac WC, Fang R, et al. Complications after fasciotomy revision and delayed compartment release in combat patients. J Trauma. 2008;64:S153–62.
54. Blick SS, Brumback RJ, Poka A, Burgess AR, Ebraheim NA. Compartment syndrome in open tibial fractures. J Bone Joint Surg Am. 1996;68:1348–53.
55. Abouezzi Z, Nassoura Z, Ivatury RR, Porter JM, Stahl WM. A critical reappraisal of indications for fasciotomy after extremity vascular trauma. Arch Surg. 1998;133:547–51.

56. Gonzalez RP, Scott W, Wright A, Phelan HA, Rodning CB. Anatomic location of penetrating lower extremity trauma predicts compartment syndrome development. Am J Surg. 2009;197:371–5.
57. Cargile JS, Hurt JL, Perdue GF. Acute trauma of the femoral artery vein. J Trauma. 1992;32:364–71.
58. Gulli B, Templeman D. Compartment syndrome of the lower extremity. Orthop Clin North Am. 1994;25:677–84.
59. Heemskerk J, Kitslaar P. Acute compartment syndrome of the lower leg: retrospective study on prevalence, technique, and outcome of fasciotomies. World J Surg. 2003;27(6):744–77.
60. Matsen III FA, Winquist RA, Krugmire Jr RB. Diagnosis and management of compartmental syndromes. J Bone Joint Surg Am. 1980;62A:286–91.
61. Hayden JW. Compartment syndromes: early recognition and treatment. Postgrad Med. 1983;74:191–202.
62. Kim JY, Buck II DW, Forte AJ, Subramanian VS, Birman MV, Schierle CF, et al. Risk factors for compartment syndrome in traumatic brachial artery injuries: an institutional experience in 139 patients. J Trauma. 2009;67:1339–44.
63. McQueen MM, Court-Brown CM. Compartment monitoring in tibial fractures. The pressure threshold for decompression. J Bone Joint Surg Br. 1996;78:99–104.
64. Mubarak SJ, Owen CA, Hargens AR, Garetto LP, Akeson WH. Acute compartment syndromes: diagnosis and treatment with the aid of the wick catheter. J Bone Joint Surg Br. 1978;60:1091–5.
65. Rorabeck CH, Macnab I. Anterior tibial compartment syndrome complicating fractures of the shaft of the tibia. J Bone Joint Surg Am. 1976;58:549–50.
66. Allen MJ, Stirling AJ, Cranshaw CV, et al. Intracompartmental pressure monitoring of leg injuries. J Bone Joint Surg Br. 1985; 67:53–7.
67. Gibson JJ, Barnes MR, Allen MJ, Chan RN. Weakness of foot dorsiflexion and changes in compartment pressures after tibial osteotomy. J Bone Joint Surg Br. 1986;62:471–5.
68. McQueen MM, Christie J, Court-Brown CM. Compartment pressures after intramedullary nailing of the tibia. J Bone Joint Surg Br. 1990;72:395–7.
69. Triffitt PD, Konig D, Harper WM, Barnes MR, Allen MJ, Gregg PJ. Compartment pressures after closed tibial shaft fracture. J Bone Joint Surg Br. 1992;74:195–8.
70. Heckman MM, Whitesides Jr TE, Grewe SR, Rooks MD. Compartment pressure in association with closed tibial fractures: the relationship between tissue pressure, compartment, and the distance from the site of the fracture. J Bone Joint Surg Am. 1994;76:1285–92.
71. Ovre S, Hvaal K, Holm I, Strømsøe K, Nordsletten L, Skjedal S. Compartment pressure in nailed tibial fractures: a threshold of 30 mmHg for decompression gives 29 % fasciotomies. Arch Orthop Trauma Surg. 1998;118:29–31.
72. Ouellette EA. Compartment syndromes in obtunded patients. Hand Clin. 1998;14:431–50.
73. Whitesides TE, Haney TC, Morimoto K, Harada H. Tissue pressure measurements as a determinant for the need for fasciotomy. Clin Orthop. 1975;113:43–51.
74. Whitesides Jr TE, Haney TC, Harada H, Holmes HE, Morimoto K. A simple method for tissue pressure determination. Arch Surg. 1975;110:1311–13.
75. Rorabeck CH, Castle GSP, Hardie R, Logan J. Compartmental pressure measurements: an experimental investigation using the slit catheter. J Trauma. 1981;21:446–9.
76. Odland RM, Schmidt AH. Compartment syndrome ultrafiltration catheters: report of a clinical pilot study of a novel method for managing patients at risk of compartment syndrome. J Orthop Trauma. 2011;25:358–65.
77. Seiler III JG, Womack S, De L'Aune WR, Whitesides TE, Hutton WC. Intracompartmental pressure measurements in the normal forearm. J Orthop Trauma. 1993;7:414–16.
78. Arbabi S, Brundage SI, Gentilello LM. Near-infrared spectroscopy: a potential method for continuous, transcutaneous monitoring for compartmental syndrome in critically injured patients. J Trauma. 1999;47:829–33.
79. Gentilello LM, Sanzone A, Wang L, Liu PY, Robinson L. Near-infrared spectroscopy versus compartment pressure for the diagnosis of lower extremity compartmental syndrome using electromyography-determined measurements of neuromuscular function. J Trauma. 2001;51:1–8.
80. Giannotti G, Cohn SM, Brown M, Varela JE, McKenney WG, Wiseberg JA. Utility of near-infrared spectroscopy in the diagnosis of lower extremity compartment syndrome. J Trauma. 2000;48:396–9.
81. Abraham P, Leftheriotis G, Saumet JL. Laser Doppler flowmetry in the diagnosis of chronic compartment syndrome. J Bone Joint Surg Br. 1998;80:365–9.
82. Jerosch J, Geske B, Sons HU, Winkelmann W. The value of sonography in assessing intracompartmental pressure in the anterior tibial compartment. Ultraschall Med. 1989;10:206–10.
83. Lynch JE, Heyman JS, Hargens AR. Ultrasonic device for the noninvasive diagnosis of compartment syndrome. Physiol Meas. 2004;25:N1–9.
84. Wiemann JM, Ueno T, Leek BT, Yost WT, Schwartz AK, Hargens AR. Noninvasive measurements of intramuscular pressure using pulsed phase-locked loop ultrasound for detecting compartment syndromes: a preliminary report. J Orthop Trauma. 2006;20:458–63.
85. Rominger M, Lukosch C, Bachmann G. Compartment syndrome: value of MR imaging. Radiology. 1995;197:296.
86. Rominger MB, Lukosch CJ, Bachmann GF. MR imaging of compartment syndrome of the lower leg: a case control study. Eur Radiol. 2004;14:1432–9.
87. Arokoski JP, Surakka J, Ojala T, Kolari P, Jurvelin JS. Feasibility of the use of a novel soft tissue stiffness meter. Physiol Meas. 2005;26:215–28.
88. Steinberg BD, Gelberman RH. Evaluation of limb compartment with suspected increased interstitial pressure: a noninvasive method for determining quantitative hardness. Clin Orthop Relat Res. 1994;300:248–53.
89. Dellon AL, Schneider RJ, Burke R. Effect of acute compartmental pressure change on response to vibratory stimuli in primates. Plast Reconstr Surg. 1983;72:208–16.
90. Phillips JH, Mackinnon SE, Beatty SE, Dellon AL, O'Brien JP. Vibratory sensory testing in acute compartment syndromes: a clinical and experimental study. Plast Reconstr Surg. 1987;79:796–801.
91. Edwards PD, Miles KA, Qwens SJ, Kemp PM, Jenner JR. A new noninvasive test for the detection of compartment syndromes. Nucl Med Commun. 1999;20:215–18.
92. Shadgan B, Menon M, O'Brien PJ, Reid WD. Diagnostic techniques in acute compartment syndrome of the leg. J Orthop Trauma. 2008;22:581–7.
93. De Bakey ME, Simeone FA. Battle injuries of the arteries in World War II. An analysis of 2,471 cases. Ann Surg. 1946;123:534–79.
94. Kelly RP, Whitesides Jr RE. Transfibular route for fasciotomy of the leg. In: Proceedings of the American Academy of Orthopaedic Surgeons. J Bone and Joint Surg. 1967;49-A:1022–3.
95. Singh N, Bluman E, Starnes B, Andersen C. Delayed primary closure for decompressive leg fasciotomy wounds. Am Surg. 2008;74:217–20.
96. Berman SS, Schilling JD, McIntyre KE, Hunter GC, Bernhard VM. Shoelace technique for delayed primary closure of fasciotomies. Am J Surg. 1994;167:435–6.

97. Zorilla P, Marin A, Gómez LA, Salido JA. Shoelace technique for gradual closure of fasciotomy wounds. J Trauma. 2005;59: 1515–17.
98. Janzing HMJ, Broos PLO. Dermatotraction: an effective technique for the closure of fasciotomy wounds: a preliminary report of fifteen patients. J Orthop Trauma. 2001;15:438–41.
99. Chiverton N, Redden JF. A new technique for delayed primary closure of fasciotomy wounds. Injury. 2000;31:21–4.
100. Zannis J, Angobaldo J, Marks M, DeFranzo A, David L, Molnar J, et al. Comparison of fasciotomy wound closures using traditional dressing changes and the vacuum-assisted closure device. Ann Plast Surg. 2009;62:407–9.
101. Dedmond BT, Kortesis B, Punger K, Simpson J, Argenta J, Kulp B, et al. The use of Negative-Pressure Wound Therapy (NPWT) in the temporary treatment of soft-tissue injuries associated with high-energy open tibial shaft fractures. J Orthop Trauma. 2007; 21:11–7.
102. Finkelstein JA, Hunter GA, Hu RW. Lower limb compartment syndrome: course after delayed fasciotomy. J Trauma. 1996;40:342–4.
103. Williams AB, Luchette FA, Papaconstantinou HT, Lim E, Hurst JM, Johannigman JA, Davis Jr K. The effect of early versus late fasciotomy in the management of extremity trauma. Surgery. 1997;122:861–6.
104. Rush DS, Frame SB, Bell RM, Berg EE, Kerstein MD, Haynes JL. Does open fasciotomy contribute to morbidity and mortality after acute lower extremity ischemia and revascularization. J Vasc Surg. 1989;10:343–50.
105. Jensen SL, Sandermann J. Compartment syndrome and fasciotomy in vascular surgery. A review of 57 cases. Eur J Vasc Endovasc Surg. 1997;13:48–53.
106. Fitzgerald A, Gaston P, Wilson Y, Quaba A, McQueen M. Long-term sequelae of fasciotomy wounds. Br J Plast Surg. 2000;53(8):690–3.
107. Fröber R, Linss W. Anatomic bases of the forearm compartment syndrome. Surg Radiol Anat. 1994;16:341–7.
108. Botte M, Gelberman R. Acute compartment syndrome of the forearm. Hand Clin. 1998;14:391–403.
109. Dente CJ, Feliciano DV, Rozycki GS, Cava RA, Ingram WL, Salomone JP, et al. A review of upper extremity fasciotomies in a level I trauma center. Am Surg. 2004;70:1088–93.
110. Kalyani BS, Fisher BE, Roberts CS, Giannoudis PV. Compartment syndrome of the forearm: a systematic review. J Hand Surg Am. 2011;36:535–43.
111. Schwartz JJ, Brumback R, Lakatos R, Poka A, Bathon G, Burgess A. Acute compartment syndrome of the thigh. J Bone Joint Surg Am. 1998;71:392–400.
112. Mithöfer K, Lhowe D, Vrahas M, Altman DT, Altman GT. Clinical spectrum of acute compartment syndrome of the thigh and its relation to associated injuries. Clin Orthop Relat Res. 2004;425:223–9.
113. Ojike N, Roberts C, Giannoudis P. Compartment syndrome of the thigh: a systematic review. Injury. 2010;41:133–6.

Diabetic Foot Infection

5

Richard F. Neville, Afsoon D. Roberts, and Gary L. Simon

Introduction

Diabetes mellitus represents a major risk factor for the development of foot infections. In patients with diabetes, foot infections rank among the most common infectious complications requiring hospitalization and are a frequent cause of lower extremity amputation [1]. A study of 1,666 diabetic patients reported a 50-fold increase in the risk of hospitalization and a 150-fold increase in the risk of amputation in patients who developed foot infections [2]. Diabetic foot infections are soft-tissue infections with approximately one fifth involving osteomyelitis proven by bone culture. Infected diabetic foot wounds precede two-thirds of lower extremity amputations, and diabetics have at least a tenfold greater risk of being hospitalized for soft-tissue and bone infections of the foot compared to individuals without diabetes.

Risk Factors

Neuropathy, ischemia, and an abnormal immune response form a triad of underlying risk factors that contribute to diabetic foot infections. Diabetic neuropathy encompassing sensory, motor, and autonomic nerves causes a series of structural changes that predispose the diabetic foot to ulceration and infection [3]. Sensory neuropathy blunts the response of small pain and temperature fibers allowing minor injuries to go unnoticed. In the desensitized diabetic foot, a small traumatic injury or pressure point can progress to a deep ulcer without warning symptoms. Motor neuropathy alters the tone of leg and intrinsic foot muscles which leads to progressive changes in the architecture of the foot and the emergence of new pressure points [4]. Autonomic neuropathy decreases sweat and oil gland production creating dry, brittle skin which is susceptible to ulceration and bacterial invasion.

Ischemia, the second part of the risk factor triad, compromises healing by restricting the supply of oxygen, immune cells, and antibiotics to the site of injury or infection. In the past, diabetic foot ischemia was erroneously ascribed to occlusion of the arterioles, and the notion of "small vessel disease" discouraged attempts at revascularization in favor of primary amputation. More recent evidence shows that macrovascular, not microvascular, occlusive disease causes ischemia in diabetic patients. The most common disease pattern in diabetes involves occlusive lesions of the tibial and peroneal arteries with relative sparing of the pedal arteries and arterioles which remain patent. Successful surgical bypasses using distal tibial and pedal artery targets prove that limb loss is not a foregone conclusion in diabetic patients with ischemia. Although microcirculatory dysfunction is present in the diabetic foot, it impairs healing via mechanisms other than occlusive disease. Neuropathy decreases the microcirculation by shunting blood away from the tissues through arteriovenous connections, while basement membrane thickening in the arterioles and capillaries impedes leukocyte migration.

Immune dysfunction increases the risk of diabetic foot infections especially in patients with high serum glucose concentrations. Hyperglycemia negatively affects nearly every component of the immune system and wound healing. Poor adherence and impaired chemotaxis decrease the number of neutrophils and macrophages migrating to the site of infection [5]. Immune cells that do migrate suffer from interruptions in intracellular signaling necessary for bactericidal and phagocytic activity. When serum glucose exceeds 200 mg/dl, glycosylation increases collagenase activity which impairs wound healing by reducing the collagen content at the site of tissue injury. Tight blood glucose control reduces morbidity

R.F. Neville, MD (✉)
Division of Vascular Surgery, The George Washington University MFA, 2150 Pennsylvania Avenue, 6B-407, Washington, DC 20037, USA
e-mail: rneville@mfa.gwu.edu

A.D. Roberts, MD • G.L. Simon, MD, PhD
Division of Infectious Diseases, The George Washington University MFA, Washington, DC, USA

V. Gahtan and M.J. Costanza (eds.), *Essentials of Vascular Surgery for the General Surgeon*,
DOI 10.1007/978-1-4939-1326-8_5,

and mortality and plays an important role in the management of diabetic foot infections [6].

The overall pathophysiology of the diabetic foot involves neuropathy, ischemia, and immune dysfunction which conspire to dismantle several lines of defense against infection. Diabetic patients often fail to mount a normal hyperemic and vasodilatory response to an injury or ulcer, and this blunted neuroinflammatory reaction allows infections to go undetected. Unrecognized and untreated diabetic foot infections progressively spread to deeper layers ultimately resulting in limb-threatening abscesses or contiguous osteomyelitis.

Physical Exam

An accurate physical exam requires knowledge of the unique manifestations of neuropathy, ischemia, and infection that occur in the diabetic foot. Progressive denervation from neuropathy alters the physical appearance and musculoskeletal architecture of the foot. Wasting of the intrinsic foot muscles allows the flexor muscles to draw up the toes into a clawed position creating pressure points on the tips of the toes and over the plantar aspect of the metatarsal heads. Charcot foot represents an advanced form of degenerative arthropathy characterized by complete loss of the foot architecture including arch collapse and rocker bottom deformity (Fig. 5.1). Autonomic neuropathy creates dry, brittle skin due to the loss of sweating and oil secretion, while thick calluses prone to ulceration accumulate over pressure points and weight-bearing areas. Although a pale, cool foot suggests underlying ischemia, warmth and hyperemia do not always indicate adequate arterial perfusion. A warm, pink foot may result from inappropriate arteriovenous shunting due to neuropathy or an acute fracture in a patient with Charcot foot. Likewise, physical signs can be misleading in a diabetic foot infection. Localized inflammatory signs of infection including erythema, rubor, cellulitis, and tenderness may be subtle or completely absent. A thorough search for infection must include careful palpation of the foot for areas of tenderness or fluctulance overlying an undrained abscess. Superficial eschars should be unroofed, and all ulcers should be inspected to search for deep space infections. Systemic signs of infection such as fever, tachycardia, and leukocytosis are not reliable in diabetic patients. Unexplained hyperglycemia may be the only indication of an advanced, underlying infection.

Classification

The International Working Group on the Diabetic Foot (IWGDF) and the Infectious Disease Society of America (IDSA) outlined clinical criteria for diagnosing and classifying the severity of diabetic foot infections [7, 8]. This classification can serve as a guide for the type treatment, duration of therapy, and outcome predictions. Grade 1 wounds lack purulence or any manifestation of inflammation and are considered uninfected. Grade 2 indicates the presence of two or more manifestations of inflammation such as purulence, erythema, pain, warmth, or induration. At this severity level cellulitis does not extend beyond 2 cm around any ulcer site, inflammation is limited to skin or superficial subcutaneous tissues, and there is no associated systemic illness. Grade 3 infections occur in systemically and metabolically stable patients who have cellulitis that extends more than 2 cm around any ulcer site, lymphangitic streaking, or infection that spreads below the superficial fascia. Other features of a Grade 3 infection include deep-tissue abscesses, gangrene, or involvement of the muscle, tendon, joint, or bone. Finally, severe or Grade 4 infections are those accompanied by systemic toxicity or metabolic instability such as fever, hypotension, tachycardia, confusion, leukocytosis, acidosis, hyperglycemia, and azotemia.

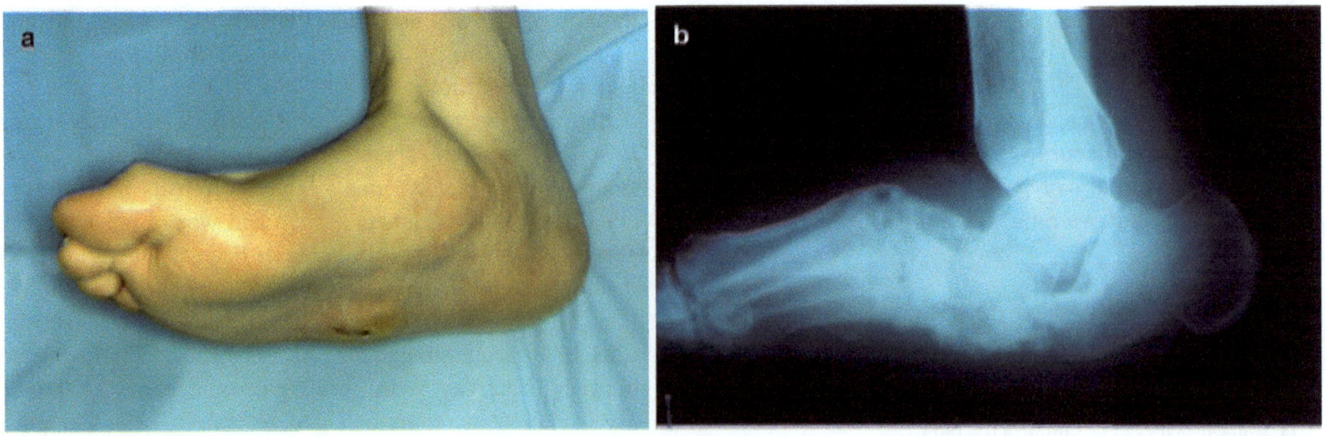

Fig. 5.1 (**a**) Charcot foot demonstrating characteristic loss of the plantar arch with a "rocker bottom" deformity. (**b**) Radiographic image of Charcot foot demonstrating bone destruction and loss of the normal architecture of the foot

A prospective study validated this classification system by following 199 infections: 48 % classified as mild, 34 % moderate, and 18 % severe [9]. The study reported a statistically significant correlation between the defined severity of infection and the risk of amputation, anatomic level of amputation, and need for hospitalization. Patients with mild infections are unlikely to develop osteomyelitis and do not require hospitalization or amputations, whereas those with more severe disease warrant aggressive medical and surgical care. The accuracy of clinical assessment decreases in patients with neuropathy, ischemia, and immune dysfunction. This triad of complications can diminish the neuroinflammatory response to infection in patients with diabetes masking the classic physical findings of inflammation and infection.

Diagnosis of Diabetic Foot Infection

Several factors influence the microbiology of diabetic foot infections including the prior use of antibiotics and whether the infection is acute versus chronic and superficial versus deep [3]. Drawing a line between infection and bacterial colonization helps define the potentially complex and polymicrobial microbiology. The mere presence of organisms in a wound does not translate into a clinical infection as all chronic wounds and ulcers open to skin commensals become colonized with multitudes of bacteria. Infection develops as bacteria multiply within the wound, overwhelming host defenses as a result of critical numbers, microbial enzymes, or impaired host immunity. Although a colony count of 10^5 bacteria per gram of tissue often defines infection, this number may vary depending on the organism [10]. Virulent bacteria such as beta-hemolytic streptococci have enzymes that promote tissue invasion leading to rapidly progressive infections despite quantitatively low bacterial burdens. This clinical scenario demonstrates that infection depends on the type of organism and its characteristics in addition to the absolute number of bacteria present.

The technique used to collect wound cultures plays an important role in defining the microbial etiology of a diabetic foot infection. Culturing the surface of a purulent ulcer should be avoided since it will reflect wound colonization and fail to isolate the causative bacteria. Recommended modalities for obtaining cultures include: scraping or curetting the wound base after debridement, aspirating an abscess, or tissue biopsy. A properly obtained wound culture specimen ensures appropriate antibiotic coverage for the organisms involved based on their susceptibility.

The diagnosis of diabetic wound infections cannot rely on wound culture results alone; it also requires clinical findings consistent with infection. Sotto et al. examined the importance of pathogens versus colonizers in patients with foot ulcers not on prior antibiotics who were growing *Staphylococcus aureus* as the sole organism from wound cultures [11]. Using the IDSA classification system and oligonucleotide arrays to detect genes encoding various virulence factors and antibiotic resistance profiles, they found that both resistance and virulence factors were more likely to be present in infected versus colonized wounds. Virulence factors were present in only 9 % of Grade 1 (uninfected) patients versus 98 % of those with infected ulcers. Jeandrot examined inflammatory markers, serum procalcitonin, and C-reactive protein as a means of distinguishing mildly infected from noninfected diabetic foot ulcers [12]. C-reactive protein had the highest sensitivity and specificity for distinguishing Grade 2 (mild) from Grade 1 (uninfected) ulcers. Combining C-reactive protein and procalcitonin levels increased the accuracy of predicting infection.

Although it can be challenging, diagnosing osteomyelitis is essential to ensure appropriate treatment. The presence or absence of osteomyelitis often determines the duration of antibiotic therapy and the need for surgical debridement. A bone biopsy provides the most reliable test for osteomyelitis. The diagnosis of osteomyelitis can be made by isolating bacteria from an aseptically obtained bone sample which has histologic features of infection (inflammatory cells, necrosis). Stopping antibiotics 2 weeks in advance of the biopsy can decrease the probability of a false-negative result. A CT or fluoroscopically guided percutaneous bone biopsy has proven to be a safe and accurate alternative to a surgical biopsy. The presence of ischemia increases the risk of non-healing making an invasive procedure such as a bone biopsy less appealing. If a bone biopsy is not available or contraindicated by ischemia, the diagnosis of osteomyelitis depends on surrogate markers including clinical, laboratory, and imaging findings.

Nonhealing ulcers over bony prominences should raise the suspicion of underlying osteomyelitis. Other clinical findings associated with osteomyelitis include exposed bone and large ulcers. In the appropriate clinical setting, probing to bone can help make the diagnosis at the bedside. The technique involves gently inserting a sterile, blunt metal probe through the ulcer. Striking bone increases the likelihood of osteomyelitis if the prevalence of bone infection is high (>60 %). If the prevalence of bone infection is low (<20 %), failure to probe to bone can eliminate the diagnosis of osteomyelitis.

Osteomyelitis usually causes the erythrocyte sedimentation rate (ESR) to rise. An ESR greater than 70 increases the likelihood of osteomyelitis, while a low ESR can help rule out the diagnosis. Other laboratory values such as C-reactive protein, procalcitonin, and blood leukocyte count have less accumulated evidence linking them to osteomyelitis.

Radiologic evaluation for osteomyelitis usually begins with plain films of the foot in two or three views. Table 5.1

Table 5.1 Plain X-ray findings suggesting osteomyelitis

Periosteal reaction or elevation
Loss of cortex with bony erosion
Focal loss of trabecular pattern or marrow radiolucency
New bone formation
Bone sclerosis with or without erosion
Sequestrum: devitalized bone with radiodense appearance that has become separated from normal bone
Involucrum: a layer of new bone growth outside existing bone resulting from the stripping off of the periosteum and new bone growing from the periosteum
Cloacae: opening in involucrum or cortex through which sequestra or granulation tissue may be discharged

lists X-ray findings consistent with osteomyelitis. The sensitivity of plain X-rays ranges from 28 to 75 % and seems to depend on the timing of the imaging. Long-standing cases are more likely to show radiographic signs of osteomyelitis compared to cases that have only been present for 1 or 2 weeks. Overall the presence or absence of plain X-ray findings can neither confirm nor eliminate the diagnosis of osteomyelitis. Plain X-rays may be more predictive when they document sequential changes over time (greater than 2-week interval between films).

Magnetic resonance imaging relies on the presence of marrow edema to provide a faster and potentially more accurate diagnosis of osteomyelitis. Unfortunately, marrow edema is not specific to infection and may be seen with other conditions including gout and neuropathic osteoarthropathy such as Charcot foot which can complicate diabetes mellitus. Distinguishing Charcot arthropathy from infection can be difficult, and this may explain why some MRI studies have reported a specificity of only 60 % [13].

Nuclear medicine offers a variety of techniques for detecting osteomyelitis. Technetium radionuclide bone scans suggest osteomyelitis when increased blood pool activity and radionuclide intensity localizes to the bone. Although these exams are sensitive, the incidence of false-positive bone scans exceeds 50 % in many studies [14]. Combining technetium scans with indium^{111} white blood cell scans may improve diagnostic accuracy [15]. Recent reports using ^{18}F-fluorodeoxyglucose positron emission tomography as a means of differentiating soft-tissue infections from osteomyelitis have been promising, but larger studies are needed to evaluate this approach [16].

Microbiology of Diabetic Foot Infections

Aerobic gram-positive cocci colonize the skin and frequently cause acute infections. In acutely infected patients, commonly isolated pathogens include *Staphylococcus aureus* and beta-hemolytic streptococci (groups A, B, C, and G) [17]. In contrast, chronic wounds tend to be polymicrobial with a mixture of aerobic and anaerobic bacteria [17, 18]. The recovery of anaerobes requires appropriate methods of sampling, transportation, and processing of the tissue. Aerobic organisms frequently include gram-positive cocci, namely, staphylococci, streptococci, and enterococci. A wide variety of aerobic gram-negative bacilli can also be isolated from chronic diabetic foot infections including *Enterobacteriaceae (Escherichia coli), Proteus, Klebsiella,* and *Pseudomonas. Pseudomonas aeruginosa* is especially prominent in ulcers that are macerated, and anaerobic organisms (*Peptococcus, Peptostreptococcus, Clostridia, Fusobacterium, Bacteroides*) are often found in the setting of ischemia and gangrene [19].

Hospitalization and prolonged antibiotic therapy can alter the sensitivity profile of organisms. Antibiotic naïve patients tend to have wounds with predominantly gram-positive organisms, whereas patients previously treated with antibiotics have wounds harboring gram negatives with increased antibiotic resistance requiring broader and longer courses of therapy. Richards et al. studied 188 patients with diabetic foot infections and identified 45 individuals with multidrug-resistant organisms [20]. The risk factors for developing multidrug resistance were deep and recurrent ulcers, prior hospitalization, elevated hemoglobin A1C levels, and proliferative retinopathy. After multivariate analysis, only prior hospitalization and proliferative retinopathy remained as significant risk factors for multidrug-resistant organisms. Interestingly, the presence of multidrug-resistant organisms did not affect the time to wound healing.

Osteomyelitis in patients with diabetes usually results from the spread of a contiguous soft-tissue infection. As such, osteomyelitis and diabetic foot infections share a similar microbiologic spectrum. *Staphylococcus aureus* is the predominant organism with *Enterobacteriaceae* being more common than *Pseudomonas* species [21]. In addition to these traditional pathogens, impaired host defenses and necrotic soft tissue and bone may allow low virulence, colonizing organisms such as coagulase-negative staphylococci or *Corynebacterium* species to become pathogens [6].

Treatment of Diabetic Foot Infections

The treatment of diabetic infections depends on the severity and extent of infection. The current recommendations for treatment of diabetic foot infections are based on expert opinion and consensus rather than well-controlled clinical trials. Nevertheless, it is clear that comprehensive management of diabetic foot infections requires a multidisciplinary team approach. Ideally the team managing these complex infections should include surgeons, podiatrists, infectious disease specialists, endocrinologists, and radiologists.

The absence of well-controlled clinical trials and other factors have made it difficult to provide clear-cut recommendations regarding antimicrobial therapy. There is a lack of standardized definitions for infection, improvement, and cure especially when surgical intervention is included in the protocol. The heterogeneity of the patient population has made study design challenging. Patients vary widely with respect to arterial supply, duration of infection, and preexisting comorbidities. Crouzet et al. reviewed antibiotic regimens for diabetic foot infections to assess the quality of randomized trials conducted between 1999 and 2009. They found great heterogeneity with respect to study design, selection criteria, duration of therapy, and microbiological end points and concluded that further studies were needed to develop standardized outcome definitions and guidelines for therapy.

Since there are no standardized recommendations, treatment decisions for diabetic foot infection must rely on knowledge of the likely pathogens and the spectrum of antibiotics that can reliably provide coverage. Noninfected ulcerations of a diabetic foot do not require antibiotic treatment. An ulcer with a clean base and healthy granulation tissue that does not probe to bone, and has no evidence of erythema, edema, or other signs of inflammation, does not warrant antibiotic therapy. Chantelau et al. studied the effect of oral antibiotics on neuropathic diabetic foot ulcers and found no added benefit from antibiotic treatment as a supplement to standardized therapy of pressure relief and wound care [22].

Mild infections (IDSA classification Grade 2) are usually caused by aerobic gram-positive cocci, predominantly *Staphylococcus aureus*, and Group B streptococci [23]. Anaerobic organisms are rarely isolated in these patients. Therefore, mild skin and soft-tissue infections can be treated similarly to those in the nondiabetic patient population using antibiotics with activity against gram-positive organisms. Moderate to severe infections (IDSA classification Grade 3 and 4) are likely to be polymicrobial with a mixture of aerobic gram-positive cocci, aerobic gram-negative rods, and anaerobes. In this setting, antibiotics with a broader spectrum of antimicrobial activity are warranted. In one of the largest studies of moderate and severe diabetic foot infections, Lipsky and coworkers conducted a randomized, double-blinded, multicenter trial comparing ertapenem to piperacillin/tazobactam [24]. The clinical success rates for ertapanem and piperacillin/tazobactam were similar (94 % vs. 92 %). Interestingly, although ertapenem does not provide coverage for *Pseudomonas* or enterococci, the clinical response for patients from whom these organisms were isolated was similar. This result suggests that either these bacteria are not particularly pathogenic in this clinical situation or that their role in polymicrobial infections may be dependent upon the microbial milieu. These findings support the theory that providing coverage for most, if not all of the bacteria present, when combined with appropriate surgical intervention, may be adequate treatment for moderate to severe diabetic foot infections.

Antibiotic Options for Gram-Positive Coverage

Although enterococci and streptococci may be isolated from a diabetic foot infection, it is important to provide coverage for *Staphylococcus aureus* unless the absence of this organism can be confirmed. Semisynthetic penicillins such as nafcillin or oxacillin are excellent drugs for the treatment of methicillin-sensitive *Staphylococcus aureus* (MSSA). Although cefazolin can also be used, it may suffer from an inoculum effect that results in clinical failure despite apparent in vitro susceptibility. Vancomycin has emerged as the mainstay for empiric antimicrobial coverage in this setting because of the prevalence of methicillin-resistant *Staphylococcus aureus* (MRSA). Vancomycin also has activity against streptococci and most isolates of *Enterococcus faecalis*. Monitoring the serum concentration of vancomycin ensures that the level of drug falls within an optimal therapeutic window and provides a means for adjusting the dose in patients with renal insufficiency.

Linezolid is an oxazolidinone with activity against gram-positive organisms such as staphylococci (including both MSSA and MRSA isolates), streptococci, and enterococci including vancomycin-resistant isolates (VRE). Linezolid has 100 % bioavailability after oral administration. The drug has FDA indications for complicated skin and soft-tissue infections, including diabetic foot infections. Itani compared outcomes of patients with skin and soft-tissue infections receiving vancomycin versus linezolid [25]. Linezolid was associated with a shorter length of stay and duration of antibiotics. Another study compared oral linezolid to vancomycin on patients requiring surgical intervention for complicated skin infections due to MRSA [26]. Linezolid achieved a higher clinical cure rate compared to vancomycin which was associated with more treatment failures and amputations. Although linezolid does not have an FDA indication for osteomyelitis, it does penetrate the bone.

Daptomycin is a lipopeptide with bactericidal activity against gram-positive organisms including MRSA, MSSA, streptococci, enterococci, and VRE. Administered daily, the drug requires weight-based dosing and only comes in a parenteral formulation. Using a rat model of chronic osteomyelitis, Rouse found that parenteral daptomycin or vancomycin significantly decreased the number of bacteria in the bone surrounding the infection site [27]. Another study used microdialysis to investigate the ability of daptomycin to penetrate the soft tissue and bone in diabetic patients with foot infections [28]. They found that multiple administrations of daptomycin achieved a sufficient free concentration in adipose tissue and bone to eradicate gram-positive organisms in diabetic foot infections including those complicated by osteomyelitis.

Antibiotic Options for Polymicrobial Coverage

Tigecycline is a glycylcycline with a broad spectrum of antimicrobial activity covering gram-positive organisms such as staphylococci (including MRSA), streptococci, and enterococci (including VRE) that is used for the treatment of skin and soft-tissue infections as well as intra-abdominal infections. Tigecycline also covers a range of gram-negative organisms; however, it is not active against *Pseudomonas aeruginosa* or anaerobic microorganisms including *Bacteroides fragilis*. Based on its wide spectrum of activity, tigecycline has a potentially useful role in treating diabetic foot infections that warrant polymicrobial coverage. Tigecycline significantly reduced bacterial growth in a rat model of osteomyelitis in which bone infection was induced with intramedullary injections of MRSA [29].

Carbapenem antibiotics such as meropenem, imipenem, and doripenem have very broad-spectrum antimicrobial activity and can be used as single-agent therapy in the treatment of diabetic foot infections. These drugs have broad-spectrum activity against gram-positive, gram-negative, and anaerobic organisms; however, they do not have activity against MRSA. Ertapenem has a pharmacokinetic advantage over other carbapenems allowing once daily dosing; however, it has a narrower spectrum of activity than other members of the carbapenem group and does not have activity against *Pseudomonas aeruginosa*. The results of the SIDESTEP trial comparing piperacillin/tazobactam to ertapenem were already discussed above [24]. A recent case series studied outcomes in the empiric use of ertapenem in 12 cases of osteomyelitis treated for an average of 6 weeks with ertapenem [30]. The investigators reported resolution of clinical signs and symptoms in 50 % of the cases, a success rate similar to that found in retrospective studies of conservatively treated osteomyelitis. In another study, Boselli measured the bone and synovial tissue concentration following a 1 g infusion of ertapenem in 18 patients who were undergoing total hip replacement [31]. They found that the concentrations achieved in cancellous and cortical bone and synovial tissue exceeded the ertapenem MIC_{90} for at least 24 h for most aerobic organisms and 12–24 h for anaerobes.

Levofloxacin, ciprofloxacin, and ofloxacin are quinolone antibiotics that have broad-spectrum activity against gram-negative aerobic organisms. Their activity against gram-positive organisms is sporadic, and resistance for both MSSA and MRSA has been increasing. Newer-generation quinolones such as moxifloxacin have the added advantage of improved activity against gram-positive and anaerobic pathogens. Moxifloxacin has very high bioavailability after oral administration and does not require adjustment for patients with renal impairment. Several studies examined the use of quinolones in bone and joint infections including a recent review which confirmed the therapeutic efficacy of quinolones in the treatment of osteomyelitis [32].

There are numerous beta-lactam antibiotic options that can be used in the setting of diabetic foot infections, and a discussion of all possible options is beyond the scope of this review. Beta-lactam/beta-lactamase inhibitors such as piperacillin/tazobactam or ticarcillin-clavulanate offer activity against a broad range of organisms including gram-positive organisms (except MRSA and VRE) and gram-negative bacteria including *Pseudomonas* species and anaerobes.

Other antibiotics such as those in the cephalosporin class (e.g., cefepime or ceftazidime) do not provide adequate anaerobic coverage, but can be combined with other agents such as clindamycin or metronidazole which have excellent activity against anaerobic pathogens. Ceftobiprole, a fifth-generation extended-spectrum cephalosporin, is the first cephalosporin with activity against MRSA. It covers other aerobic gram-positive cocci except VRE, and its gram-negative coverage is similar to that of third-generation cephalosporins. Like other cephalosporins, ceftobiprole cannot be used against beta-lactamase-producing *Enterobacteriaceae*. Ceftobiprole exhibits activity against anaerobic gram-positive organisms and selective gram-negative anaerobes but does not cover *Bacteroides fragilis*. Noel et al. found that ceftobiprole was not inferior to vancomycin in a randomized, double-blind trial of ceftobiprole versus vancomycin for the treatment of complicated skin and skin structure infections caused by gram-positive bacteria [33].

Parenteral Versus Oral Antibiotic Therapy

Most mild and many moderate diabetic infections can be treated with oral regimens such as trimethoprim-sulfamethoxazole, clindamycin, or quinolones. In the case of moderate to severe infections, most clinicians favor parenteral therapy initially; however, the necessity of using parenteral therapy in all patients, even in those with more severe infections, may not be warranted. Linezolid, trimethoprim-sulfamethoxazole, and quinolones achieve comparable serum concentrations when given orally or parenterally. Although there is little well-controlled comparative data, it is likely that some patients can be successfully treated with oral instead of intravenous antibiotic therapy.

Duration of Antibiotic Therapy

The optimal duration of therapy for diabetic foot infections remains unclear and depends on several variables. The IDSA guidelines base the duration of therapy on the extent tissue necrosis and whether the necrotic tissue has been surgically debrided. The guidelines recommend a short course of therapy (1–2 weeks) for mild infections and 2–4 weeks for moderate to severe infections. The duration of therapy for osteomyelitis varies according to the viability of the bone. Viable bone with osteomyelitis requires 4–6 weeks of therapy, while necrotic bone should receive 3 or more months of therapy. Clearing infection from necrotic bone may be difficult regardless of antibiotic duration, and surgical debridement of all necrotic material with viable tissue/bone at the margin often provides the best opportunity for cure. After debridement, if histologic examination of tissue or bone at the proximal margin reveals no evidence of infection or inflammation, a short course of postoperative antibiotics is all that is necessary.

The use of inflammatory markers can help define the length of antibiotic therapy. Patients with persistent elevation of C-reactive protein or sedimentation rate are at increased risk for recurrence of infection. On the other hand, prompt normalization of these markers is encouraging and supports a shorter course of therapy.

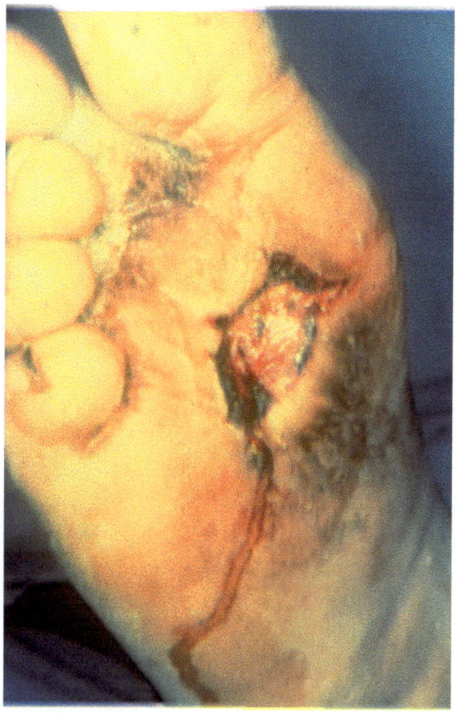

Fig. 5.2 Deep diabetic foot ulcer on the plantar aspect of the foot. The ulcer has characteristic findings of a severe infection including surrounding erythema and purulent drainage

Surgical Therapy

Surgery and antibiotic therapy serve as complementary treatment modalities in the management of moderate and severe diabetic foot infections. An infection that penetrates the superficial fascia of the foot mandates surgical exploration to evacuate the deep space abscess, excise necrotic tissue, and minimize the risk for further spread (Fig. 5.2). Prompt surgical intervention with aggressive debridement back to viable tissue offers the best opportunity for limb salvage and sustained function. Even patients with diabetes can heal long foot incisions and minor amputations if the infection is well controlled and arterial perfusion is adequate. In this clinical setting, limb salvage rates of 90 and 82 % can be achieved at 1 and 5 years, respectively [34].

Determining the need for surgical intervention requires a thorough search for infection and its sequelae as part of the diabetic foot evaluation. The physical exam should focus on "hidden" spaces (toe web spaces, under calluses or encrusted areas) and pressure points that can harbor infection. Often the presentation of an infected diabetic foot will be underwhelming, as up to two-thirds of diabetic patients do not have the traditional systemic signs of infection such as pain, chills, leukocytosis, and fever. Serious diabetic foot infections (fasciitis, osteomyelitis) may manifest first as an area of cellulitis or a sinus tract that belies the extent and severity of the underlying infection (Fig. 5.3). Ulcers should be unroofed of necrotic crusts or debris to assess the base. Purulence, foul odor, or surrounding erythema of an ulcer indicates infection.

Necrotizing soft-tissue infections occur more commonly in diabetics, and knowledge of the anatomy and muscular compartments of the foot can help anticipate the pattern of spread and achieve proximal control. The plantar aspect of the foot has four major plantar spaces: medial, central (deep and superficial), and lateral (Fig. 5.4). Plantar-based incisions provide the most direct access to infections in the forefoot and midfoot. The incision should start at the distal most extent of the infection and extend proximally until encountering healthy, viable tissue. In the setting of wet toe gangrene or a web space abscess, the plantar incision can be a direct continuation of the open-toe amputation. A longitudinally oriented plantar incision follows the natural anatomy of the flexor tendons and soft tissues and has the flexibility to extend proximally toward the medial malleolus or distally into each of the affected interspaces if necessary (Fig. 5.5).

Successful surgery for diabetic foot infections involves thoroughly exploring the wound and aggressively excising infected tissue. Careful wound exploration can identify foreign bodies, abscesses, or sinus tracts that could prolong the infection if they were not recognized and treated. Severe cases of necrotizing fasciitis often require opening adjacent fascial compartments and exploring any tissue planes that easily separate to gain control of the infection. Once adequate exposure has been achieved, debridement begins by removing all ischemic appearing and grossly necrotic soft tissue.

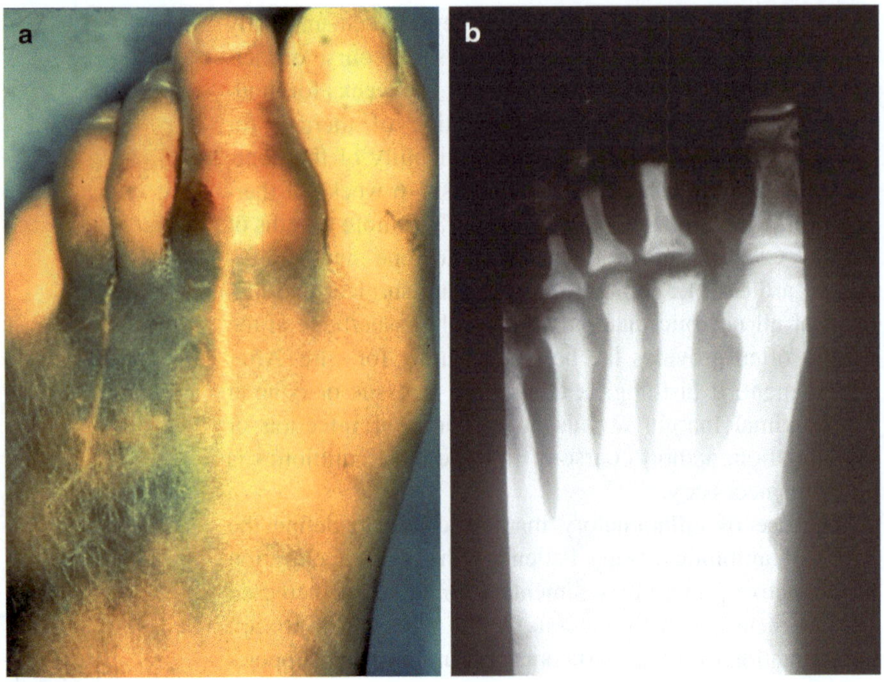

Fig. 5.3 (**a**) Severe diabetic foot infection manifesting as cellulitis and induration of the 2nd toe. (**b**) Radiographic image of the foot showing gas in the soft tissue consistent with advance infection

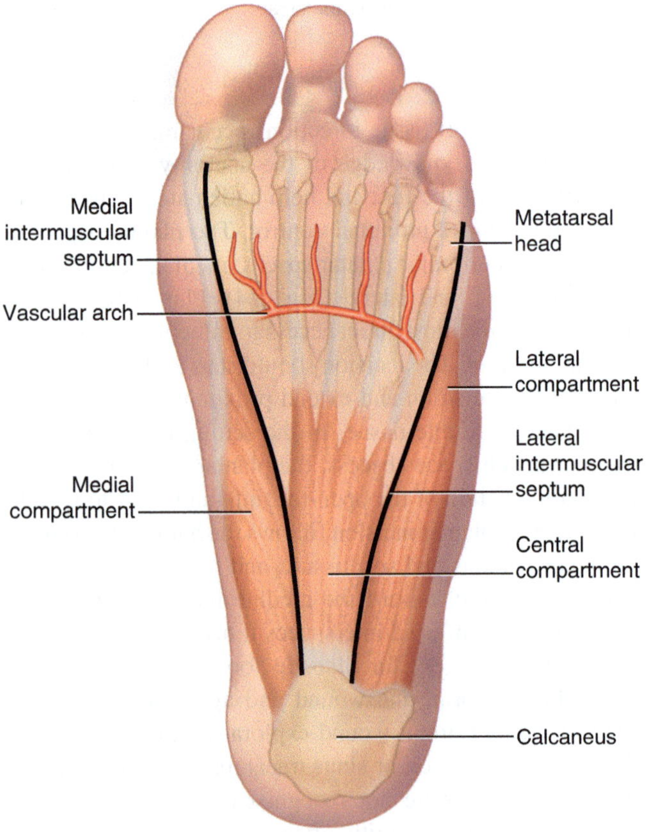

Fig. 5.4 The plantar spaces of the foot

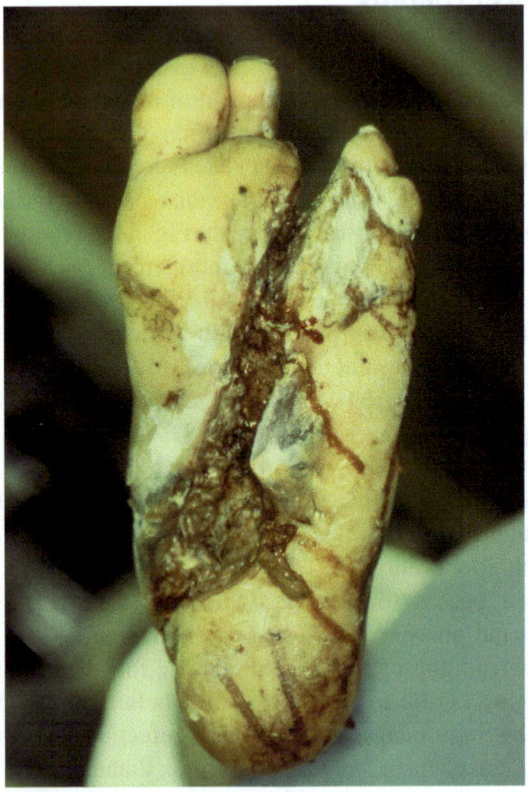

Fig. 5.5 Intraoperative image of a severe diabetic foot infection that has been exposed for debridement with a longitudinal plantar incision extending from the site of the 3rd toe amputation to the medial malleolus

Tendons and their sheaths should also be resected as they often act as pathways tracking purulent material into the more proximal foot. The severity of infection dictates the extent of debridement which should continue until viable tissue is encountered. Performing these cases without the use of a tourniquet makes viable tissue easier to recognize and may help avoid over debridement. Exposed bone within the debrided wound should be removed if possible to facilitate future soft-tissue coverage as necessary. Although it lacks supporting evidence, antibiotic irrigation appears to be a reasonable adjunct to surgery that may help speed the resolution of infection.

The surgical wound should then be packed open with saline-moistened gauze and allowed to heal by secondary intention. Dressing changes two or three times a day allow for regular wound inspection and further bedside debridement to remove residual necrotic material if necessary. Negative pressure wound therapy can simplify the care of postoperative diabetic foot infections by decreasing the frequency of dressing changes and accelerating the rate of wound closure. In a randomized trial comparing vacuum-assisted closure negative wound therapy (VAC) to standard moist gauze dressings, VAC therapy resulted in a higher proportion of healed wounds, faster healing rates, and fewer subsequent amputations [35]. VAC therapy achieved superior results at a lower average total cost mainly due to fewer dressing changes and a reduced need for further surgical debridement or amputation [36]. Adjunctive procedures to achieve wound closure including skin grafts and a variety of flaps (local, muscle, pedicle, and musculotedinous) usually require participation by a multidisciplinary team of specialists (Fig. 5.6).

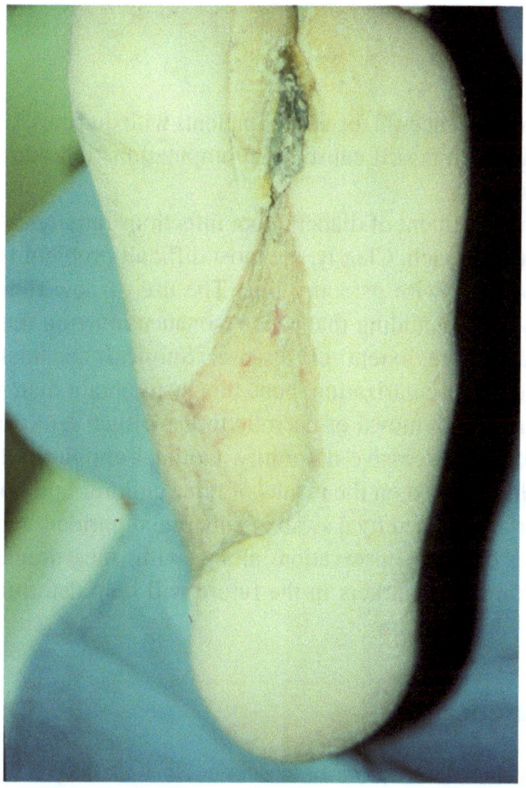

Fig. 5.6 The foot depicted in Fig. 5.5 after debridement, wound care, and skin grafting

A universal, widely accepted algorithm for the management of osteomyelitis does not exist. Treatment strategies range from antibiotics alone to complete resection of the infected bone to some combination of the two approaches. Important factors to consider in cases of osteomyelitis include the anatomic site of infection, the local vascular supply, the extent of soft-tissue and bone destruction, the presence of systemic signs of infection, and the patient's preferences. Using antibiotics alone to treat osteomyelitis may benefit from prolonged, parenteral medications at higher than the recommended doses; however, supporting evidence for this approach is scarce. Senneville conducted a small retrospective study on diabetic patients treated with antibiotics alone and no surgery for osteomyelitis of the toe or metatarsal head [37]. They reported that 32 of 50 patients (64 %) achieved remission of osteomyelitis as defined by the absence of any sign of infection at the initial or contiguous site. The mean duration of antibiotics was 11 ± 4 weeks, and bone culture-based antibiotic therapy was the only variable associated with remission. Conservative surgery that preserves as much of the normal foot architecture offers the best chance for maintaining a functional limb with limited disability. This strategy may translate into limited resection of a digit or metatarsal bone combined with 4–6 weeks of culture directed antibiotics postoperatively.

Regardless of antibiotic choices and surgical technique, eradication of infection and healing cannot be achieved without adequate perfusion. Although minor infections and superficial ulcers often heal with wound care alone, deep infections and significant tissue loss will not resolve in patients with arterial disease. In patients with advanced diabetic foot infections, absent palpable pedal pulses should prompt vascular imaging studies to confirm the diagnosis and plan for treatment. Revascularization options include endovascular interventions and surgical bypasses, the details of which are beyond the scope of this chapter. Active infection should be controlled with drainage, debridement, and antibiotics before proceeding with a surgical bypass. Controlling the infection and preparing for surgery should take only a few days. Putting off surgery in an attempt to sterilize the wound is not beneficial, and the delay in revascularization may lead to further necrosis rendering the foot unsalvageable.

Conclusion

Despite advances in the care of patients with diabetes, diabetic foot infections still cause more amputations than any other condition.

The treatment of diabetic foot infections requires a multimodal approach. Clearly, the most difficult problem is treating patients with osteomyelitis. The use of new radiologic techniques including magnetic resonance imaging may help to define the extent of disease. Surgical considerations include revascularization, bone biopsy to obtain material for culture, and removal of necrotic tissue if such removal does not lead to excessive deformity. Optimal antibiotic therapy should be based on the results of bone cultures and not from material obtained by a swab of superficial purulent material. Close clinical observation along with measurement of inflammatory markers in the future will help determine the duration of therapy.

References

1. Boulton AJ, Vileikyte L, Ragnarson-Tennvall G, Apelvist J. The global burden of diabetic foot disease. Lancet. 2005;366:1719–24.
2. Lavery LA, Armstrong DG, Wunderlich RP, Mohler MJ, Wendel CS, Lipsky BA. Risk factors for foot infections in individuals with diabetes. Diabetes Care. 2006;29:1288–93.
3. Kalish J, Hamdan A. Management of diabetic foot problems. J Vasc Surg. 2010;51(2):476–86.
4. Powlson AS, Coll AP. The treatment of diabetic foot infections. J Antimicrob Chemother. 2010;65 Suppl 3:iii3–9.
5. Joshi N, Caputo G, Weitecamp M, Karchmer A. Infections in patients with diabetes. N Engl J Med. 1999;34:1906–12.
6. Delmaire M, Maugendre D, Moreno M, Le Goff MC, Allanic H, Genetet B. Impaired leukocyte functions in diabetic patients. Diabet Med. 1997;14:29–34.
7. Lipsky BA, Berendt AR, Deery HG, Embil JW, Joseph WS, Karchmer AW, LeFrock JL, Lew DP, Mader JT, Norden C, Tan JS. Diagnosis and treatment of diabetic foot infections. Clin Infect Dis. 2004;39:885–910.
8. Lipsky BA. A report from the international consensus on diagnosing and treating the infected diabetic foot. Diabetes Metab Res Rev. 2004;20 Suppl 1:S68–77.
9. Lavery LA, Armstrong DG, Murdoch DP, Peters EJ, Lipsky BA. Validation of the Infectious Disease Society of America's diabetic foot infection classification system. Clin Infect Dis. 2007;44: 562–5.
10. Robson MC, Mannari RJ, Smith PD, Payne WG. Maintenance of wound bacterial balance. Am J Surg. 1999;178:399–402.
11. Sotto A, Richard JL, Jordan N, Combescure C, Bouziges N, Lavigne JP. Miniaturized oligonucleotide arrays. A new tool for discriminating colonization from infection due to Staphylococcus in diabetic foot ulcers. Diabetes Care. 2007;30:2051–6.
12. Jeandrot A, Richard JL, Combescure C, Jourdan N, Finge S, Rodier M, Corbeau P, Sotto A, Lavigne JP. Serum procalcitonin and C-reactive protein concentrations to distinguish mildly infected from non-infected diabetic foot ulcers: a pilot study. Diabetologia. 2008; 5:347–52.
13. Termaat MF, Raijmakers PG, Scholten HJ, Bakker FC, Patka P, Haarman HJ. The accuracy of diagnostic imaging for the assessment of chronic osteomyelitis: a systematic review and meta-analysis. J Bone Joint Surg Am. 2005;87:2464–71.
14. Keenan AM, Tindel NL, Alavi A. Diagnosis of pedal osteomyelitis in diabetic patients using current scintigraphic techniques. Arch Intern Med. 1989;149:2262–6.
15. Yuh WTC, Corson JD, Baraniewski HM, Rezai K, Shamma AR, Kathol MH, Sato Y, El-Khoury GY, Hawes DR, Platz CE, Cooper RR, Corry RJ. Osteomyelitis of the foot in diabetic patients: evaluation with plain film, 99m Tc-MDP bone scintigraphy and MR imaging. AJR Am J Roentgenol. 1989;152:795–800.
16. Kumar R, Basu S, Torigian D, Anand V, Zhuang H, Alavi A. Role of modern imaging techniques for diagnosis of infection in the era of ^{18}F-fluorodeoxyglucose positron emission tomography. Clin Microbiol Rev. 2008;21:209–24.
17. Abdulrazak A, Bitar ZI, Al-Shamali AA, Mobasher LA. Bacteriological study of diabetic foot infections. J Diabetes Complications. 2005;19(3):138–41.
18. Ramakant P, Verma AK, Misra R, Prasad KN, Chand G, Mishra A, Agarwal G, Agarwal A, Mishra SK. Changing microbiological profile of pathogenic bacteria in diabetic foot infections: time for a rethink of which empirical therapy to choose. Diabetologia. 2011; 54:58–64.
19. Miller A, Henry M. Update in diagnosis and treatment of diabetic foot infections. Phys Med Rehabil Clin N Am. 2009;20:611–25.
20. Richard JL, Sotto A, Jourdan N, Combescure C, Vannereau D, Rodier M, Lavigne JP. Risk factors and healing impact of multidrug resistant bacteria in diabetic foot ulcers. Diabetes Metab. 2008;34:363–9.
21. Lipsky BA. Osteomyelitis of the foot in the diabetic patient. Clin Infect Dis. 1997;25:1318–26.
22. Chantelau E, Tanudjaja T, Altenhofer F, Ersanli Z, Lacigova S, Metzger C. Antibiotic treatment for uncomplicated neuropathic foot ulcers in diabetes: a controlled trial. Diabet Med. 1996;13:156–9.
23. Kosinski MA, Joseph WS. Update on the treatment of diabetic foot infections. Clin Podiatr Med Surg. 2007;24:383–96.
24. Lipsky BA, Armstrong DG, Citron DM, Morgenstern DE, Abramson MA. Ertapenem versus piperacillin/tazobactam for diabetic foot infections (SIDESTEP): prospective, randomized, controlled, double-blinded, multicenter trial. Lancet. 2005;366: 1695–703.
25. Itani KM, Eigelt L, Li JZ. Linezolid reduces length of stay and duration of intravenous treatment compared with vancomycin for complicated skin and soft tissue infections due to suspected or proven methicilin-resistant Staphylococcus aureus (MRSA). Int J Antimicrob Agents. 2005;26(6):442–8.
26. Sharpe JN, Shively EH, Polk HC. Clinical and economic outcomes of oral linezolid versus intravenous vancomycin in the treatment of MRSA-complicated lower extremity skin and soft tissue infections caused by methicillin-resistant Staphylococcus aureus. Am J Surg. 2005;189(4):425–8.
27. Rouse MS, Piper KE, Jacobson M, Jacofsky DJ, Steckelberg JM, Patel R. Daptomycin treatment of Staphylococcal aureus experimental chronic osteomyelitis. J Antimicrob Chemother. 2006;57:301–5.
28. Traunmuller F, Schintler MV, Metzler J, Spendel S, Mauric O, Popovic M, Konz KH, Scharnagl E, Joukhadar C. Soft tissue and bone penetration abilities of daptomycin in diabetic patients with bacterial foot infections. J Antimicrob Chemother. 2010;65(6): 1252–7.
29. Kandemir O, Oztuna V, Colak M, Akdag A, Camdeviren H. Comparison of the efficacy of tigecycline and teicoplanin in an experimental methicillin resistant Staphylococcus aureus osteomyelitis model. J Chemother. 2008;20(1):53–7.

30. Goswami ND, Johnson MD, Chu VH. Ertapenem for treatment of osteomyelitis: a case series. BMC Res Notes. 2011;4:478.
31. Boselli E, Breith D, Djabarouti S, Bel JC, Saux MC, Allaouchiche B. Diffusion of ertapenem into bone and synovial tissues. J Antimicrob Chemother. 2007;60:893–6.
32. Rissing JP. Antimicrobial therapy for chronic osteomyelitis in adults: role of quinolones. Clin Infect Dis. 1997;25:1327–33.
33. Noel GJ, Strauss RS, Amsler K, Heep M, Pypstra R, Solomkin J. Results of a double-blind, randomized trial of ceftobiprole treatment of complicated skin and skin structure infections caused by gram-positive bacteria. Antimicrob Agents Chemother. 2008;52(1):37–44.
34. Lipsky BA. Medical treatment of diabetic foot infections. Clin Infect Dis. 2004;39 Suppl 2:S104–14.
35. Blume PA, Walters J, Payne W, Ayala J, Lantis J. Comparison of negative pressure wound therapy using vacuum-assisted closure with advanced moist wound therapy in the treatment of diabetic foot ulcers: a multicenter randomized controlled trial. Diabetes Care. 2008;31:631–6.
36. Armstrong DG, Lavery LA. Diabetic Foot Study Consortium. Negative pressure wound therapy after partial diabetic foot amputation: a multicentre, randomised controlled trial. Lancet. 2005;366: 1704–10.
37. Senneville E, Lombart A, Beltrand E, Valette M, Legout L, Cazaubiel M, Yazdanpanah Y, Fontaine P. Outcome of diabetic foot osteomyelitis treated non-surgically. Diabetes Care. 2008;31: 637–42.

Part III

Chronic Arterial Disease

PAD and Claudication

6

Hasan Haldun Dosluoglu and Purandath Lall

Peripheral arterial disease (PAD) refers to occlusive arterial lesions which decrease blood flow to the extremities. Although PAD rarely leads to limb-threatening ischemia, it can cause significant disability in the form of limited walking and decreased quality of life. In the majority of patients, atherosclerosis causes PAD; however, other conditions can result in arterial occlusive lesions. These rare non-atherosclerotic causes of PAD include thromboembolism, inflammatory diseases, aneurysms, traumatic injuries, adventitial cysts, popliteal artery entrapment syndrome, and congenital anomalies [1, 2]. PAD, defined by an ankle-brachial index (ABI) less than 0.90, affects over ten million people in the USA with an increasing prevalence among older adults. In the US National Health and Nutrition Examination Survey (NHANES) of an unselected population over age 40, the prevalence of PAD increased from 2.5 % at age 50–59 to 14.5 % in people over the age of 70 [2]. The ABI provides an accurate initial screening test for PAD that has the advantage of being noninvasive and objective. An ABI of 0.9 or less has a sensitivity of 95 % for detecting angiographically proven PAD in patients with claudication, while an ABI greater than 0.9 is 100 % specific for identifying individuals who do not have PAD [3]. The revised American College of Cardiology/American Heart Association (ACC/AHA) guidelines recommend a resting ABI to screen for PAD in all patients 65 and older (decreased from age 70 in the previous recommendations) and in patients age 50 and older who have a smoking history or diabetes [4]. Because PAD, coronary artery disease, and cerebrovascular disease all share the same risk factors, patients with PAD may harbor atherosclerotic disease in other arterial territories and body systems.

Intermittent claudication (IC) is the most common symptom of PAD and its prevalence increases with age from approximately 3 % at age 40 to 6 % at age 60 [5]. Patients with IC describe pain or weakness in the legs brought on by walking and relieved by rest. These symptoms result from transient exertional ischemia of the muscle groups involved in ambulation. Walking increases the workload and energy demands of lower extremity muscles, especially in the calf. Normally, blood flow increases to meet the demand for more energy. In patients with PAD, fixed arterial occlusions prevent an increase in blood flow, and this supply-demand mismatch creates relative ischemia in the muscle. The muscle switches over to inefficient anaerobic metabolism which results in decreased muscle performance, cramping, weakness, and pain. When the patient stops walking, the energy demands and blood supply equalize and the pain and weakness resolve.

Risk Factors for the Development of PAD

Smoking

Cigarette smoking induces endothelial cell injury and increases the risk of atherosclerosis, PAD, and IC fourfold compared to nonsmokers [6] (Fig. 6.1). Smoking has a stronger association with PAD than coronary artery disease (CAD), and the severity of PAD increases with the number of cigarettes smoked. A lifetime of smoking over 25 pack years increases the risk of PAD (HR 2.72), while smoking cessation significantly decreases the incidence of intermittent claudication, the primary symptom of PAD [7, 8]. Although the exact toxic components of cigarette smoke and the mechanisms involved in smoking-related cardiovascular dysfunction remain unclear, smoking increases inflammation, thrombosis, and oxidation of low-density lipoprotein (LDL) cholesterol. Even low-tar cigarettes and smokeless

H.H. Dosluoglu, MD, FACS (✉)
State University of New York at Buffalo, Buffalo, NY, USA

Department of Surgery, Division of Vascular Surgery,
VA Western New York Healthcare System, 3495 Bailey Avenue,
Buffalo, NY 14215, USA
e-mail: dosluoglu@yahoo.com; hdosluog@buffalo.edu

P. Lall, MBBS, FRCS(Ed), FACS
Department of Surgery, Division of Vascular Surgery, South West
Regional Health Authority, San Fernando, Trinidad and Tobago

V. Gahtan and M.J. Costanza (eds.), *Essentials of Vascular Surgery for the General Surgeon*,
DOI 10.1007/978-1-4939-1326-8_6,

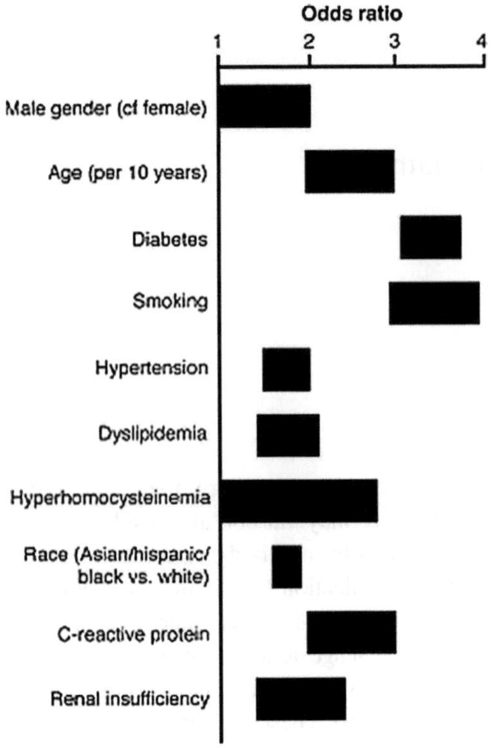

Fig. 6.1 Approximate range of odds ratios for risk factors for symptomatic peripheral arterial disease (Reproduced, with permission, from Elsevier, Norgren et al. [3])

tobacco increase the risk of cardiovascular events compared to nonsmokers [9].

Diabetes Mellitus (DM)

DM increases the risk of PAD three- to fourfold, doubles the risk of IC, and increases the risk of amputation several fold compared to nondiabetics [10]. The pathophysiology of diabetes includes abnormalities in the endothelium, vascular smooth muscle cells, and platelet as well as metabolic abnormalities such as hyperglycemia, increased free fatty acids, and insulin resistance [11]. Increased hemoglobin A1c (HbA1c) levels reflect chronic hyperglycemia and poorly controlled diabetes. Every 1 % increase in HbA1c level increases the risk of PAD by 26 % [3, 12].

Hypertension

Elevated blood pressure increases the risk of PAD twofold to threefold [13]. Approximately 2–5 % of patients presenting with hypertension have intermittent claudication and the prevalence increases with age. Conversely, an estimated 35–55 % of patients with PAD require treatment for hypertension [14]. Although the exact mechanism remains undefined, recent studies suggest that hypertension facilitates the development and progression of atherosclerosis by causing oxidative stress or injury to the endothelium which leads to inflammation of the arterial wall [15].

Dyslipidemia

Independent lipid risk factors for PAD include elevated levels of total cholesterol, LDL cholesterol, triglycerides, and lipoprotein(a). Extensive research suggests that the deposition, modification, and cellular uptake of cholesterol play an important role in the pathophysiology of atherosclerosis. Cholesterol injures the vascular endothelium which leads to inflammation and vessel remodeling. Vascular endothelium actively regulates vascular tone, lipid breakdown, thrombogenesis, inflammation, and vessel growth, all of which contribute to the development of atherosclerosis [16]. Elevated levels of high-density lipoprotein (HDL) cholesterol and apolipoprotein (a-1) appear to be lipid factors which protect against the development of PAD [3]. Several studies have shown that lowering cholesterol improves endothelial function, which may at least in part explain the early and substantial reduction in major cardiovascular events associated with lowering cholesterol.

Inflammatory Markers

Arterial inflammation appears to be present well before atherosclerosis is grossly visible. C-reactive protein (CRP) has been identified as a stable, easily detected marker for inflammation. Recent studies showed that higher CRP levels were positively associated with PAD, independent of other confounding risk factors including smoking, waist circumference, body mass index, blood pressure, glycosylated hemoglobin, and serum total cholesterol [17].

Hyperhomocysteinemia

An elevation in plasma homocysteine, an amino acid byproduct of the demethylation of methionine, is an independent risk factor for PAD. Hyperhomocysteinemia is present in about 30 % of young patients with PAD compared to only 1 % in the general population [3].

Chronic Kidney Disease (CKD)

Patients with CKD defined by an estimated glomerular filtration rate (eGFR) between 15 and 59 ml/min per 1.73 m^2 are at increased risk for developing PAD. After adjustment for cardiovascular disease risk factors, individuals with CKD had a 1.5-fold higher risk for developing PAD compared to those with normal kidney function [18].

Race

According to the NHANES (National Health and Nutrition Examination Survey) [2] and GENOA (Genetic Epidemiology Network of Arteriopathy) [19] studies, PAD is twice as common among the black population even when other risk factors such as elevated blood pressure, diabetes, and obesity are considered.,

Age and Gender

The risk of PAD increases in patients 50 years or older. Although PAD affects slightly more men than women, gender differences decrease in advanced age groups.

Diagnosis

The diagnosis of PAD usually relies on a problem-oriented history and a detailed physical examination of the vascular system. Objective, noninvasive vascular testing can then verify the clinical findings. One-third of patients with PAD present with intermittent claudication which consists of lower extremity aches, cramps, numbness, or fatigue that is induced by exercise and relieved by a short period of rest (usually less than 10 min). Although claudication symptoms usually affect the calf muscles, they may also occur in the thighs and buttocks depending on the location of the occlusive disease. Upper extremity muscle fatigue with exertion can occur in the setting of subclavian or axillary artery occlusive disease. In general, the claudication symptoms localize to one level distal to the occlusive lesion. Hence, calf claudication usually results from superficial femoral artery occlusion, while buttock and thigh claudication suggest more proximal disease of the aorta or iliac arteries.

Differentiating the symptoms of claudication from other causes of limb pain requires a thorough history including pain location and sites of radiation, relieving and aggravating factors, symptom duration, and reproducibility. A past medical history focusing on smoking and other risk factors for atherosclerosis should be obtained in addition to the social history to determine the functional and quality-of-life impact of claudication. Note that some patients with PAD do not complain of typical claudication because their severe medical comorbidities prevent them from walking enough to produce symptoms. Other uncommon vascular pathologies (e.g., popliteal artery entrapment) may also present with claudication in young patients who do not have atherosclerotic risk factors. Table 6.1 shows the differential diagnosis for intermittent claudication.

The physical examination should include a comprehensive vascular assessment because patients often have arterial disease affecting more than one area. Essential components of the exam include blood pressure measurements in both arms, a cardiac assessment, and a detailed abdominal examination to evaluate for an abdominal aortic aneurysm. Both lower extremities should be examined and compared to each other. Some less specific findings of PAD include pallor with elevation/dependent rubor (associated with critical limb ischemia), decreased hair growth, coolness in the most distal aspect of the extremity, dystrophic nails, and occasionally muscle atrophy. Bruits suggesting turbulent arterial flow may be heard over the carotid arteries, abdominal aorta or its branches, and femoral arteries. A detailed examination of the right and left radial, ulnar, brachial, carotid, femoral, popliteal, dorsalis pedis, and posterior tibial pulses should be done and compared side to side. Vessel wall calcification may be palpable (i.e., firm vessel with limited pulsatility) in patients with long-standing renal failure and diabetes, while patients with arteritis may have vessels that are tender to palpation. Pulse strength should be graded as absent, weak, normal, or aneurysmal, and the capillary refill time noted. In patients who present with severe PAD, Buerger's elevation test usually demonstrates pallor on elevation and dependent rubor ("sunset sign"). A key component of the examination is determining the presence or absence of a femoral pulse. A non-palpable femoral pulse usually indicates aortoiliac disease or common femoral artery occlusion, and this finding often helps to determine further imaging choices and treatment options. A normal femoral pulse with absent popliteal and pedal pulses typically indicates superficial femoral arterial disease, while palpable femoral and popliteal pulses with absent pedal pulses often indicate infrapopliteal occlusive disease (the latter frequently occurring in diabetic patients). A handheld Doppler probe should be used for documentation if pulses are not palpable.

Work-Up

Although the clinical history often suggests the diagnosis of PAD, physical exam and pulse evaluation may not be reliable enough to make the diagnosis with confidence. Criqui et al. showed that only 18 % of patients with abnormal posterior tibial pulses had additional objective evidence of PAD [20]. Noninvasive screening tests and imaging studies help confirm the diagnosis by providing accurate and reproducible findings which support the diagnosis of PAD.

Table 6.1 Differential diagnosis of intermittent claudication

Condition	Location	Prevalence	Characteristic	Effect of exercise	Effect of rest	Effect of position	Other characteristics
Calf IC	Calf muscles	3–5 % of adult population	Cramping, aching discomfort	Reproducible onset	Quickly relieved	None	May have atypical limb symptoms on exercise
Thigh and buttock IC	Buttock, hip, thigh	Rare	Cramping, aching discomfort	Reproducible onset	Quickly relieved	None	Impotence May have normal pedal pulses with isolated aortoiliac disease
Foot IC	Foot arch	Rare	Severe pain on exercise	Reproducible onset	Quickly relieved	None	Also may present as numbness
Chronic compartment syndrome	Calf muscles	Rare	Tight, bursting pain	After significant exercise (e.g., jogging)	Subsides very slowly	Relief with elevation	Typically affects heavily muscled athletes
Venous claudication	Entire leg, worse in calf	Rare	Tight, bursting pain	After walking	Subsides slowly	Relief speeded by elevation	History of iliofemoral deep venous thrombosis, signs of venous congestion, edema
Nerve root compression	Radiates down leg	Common	Sharp lancinating pain	Induced by sitting, standing, or walking	Often present at rest	Improved by change in position	History of back problems Worse with sitting Relief when supine or sitting
Symptomatic Baker's cyst	Behind knee, down calf	Rare	Swelling, tenderness	With exercise	Present at rest	None	Not intermittent
Hip arthritis	Lateral hip, thigh	Common	Aching discomfort	After variable degrees of exercise	Not quickly relieved	Improved when not weight bearing	Symptoms variable History of degenerative arthritis
Spinal stenosis	Often bilateral buttocks, posterior leg	Common	Pain and weakness	May mimic IC	Variable relief, but can take a long time to recover	Relief by lumbar spine flexion	Worse with standing and spine extension
Foot/ankle arthritis	Ankle, foot arch	Common	Aching pain	After variable degrees of exercise	Not quickly relieved	May be relieved by not bearing weight	Variable; may relate to activity level and present at rest

Adapted from Norgren et al. [3]

The ankle-brachial index (ABI) is a simple and accurate test for detecting PAD that can be performed in the office or at the bedside. Measuring the ABI involves using a handheld Doppler probe and manual blood pressure cuff to record the systolic blood pressure at the ankle and in the arm. The blood pressure cuff should be placed just above the ankle while locating the posterior tibial artery or dorsalis pedis artery with the Doppler probe. While maintaining the Doppler signal, the blood pressure cuff is inflated until the signal is obliterated. The cuff is then slowly deflated and the pressure at which the Doppler signal returns is the systolic ankle pressure. The same steps are repeated for the remaining pedal artery. The brachial pressure is obtained in the same manner with a blood pressure cuff on the upper arm and a Doppler probe on the radial or ulnar pulse. To calculate the ABI, the highest systolic pressure measured at the ankle is divided by the higher of the two systolic brachial pressures (Fig. 6.2). Using the higher brachial pressure for both lower extremities ensures that the ABI will not be underestimated in patients with upper extremity blood pressure discrepancy due to subclavian artery stenosis.

The ABI correlates with the presence and severity of occlusive disease with a normal ABI ranging from 0.90 to 1.3; an ABI of 0.70–0.90 indicates mild disease; 0.40–0.70 moderate disease; and an ABI less than 0.40 indicates severe occlusive disease [21]. An ABI greater than 1.3 should raise suspicion that the arterial wall is stiffened by medial calcinosis, as often occurs in diabetics. In some patients with moderate wall calcification, a normal ABI may not reflect the true perfusion to the lower extremities. A falsely elevated ABI should

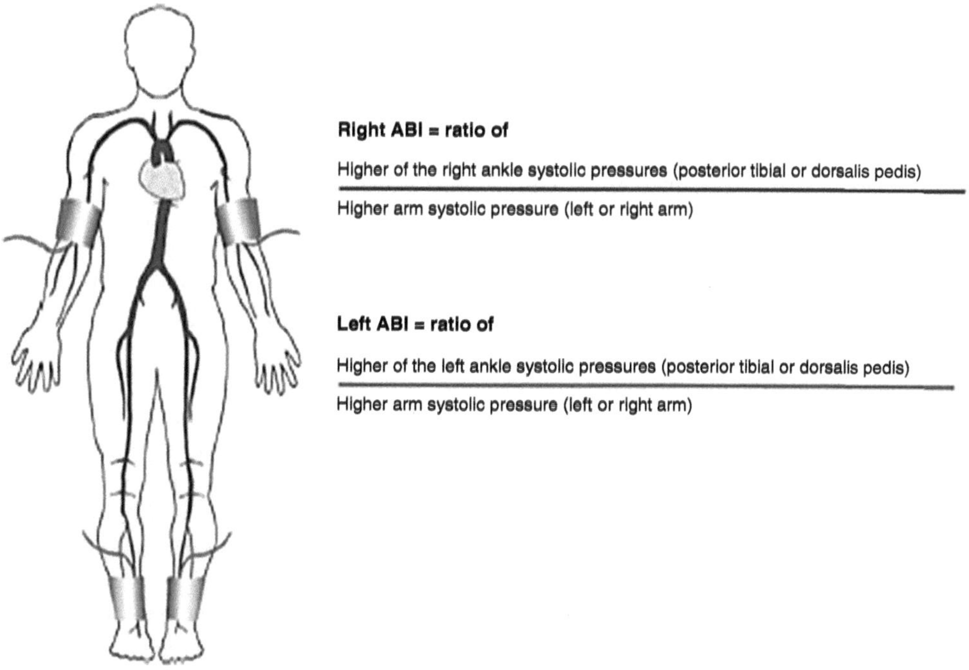

Fig. 6.2 Calculation of the ankle-brachial index (*ABI*)

be suspected in patients with a strong clinical suspicion for PAD or typical claudication symptoms who have absent palpable pedal pulses despite a normal or near normal ABI. This finding should prompt further testing with waveform analyses or imaging studies.

Most patients with intermittent claudication have an ABI between 0.5 and 0.9, while those with ischemic rest pain have an ABI less than 0.4, and patients with impending gangrene have an ABI less than 0.3. Common mistakes to avoid when taking an ABI include not using the higher of the two arm pressures as the denominator, failure to have the patient supine for at least 5 min to allow stabilization of blood pressure and failure to choose an appropriately sized cuff (the bladder length of the cuff should be 80 %, and the width should be 40 % of the circumference of the extremity).

The noninvasive vascular lab can perform several tests that evaluate PAD in more detail and may help confirm the diagnosis in patients with atypical clinical presentations. Segmental limb pressures can detect and localize arterial occlusive lesions by using cuffs placed at the arm, at the upper thigh, above the knee, below the knee, and at the ankle. A pressure drop of 20 mmHg or more at any level in comparison to the proximal or contralateral level indicates significant arterial disease. Occasionally, well-developed collateral vessels can compensate for occlusive disease and minimize the pressure disparity. Inaccurate readings may also result from using an undersized cuff on the thigh which falsely elevates the pressure, masking iliac artery stenosis.

Pulse volume recording (PVR) offers another alternative to detect and localize PAD. Cuffs placed on the lower extremity at multiple levels are inflated to 65 mmHg and the pulse waveforms are recorded. A normal pulse waveform consists of a rapid upslope, a sharp systolic peak, a dicrotic notch, and a gentle bow toward the baseline. In the presence of PAD, the waveform becomes dampened and the degree of dampening usually correlates with the severity of the stenosis. Compared to segmental pressure measurements, PVR is less affected by arterial calcification and combining PVR and segmental pressure measurements increases the overall accuracy for detecting PAD [22].

Although exercise testing is rarely required to diagnose PAD, it can distinguish arterial claudication from pseudoclaudication. As a physiologic study, exercise testing can also determine the extent to which underlying conditions such cardiopulmonary, orthopedic, or muscular disease contribute to the patient's symptoms. The patient usually rests for 20 min before measuring the resting ABI. The patient then walks on a treadmill at a fixed speed (2 mph) and inclination (10–12°) for 5 min or until claudication symptoms develop. Repeated toe raises can substitute for walking when a treadmill is not available. The patient then reclines and the ankle and arm pressures are measured immediately and repeated every 2 min for 10 min or until the pressure returns to resting levels. In the supine position, a decrease in ABI of 15–20 % is diagnostic for PAD. Patients with severe aortic stenosis, uncontrolled hypertension, severe congestive heart failure, unstable angina, or chronic obstructive pulmonary disease should not undergo exercise testing.

Digital pressure measurements can be used to detect PAD in patients who have noncompressible vessels or falsely elevated ABI's (typically due to diabetes or ESRD). The toe-brachial index (TBI) helps to provide a frame of reference as the normal toe pressure is 20–40 mmHg lower than the ankle pressure. A normal TBI is greater than 0.7, a TBI of 0.64–0.7 is borderline, and a TBI less than 0.64 is clearly abnormal [23]. A toe pressure less than 30 mmHg is associated with ischemic symptoms.

In most patients, the combination of clinical history, physical exam, and noninvasive tests can establish the diagnosis of PAD and determine the level of occlusive disease. Imaging studies are not required to confirm the diagnosis of PAD, nor should they be used as first line screening tests as they do not alter the natural history of the disease or the initial management strategy. The primary role of imaging studies involves treatment planning for patients who are being considered for revascularization. Chapter 8 has a more detailed description of the most common imaging modalities including duplex ultrasound, computed tomography angiography (CTA), magnetic resonance angiography (MRA), and catheter-directed angiography.

Treatment Indications and Options

The management of PAD poses a challenge because it represents a systemic disease with a wide range of clinical severity. Developing an individualized treatment plan for patients with claudication requires knowledge of the natural history of PAD, as well as a thorough evaluation of each patient's unique comorbidities, including extent of systemic atherosclerosis, functional capacity, and cardiovascular risk factors (Fig. 6.3). Most patients with intermittent claudication have a slow decrease in walking distances and rarely progress to limb-threatening ischemia (rest pain, ischemic ulcer, or gangrene) especially when risk factors are controlled. Only 25 % of patients with claudication demonstrate any clinical deterioration of the limb perfusion, and the risk of major amputation in a claudicant ranges from 1 to 7 % over 5 years [24–26]. Decisions on the timing and type of intervention depend on the extent of anatomic involvement, the available revascularization options, and the expected benefits of intervention balanced against early and late risk. The patient with claudication should clearly understand that they do not have limb-threatening ischemia and that intervention is not required for immediate limb salvage or prevention of amputation in the future. Treatment strategies for patients with claudication should focus on controlling cardiovascular risk factors, increasing walking distance, and improving the quality of life. Achieving these goals requires an individualized treatment plan based on the extent of disability and functional needs of each patient. Success in managing patients with claudication involves education regarding what to expect from each proposed treatment and encouraging active participation in the decision-making process.

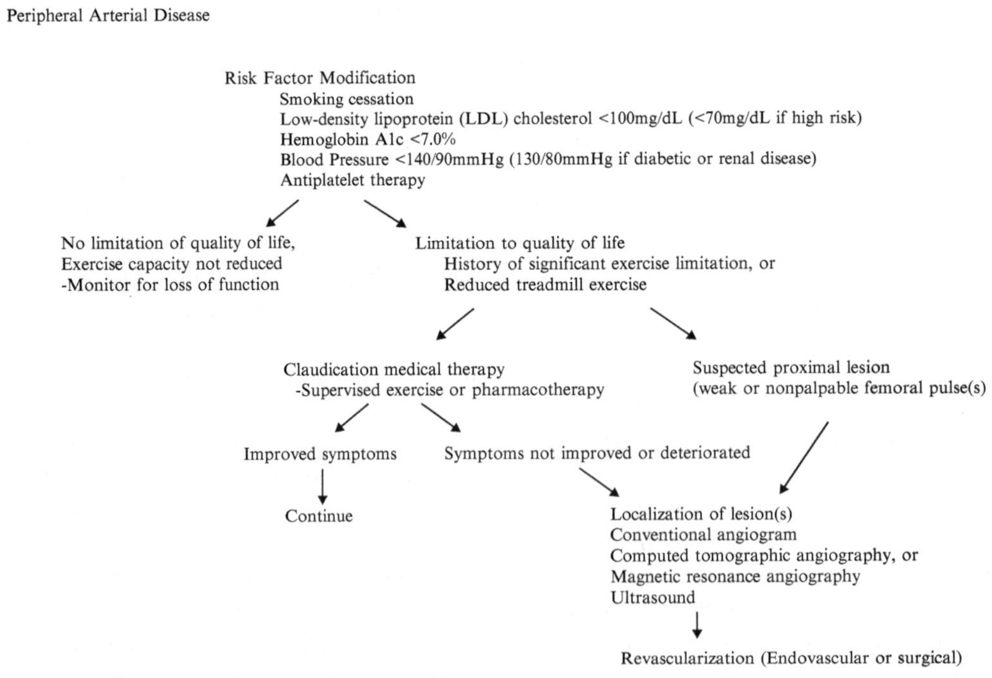

Fig. 6.3 Overall treatment strategy for peripheral arterial disease. *BP* blood pressure, *HbA1c* hemoglobin A1c, *LDL* low-density lipoprotein, *MRA* magnetic resonance angiography, *CTA* computed tomographic angiography

Since PAD (ABI < 0.9) is a manifestation of systemic atherosclerosis, it is not surprising that it has a strong association with CAD and stroke. In a study on the fate of 2,777 male claudicants, the mortality rate was 42 and 65 % at 5 and 10 years, respectively, with myocardial infarction accounting for two-thirds of the 1,363 deaths [26]. A decrease in ABI correlated with an increase in the incidence of cardiac and cerebrovascular disease in a population study of 13,678 patients over a 13-year period [26]. In another large study on patients older than 70 or age 50–69 with diabetes or smoking history, 16 % of patients with an ABI less than 0.9 had symptomatic CAD or cerebrovascular disease [27]. The ACC/AHA guidelines emphasize the fact that the most significant risk facing patients with claudication is cardiac death, not limb loss. The risk of cardiac death for claudicants is 3–5 % per year compared to a 1 % risk of amputation [28].

Medical Management

Risk Factor Modification:

All patients with PAD require cardiovascular risk factor modification irrespective of the treatment plan for their claudication symptoms.

Smoking

Smoking cessation is the cornerstone of any treatment plan for claudication. Active smokers should be educated so that they understand that none of their other medications surpasses the importance of smoking cessation. Smoking cessation decreases the risk of death, myocardial infarction, amputation, and lower extremity intervention. Patients who quit smoking significantly improve their exercise time compared to those who continue to smoke [4, 29]. The issue of smoking cessation should be discussed at each clinical encounter with patients who smoke. Unfortunately, physician advice and frequent follow-up achieved a quit smoking rate of only 5 %. Not surprisingly an intensive smoking cessation program with individual counseling and pharmacologic therapy resulted in better quit rates compared to verbal advice alone (21 % vs. 7 %) [30, 31]. The addition of medications such as bupropion and varenicline or nicotine replacement can provide valuable assistance to patients attempting smoking cessation. Varenicline acts as a partial agonist of $\alpha 4\beta 2$ nicotine acetylcholine receptor, which minimizes the effect of withdrawal by releasing dopamine to reduce craving. In randomized clinical trials, varenicline had superior quit rates compared to nicotine replacement and bupropion [32]. At 9 weeks, varenicline had a quit rate of 44 % versus 16 % for nicotine replacement, 30 % with bupropion, and 35 % with both bupropion and nicotine replacement [33].

Hyperlipidemia

The current guidelines by ACC/AHA recommend an LDL cholesterol level of less than 100 mg/dl in patients with PAD and less than 70 mg/dl in those with evidence of generalized atherosclerosis. Lipid-lowering agents, especially statins (3-hydroxy-3-methyglutaryl coenzyme A (HMG-CoA)), have been increasingly used as they have been shown to decrease cardiac-related events. The beneficial effects of statins appear to extend beyond their lipid-lowering properties. These pleiotropic properties include the ability to stabilize atherosclerotic plaque while decreasing oxidative stress, vascular inflammation, and platelet aggregability [34].

The Heart Protection Study (HPS) [35] randomized 20,500 patients (6,748 with PAD) to simvastatin 40 mg, antioxidant vitamins, a combination of the two, or placebo. Patients who received 40 mg of simvastatin had a significant reduction in overall mortality (12 %), vascular mortality (17 %), coronary events (24 %), all strokes (27 %), and noncoronary revascularization (16 %). Results were similar in the PAD subgroup. In a meta-analysis of statin therapy [36], a 39 mg/dl reduction in LDL was associated with a 20 % decrease in major cardiovascular event risk independent of the initial lipid levels, including those with normal lipid levels.

Patients with PAD may also have abnormal HDL and triglyceride metabolism. Increasing low HDL levels (<40 mg/dl) using fibrates or niacin benefits patients with coronary artery disease by reducing the risk of nonfatal MI, cardiovascular death, and progression of coronary atherosclerosis [37–39].

Dietary modification should be the initial intervention to control abnormal lipid levels. In addition, patients who are overweight (BMI 25–30) or obese (BMI >30) should be counseled for weight reduction and referred for weight reduction programs if available.

Diabetes Mellitus

Although the microvascular complications of diabetes (retinopathy, nephropathy) increase with uncontrolled blood glucose levels, strict glucose control does not seem to decrease the rate of macrovascular complications, particularly PAD. Nevertheless, the current American Diabetes Association guidelines recommend hemoglobin A_{1c} <7 % as a treatment goal for all patients with DM [39, 40].

Hypertension

The current guidelines recommend a target blood pressure of less than 140/90 mmHg in high risk groups such as those with PAD and less than 130/80 mmHg in patients who also have diabetes or renal insufficiency [41, 42]. The benefit of blood pressure control on decreasing the risk of cardiovascular events does not seem to be linked to the specific medication used. Often more than one medication is needed to achieve this goal. Thiazide diuretics are first line agents, and ACE inhibitors or angiotensin receptor blockers are recommended in patients with diabetic renal disease or congestive heart failure. A subgroup analysis of the 4,046 patients with PAD in the Heart Outcomes Prevention Evaluation (HOPE) study showed a 22 % decrease in the risk of stroke, MI, and vascular mortality in patients randomized to receive an ACE inhibitor (ramipril) [43]. This finding which was independent of the absolute reduction in blood pressure provides support for the use of ACE inhibitors as a treatment for hypertension in patients with PAD. Beta-adrenergic blocking medications can also be used for patients with PAD, especially those with coronary artery disease. Randomized trials have refuted the previously held belief that these medications could exacerbate claudication symptoms.

Homocysteine

Although an elevated homocysteine level is associated with PAD, treatment of patients with high doses of folic acid is not recommended as it has failed to show any benefit [3]. Checking homocysteine levels and giving supplemental folic acid or B vitamins may be appropriate in patients with a family history of multiple thrombotic events or premature cardiovascular events in the absence of conventional atherosclerotic risk factors.

Antiplatelet Drug Therapy

All patients with claudication should receive antiplatelet therapy because it reduces the risk of MI, ischemic stroke, and vascular mortality. The Antithrombotic Trialists' Collaboration which included 102,459 patients with cardiovascular disease showed that the risk of cardiovascular events in patients treated with aspirin-(acetylsalicylic acid, ASA) was 9.5 % versus 11.9 % in the control group. Patients with claudication had an 18–23 % decrease in cardiovascular events in a subgroup analysis [44]. Low dose (75–150 mg) ASA has proved to be as effective as higher dose aspirin, without the increased risk of gastrointestinal bleeding.

Clopidogrel remains the only FDA-approved antiplatelet medication for the secondary prevention of atherosclerotic vascular disease. In the CAPRIE Trial (Clopidogrel vs. Aspirin in Patients at Risk of Ischemic Events) [45] patients who received clopidogrel (75 mg daily) had a 24 % relative risk reduction for MI, stroke, and death compared to patients receiving ASA (325 mg). Although combination therapy with clopidogrel and ASA may be more effective in acute coronary syndromes, this benefit was not demonstrated in other high risk populations including patients with PAD. Combination therapy increases the risk of bleeding and is not currently recommended as a long-term antiplatelet regimen except in patients with other indications such as drug-eluting coronary stents.

Treatment of Claudication Symptoms

In addition to cardiovascular risk reduction, medical management includes improvement in walking ability and hence the quality of life of patients with claudication. Pharmacologic agents and exercise therapy are the major components of this aspect of medical treatment for claudication.

Pharmacologic Agents

Cilostazol

Cilostazol is one of two currently FDA-approved drugs for intermittent claudication and the only one with evidence of significant clinical efficacy. As a phosphodiesterase III inhibitor, cilostazol acts as a vasodilator with antiplatelet properties. It also inhibits smooth muscle cell contraction, decreases serum triglycerides, and increases HDL. In a meta-analysis of 6 randomized controlled trials including 1,751 patients (740 on placebo, 281 on cilostazol 50 mg bid, 730 on cilostazol 100 mg bid), peak treadmill performance increased 50–70 m in patients on cilostazol compared to those on placebo [46]. Quality of life measures as tested by WIQ and SF-36 also significantly improved. In a randomized controlled trial, cilostazol therapy increased the maximal walking distance by 107 m (54 % increase), compared to an increase of 64 m in those taking pentoxifylline (30 % increase and statistically the same as placebo) [47]. Cilostazol is contraindicated in patients with congestive heart failure because it is a phosphodiesterase inhibitor and could potentially exacerbate heart failure; however, no direct adverse events have been reported with cilostazol. Rare side effects of cilostazol including headache, diarrhea, and gastrointestinal discomfort can be minimized by starting at a lower dose of 50 mg bid for 1–2 weeks, then increasing to the full dose of 100 mg bid. Patients and prescribing physicians should understand that the full dose should be the goal as the lower dose is not as effective in achieving results.

Pentoxifylline

The first and only other FDA-approved drug for claudication, pentoxifylline is a methylxanthine derivative which improves oxygen delivery by its rheolytic effect on red blood cells and its inhibitory effect on platelet aggregation and fibrinogen levels. Clinical studies showed only a modest and inconsistent improvement in claudication symptoms and walking distance [48, 49]. Pentoxifylline is currently offered to patients who have benefited from the drug before or in patients who cannot receive cilostazol because of a history of CHF or intolerable side effects. Pentoxifylline has an excellent safety profile with elevated blood pressure being one of its few side effects. The standard dose is 400 mg tid, which can be increased to 600 mg tid.

Statins

Statin drugs have been reported to improve pain-free walking time and walking distance in patients with claudication [50]. These results may reflect the ability of statins to improve vasomotor blood flow and stimulate angiogenesis [51].

Other Medications

A number of agents and classes of drugs (naftidrofuryl, propionyl-L-carnitine, buflomedil, defibrotide, prostaglandins, L-arginine, vasodilators) have been studied but will not be discussed here due to unavailability or lack of proven efficacy.

Exercise Therapy

Exercise remains an effective form of therapy for patients with claudication [52]. Structured exercise programs improve pain-free ambulation distance and overall walking performance [25, 52–54]. In addition, exercise reduces cardiovascular morbidity and mortality by lowering blood pressure and cholesterol levels and controlling glucose levels in diabetics. ACC/AHA guidelines give a strong recommendation with solid supporting evidence (level IA) for supervised exercise in the treatment of intermittent claudication. Specifically the guidelines suggest walking for a minimum of 30–45 min per session, three to four times per week for at least 12 weeks. Walking should continue until reaching pain tolerance (rather than the onset of pain). Patients should then stop for a brief rest and resume walking as soon as the pain resolves.

A recent meta-analysis including 9 studies with 873 participants compared the outcome of medical therapy, supervised exercise, and endovascular intervention. Endovascular therapy increased ABI, initial claudication distance, and maximum claudication distance compared to medical therapy during early follow-up [54].Patients treated with endovascular intervention had significantly better ABIs at immediate and early follow-up compared to supervised exercise; however, the mean differences were small, and treadmill walking distances were the same. Endovascular intervention plus supervised exercise improved early and intermediate results compared to those who had supervised exercise alone.

The main drawback of exercise therapy is that about a third of patients are not medically fit to participate and another third are simply resistant to the treatment regimen. Lack of reimbursement by Medicare or insurers for supervised programs, the most effective form of exercise therapy, creates another hurdle. Nevertheless, all patients should be informed about the benefits of a regular walking regimen as a primary component of medical management for claudication.

Endovascular or Surgical Revascularization

The TASC II document proposed a decision-making algorithm for managing patients with claudication (Fig. 6.3) which recommends revascularization (endovascular or surgical) only after failure of medical therapy for those with infrainguinal disease. Patients with proximal (aortoiliac) occlusive lesions may be considered for revascularization earlier.

Advances in endovascular technology have triggered an increase in the number of endovascular procedures performed to treat claudication. It is still unclear whether this trend represents an evolution of therapy that translates into improved patient outcomes. A number of studies comparing medical therapy and endovascular intervention have shown equivalent outcomes, especially in long-term follow-up. In the Edinburgh Study, 62 out of over 600 screened patients (47 with SFA stenoses or occlusions, 15 with iliac stenoses) were randomized to either balloon angioplasty or medical management (low dose EC-ASA, lifestyle modification). After 2 years, there was no difference in maximal walking distance, claudication onset distance, and quality of life (QoL) measures [55]. The Oxford trial randomized 56 patients to exercise training or percutaneous transluminal angioplasty (PTA). In patients with disease confined to the superficial femoral artery, exercise training conferred a greater improvement in claudication and maximum walking distance compared to PTA. In contrast, patients with iliac occlusive lesions had better results with PTA which may reflect the 20 % better patency rate achieved in this subgroup [56].

Evidence favoring revascularization over exercise therapy includes the prospective study by Gelin et al. involving 264 patients randomized to exercise or revascularization (endovascular or surgical) [57]. After 1 year patients randomized to revascularization had significant functional improvement and a patency rate of 76 %. In a review of 4,888 PTAs and 4,511 bypasses, Hunink et al. developed a decision analytic model to compare no treatment, initial PTA without further intervention, initial PTA with repeat endovascular intervention, initial PTA with subsequent surgical bypass, bypass surgery with no further therapy, and bypass surgery followed by graft revision [58]. Their decision and cost-effectiveness analysis suggested that a "PTA first strategy" increased quality adjusted life expectancy by 2–13 months in a typical 65-year-old patient with claudication and resulted in decreased lifetime expenditures compared to bypass surgery. Sensitivity analysis showed that PTA was the preferred initial treatment as long as the 5-year-patency exceeded 30 %.

Taylor et al. make a persuasive argument for endovascular therapy to treat aortoiliac disease in their series of 669 patients (1,000 limbs), 70 % of whom had aortoiliac occlusive disease [59]. Over 60 % of the limbs had a successful endovascular intervention, with symptomatic relief achieved in 78 % of patients. They reported a 5-year secondary patency rate of 94 %, a limb salvage of 99 %, and an overall survival of 77 %. The clinical success and minimal morbidity of endovascular interventions compares favorably with medical therapy which suffers from a relatively high failure rate and a lack of insurance coverage for supervised exercise programs. These authors advocated a more liberal approach to intervention in patients with claudication, challenging the recommendation that revascularization be offered only after a trial and failure of medical therapy.

Medical therapy, exercise, and endovascular intervention do not necessarily represent mutually exclusive management strategies for claudication. The CLEVER Study examined combinations of therapy by randomizing 111 patients with aortoiliac disease to: optimal medical care (OMC) including cilostazol and self-directed exercise; medical care plus supervised exercise (SE); or medical care plus endovascular stenting (ST) [60]. At the 6-month follow-up, change in peak walking time was greatest for SE, intermediate for ST, and least with OMC (mean change versus baseline, 5.8 ± 4.6, 3.7 ± 4.9, and 1.2 ± 2.6 min, respectively). Disease-specific quality of life also improved with both SE and ST compared with OMC. It is important to note that the patients in the CLEVER Study had relatively limited lesions (mean lesion length 3.9 cm, 38 % occlusions) and more than twice as many patients (43 %) in the stented group had complete relief of claudication symptoms compared to patients in supervised exercise group (21 %).

Since supervised exercise therapy likely benefits patients by improving their cardiopulmonary fitness, it may function as a valuable adjunct to revascularization. A recent meta-analysis included eight randomized clinical trials comparing PTA and supervised exercise therapy (SET) and found that while PTA and SET were equally effective, PTA plus SET improved walking distance and some domains of quality of life scales compared to PTA alone [61].

Although endovascular interventions have low morbidity and essentially no mortality, achieving optimal long-term outcomes requires knowledge of the disease complexity and the expected durability of the revascularization procedure. Lesion anatomy may be the most important factor in determining which type of revascularization will yield the longest patency. The TASC working group classified anatomic patterns of disease for aortoiliac and femoropopliteal segments (type A to D) and made revascularization recommendations for each subgroup [62]. The current guidelines published in 2007 and known as TASC II recommend endovascular therapy for TASC type A lesions and surgery for type D lesions [3]. Endovascular treatment is also the preferred treatment for type B lesions with surgery being preferred for good risk patients with type C lesions. The guidelines suggest considering the patient's comorbidities and personal preference as well as the local operator's long-term success when making treatment choices for type B and C lesions both in aortoiliac and femoropopliteal segments. Figures 6.4 and 6.5 show the TASC classification of aortoiliac and femoropopliteal lesions.

Multilevel arterial disease occurs less commonly in patients with claudication compared to those with critical limb ischemia, and decision making regarding which segment to treat and how to treat it can be challenging. A hybrid approach has emerged as an effective technique for addressing all levels of arterial disease with one intervention involving both surgical and endovascular techniques [63–65].

Aortoiliac Disease

Endovascular interventions have had the greatest impact on aortoiliac arterial disease with angioplasty and stenting now considered by many to be first line therapy even for complex lesions (TASC C and D) [66, 67]. Endovascular aortoiliac interventions increased by 850 % between 1995 and 2000 in a NIS sample [68], whereas aortobifemoral bypass surgery decreased by 16 % during the same time period. The introduction of covered stents, reentry devices, and the increased use of brachial access has allowed patients with complex aortoiliac occlusions to be treated by endovascular means, while open reconstructions using direct (aortobifemoral) or extraanatomic bypasses (axillobifemoral, femorofemoral) are less commonly required.

Successful endovascular intervention for patients with aortoiliac occlusive disease requires careful pre-procedure assessment of anatomy and revascularization options. When treating a patient with disabling claudication and weak or absent femoral pulses, a noninvasive imaging study (CTA or MRA) performed preoperatively can help plan the procedure. The extent of occlusive disease, amount and location of calcification, and the common femoral artery plaque burden can determine the access site (femoral vs. brachial), the use of covered stents, and the need for common femoral endarterectomy in addition to the iliac intervention (hybrid procedure).

Balloon angioplasty of focal iliac artery stenoses has a 4-year patency of 44–65 %, while complete iliac artery occlusions have higher failure rates after balloon angioplasty alone [69, 70]. The Dutch Iliac Stent Trial Study Group [71] randomized patients with iliac artery lesions to primary PTA versus primary balloon expandable stent placement. Although the two groups had similar outcomes, nearly half (43 %) the patients in the PTA group required stent placement. A meta-analysis comparing primary stenting to selective stenting in more than 1,300 patients found a better initial success rate (>90 %) and primary patency rate (>70 % at 5 years) in the primary stent group. Most interventionists primarily stent iliac artery lesions; however, balloon angioplasty with selective stenting is reasonable in iliac stenoses confined to one artery segment [70].

Type A lesions

- Unilateral or bilateral stenoses of CIA
- Unilateral or bilateral single short (≤3 cm) stenosis of EIA

Type B lesions:

- Short (≤3 cm) stenosis of infrarenal aorta
- Unilateral CIA occlusion
- Single or multiple stenosis totaling 3–10 cm involving the EIA not extending into the CFA
- Unilateral EIA occlusion not involving the origins of internal iliac or CFA

Type C lesions

- Bilateral CIA occlusions
- Bilateral EIA stenoses 3–10 cm long not extending into the CFA
- Unilateral EIA stenosis extending into the CFA
- Unilateral EIA occlusion that involves the origins of internal iliac and/or CFA
- Heavily calcified unilateral EIA occlusion with or without involvement of origins of internal iliac and/or CFA

Type D lesions

- Infra-renal aortoiliac occlusion
- Diffuse disease involving the aorta and both iliac arteries requiring treatment
- Diffuse multiple stenoses involving the unilateral CIA, EIA, and CFA
- Unilateral occlusions of both CIA and EIA
- Bilateral occlusions of EIA
- Iliac stenoses in patients with AAA requiring treatment and not amenable to endograft placement or other lesions requiring open aortic or iliac surgery

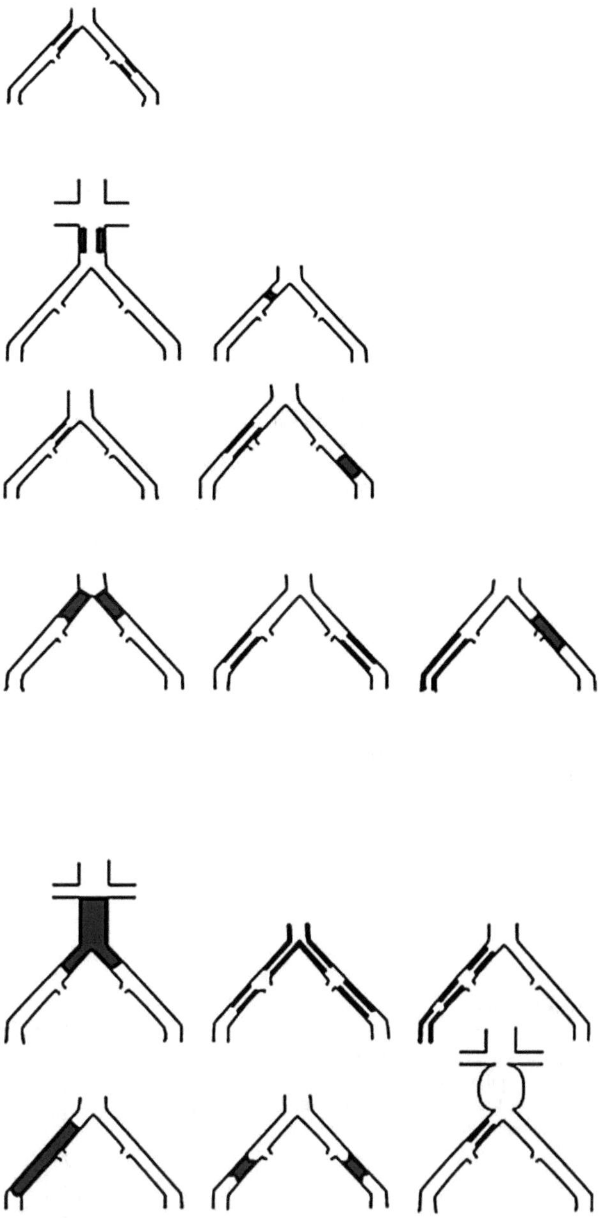

Fig. 6.4 TASC classification of aortoiliac lesions. *CIA* common iliac artery, *EIA* external iliac artery, *CFA* common femoral artery, *AAA* abdominal aortic aneurysm (Reproduced with permission from Elsevier, Norgren et al. [3])

Endovascular interventions for aortoiliac TASC A and B lesions have consistently achieved 80–85 % patency at 5 years [72]. Although the earlier studies reported lower patency rates for TASC C and D lesions, more recent studies have reported patency rates comparable to those achieved with less severe lesions. Kashyap et al. found that patients with TASC C and D lesions treated with aortobifemoral bypass had higher primary patency rates compared to patients treated with endovascular therapy; however, secondary patency rates were similar for both groups (95 % and 97 % at 3 years in endovascular and direct reconstructions, respectively) [66]. Of note, a femoral endarterectomy is required in combination with iliac stenting in 10–20 % of patients especially in series reported by vascular surgeons [64, 65].

Surgical Treatment

The safety and efficacy of endovascular therapy has relegated direct aortoiliac reconstruction to a second or third line treatment option usually reserved for occlusive lesions that cannot be recanalized. Patients with juxtarenal aortic occlusions and

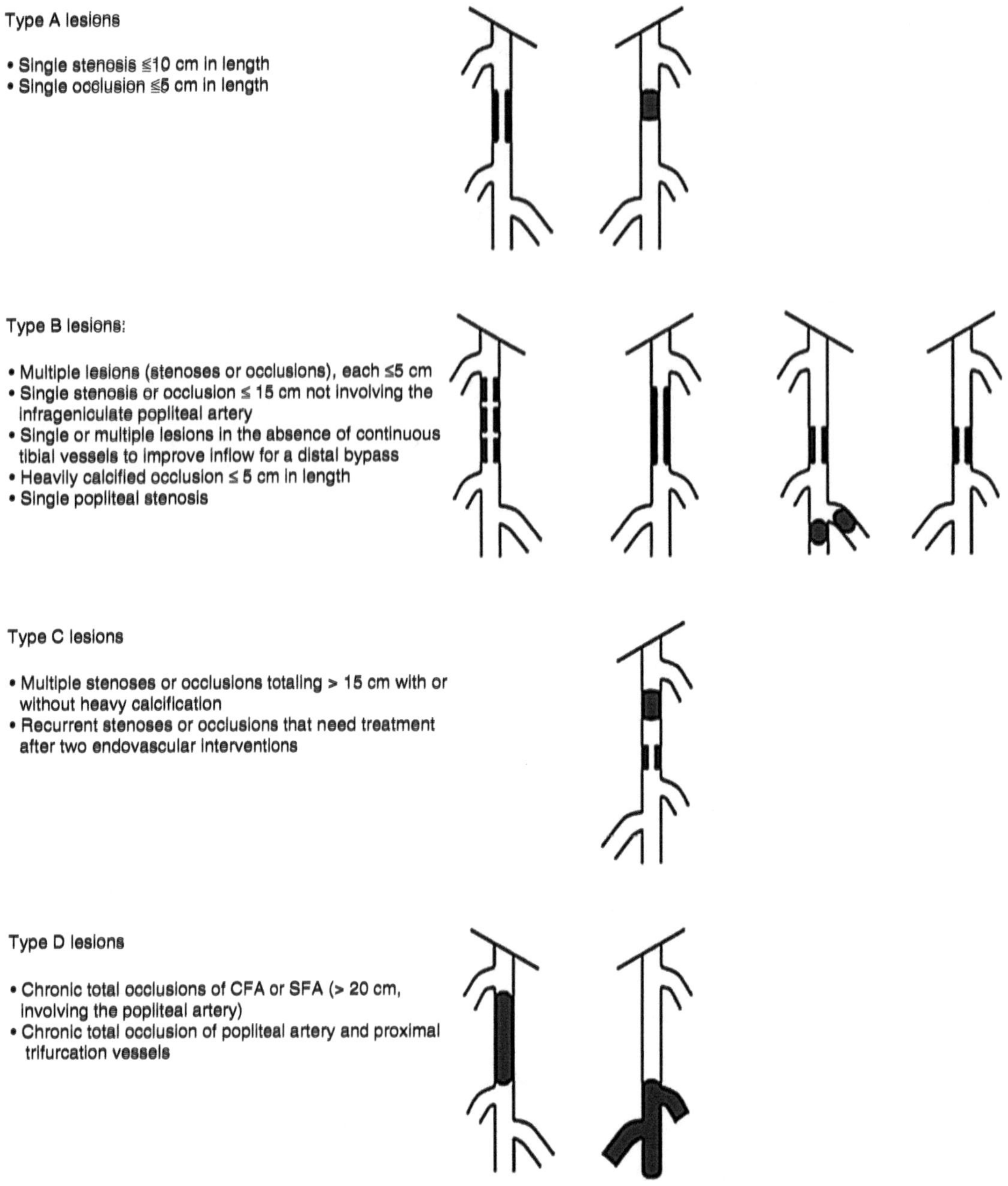

Fig. 6.5 TASC classification of femoral popliteal lesions. *CFA* common femoral artery, *SFA* superficial femoral artery (Reproduced with permission from Elsevier, Norgren et al. [3])

those with aneurysmal and occlusive aortic disease may still be better served with direct surgical reconstruction which usually entails suprarenal aortic clamping and aortic endarterectomy. These indications for surgery have become less absolute with the increasing use of stent grafts and other adjunctive techniques which have expanded endovascular treatment options for patients at high risk for major surgery. Heavy calcification in the iliac and aortic segments are no longer contraindications to endovascular interventions, as the use of stent grafts enables dilation of a severely atherosclerotic artery with protection from uncontrolled hemorrhage if the artery ruptures. Surgeries for aortoiliac occlusive disease including aortobifemoral bypass, aortic endarterectomy, and extraanatomic bypass are described in Chapter 8.

Infrainguinal Disease

Intervening on patients with claudication due to infrainguinal disease involves a more complicated decision-making process than choosing to revascularize patients with aortoiliac occlusive disease. Medical management remains the preferred initial treatment for claudication due to infrainguinal disease, with revascularization reserved for those who fail non-interventional therapy. Several factors can influence the decision to intervene including the disease location, the degree of disability, and the expected durability of revascularization. Once a decision to intervene has been made, noninvasive imaging with duplex ultrasonography, CTA, or MRA can anatomically characterize the disease to help determine the interventional options. Patients with TASC A or B anatomy are usually amenable to endovascular revascularization, while patients with more advanced disease (TASC C or D) disease require a more complex decision-making process. Strict adherence to the TASC recommendations would mandate surgery for these patients; however, most vascular specialists individualize their treatment decisions and initially pursue an endovascular intervention if it seems feasible.

Bypass surgery for patients with claudication due to infrainguinal disease can be a source of disagreement among vascular specialists. Although claudication limits walking and decreases quality of life, it is not a limb-threatening condition nor does it require surgery for limb salvage. The desire to improve a patient's walking ability with a surgical bypass must be balanced against the small but real risk of limb loss if the bypass fails or becomes infected. Physicians and patients must acknowledge and discuss these issues before embarking on lower extremity bypass surgery for claudication.

Some practitioners advocate an expanded role for bypass procedures in patients with claudication. The fact that patients with claudication live longer than those with CLI places a premium on the durability of revascularization procedures. Recent studies suggest that good surgical risk patients with adequate caliber great saphenous vein available should be considered for surgical revascularization before attempting endovascular recanalization of long, complicated arterial occlusions. Preference is given to the great saphenous vein because surgical revascularization using synthetic grafts (PTFE) even in the above-knee position appears to have inferior outcomes in patients with TASC C and D disease [73]. In a meta-analysis of 73 studies on femoropopliteal bypass grafts from 1986 to 2004, Perreira et al. [74] reported 5-year primary patency rate for claudicants of 57 % for above-knee PTFE, 77 % for above-knee vein, and 65 % for below-knee vein. These findings lend support to a strategy of pursuing endovascular revascularization when the surgical alternative involves an infrainguinal bypass using a synthetic graft. In contrast to femoropopliteal occlusive disease, infrapopliteal interventions should generally be avoided in patients with claudication. More aggressive medical therapy should be considered before performing open or endovascular interventions in patients with claudication due to below-knee occlusive lesions.

The variety of endovascular tools being marketed for femoropopliteal disease highlights the fact that a widely accepted treatment strategy does not exist. Although percutaneous balloon angioplasty (PTA), stenting (plain or drug-eluting), stent grafting, cryoplasty, and debulking procedures (laser-assisted PTA, atherectomy) appear to be safe and moderately effective, none of these techniques has proven to be superior in the treatment of femoropopliteal occlusive lesions. Balloon angioplasty with selective stenting remains the most commonly performed endovascular intervention. Indications for stenting after PTA of the SFA include suboptimal technical results such as flow limiting dissections, elastic recoil, or residual stenosis greater than 30 %.

Over the last decade, primary stenting has emerged as a common technique especially in patients with greater than 5 cm occlusions (TASC B and above) [75]. Earlier studies that showed comparable patency rates for balloon angioplasty with selective stenting versus primary stenting were conducted before nitinol-based stents were available. Randomized trials showed primary stenting with nitinol stents improved 1 year patency rates compared to balloon angioplasty (65–80 % vs. 30–40 %) in patients with TASC B femoropopliteal lesions (mean lesion length 71–101 mm) [76–80]. A drug-eluting stent recently approved in the USA has also shown promise in the treatment of femoropopliteal lesions. In a randomized study of 120 patients the paclitaxel-coated stent improved 1- and 2-year patency rates compared to bare metal stents following failed balloon angioplasty [81].

The optimal treatment for TASC C and D lesions remains controversial. Although the TASC document recommends surgical bypass for medically good risk patients with TASC II C and D lesions (occlusion and stenosis length >15 cm), real-world practice often favors endovascular therapy as a first line intervention. An individualized approach may offer the best treatment strategy. Patient factors to consider when deciding between interventional options include medical comorbidities, life expectancy, lesion anatomy, and autogenous conduit availability.

Conclusion

PAD and claudication decrease the quality and quantity of life. Not only do patients with claudication have difficulty walking; they also have an increased 5-year mortality rate of 30–40 % largely due to cardiovascular events. Although endovascular interventions can extend walking distance by increasing arterial perfusion, they do not improve survival. To live longer, patients with PAD and claudication must adopt lifestyle changes aimed at reducing cardiovascular risk including smoking cessation, regular exercise, antithrombotic medication, and cholesterol lowering. Assessing the outcome of patients treated for claudication therefore requires more than just reporting the patency rates after an intervention. Quality of life parameters, functional capacity, and long-term survival more accurately measure the overall success of the various treatment strategies for PAD and claudication.

References

1. Rosamond W, Flegal K, Furie K, et al. Heart disease and stroke statistics—2008 update: a report from the American Heart Association Statistics Committee and Stroke Statistics Subcommittee. Circulation. 2008;117:e25–146.
2. Selvin E, Erlinger TP. Prevalence of and risk factors for peripheral arterial disease in the United States: results from the National Health and Nutrition Examination Survey, 1999–2000. Circulation. 2004;110(6):738–43.
3. Norgren L, Hiatt WR, Dormandy JA, Nehler MR, Harris KA, Fowkes FG, TASC II Working Group. Inter-Society Consensus for the Management of Peripheral Arterial Disease (TASC II). J Vasc Surg. 2007;45(Suppl S):S5–67.
4. Rooke TW, Hirsch AT, Misra S, Sidawy AN, Beckman JA, Findeiss LK, Golzarian J, Gornik HL, Halperin JL, Jaff MR, Moneta GL, Olin JW, Stanley JC, White CJ, White JV, Zierler RE. American College of Cardiology Foundation/American Heart Association Task Force on Practice Guidelines; Society for Cardiovascular Angiography and Interventions; Society of Interventional Radiology; Society for Vascular Medicine; Society for Vascular Surgery. 2011 ACCF/AHA focused update of the guideline for the management of patients with peripheral artery disease (updating the 2005 guideline): a report of the American College of Cardiology Foundation/American Heart Association Task Force on Practice Guidelines: developed in collaboration with the Society for Cardiovascular Angiography and Interventions, Society of Interventional Radiology, Society for Vascular Medicine, and Society for Vascular Surgery. J Vasc Surg. 2011;54(5):e32–58.
5. Dormandy J, Heeck L, Vig S. Intermittent claudication: a condition with underrated risks. Semin Vasc Surg. 1999;12:96–108.
6. Fowkes FG, Housley E, Riemersma RA, et al. Smoking, lipids, glucose intolerance, and blood pressure as risk factors for peripheral atherosclerosis compared with ischemic heart disease in the Edinburgh Artery Study. Am J Epidemiol. 1992;135:331–40.
7. Conen D, Everett BM, Kurth T, Creager MA, Buring JE, Ridker PM, Pradhan AD. Smoking, smoking cessation, and risk for symptomatic peripheral artery disease in women: a cohort study. Ann Intern Med. 2011;154(11):719–26.
8. Fowkes FG, Housley E, Cawood EH, Macintyre CC, Ruckley CV, Prescott RJ. Edinburgh Artery Study: prevalence of asymptomatic and symptomatic peripheral arterial disease in the general population. Int J Epidemiol. 1991;20(2):384–92.
9. Ambrose JA, Barua RS. The pathophysiology of cigarette smoking and cardiovascular disease. J Am Coll Cardiol. 2004;43(10):1731–7.
10. Clark N. Peripheral arterial disease in people with diabetes. Diabetes Care. 2003;26:3333–41.
11. Creager MA, Lüscher TF, Cosentino F, Beckman JA. Diabetes and vascular disease: pathophysiology, clinical consequences, and medical therapy: part I. Circulation. 2003;108:1527–32.
12. Selvin E, Marinopoulos S, Berkenblit G, Rami T, Brancati FL, Powe NR, et al. Metaanalysis: glycosylated hemoglobin and cardiovascular disease in diabetes mellitus. Ann Intern Med. 2004;141:421–31.
13. Murabito JM, D'Agostino RB, Silbershatz H, et al. Intermittent claudication. A risk profile from The Framingham Heart Study. Circulation. 1997;96:44–9.
14. Clement DL, De Buyzere ML, Duprez DA. Hypertension in peripheral arterial disease. Curr Pharm Des. 2004;10(29):3615–20.
15. Alexander RW. Hypertension and the pathogenesis of atherosclerosis oxidative stress and the mediation of arterial inflammatory response: a new perspective. Hypertension. 1995;25:155–61.
16. Vogel RA. Cholesterol lowering and endothelial function. Am J Med. 1999;107(5):479–87.
17. Shankar A, Li J, Nieto FJ, Klein BE, Klein R. Association between C-reactive protein level and peripheral arterial disease among US adults without cardiovascular disease, diabetes, or hypertension. Am Heart J. 2007;154(3):495–501.
18. Wattanakit K, Folsom AR, Selvin E, Coresh J, Hirsch AT, Weatherley BD. Kidney function and risk of peripheral arterial disease: results from the Atherosclerosis Risk in Communities (ARIC) Study. Am Soc Nephrol. 2007;18(2):629–36.
19. Kullo IJ, Bailey KR, Kardia SL, Mosley TH, Boerwinkle E, Turner ST. Ethnic differences in peripheral arterial disease in the NHLBI Genetic Epidemiology Network of Arteriopathy (GENOA) study. Vasc Med. 2003;8(4):237–42.
20. Criqui MH, Fronek A, Klauber MR, Barrett-Connor E, Gabriel S. The sensitivity, specificity, and predictive value of traditional clinical evaluation of peripheral arterial disease: results from non-invasive testing in a defined population. Circulation. 1985;71(3):516–22.
21. Hiatt WR. Medical treatment of peripheral arterial disease and claudication. N Engl J Med. 2001;344:1608–21.
22. Kohler TR, Sumner DS. Chapter 14. Vascular laboratory: arterial physiologic assessment. In: Cronenwett JL, Wayne Johnston K, editors. Rutherford's vascular surgery. 7th Edition, 2010, Elsevier, Philadelphia.
23. Carter SA. Role of pressure measurements in vascular disease. In: Bernstein EF, editor. Vascular diagnosis. 4th ed. St Louis: CV Mosby; 1993. p. 486–512.
24. O'Riordan DS, O'Donnell JA. Realistic expectations for the patient with intermittent claudication. Br J Surg. 1991;78:861–3.
25. Cox GS, Hertzer NR, Young JR, et al. Non-operative treatment of superficial femoral artery disease: long term follow-up. J Vasc Surg. 1993;17:172–81.
26. Muluk SC, Muluk VS, Kelley ME, et al. Outcome events in patients with claudication: a 15 year study in 2777 patients. J Vasc Surg. 2001;33:251–7.
27. Hirsch AT, Criqui MH, Treat-Jacobson D, et al. Peripheral arterial disease detection, awareness, and treatment in primary care. JAMA. 2001;286:1317–24.
28. Hirsch AT, Haskal ZJ, Hertzer NR, et al. ACC/AHA 2005 guidelines for the management of patients with peripheral arterial disease (lower extremity, renal, mesenteric and abdominal aortic): executive summary a collaborative report from the American Association for Vascular Surgery, Society for Vascular Surgery, Society for Cardiovascular Angiography and Intervention, Society for Vascular Medicine and Biology, Society for Interventional Radiology and the ACC/AHA Task Force on Practice Guidelines (Writing Committee to Develop Guidelines for the Management of Patients with Peripheral Arterial Disease) endorsed by the American Association of Cardiovascular and Pulmonary Rehabilitation; National Heart, Lung and Blood Institute; Society for Vascular Nursing; TransAtlantic Inter-Society Consensus; and Vascular Disease Foundation. J Am Coll Cardiol. 2006;47:1239–312.
29. Smith I, Franks PI, Greenhalgh RM, Poulter NR, Powell JT. The influence of smoking cessation and hypertriglyceridaernia on the progression of peripheral arterial disease and the onset of critical ischemia. Eur J Vase Endovasc Surg. 1996;11:402–8.

30. Hennrikus D, Joseph AM, Lando HA, et al. Effectiveness of a smoking cessation program for peripheral artery disease patients: a randomized controlled trial. J Am Coll Cardiol. 2010; 56:2105–12.
31. Anthonisen NR, Skeans MA, Wise RA, et al. The effects of smoking cessation intervention on 1, 4, 5-year mortality: a randomized clinical trial. Ann Intern Med. 2005;142:233–9.
32. Cahill K, Stead LF, Lancaster T. Nicotine receptor partial agonists for smoking cessation. Cochrane Database Syst Rev. 2012;4, CD006103.
33. Jorenby DE, Hays JT, Rigotti NA, et al. Efficacy of varenicline, an alpha4beta2 nicotinic acetylcholine receptor partial agonist, vs placebo or sustained release bupropion for smoking cessation: a randomized controlled trial. JAMA. 2006;296:56–63.
34. Marzilli M. Pleiotropic effects of statins. Am J Cardiovasc Drugs. 2010;10 Suppl 1:3–9.
35. HPSCG. MRC/BHF Heart Protection Study of cholesterol lowering with simvastatin in 20,536 high-risk individuals: a randomised placebo-controlled trial. Lancet. 2002;360(9326):7–22.
36. Baigent C, Keech A, Kearney PM, Blackwell L, Buck G, Pollicino C, et al. Efficacy and safety of cholesterol-lowering treatment: prospective meta-analysis of data from 90,056 participants in 14 randomised trials of statins. Lancet. 2005;366(9493):1267–78.
37. Rubins HB, Robins SJ, Collins D, Fye CL, Anderson JW, Elam MB, et al. Gemfibrozil for the secondary prevention of coronary heart disease in men with low levels of high-density lipoprotein cholesterol. Veterans Affairs High-Density Lipoprotein Cholesterol Intervention Trial Study Group. N Engl J Med. 1999; 341(6):410–18.
38. Blankenhorn DH, Azen SP, Crawford DW, Nessim SA, Sanmarco ME, Selzer RH, et al. Effects of colestipol-niacin therapy on human femoral atherosclerosis. Circulation. 1991;83(2):438–47.
39. Taylor AJ, Sullenberger LE, Lee HJ, Lee JK, Grace KA. Arterial Biology for the Investigation of the Treatment Effects of Reducing Cholesterol (ARBITER) 2: a double-blind, placebo-controlled study of extended-release niacin on atherosclerosis progression in secondary prevention patients treated with statins. Circulation. 2004;110(23):3512–17.
40. ADA. Standards of medical care in diabetes – 2006. Diabetes Care. 2006;29 Suppl 1:S4–42.
41. Chobanian AV, Bakris GL, Black HR, et al. Seventh report of the Joint National Committee on Prevention, Detection, Valuation, and Treatment of High Blood Pressure. Hypertension. 2003;42: 1206–52.
42. ESH/ESC European Society of Hypertension—European Society of Cardiology guidelines for the management of arterial hypertension. J Hypertens. 2003;21:1000–53.
43. Yusuf S, Sleight P, Pogue J, Bosch J, Davies R, Dagenais G. Effects of an angiotensin-converting-enzyme inhibitor, ramipril, on cardiovascular events in high-risk patients. The Heart Outcomes Prevention Evaluation Study Investigators. N Engl J Med. 2000;342(3):145–53.
44. ATC. Collaborative meta-analysis of randomised trials of antiplatelet therapy for prevention of death, myocardial infarction, and stroke in high risk patients. Br Med J. 2002;324(7329): 71–86.
45. CAPRIE. A randomised, blinded, trial of clopidogrel versus aspirin in patients at risk of ischaemic events (CAPRIE). CAPRIE Steering Committee. Lancet. 1996;348(9038):1329–39.
46. Regensteiner J, Ware JJ, McCarthy W, Zhang P, Forbes W, Heckman J, et al. Effect of cilostazol on treadmill walking, community-based walking ability, and health-related quality of life in patients with intermittent claudication due to peripheral arterial disease: metaanalysis of six randomized controlled trials. J Am Geriatr Soc. 2002;50(12):1939–46.
47. Dawson DL, Cutler BS, Hiatt WR, Hobson II RW, Martin JD, Bortey EB, Forbes WP, Strandness Jr DE. A comparison of cilostazol and pentoxifylline for treating intermittent claudication. Am J Med. 2000;109:523–30.
48. Girolami B, Bernardi E, Prins M, ten Cate J, Hettiarachchi R, Prandoni P, et al. Treatment of intermittent claudication with physical training, smoking cessation, pentoxifylline, or nafronyl: a meta-analysis. Arch Intern Med. 1999;159:337–45.
49. Moher D, Pham B, Ausejo M, Saenz A, Hood S, Barber G. Pharmacological management of intermittent claudication: a meta-analysis of randomised trials. Drugs. 2000;59:1057–70.
50. Mondillo S, Ballo P, Barbati R, et al. Effects of simvastatin on walking performance and symptoms of intermittent claudication in hypercholesterolemic patients with peripheral vascular disease. Am J Med. 2003;114:359–64.
51. Mohler III ER, Hiatt WR, Creager MA. Cholesterol reduction with atorvastatin improves walking distance in patients with peripheral arterial disease. Circulation. 2003;108:1481–6.
52. Gardner AW, Poehlman ET. Exercise rehabilitation programs for the treatment of claudication pain. A meta-analysis. JAMA. 1995;274:975–80.
53. Stewart KJ, Hiatt WR, Regensteiner JG, et al. Exercise training for claudication. N Engl J Med. 2002;347:1941–51.
54. Ahimastos AA, Pappas EP, Buttner PG, Walker PJ, Kingwell BA, Golledge J. A meta-analysis of the outcome of endovascular and noninvasive therapies in the treatment of intermittent claudication. J Vasc Surg. 2011;54:1511–21.
55. Whyman MR, Fowkes FG, Kerracher EM, Gillespie IN, Lee AJ, Housley E, Ruckley CV. Is intermittent claudication improved by percutaneous transluminal angioplasty? A randomized controlled trial. J Vasc Surg. 1997;26:551–7.
56. Perkins JM, Collin J, Creasy TS, Fletcher EW, Morris PJ. Exercise training versus angioplasty for stable claudication. Long and medium term results of a prospective, randomised trial. Eur J Vasc Endovasc Surg. 1996;11:409–13.
57. Gelin J, Jivegård L, Taft C, Karlsson J, Sullivan M, Dahllöf AG, Sandström R, Arfvidsson B, Lundholm K. Treatment efficacy of intermittent claudication by surgical intervention, supervised physical exercise training compared to no treatment in unselected randomised patients I: one year results of functional and physiological improvements. Eur J Vasc Endovasc Surg. 2001;22: 107–13.
58. Hunink MG, Wong JB, Donaldson MC, Meyerovitz MF, de Vries J, Harrington DP. Revascularization for femoropopliteal disease. A decision and cost-effectiveness analysis. JAMA. 1995;274: 165–71.
59. Taylor SM, Kalbaugh CA, Healy MG, Cass AL, Gray BH, Langan III EM, Cull DL, Carsten III CG, York JW, Snyder BA, Youkey JR. Do current outcomes justify more liberal use of revascularization for vasculogenic claudication? A single center experience of 1,000 consecutively treated limbs. J Am Coll Surg. 2008;206: 1053–62.
60. Murphy TP, Cutlip DE, Regensteiner JG, Mohler ER, Cohen DJ, Reynolds MR, et al. Supervised exercise versus primary stenting for claudication resulting from aortoiliac peripheral artery disease: six-month outcomes from the claudication: exercise versus endoluminal revascularization (CLEVER) study. Circulation. 2012;125:130–9.
61. Frans FA, Bipat S, Reekers JA, Legemate DA, Koelemay MJ. Systematic review of exercise training or percutaneous transluminal angioplasty for intermittent claudication. Br J Surg. 2012;99:16–28.
62. Dormandy JA, Rutherford RB. Management of peripheral arterial disease (PAD). TASC Working Group. TransAtlantic Inter-Society Consensus (TASC). J Vasc Surg. 2000;31:S1–296.

63. Nelson PR, Powell RJ, Schermerhorn ML, Fillinger MF, Zwolak RM, Walsh DB, Cronenwett JL. Early results of external iliac artery stenting combined with common femoral artery endarterectomy. J Vasc Surg. 2002;35:1107–13.
64. Dosluoglu HH, Lall P, Cherr GS, Harris LM, Dryjski ML. Role of simple and complex hybrid revascularization procedures for symptomatic lower extremity occlusive disease. J Vasc Surg. 2010;51:1425–35.
65. Ebaugh JL, Gagnon D, Owens CD, Conte MS, Raffetto JD. Comparison of costs of staged versus simultaneous lower extremity arterial hybrid procedures. Am J Surg. 2008;196:634–40.
66. Kashyap VS, Pavkov ML, Bena JF, Sarac TP, O'Hara PJ, Lyden SP, Clair DG. The management of severe aortoiliac occlusive disease: endovascular therapy rivals open reconstruction. J Vasc Surg. 2008;48:1451–7.
67. Piazza M, Ricotta II JJ, Bower TC, Kalra M, Duncan AA, Cha S, Gloviczki P. Iliac artery stenting combined with open femoral endarterectomy is as effective as open surgical reconstruction for severe iliac and common femoral occlusive disease. J Vasc Surg. 2011;54:402–11.
68. Upchurch GR, Dimick JB, Wainess RM, et al. Diffusion of new technology in health care: the case of aorto-iliac occlusive disease. Surgery. 2004;136:812.
69. Parsons RE, Suggs WD, Lee JJ, et al. Percutaneous transluminal angioplasty for the treatment of limb threatening ischemia: do the results justify an attempt before bypass grafting? J Vasc Surg. 1998;28:1066–71.
70. Bosch JL, Hunink MG. Meta-analysis of the results of percutaneous transluminal angioplasty and stent placement for aortoiliac occlusive disease. Radiology. 1997;204:87–96.
71. Klein WM, van der Graaf Y, Seegers J, et al. Long-term cardiovascular morbidity, mortality, and reintervention after endovascular treatment in patients with iliac artery disease: the Dutch Iliac Stent Trial Study. Radiology. 2004;232:491–8.
72. Galaria II, Davies MG. Percutaneous transluminal revascularization for iliac occlusive disease: long-term outcomes in TransAtlantic Inter-Society Consensus A and B lesions. Ann Vasc Surg. 2005;19:352–60.
73. Dosluoglu HH, Cherr GS, Lall P, Harris LM, Dryjski ML. Stenting vs. above-knee polytetrafluoroethylene bypass for TransAtlantic Inter-Society Consensus-II (TASC-II) C and D superficial femoral artery disease. J Vasc Surg. 2008;48:1166–74.
74. Pereira CE, Albers M, Romiti M, Brochado-Neto FC, Pereira CAB. Meta-analysis of femoropopliteal bypass grafts for lower extremity arterial insufficiency. J Vasc Surg. 2006;44:510–17.
75. Scott EC, Biuckians A, Light RE, Scibelli CD, Milner TP, Meier III GH, Panneton JM. Subintimal angioplasty for the treatment of claudication and critical limb ischemia: 3-year results. J Vasc Surg. 2007;46:959–64.
76. Schillinger M, Sabeti S, Dick P, Amighi J, Mlekusch W, Schlager O, et al. Sustained benefit at 2 years of primary femoropopliteal stenting compared with balloon angioplasty with optional stenting. Circulation. 2007;115:2745–9.
77. Krankenberg H, Schlüter M, Steinkamp HJ, Bürgelin K, Scheinert D, Schulte KL, Minar E, Peeters P, Bosiers M, Tepe G, Reimers B, Mahler F, Tübler T, Zeller T. Nitinol stent implantation versus percutaneous transluminal angioplasty in superficial femoral artery lesions up to 10 cm in length: the femoral artery stenting trial (FAST). Circulation. 2007;116:285–92.
78. Dick P, Wallner H, Sabeti S, Loewe C, Mlekusch W, Lammer J, Koppensteiner R, Minar E, Schillinger M. Balloon angioplasty versus stenting with nitinol stents in intermediate length superficial femoral artery lesions. Catheter Cardiovasc Interv. 2009; 74:1090–5.
79. Bosiers M, Torsello G, Gissler HM, Ruef J, Müller-Hülsbeck S, Jahnke T, Peeters P, Daenens K, Lammer J, Schroë H, Mathias K, Koppensteiner R, Vermassen F, Scheinert D. Nitinol stent implantation in long superficial femoral artery lesions: 12-month results of the DURABILITY I study. J Endovasc Ther. 2009;16: 261–9.
80. Laird JR, Katzen BT, Scheinert D, Lammer J, Carpenter J, Buchbinder M, Dave R, Ansel G, Lansky A, Cristea E, Collins TJ, Goldstein J, Cao AY, Jaff MR, RESILIENT Investigators. Nitinol stent implantation vs balloon angioplasty for lesions in the superficial femoral and proximal popliteal arteries of patients with claudication: three-year follow-up from the RESILIENT randomized trial. J Endovasc Ther. 2012;19:1–9.
81. Dake MD, Ansel GM, Jaff MR, Ohki T, Saxon RR, Smouse HB, Zeller T, Roubin GS, Burket MW, Khatib Y, Snyder SA, Ragheb AO, White JK, Machan LS, Zilver PTX Investigators. Paclitaxel-eluting stents show superiority to balloon angioplasty and bare metal stents in femoropopliteal disease: twelve-month Zilver PTX randomized study results. Circ Cardiovasc Interv. 2011;4: 495–504.

7 Critical Limb Ischemia

Michael A. Golden and Brant W. Ullery

Introduction

Critical limb ischemia (CLI) represents the most severe clinical manifestation of lower extremity peripheral arterial disease (PAD) and is defined as the presence of ischemic rest pain, nonhealing ulcers, or gangrene attributable to objectively proven arterial occlusive disease [1]. Patients with CLI occupy the extreme end of the PAD spectrum and fall into the severe disease categories according to the Fontaine (stages III or IV) and Rutherford (category 4–6) clinical staging systems for PAD (Table 7.1). Symptoms lasting longer than 2 weeks distinguish CLI from acute limb ischemia.

While the presence of PAD implies an imbalance of arterial blood supply versus demand, the arterial disease observed in CLI is severe enough that perfusion fails to meet the resting metabolic requirements of the tissues. The chronic lack of blood flow initiates a cascade of pathophysiologic events that ultimately leads to rest pain or trophic changes of the lower extremity or both. Critical limb ischemia usually results from severe atherosclerotic stenoses or occlusions at two or more levels of the lower extremity arterial tree. This multi-level disease pattern severely diminishes flow through collateral beds leading to limb-threatening ischemia. Other less common etiologies of CLI include atheroembolic or thromboembolic diseases, vasculitis, in situ thrombosis related to hypercoagulable states, popliteal artery entrapment, trauma, cystic adventitial disease, and thromboangiitis obliterans [2]. Regardless of the underlying cause, the pathogenesis of CLI involves a complex array of changes to the macrovascular and microvascular systems and surrounding tissues of the lower extremity [3].

M.A. Golden, MD (✉)
Division of Vascular Surgery and Endovascular Therapy,
Department of Surgery, Penn Presbyterian Medical Center,
51 North 39th Street, Wright-Saunders, Suite 266, Philadelphia,
PA 19104, USA
e-mail: Michael.Golden@uphs.upenn.edu

B.W. Ullery, MD
Division of Vascular Surgery and Endovascular Therapy,
Department of Surgery, University of Pennsylvania,
Philadelphia, PA, USA

Clinical Manifestations

Claudication

Intermittent claudication occurs due to relative muscle ischemia from a transient imbalance between arterial blood supply and demand. Patients with claudication have reproducible discomfort of a defined group of muscles that is induced by exercise and relieved with rest. The lower extremity discomfort predictably occurs one level distal to the anatomic location of arterial occlusive lesions; however, symptoms can vary widely in distribution and severity. Buttock and hip discomfort usually correlates to aortoiliac disease, whereas thigh discomfort is associated with aortoiliac or common femoral artery disease, upper calf discomfort is associated with superficial femoral artery disease, lower calf pain is associated with popliteal artery disease, and discomfort at the level of the foot or instep is associated with tibioperoneal arterial disease. Claudication, even in its most severe form, does not imply limb-threatening ischemia or impending CLI. Symptoms of claudication usually remain stable over time, and very few patients with claudication progress to CLI. The majority of patients with CLI do not have a history of slowly worsening claudication. Instead, they have debilitating ischemic ulcers and gangrene at the time of their initial presentation.

Rest Pain

Ischemic rest pain is characterized by severe burning pain localized to the forefoot and toes of a chronically ischemic lower extremity. Such diffuse pedal ischemia is associated with a systolic arterial blood pressure less than 40 mmHg at the

V. Gahtan and M.J. Costanza (eds.), *Essentials of Vascular Surgery for the General Surgeon*,
DOI 10.1007/978-1-4939-1326-8_7, © Springer Science+Business Media New York 2015

Table 7.1 Classification of peripheral arterial disease: Fontaine's stages and Rutherford's categories

Fontaine		Rutherford			
Stage	Clinical	Grade	Category	Clinical	
I	Asymptomatic	0	0	Asymptomatic	
IIa	Mild claudication	I	1	Mild claudication	
IIb	Moderate to severe claudication	I	2	Moderate claudication	
		I	3	Severe claudication	
III	Ischemic rest pain	II	4	Ischemic rest pain	*Critical limb ischemia*
IV	Ulceration or gangrene	III	5	Minor tissue loss	
		III	6	Major tissue loss	

Modified from Norgren et al. [1]

ankle and less than 30 mmHg at the toes [4]. The discomfort associated with rest pain is often refractory to analgesics and can be prompted or aggravated by elevation of the lower extremity. Patients frequently experience ischemic rest pain at night owing to the relative elevation of the lower extremity during the recumbent or reclining position assumed while trying to sleep. Limb dependency, on the other hand, typically results in symptomatic improvement or sometimes complete resolution of discomfort in the lower extremity. This tendency to keep the ischemic lower extremity in a dependent position explains why some patients with CLI present with symptoms of lower extremity edema.

Ischemic Ulcer

An ischemic ulcer forms after an initial break in the integrity of the skin as a result of soft tissue trauma. Such trauma is typically mild and occurs at sites of increased focal pressure in the lower extremity such as the lateral malleolus, metatarsal heads, or distal extent of the toes. Due to impaired oxygenation and inadequate blood flow to the site of injury, breaks in the skin fail to heal and persist as chronic, painful erosions [5]. Ischemic ulcers are usually dry and punctate and may be associated with other signs of chronic lower extremity ischemia, including rest pain, hair loss, skin atrophy, nail hypertrophy, and pallor. The aching or burning pain that patients with ischemic ulcers experience results from both chronic severe ischemic neuropathy and the presence of sensory nerves at the site of the ulcer.

Gangrene

Tissue necrosis, or gangrene, occurs when the vascular supply of the lower extremity fails to maintain cellular viability. The lower extremity may appear cyanotic with anesthetic tissue that is associated with or progresses to frank necrosis. The extent of gangrene can range from a single digit to the entire lower extremity depending on the severity of underlying PAD and local resting metabolic requirements. Patients may initially describe severe pain due to a variety of factors, including ischemic neuropathy, osteomyelitis, coexisting ascending infection, or associated ischemic injury to the skin and subcutaneous sensory nerves. Pain typically abates with the progression of gangrene due to ischemic necrosis of the sensory nerves and surrounding tissues.

Gangrene is described as either dry or wet based on clinical examination. Dry gangrene appears gradually and progresses slowly. Tissue becomes cold and has a characteristic hard, dry texture that ultimately sloughs off. Dry gangrene can result from embolization to the toe or forefoot and usually produces a clear demarcation between viable and necrotic tissue. A clearly demarcated digit or forefoot may autoamputate without proximal progression of gangrene. Due to the rather slow and emotionally disturbing nature of demarcation, an elective amputation of the involved portion of the lower extremity provides a more acceptable alternative. Most patients have inadequate arterial perfusion to heal the distal amputation site and therefore require a revascularization procedure for limb salvage.

Wet gangrene is a life-threatening complication of an untreated infected wound, which requires emergency surgery. Infection of the extremity by saprogenic microorganisms such as *Clostridium perfringens* produces soft tissue edema and cessation of local arterial and venous blood flow. The stagnant blood pools in the lower extremity and promotes further rapid bacterial proliferation. Bacterial toxins are absorbed by the surrounding tissue of the lower extremity resulting in fulminant sepsis and death if not treated promptly with intravenous antibiotics and debridement or amputation. Wet gangrene represents the progression of coagulative necrosis to liquefactive necrosis, with the affected limb featuring a moist, edematous, soft, and often blistering appearance.

Patient Evaluation

Diagnosis

Clinical History

The evaluation of a patient with PAD begins with a detailed history and careful physical examination. Although patients with PAD may report limitations in exercise performance and walking ability, the 2005 American College of Cardiology/American Heart Association (ACC/AHA) guidelines on PAD suggest that only 10–35 % of patients present with classic claudication symptoms (Fig. 7.1) [2]. Less than 3 % of patients present with symptoms of CLI. Instead, the majority of patients with PAD are either asymptomatic or complain of atypical leg pain at initial clinical presentation. An estimated 5–10 % of patients with asymptomatic PAD or claudication will progress to CLI within 5 years.

Identification of risk factors for PAD can aid in distinguishing symptoms of PAD from other less common causes of lower extremity ischemia such as radiation fibrosis, fibromuscular dysplasia, popliteal entrapment, vasculitis, and adventitial cystic disease. Non-arterial and nonvascular pathologies should also be considered in the differential diagnosis of lower extremity discomfort, including deep venous thrombosis, peripheral neuropathy, spinal stenosis, and musculoskeletal disorders. Because atherosclerosis is a systemic disease, the risk factors for PAD mirror those of coronary artery disease. In patients with a history of hypertension, tobacco use, diabetes mellitus, chronic renal failure, and dyslipidemia, PAD is more likely to be the underlying cause of their lower extremity complaints [6–9]. The 2005 ACC/AHA guidelines also identified the following groups to be at increased risk for lower extremity PAD: age ≥70 years, age 50–69 years with a history of smoking or diabetes, and age 40–49 with diabetes and at least one additional risk factor for atherosclerosis, leg symptoms suggestive of claudication with exertion or ischemic pain at rest, abnormal lower extremity pulse examination, and those patients with known atherosclerosis at other anatomic sites (e.g., coronary, carotid, or renal artery disease) [2].

Physical Examination

Clinical findings consistent with PAD include cool temperature of the leg, absent or diminished pulses in the legs or feet, thin or shiny appearance of the skin, hair loss, nonhealing wounds or gangrene, pallor with elevation of the extremity, dependent rubor (foot redness with dependent position), and hypertrophic changes of the toenails. Patients may also demonstrate restricted mobility as a result of numbness, weakness, or heaviness in the muscles of the leg. Examination in patients with suspected lower extremity arterial disease should include a thorough search for the presence and strength of all lower extremity pulses, as well as evaluation for cardiac murmurs, bruits, and aneurysms. Pulses should be assessed on both legs at all levels and any abnormalities correlated with lower extremity symptoms to determine lateralization of occlusive disease. A diminished or absent femoral pulse suggests inflow disease due to aortoiliac occlusive lesions. A normal femoral but absent distal pulse suggests preserved inflow but impaired infrainguinal outflow to the leg.

Despite the utility of the pulse examination, physical exam of the femoral artery pulse has been shown to be little better than relying on subjective symptoms of claudication to diagnose large-vessel PAD. Moreover, the absence of pedal pulses tends to overdiagnose PAD as evidenced by the fact that only 18 % of patients with abnormal posterior tibial pulses have additional objective evidence of PAD [10]. The diagnosis of PAD in suspected patients must therefore be confirmed using noninvasive screening tests and, if needed, other hemodynamic or imaging studies.

Routine Noninvasive Vascular Screening Studies

The resting ankle-brachial systolic pressure index (ABI) should be performed in all patients with a clinical history and/or physical exam suggestive of PAD. This chapter describes the technique for measuring an ABI.

The normal reference range for ABI is 0.90–1.2. A decreased ABI in symptomatic patients confirms the presence of hemodynamically significant peripheral arterial occlusive disease between the heart and ankle, with a lower ABI correlating with more severe occlusive disease. An ABI of less than 0.90 is 95 % sensitive in identifying

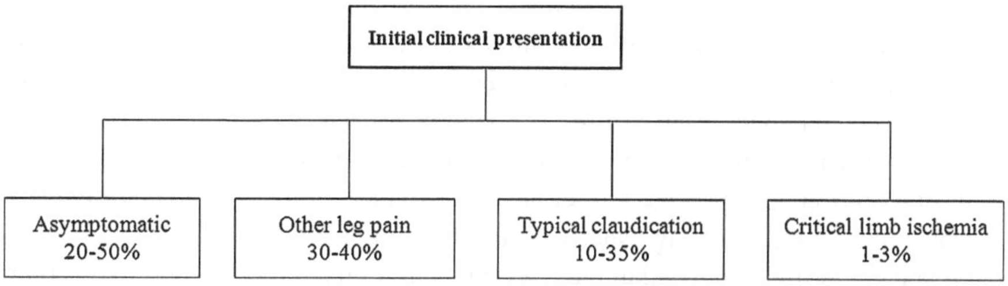

Fig. 7.1 Initial clinical presentation of patients with peripheral arterial disease (PAD)

angiographically confirmed PAD [1, 11]. Patients with claudication generally have an ABI in the range of 0.40–0.90, whereas those with rest pain or tissue loss have an ABI in the range of 0.20–0.50 and zero to 0.40, respectively. It is important to note, however, that over 50 % of patients with an abnormal ABI will fail to demonstrate typical symptoms of claudication or CLI due to the presence of other major comorbidities [1]. In addition to its ability to detect PAD, the ABI may also function as a marker for systemic atherosclerotic disease. Several studies have noted a strong correlation between ABI and mortality [12–14], with one report even noting a near linear relationship between ABI and fatal and nonfatal cardiovascular events [13].

Significant arterial calcification causes blood vessel incompressibility which will falsely elevate the ABI. In such cases, a toe-brachial index may be used to diagnose PAD as digital vessels are often spared from calcification. The toe-brachial index is calculated by dividing the toe systolic pressure by the highest brachial systolic pressure and can be measured by a noninvasive vascular lab using small blood pressure cuffs. A normal toe-brachial index is greater than 0.70. Most cases of CLI are associated with ankle systolic blood pressures less than 50 mmHg or toe systolic blood pressures less than 30 mmHg. Foot lesions usually heal when toe pressure exceeds 30–40 mmHg (or slightly higher in diabetic patients).

To evaluate PAD in more detail, the noninvasive vascular lab can perform segmental limb systolic pressures, plethysmography, Doppler waveform analysis, and exercise testing. More details of these exams can be found in this chapter.

Pre-intervention Imaging

Imaging studies are not required to confirm the diagnosis nor should they be used as first-line screening tests for CLI or PAD. The primary role of imaging studies involves treatment planning for patients who require revascularization for limb salvage. Imaging exams create an arterial road map that helps determine what, if any, endovascular and surgical therapy options are feasible.

Duplex Ultrasound

Duplex ultrasound provides a reliable and inexpensive imaging option to evaluate arterial occlusive disease and other vascular pathologies. Capabilities of duplex ultrasonography include the ability to differentiate stenoses from occlusions, characterize the occlusive nature of specific arterial segments, evaluate for arterial trauma, assess adequacy of surgical intervention, and provide surveillance for bypass grafts. Duplex ultrasound scanning usually proceeds from proximal to distal, recording artery diameter, presence and character of atherosclerosis, and velocity spectral waveform. In stenotic lesions that significantly reduce the vessel diameter, arterial flow becomes turbulent with increased systolic and diastolic velocities. Velocity criteria can classify the severity of the lesion with greater than 80 % accuracy depending on the arterial segment scanned.

Although the exam quality depends on the technical skill of the sonographer, duplex ultrasound has proven to be a sensitive and specific test for arterial occlusive disease. A meta-analysis of 14 studies demonstrated the sensitivity and specificity of duplex scanning for ≥50 % stenosis or occlusion to be 86 and 97 % for aortoiliac disease and 80 and 98 % for femoropopliteal disease [15]. In a recent prospective, blinded study, Eiberg et al. [16] compared duplex ultrasound scans to the angiographic findings in 42 patients with claudication and 127 patients with CLI. The interobserver agreement between duplex ultrasound and angiography was generally good with both techniques independent of the severity of PAD. Duplex ultrasound was noted to perform better in the supragenicular arteries than in the infragenicular arteries but still compared favorably with angiography down to the level of the tibial vessels. Several additional studies reported a similar correlation between these two imaging studies [17–19]. Such findings support duplex ultrasound as a useful noninvasive alternative to conventional contrast angiography, particularly among those patients with renal failure and contrast allergies.

Computed Tomographic Angiography

Multidetector computed tomographic angiography (CTA) allows for the rapid acquisition of high-resolution, contrast-enhanced arterial images. The CTA images can then be reviewed in multiple projections and reconstructions to illustrate artertial anatomy, localize occlusive disease, and detect vessel wall calcification. The abundance of information gained from CTA has made it a widely used exam for treatment planning. A meta-analysis of 12 studies evaluating 9,541 arterial segments in 436 patients showed that multidetector CTA detected greater than 50 % segmental stenosis with a pooled sensitivity and specificity of 92 and 93 %, respectively [20]. The diagnostic performance of CTA was noted to be lower in the infrapopliteal arteries but not significantly different from that observed in the aortoiliac or femoropopliteal arterial systems. More recently, a meta-analysis published in 2009 of 20 studies similarly compared the diagnostic performance of CTA to the reference standard contrast angiography for the evaluation of 19,092 lower extremity arterial segments in 957 symptomatic patients [21]. The overall sensitivity and specificity of CTA in that analysis was 95 and 96 %, respectively.

The drawbacks of CTA include its high cost and the associated exposure to both ionizing radiation and intravenous nephrotoxic contrast agents. CTA requires an intravenous bolus of more than 100 mL of iodinated contrast in the average adult, making it less desirable for patients with chronic renal insufficiency (estimated glomerular filtration rate (eGFR) <60 ml/kg/min). An imaging pitfall specific to CTA involves the use of narrow window settings to optimize image quality in the presence of arterial wall calcifications or previously placed stents. These imaging settings may overestimate the degree of stenosis or suggest a spurious arterial occlusion. In patients with diabetes or ESRD, extensive atherosclerotic calcification within small crural or pedal arteries may make it impossible to detect a patent vessel lumen regardless of the window/level selection. Fortunately, most of these artifacts are easily identified by examining additional views, complementary imaging modalities, or source images [22].

Magnetic Resonance Angiography

Three-dimensional gadolinium-enhanced magnetic resonance angiography (MRA) offers an increasingly common noninvasive option to assess the peripheral vasculature without the need for sedation, catheterization, ionizing radiation, or iodinated contrast agents. The sensitivity and specificity for the detection of greater than 50 % arterial stenoses or occlusions using this modality exceed 90 % [23–25]. Owen and colleagues [26] conducted a prospective comparative study of 30 patients who underwent both MRA and contrast angiography. Evaluation of 390 arterial segments in these patients demonstrated a higher sensitivity in distal segments (92–96 %) compared with more proximal segments (69–79 %). Specificity was similar in both distal (90–91 %) and proximal segments (86–96 %).

Magnetic resonance angiography generates a three-dimensional data set that can be reformatted to reproduce digital subtraction angiography-like vascular images that feature details pertinent to prognosis and treatment planning, including those related to the thrombus characteristics, plaque composition, presence of dissection, or extent of arterial wall inflammation. An MRA's ability to image arteries and the surrounding musculoskeletal structures also makes it ideal for evaluating patients with popliteal artery entrapment syndrome.

There is increasing evidence to suggest that some patients with renal failure who are exposed to gadolinium-based magnetic resonance imaging contrast agents may develop a rare but serious fibrosing disorder referred to as nephrogenic systemic fibrosis (NSF). This disorder is characterized by hardening of the skin and development of fibrotic nodules and plaques. In its most severe form, NSF may result in systemic fibrosis affecting solid organs such as the lungs, heart, and liver [27, 28]. Current clinical guidelines advise against the use of gadolinium in patients with an eGFR less than 30 ml/kg/min. An MRA is also not appropriate for claustrophobic patients or patients with pacemakers or metallic implants.

Contrast Angiography

Digital subtraction angiography (DSA) remains the gold standard imaging modality in peripheral vascular surgery. Angiography should usually be reserved for patients who are expected to undergo attempted revascularization. The exam begins with percutaneous needle access to the common femoral artery in the contralateral limb to allow complete imaging of the inflow, diseased segment, and outflow vessels. DSA involves the generation of fluoroscopic images by subtracting a pre-contrast image from images taken after the administration of an intra-arterial contrast medium, thereby producing a net image showing only contrast-filled blood vessels. The combination of excellent spatial and temporal resolution and a large field of view allows for rapid imaging of the entire peripheral arterial tree. A complete evaluation of the aorta, iliac, femoral, popliteal, and tibioperoneal vessels may be performed simultaneously or, more commonly, sequentially with overlapping runs. In addition, the presence and extent of collateral blood flow can be readily evaluated with this form of imaging. In some cases, measuring the pressure gradients across an arterial lesion (usually in the aortoiliac segment) can increase the arteriogram's sensitivity and gauge the response to intervention. Hemodynamically significant lesions have a resting systolic pressure gradient which exceeds 20 mmHg.

The clinical utility of angiography must be balanced against the fact that it represents an invasive form of imaging. Angiography requires arterial access, ionizing radiation, and nephrotoxic contrast exposure. Potential complications of angiography include distal atheroembolization, arterial dissection, and access site complications (e.g., pseudoaneurysm, hematoma, thrombosis, arteriovenous fistula). DSA imaging requires a stationary target, and any patient movement will produce significant artifact. Optimizing technical factors such as frame rate, contrast injection volume, and C-arm projection angle will also produce the highest-quality images.

Cardiac Risk Stratification

Cardiovascular events are the most significant complication in patients undergoing vascular surgery. Lower extremity revascularization is classified as a high-risk surgery according to the ACC/AHA preoperative assessment guidelines and carries a combined incidence of cardiac death and nonfatal myocardial infarction of greater than 5 % [2]. The increased rate of cardiovascular complications stems from the fact that patients in need of revascularization belong to a subgroup of high-risk patients who have a corresponding high incidence of CAD and left ventricular systolic dysfunction compared to matched controls [29–31]. Additional clinical predictors of increased perioperative cardiovascular risk include unstable coronary syndromes, decompensated congestive heart failure, significant arrhythmias, and severe valvular heart disease [32]. In this patient population with compromised baseline cardiac function, physiologic stressors associated with vascular surgery such as blood loss, volume shifts, and hemodynamic fluctuations may have a greater impact which further increases their risk of perioperative myocardial ischemia.

The 2007 ACC/AHA guidelines recommend that the estimation of perioperative risk should integrate major, intermediate, and minor predictors of cardiac risk, functional capacity, surgery-specific risk, and, when indicated, the results of noninvasive tests, including stress testing and echocardiography (Table 7.2) [1, 32]. This systematic approach subjects only a minority of patients ultimately to invasive preoperative evaluation, while some patients can forego noninvasive evaluation completely. According to the ACC/AHA guidelines, patients without active cardiac symptoms scheduled for low-risk vascular surgery and those with good functional capacity require no preoperative testing beyond a 12-lead electrocardiogram [2, 33]. Patients with poor or unknown functional capacity or cardiac symptoms are managed according to the number of clinical risk factors. Patients with one or two risk factors can proceed with surgery unless testing will alter management, whereas noninvasive testing is generally recommended for patients with three or more risk factors. Additional evaluation allows refinement of the initial risk estimate and may include exercise or pharmacologic stress testing, resting echocardiography, and/or preoperative cardiac catheterization and coronary revascularization. The aforementioned guidelines are based on preoperative evaluation of patients undergoing elective surgery. Patients requiring urgent or emergent vascular procedures are unlikely to derive benefit from delaying surgery for additional testing and medical management and should proceed directly to surgery.

Table 7.2 Clinical predictors of cardiac risk

Major	Unstable coronary syndromes
	Unstable or severe angina
	Recent myocardial infarction
	Decompensated heart failure
	Significant arrhythmias
	Severe valvular disease
Intermediate	History of heart disease
	History of compensated or prior heart failure
	History of cerebrovascular disease
	Diabetes mellitus
	Renal insufficiency
Minor	Advanced age (>70 years)
	Abnormal electrocardiogram,
	e.g., left ventricular hypertrophy, ST-T abnormalities
	Rhythm other than sinus
	Uncontrolled systemic hypertension

Modified from Fleisher et al. [32]

Treatment

Information pertaining to the natural history of nonrevascularized lower extremities in patients with CLI is extrapolated from the placebo arms of pharmacotherapy trials performed on patients with unreconstructable peripheral arterial occlusive disease. Unlike the often benign nature of intermittent claudication, nearly 40 % of patients with CLI will progress to amputation within 6 months in the absence of revascularization [34]. Given this dismal prognosis, revascularization plays a prominent role in the overall treatment plan for functional patients with CLI (Fig. 7.2). The primary treatment goals for CLI include relief of ischemic rest pain, healing of ischemic ulcers, limb salvage, improvement of patient function and quality of life, and increased survival.

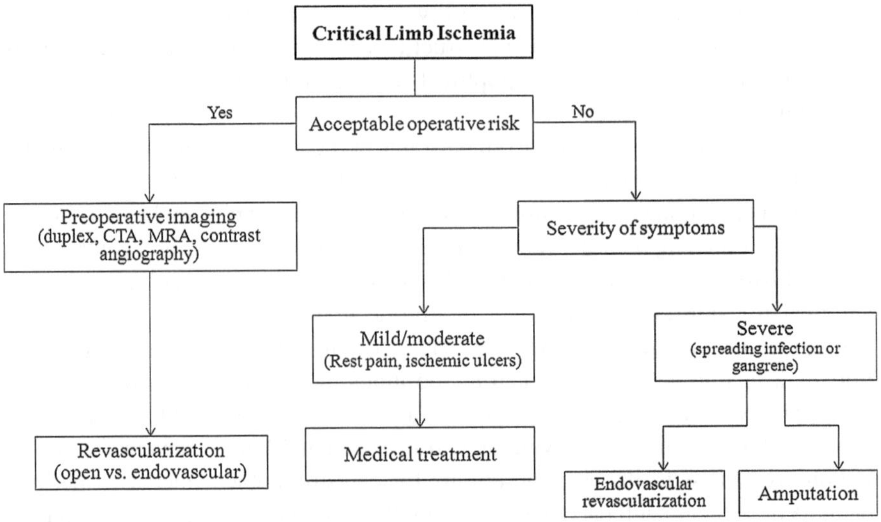

Fig. 7.2 Algorithm for managing patients with critical limb ischemia

Concomitant medical therapy provides an important adjunct to revascularization as it plays an essential role in controlling ischemic neuropathy, treating or preventing coexisting infections in critically ischemic lower extremities, halting progression of systemic atherosclerosis, and managing the underlying cardiovascular risk profile of patients.

It is important to emphasize that medical and surgical treatments for CLI are not mutually exclusive. In fact, it is imperative that all patients with CLI receive medical therapy, whether or not they are candidates to undergo invasive revascularization. To the extent possible, patients should commit to regular exercise, healthy eating habits, and aggressive risk factor modification, including smoking cessation, blood pressure control, reduction in fasting blood glucose levels, and lipid-lowering therapy, as indicated. Antiplatelet and statin therapy also appears to be beneficial. Strict compliance with medical therapy will have a profound impact on the patient's prognosis and the ultimate success of any revascularization strategy.

Revascularization

Despite a paucity of level I evidence to support proposed treatment algorithms in PAD, surgical bypass has long been considered the gold standard method of revascularization across the PAD spectrum. Continued development of catheter-based technology has expanded the revascularization options such that endovascular intervention is now considered to be a suitable primary therapeutic alternative. The utilization of one approach over another may reflect a generational change in the treatment of lower extremity ischemia, with recently trained vascular surgeons performing a disproportionately higher number of endovascular procedures compared to their older colleagues. The role of endovascular therapy in the treatment of CLI continues to evolve, and its ultimate role will be determined by ongoing technical refinements, growing clinical experience, and the clarification of long-term outcomes and costs.

The Bypass versus Angioplasty in Severe Ischemia of the Leg (BASIL) trial is the only randomized controlled trial to date comparing the efficacy of balloon angioplasty-first versus bypass surgery-first treatment strategies in patients with CLI [35]. In their initial 2005 report, BASIL investigators noted no difference in short-term clinical outcomes but did find that surgery was associated with increased morbidity (57 % vs. 41 %) and greater expense during the first 12 months. Post hoc analysis showed that beyond 2 years from intervention, patients initially randomized to bypass surgery were more likely to be alive and without limb amputation. To further explore this finding, patients were monitored for an additional 2.5 years and analyzed on an intent-to-treat basis, and results were published in 2010 as an extension of the BASIL study [36]. This analysis revealed that patients who survived for 2 years and who were initially randomized to bypass surgery gained a significant 7.3 months (95 % CI, 1.2–13.4 months, $P=0.02$) of additional life expectancy and an additional nearly significant 5.9 months (95 % CI, 0.2–12.0 months, $P=0.06$) of amputation-free survival over the subsequent follow-up period compared to those initially randomized to the angioplasty-first treatment strategy.

It is important to note several limitations in the BASIL study. First, the study cohort in the BASIL trial was limited to those with CLI due to infrainguinal occlusive disease. Results in such patients cannot be generalized to those with CLI resulting from aortoiliac occlusive disease. Second, the BASIL trial began its 5-year enrollment in 1999, and the results must be interpreted with caution given that over a decade of technological advancement has passed since the study began. Moreover, stenting of the infrainguinal arteries was not considered standard of care in the United Kingdom at the time of the trial, evidenced by the fact that only 9 out of 224 patients randomized to the angioplasty-first strategy had angioplasty combined with stent placement.

The updated ACC/AHA guidelines for the management of PAD stem from the BASIL trial and are consistent with recommendations made by the BASIL trial investigators [33]. Patients with CLI who have a life expectancy or course of disease projected to exceed 2 years are probably better served with a bypass surgery-first strategy, preferably using autogenous vein. Those with CLI who have a life expectancy of less than 2 years, and potentially those who do not have autogenous vein for use as a conduit, are probably better served with an angioplasty-first strategy given that their limited survival precludes them from achieving the potential longer-term benefits of surgery. Moreover, patients deemed to have limited preoperative survival may be more vulnerable to suffer postoperative morbidity and mortality, thereby making the less expensive, minimally invasive nature of endovascular therapy a more appropriate option in this subgroup of patients.

Determining the optimal method of revascularization in CLI is based on a balance between the risks of the specific intervention and the degree and durability of improvement that can be expected from the intervention [1]. The efficacy of any revascularization attempt depends on the arterial inflow, distal outflow, size and length of the diseased arterial segment, degree of systemic disease, and type of procedure performed. Adequate inflow and sufficient outflow are essential in order to maintain long-term patency of any arterial reconstruction. Among patients with concomitant inflow (suprainguinal) and outflow (infrainguinal) disease, the ACC/AHA guidelines recommend that inflow lesions be treated first independent of the chosen treatment strategy [2]. Subsequent revascularization of outflow disease is indicated if the ABI remains less than 0.8 in the presence of ongoing infection, ischemic ulcers, or gangrene.

The Lower Extremity Grading System (LEGS) score offers an outcome-based standardization tool for lower extremity arterial interventions in patients with either claudication or CLI [37]. The score consists of five objective criteria: angiographic pattern of disease, presenting complaints, functional status of the patient, medical comorbidities, and technical factors. The composite LEGS score determines the recommended interventional treatment strategy which may involve endovascular therapy, open surgery, or major limb amputation. Prospective studies demonstrated that patients treated according to the LEGS algorithm had higher rates of limb salvage, patency of arterial reconstruction, and maintenance of ambulation compared to those treated with strategies contrary to LEGS.

Patients with claudication generally have superior patency rates compared to patients with CLI across nearly all forms of arterial reconstruction for chronic lower extremity arterial disease. Since claudicants have less severe arterial occlusive disease and longer life expectancy relative to those with CLI, these patients tend to contribute more to data directed at long-term clinical outcomes. As a result, studies focused primarily on cohorts with low-risk claudicants will report disproportionately better patency and survival data compared to those limited to higher-risk patients with CLI. Most studies report success of revascularization as a function of primary patency, implying uninterrupted patency without the need for re-intervention, or secondary patency, defined as patency of the initially treated vessel following a re-intervention to restore patency after occlusion.

Aortoiliac (Suprainguinal) Revascularization

Severe aortoiliac occlusive disease has been traditionally treated using a variety of open surgical approaches, including aortobifemoral bypass, aortoiliac endarterectomy, iliofemoral bypass, and extra-anatomic bypass. Of these, aortobifemoral bypass has long been considered to be the gold standard treatment for hemodynamically significant aorto-bi-iliac disease in low-risk patients given its safety and efficacy (mortality rate less than 5 %; 5-year patency rates greater than 80 %) [38–41]. The bifurcated bypass graft in this procedure originates from the infrarenal abdominal aorta and routes one limb to each femoral artery via either a transperitoneal or retroperitoneal approach. A preoperative CTA is essential to assess the calcium and thrombus content of the proximal aorta. An aorta with thrombus and plaque extending to the level of renal arteries requires a proximal thromboendarterectomy with a suprarenal aortic clamp in place and the renal arteries controlled with clamps or vessel loops. Once the proximal aortic cuff has been cleared, the clamp can be moved to an infrarenal position and the proximal anastomosis can be performed in an end-to-end or end-to-side fashion. An end-to-end configuration is favored when the aorta is completely occluded to the level of the renal arteries or when severe aortic calcification precludes safe placement of a side-biting clamp. Aortic occlusive disease associated with aneurysmal dilatation also requires an end-to-end reconstruction. An end-to-side configuration has the advantage of maintaining pelvic perfusion in patients with occluded or diseased bilateral external iliac arteries. Preserving distal aortic flow may also be important in patients with a large patent inferior mesenteric artery or accessory renal arteries arising from the infrarenal aorta. The presence of femoral artery occlusive disease requires the addition of a common femoral endarterectomy and profundoplasty. Late complications include graft thrombosis (5–30 %), graft infection (0.5–3.0 %), aortoenteric fistula (<3 %), and anastomotic pseudoaneurysm (1–5 %), which is more common in patients with an end-to-side anastomosis.

More recently, a laparoscopic aortobifemoral bypass has been described as a less invasive alternative to open surgery. Tiek et al. [42] conducted a multicenter randomized controlled trial of 28 patients with TASC C or D aortoiliac occlusive lesions who underwent either open or laparoscopic aortobifemoral bypass. The laparoscopic group had a shorter mean hospital length of stay (5.5 vs. 13.0 days), earlier return to normal daily activities, and fewer postoperative complications compared to the open group. While early studies confirmed the safety of the laparoscopic aortobifemoral bypass, it has not been widely performed and the long-term patency of this approach remains unclear. Future studies may help determine whether laparoscopic aortic surgery is appropriate for a subset of patients with aortoiliac occlusive disease.

Prior to the availability of prosthetic graft material in the 1970s, aortoiliac endarterectomy served as the standard procedure for the treatment of aortoiliac occlusive disease. In a large single-center series of patients who survived over a decade after undergoing either aortoiliac endarterectomy ($n=39$) or aortobifemoral bypass ($n=166$), 10-year primary patency rates were 89 % for aortoiliac endarterectomy and 78 % for aortobifemoral bypass [43]. Graft infection or aneurysmal formation occurred in 5 % of aortobifemoral bypass cases. Aortoiliac endarterectomy has the advantage of potentially avoiding the need for prosthetic material; however, external iliac arteries often prove difficult to endarterectomize. Investigators therefore concluded that aortoiliac endarterectomy is preferable to aortobifemoral bypass in the following circumstances: (1) patients whose aortoiliac occlusive disease does not involve the external iliac arteries; (2) male patients with aortoiliac occlusive disease who, in addition to claudication, have erectile dysfunction and stenotic internal iliac origins; (3) patients with aortoiliac disease including the external iliac arteries who are not candidates for aortobifemoral bypass because of infection risk or small vessels; (4) patients with localized aortoiliac disease; and (5) patients after removal of an infected aortobifemoral bypass graft (with or without an enteric fistula) that had initially been placed end to side for aortoiliac occlusive disease.

Iliofemoral bypass and femorofemoral crossover bypass are additional open surgical options in patients with aortoiliac occlusive disease and are typically indicated in patients with unilateral iliac disease or in patients deemed not suitable for aortobifemoral bypass. In cases of bilateral iliac disease, a femorofemoral bypass may also be constructed as an adjunct to aortoiliac endarterectomy, iliofemoral bypass, or successful unilateral iliac angioplasty and stenting. Iliofemoral bypass appears to be a safe, effective, and durable bypass. Carsten and colleagues [44] reported a 10-year experience comprising 40 patients who underwent iliofemoral bypass grafting for unilateral aortoiliac disease, 58 % of whom had CLI. There were no perioperative deaths in their series, and limb salvage rates in patients with CLI were 85 and 79 % at 1 and 5 years. In addition, a multicenter randomized trial involving 143 patients with TASC type C or D aortoiliac lesions found that late patency was higher after direct iliofemoral bypass compared to femorofemoral crossover bypass in good-risk patients with unilateral iliac occlusive disease not amenable to angioplasty (93 % vs. 73 %). This study underscores the effectiveness of iliofemoral bypass, and the authors concluded that crossover bypass grafting should be reserved for high-risk patients with unilateral iliac occlusion not amenable to percutaneous intervention.

Axillofemoral-femoral bypass consists of a prosthetic bypass originating from the axillary artery and tunneled subcutaneously to the ipsilateral femoral artery with an extension crossing over to the other femoral artery. The primary advantage of this bypass rests in its ability to achieve lower extremity arterial inflow without opening a body cavity or incurring a large blood loss or fluid shift. The procedure can be done under local anesthesia if necessary, and its minimal physiologic impact makes it ideal for critically ill patients who require arterial inflow for limb salvage. It is important to measure blood pressure in both arms before choosing the donor axillary artery. Various configurations of grafts have been used, but none seems to provide a significant advantage over the others.

Although axillofemoral-femoral bypass represents a hemodynamically inferior form of arterial reconstruction, it can achieve a reasonable rate of patency and limb salvage for a challenging subset of high-risk patients. Schneider and colleagues [45] reported primary patency rates of 63 % for axillofemoral bypass and 85 % for aortofemoral bypass ($p=0.032$), with similar trends observed in secondary patency (74 % vs. 94 %, $p<0.001$). Limb salvage at 3 years was 76 % for axillofemoral bypass versus 97 % for aortofemoral bypass ($p=0.065$). As expected with the cohort of higher-risk patients, survival at 3 years was significantly lower in those who underwent axillofemoral bypass compared to aortofemoral bypass (35 % vs. 91 %, $p<0.001$).

Less frequently used extra-anatomic bypasses include the obturator bypass and thoracic aorta to bifemoral (thoracobifemoral) bypass. An obturator bypass avoids an infected or heavily fibrotic groin to provide lower extremity inflow in the setting of unilateral iliac artery occlusion. Thoracobifemoral bypass can provide bilateral lower extremity arterial inflow in patients with a hostile abdomen or multiple previous abdominal aortic procedures.

A recent review encompassing 45 studies and more than 35 years of experience with direct anatomic open surgical revascularization (excluding extra-anatomic reconstruction) for lower extremity arterial occlusive disease found that aortoiliac endarterectomy was associated with significantly lower perioperative local (3.3 %) and systemic (12.5 %) complications and mortality (2.7 %) compared to either aortofemoral or iliofemoral bypass grafting [46]. All three direct revascularization techniques in their analysis proved to be equally effective in terms of 5-year primary patency. The severity of aortoiliac disease influenced the long-term patency following these procedures, with claudication patients experiencing significantly improved 5-year primary patency rates in all three operative approaches compared to patients with CLI (aortobifemoral bypass, 90 % vs. 80 %; iliofemoral bypass, 87 % vs. 74 %; and aortoiliac endarterectomy, 91 % vs. 82 %).

Advances in endovascular therapy have made it an attractive intervention for lower extremity arterial disease that is associated with high technical success rates and low morbidity. Balloon angioplasty and stenting now represents the primary treatment modality in an ever-expanding array of aortoiliac occlusive lesions. Endovascular therapy for CLI attempts to improve arterial inflow to the infrapopliteal vessels by means of revascularization of the aortoiliac and femoropopliteal arterial segments. Ideally, endovascular intervention establishes uninterrupted, straight-line flow to at least one tibial artery that supplies the area of the foot that has rest pain or tissue loss [47]. In contrast to treatment of patients with intermittent claudication, the goal of endovascular therapy for CLI is to simply maintain patency of the occlusive lesion until the area of lower extremity tissue loss is fully healed. Once wound healing is complete, the metabolic demands sharply decrease, and less blood flow will be required to maintain tissue integrity as opposed to the heightened demands required during the healing phase. Any future restenosis of the treated occlusive lesion is likely to be clinically silent in the healed limb. As a result, most studies to date report a similar rate of limb salvage with either surgical or endovascular revascularization despite the superior patency rates observed with open surgical bypass procedures.

A recent systematic review analyzing 19 nonrandomized cohort studies involving 1,711 patients confirmed the safety and efficacy of endovascular treatment for extensive aortoiliac occlusive disease [48]. Technical success, most commonly defined as less than 30 % residual diameter stenosis and/or residual trans-lesion pressure gradient of less than 5–10 mmHg, ranged from 86 to 100 %. Reasons for technical failure included inability to cross an occluded arterial segment, thrombosis following recanalization, or iliac artery rupture. One-year primary and secondary patency ranged from 70 to 97 % and 88 to 100 %, respectively, and clinical symptomatic improvement was reported in 83–100 % of patients across all studies. Longer-term (4- or 5-year) primary and secondary patency rates ranged from 60 to 86 % and 80 to 98 %, respectively. Nearly two-thirds of the studies in this review reported a perioperative morality rate of 0 %, with the remaining seven studies citing a mortality rate of 1.2–6.7 %. The rate of perioperative morbidity varied considerably across studies, ranging from 3 to 45 %, and consisted of access site hematomas (range, 4–7 %), arterial dissections (2–5 %), distal embolization (1–11 %), pseudoaneurysms (0.5–3 %), and iliac artery or aortic ruptures (0.5–3 %). The majority of complications were treated using percutaneous or noninvasive techniques, including covered stent placement, percutaneous thrombus aspiration, and thrombolysis.

A retrospective review of 86 patients (161 limbs) who underwent aortobifemoral ($n = 75$) or iliofemoral ($n = 11$) bypass and 83 patients (127 limbs) who underwent percutaneous transluminal angioplasty and stenting of aortoiliac lesions found that the results of endovascular therapy rivals that of open arterial reconstruction [49]. The most common method of endovascular recanalization in this series was either intraplaque or subintimal passage of a hydrophilic wire and catheter through an antegrade or retrograde approach. The patients in both treatment groups had similar TASC lesion stratifications, and 40 % of cases were performed for either rest pain or tissue loss. Limb-based primary patency at 3 years was significantly higher for aortobifemoral bypass compared to endovascular therapy (93 % vs. 74 %, $p = .002$); however, secondary patency rates (97 % vs. 95 %), limb salvage (98 % vs. 98 %), and long-term survival (80 % vs. 80 %) were similar for open and endovascular techniques.

Infrainguinal Revascularization

Open surgical bypass using autogenous vein remains the gold standard revascularization strategy for patients with CLI due to infrainguinal disease. The ACC/AHA guidelines [2] made the following recommendations when surgery is performed for infrainguinal occlusive disease: (1) bypass to the above-knee or below-knee popliteal artery should use autogenous vein, if possible; (2) a distal bypass should originate at the most distal artery having continuous flow and with less than 20 % stenosis, with the distal anastomosis occurring at the site of whichever tibial or pedal artery can provide continuous flow to the foot; (3) femorotibial bypasses should use autogenous vein, such as the ipsilateral great saphenous vein, or, alternatively, other superficial veins from the leg or arm; (4) in the absence of available autogenous vein, a femorotibial bypass with prosthetic graft with or without an adjunctive procedure, such as arteriovenous fistula or vein interposition or cuff, may be considered.

A femoropopliteal bypass is indicated in patients with CLI who have severe stenosis or occlusion involving the superficial femoral artery or proximal popliteal artery. The construction of this form of bypass requires that the patent portion of popliteal artery that serves as the site of distal anastomosis is in direct luminal continuity with one or more of the tibioperoneal arteries. Femoropopliteal bypass grafts are typically referred to as either above knee or below knee based on the location of the distal anastomosis. A randomized controlled trial comparing the use of vein versus polytetrafluoroethylene (PTFE) for above-knee femoropopliteal bypass grafts found that a bypass with saphenous vein had better patency rates at all intervals and required fewer reoperations [50]. Five-year primary patency rates were 76 % for venous bypass grafts and 52 % for PTFE grafts, whereas secondary patency rates were 80 % for vein and 57 % for PTFE grafts. A systematic review of 25 articles published from 1966 to 2002 found similar results regarding superior patency at all time intervals with the use of autogenous vein in above-knee femoropopliteal bypass procedures [51]. The 2-year primary patency rate of venous bypasses was 81 % compared to 67 % for PTFE bypasses, and after 5 years, primary patency rates were 69 and 49 %, respectively. While PTFE may serve as a reasonable alternative when vein is absent or not suitable, the authors concluded that a venous bypass should be chosen at all times in femoropopliteal bypasses even in patients with limited life expectancy. The use of prosthetic grafts are generally avoided in below-knee bypasses owing to the potential for bending and kinking of the graft as it crosses the knee joint.

Nearly 30 % of occlusive lesions in CLI are limited to the tibioperoneal arteries, with such lesions commonly associated with diffuse disease and long-segment stenoses and occlusions [52]. A distal bypass from the femoral artery to the infrapopliteal vessels has inferior patency compared to more proximal lower extremity bypasses and should only be performed in cases where femoropopliteal bypass is either not feasible or fails to provide direct flow into patent runoff vessels. The selection of which outflow vessel to use for the distal anastomosis of an infrapopliteal bypass depends on the overall quality of the vessel, with preference given to whichever artery has direct continuity to the foot. The anterior and posterior tibial arteries are generally favored over the peroneal artery for the infrapopliteal anastomosis given that the peroneal is frequently smaller, more difficult to expose, and anatomically not directly continuous with the pedal arteries.

A recent meta-analysis involving 31 series of patients with CLI undergoing infrapopliteal bypass surgery with autogenous vein revealed 5-year primary patency, secondary patency, and limb salvage rates of 63, 71, and 78 %, respectively [53]. In addition, Okazaki et al. [54] reported their experience with 63 infrapopliteal bypasses performed in patients with CLI, including 57 with autogenous vein and 6 with composite graft. The primary graft patency, secondary graft patency, amputation-free survival, and overall survival were 73.7, 82.4, 84.7, and 88.1 %, respectively, at 1 year and 65.4, 76.3, 71.0, and 74.6 % at 3 years. Experience with infrapopliteal revascularization for CLI using PTFE demonstrated a much lower primary patency of 12–41 % at 3–5 years and a limb salvage rate of 37 % [55, 56]. As a result, prosthetic bypass grafts are avoided in infrapopliteal bypasses except as a last resort for limb salvage in patients who lack any available autologous vein.

A risk-adjusted analysis from the National Surgical Quality Improvement Program, a prospective, validated database collected between 2005 and 2008 from 211 hospitals, identified predictors of early graft failure after infrainguinal bypass surgery [57]. Of 9,217 procedures in the analysis, 49 % were performed for limb salvage, 43 % required a distal anastomosis to an infrapopliteal vessel, and 32 % involved the use of a prosthetic conduit. Multivariate predictors of graft failure within 30 days included female gender, limb salvage as the indication for procedure, infrapopliteal anastomosis, composite graft, current smoking, impaired sensorium, emergency procedure, previous vascular procedure, and platelets greater than 400,000. A separate analysis of 2,404 infrainguinal bypass surgeries (infrapopliteal distal anastomosis, 42 %; prosthetic conduit, 29 %) revealed an overall mortality of 2.7 % which correlated with patient age, lower body weight, significant preoperative dyspnea, dialysis, previous transient ischemic attack, and bleeding disorder [58]. Major systemic complications occurred in 5.9 % of patients and were associated with advanced age, previous myocardial infarction, dialysis, impaired sensorium, and general anesthesia. Knowledge of predictors of bypass failure gained from these studies may be incorporated into the clinical decision-making process for interventions on patients with CLI.

The success of endovascular treatment for aortoiliac disease has paved the way for increasing utilization of endovascular therapy in patients with infrainguinal occlusive disease. Conrad and colleagues [59] recently reported their experience with infrapopliteal angioplasty in 144 patients, 86 % of whom suffered from CLI. The investigators utilized a modified TASC classification for tibioperoneal occlusive disease. Despite 74 % of infrapopliteal lesions being classified as either TASC type C (39 %) or D (35 %), technical success was 95 %. The 40-month actuarial primary patency was 62 %, and primary-assisted patency was 90 %. Fifteen of 42 unhealed ulcers (13 %) following angioplasty required major amputations, resulting in a 40-month limb salvage rate of 86.2 %. A meta-analysis targeting comparative outcomes of angioplasty of infrapopliteal arteries ($n=2{,}557$) and popliteal-to-distal surgical bypass in patients with CLI noted more mixed results. Primary and secondary patency rates at three years were notably higher in the surgical bypass group relative to the angioplasty group (72.3 % vs. 48.6 % and 76.7 % vs.62.9 %, respectively); however, these differences in patency data failed to yield any appreciable change in limb salvage rates at 3 years between groups (82.4 % vs. 82.3 %).

The decision regarding initial treatment strategy for infrapopliteal revascularization depends on the relative favorability of available open and endovascular options. Specific atherosclerotic disease characteristics such as the length of stenotic or occlusive lesion(s), quality of inflow and outflow vessels, local and systemic risk factors, and the availability of autogenous conduit factor into the decision-making process. Equally important is defining the primary objective for each individual patient with CLI. For many patients, healing of an ischemic ulcer and limb salvage are of greater qualitative and prognostic value than the long-term patency of a bypass or endovascular intervention. If both open and endovascular treatment approaches are technically feasible and estimated to achieve the primary objective, the low-risk, minimally invasive nature of endovascular therapy makes it a reasonable first choice.

In addition to angioplasty and stenting, there are other evolving endovascular adjunctive therapies used in the treatment of CLI (Table 7.3). Multiple endovascular techniques can be used to cross a stenotic or occlusive lesion. Endovascular principles mandate that true intraluminal access must be obtained both proximal and distal to the lesion. Subintimal recanalization, also referred to as percutaneous intentional extraluminal and subintimal angioplasty, can be used in the treatment of chronic arterial occlusions that do not respond to conventional angioplasty [60, 61]. This technique involves the intentional passage of a guidewire into the subintima of the artery immediately proximal to the occlusion, thereby creating a controlled dissection plane. The guidewire is advanced distally through the dissection

Table 7.3 Endovascular options for lower extremity revascularization

Percutaneous transluminal balloon angioplasty
Endoluminal stent
Self-expandable versus balloon-expandable stent
Bare metal versus covered stent
Adjunctive techniques
Atherectomy
Cryoplasty
Subintimal recanalization
Aspiration thrombectomy
Cutting balloon
Reentry catheters
Retrograde recanalization
Crosser catheter
Frontrunner catheter

plane and reenters the true lumen of the patent distal artery beyond the occlusion. Balloon angioplasty is subsequently performed within the subintimal space, thereby generating a subintimal bypass parallel to the occluded arterial segment. This technique is particularly efficacious in the setting of long-segment (>15 cm) occlusions, highly calcified occlusions, and diffuse tandem lesions, each representing a form of complex arterial occlusive disease associated with decreased success using traditional transluminal balloon angioplasty [62].

Although subintimal recanalization is an established technique in the treatment of femoropopliteal occlusions, limited experience exists in patients with infrapopliteal disease. A recent 8-year experience of 120 patients with TASC type C or D lesions in the femoral artery distribution demonstrated a technical success rate of 91 % [63]. Primary and secondary patency rates at 1 year were 73 and 85 %, respectively, with a 1-year limb salvage rate of 98 %. Tartari and colleagues [64] examined the outcomes of 117 subintimal recanalization procedures in patients with CLI, including 27 patients with superficial femoral artery occlusion and 82 patients with infrapopliteal occlusion. Technical success was slightly higher in femoropopliteal lesions (89 %) compared to infrapopliteal lesions (83 %). Survival analysis at 6, 12, and 24 months demonstrated limb salvage rates of 90, 87, and 85 % and overall survival rates of 90, 88, and 83 %, respectively.

Atherectomy devices utilize plaque excision and other athero-ablative techniques to achieve and maintain patency in fibrocalcific atherosclerotic disease of the infrainguinal vessels [65]. Theoretically, atherectomy avoids the arterial wall stretch injury incurred by balloon angioplasty, thereby minimizing the rate of restenosis associated with arterial dissection and elastic recoil.

Nonsurgical Interventions

Pharmacologic Therapy

Antiplatelet Agents

The Antithrombotic Trialists' Collaboration analyzed the results of multiple randomized clinical trials of antiplatelet therapy in high-risk patients with cardiovascular disease and demonstrated a 23 % reduction in the risk of adverse cardiovascular events with the use of antiplatelet therapy in patients with PAD [66, 67]. There is no convincing evidence at the present time to support the superiority of one antiplatelet agent over another. In the CAPRIE study, the use of long-term clopidogrel in patients with PAD was more effective than aspirin in reducing the combined risk of ischemic stroke, myocardial infarction, or vascular death [68]. Results from the CHARISMA trial, however, found that clopidogrel plus aspirin was not significantly more effective than aspirin alone in reducing the risk of the same adverse cardiovascular events [69]. Moreover, the WAVE trial demonstrated no added benefit to adding warfarin to antiplatelet therapy in patients with PAD, but such combination therapy did result in greater risk of life-threatening hemorrhagic complications [70].

Based on the available studies to date, the American College of Chest Physicians currently recommends single rather than dual antiplatelet therapy for the majority of patients undergoing either open or endovascular peripheral revascularization procedures [71]. Dual antiplatelet therapy is recommended in select cases involving below-knee bypass surgery with prosthetic grafts. Long-term aspirin (75–100 mg/day) is generally the agent of choice in cases requiring single antiplatelet therapy due to lower cost and proven benefits in reducing myocardial infarction; however, clopidogrel (75 mg/day) may be used in subgroups of patients unable to tolerate aspirin.

Anticoagulation

Long-term anticoagulation is not routinely recommended in patients following lower extremity revascularization procedures. Unfractionated heparin is commonly used as an adjuvant treatment during revascularization procedures, but currently has only limited utility in the postoperative period. Some studies suggest that low molecular weight heparin has beneficial effects on the healing of ischemic ulcers [72].

The CHEST guidelines recommend single antiplatelet therapy over combination antiplatelet and warfarin therapy [71]. In the Dutch Bypass Oral Anticoagulants or Aspirin Study, a total of 2,690 patients who had undergone infrainguinal grafting were randomly assigned to oral anticoagulation (high-intensity warfarin with target international normalized ratio 3.0–4.5) or aspirin (80 mg daily). Oral anticoagulation showed better results for the prevention of infrainguinal vein-graft occlusion and for lowering the rate of perioperative ischemic events, whereas aspirin was better for the prevention of non-venous graft occlusion and was associated with fewer bleeding episodes [73]. A separate prospective randomized trial found that low-dose warfarin therapy provided some benefit for patients with a femoropopliteal prosthetic bypass and for patients with a vein bypass at high risk for thrombosis [74]. However, the addition of warfarin therapy significantly increased the risk of hemorrhagic complications. Given the available data, oral anticoagulation should be used only in select patients at high risk for graft thrombosis, including those with low flow velocities and no other options to improve graft flow.

Cilostazol (Pletal)

Cilostazol is a phosphodiesterase inhibitor that acts as a direct arterial vasodilator and exerts metabolic and antiplatelet activity. While no literature to date has shown any benefit in patients with CLI, cilostazol use improves maximal and pain-free walking distances among patients with intermittent claudication [75]. In the absence of heart failure, a therapeutic trial of 3–6 months of cilostazol is recommended in patients with intermittent claudication, but it is unlikely to produce any benefit in patients with CLI.

Prostaglandin E1

Prostaglandin E1 (PGE1) is a vasodilator and inhibitor of platelet aggregation. The use of prostaglandin has shown some evidence of early benefit in patients with CLI relative to wound healing and limb salvage. In a randomized trial comparing treatment with intravenous PGE1 versus no treatment with PGE1 in patients with CLI, those who received PGE1 were significantly less likely to sustain a combined endpoint of death, amputation, persistence of CLI, myocardial infarction, or stroke at time of hospital discharge. This benefit, however, was not sustained long term. The TASC II guidelines on the management of PAD do not support the use of PGE1 or any other prostanoids for the management of claudication or CLI.

Other Agents

Several studies have evaluated the role of chelation therapy omega-3 fatty acids, 5-hydroxytryptamine antagonists, and other vasodilators in the treatment of PAD. None of these pharmacologic agents have proven effective.

Aggressive Wound Care

Local Wound Care

The principles of wound care include the removal of all necrotic tissue, maintaining a local moist environment at the wound site, and the treatment and prevention of infection. Following local debridement, the selection of dressing should be based on wound characteristics, including the extent of residual necrotic tissue, amount of exudate, and presence of desiccation. A variety of dressings are available with some dressings serving to simply provide protection while others alter levels of wound hydration. Wet-to-dry dressings with sterile saline are the most commonly used form of dressing. Varying degrees of success with wound healing and limb salvage have been achieved with several noninterventional strategies, including the use of sterile maggots for debridement, hydrotherapy, negative pressure therapy, and hyperbaric oxygen [76–78].

Pressure Off-Loading

The combination of foot deformity (e.g., claw toe, Charcot's neuroarthropathy), neuropathy, and inadequate off-loading of the foot leads to local tissue damage and eventual ulceration [79]. Both retrospective and prospective studies have reliably demonstrated that increased plantar pressure serves as a causative factor in the development of plantar ulcers, particularly among diabetic patients, and that ulceration is often a precursor to lower extremity amputation [80, 81]. In the absence of off-loading, lower extremity ulcers are commonly associated with chronically delayed wound healing independent of the vascular supply to the lower extremity. A central goal of any treatment plan designed to heal wounds is the effective reduction in pressure on the involved portion of the lower extremity, otherwise referred to as pressure off-loading. Depending on the wound location and severity of underlying ischemia, off-loading may be achieved with the use of shoe modifications, orthotics, or other casting techniques.

Pneumatic Compression Boot Therapy

Sequential compression biomechanical devices, otherwise referred to as pneumatic compression boot therapy, can be used as an adjunct to wound care in patients with CLI and nonhealing amputation wounds or tissue loss. This form of therapy has been shown to improve the likelihood of wound healing and limb salvage when conventional revascularization strategies have been exhausted. A recent study reported encouraging outcomes in 35 patients with non-reconstructable CLI who underwent a 12-week treatment protocol of pneumatic boot therapy combined with medical treatment [82]. The 90-day mortality rate in this patient group was 0 %, and the limb salvage rate at 18 months was 88 %. Mean toe pressures increased from 38 to 67 mmHg. In a separate study, Kavros et al. [83] found that patients with chronic wounds attributed to CLI who underwent pneumatic compression boot therapy were seven times less likely to require amputation compared to a similar group of patients who had medical treatment alone without boot therapy.

Prevention and Treatment of Infection

Local infection is a serious complication of tissue loss associated with CLI. Systemic toxicity in these patients, manifested by fever or elevated inflammatory serum markers, is uncommon. Aggressive and meticulous local wound care should aid in both the prevention and early detection of infection. Because wound infections are frequently polymicrobial, empiric broad-spectrum antibiotics should commence immediately following the clinical diagnosis of infection and acquisition of wound cultures. Infections of the deep soft tissues of the lower extremity may mandate drainage and debridement of all involved tissues.

Nutrition

Advances in biochemistry have led to the discovery of vitamin C, zinc, and many other components essential for wound healing [84]. Much of current research efforts aim to determine which nutritional components can facilitate or enhance wound healing through supraphysiological doses, such as in the use of the amino acids like arginine and carnitine. The importance of nutrition is exemplified by the fact that nearly 50 % of patients admitted to the hospital are malnourished and require some form of dietary supplementation. Moreover, in a prospective study on patients undergoing lower extremity amputations for CLI, malnourished patients were noted to have a higher frequency of impaired wound healing and an increased risk of postoperative cardiopulmonary and septic complications [85]. As such, a detailed nutritional assessment and dietary supplementation, if needed, should serve as a cornerstone in optimal wound management.

Emerging Therapies

Therapeutic angiogenesis is a promising new investigational tool in the management of CLI. Stimulation of angiogenesis involves the intravenous or intramuscular gene transfer of plasmid DNA encoding for angiogenic growth factors with the goal of augmenting collateral circulation and enhancing overall vascular supply to ischemic areas of the lower extremity. The most commonly used growth factors include vascular endothelium growth factor (VEGF), fibroblast growth factor (FGF), hepatocyte growth factor (HGF), and angiopoietin 1 (Ang-1). Gene therapy has been shown to improve endothelial function, increase flow reserve, enhance collateralization, facilitate healing of ischemic ulcers, and achieve limb salvage for patients with CLI [86, 87].

Stem cells also play a potential role in therapeutic angiogenesis. The differentiation of bone marrow-derived endothelial progenitor cells and the migration and proliferation of local endothelial cells promote postnatal neovascularization. Circulating levels of endothelial progenitor cells increase in response to local ischemia, with various studies indicating that these progenitor cells incorporate into the capillaries and interstitial arteries in models of limb and myocardial ischemia [88, 89].

Spinal cord stimulation was suggested in early uncontrolled studies to be effective in reducing ischemic pain and preventing or delaying amputation in patients with severe PAD [90]. A more recent study, however, showed no difference in the rates of survival, need for amputation, or pain scores in patients randomly assigned to either best medical therapy or best medical therapy combined with spinal cord stimulation [91].

Follow-Up

Surveillance

Patients undergoing surgical or endovascular revascularization procedures for CLI should be followed in a clinical surveillance program with the goal of early identification of lesions that predispose to graft or in-stent thrombosis. Detecting these lesions early provides the opportunity for intervention prior to graft or stent occlusion [1]. Clinical surveillance programs should be performed in the immediate postoperative period and at regular intervals thereafter, typically every 6 months, for a minimum of 2 years. The program should include interval history with detailed information pertaining to the progression of CLI and the onset of new lower extremity symptoms. Vascular examination should evaluate the pulses proximal to the bypass, in the bypass graft, and in the outflow vessels. Periodic measurements of resting ABIs should also be performed.

There is currently no level I data to support the routine use of duplex ultrasound in the surveillance of surgical or endovascular lower extremity revascularizations. Several randomized clinical trials have shown variable results with regard to improved graft patency rates in patients undergoing routine long-term duplex surveillance; however, no trial to date has demonstrated any benefit relative to rates of limb salvage or cost-effectiveness using this surveillance strategy [92–95]. Moreover, a randomized trial examining the utility of such surveillance methods following endovascular interventions has yet to be performed. As such, TASC II guidelines emphasize the importance of close clinical surveillance of patients with CLI undergoing revascularization procedures but do not recommend the use of routine duplex surveillance. Duplex surveillance does have an accepted role in defined subgroups of patients with "high-risk" grafts, such as those with early flow disturbances or in those with arm vein or spliced vein grafts.

Currently available research suggests that a single follow-up duplex ultrasound is justified in all patients who have had any form of open or endovascular revascularization for CLI [96]. The duplex imaging provides measurement of peak systolic velocity and calculates the velocity ratio across all lesions. The overwhelming majority of patients will have normal duplex findings within the first 6 months of intervention and be suitable for future clinical surveillance only. Subsequent clinical deterioration or decreasing ABIs should prompt additional screening with duplex ultrasound. Patients with abnormal early duplex findings (e.g., global flow velocity less than 45 cm/s, peak systolic velocity greater than 300 cm/s at any segment, or velocity ratio of more than 3.5 across an area of stenosis) and patients with high-risk arterial reconstructions will likely benefit from continued routine duplex surveillance.

Patient-Oriented Outcomes

The natural history of CLI is progressive and carries with it a significant risk for amputation and death. Patients with CLI have the most severe form of PAD characterized by involvement of multiple arterial segments that is particularly pronounced in the infrapopliteal distribution. Based on available data, outcomes at 1 year among patients with CLI include the following: 25 % will die, 30 % will undergo an amputation, and only 45 % will be alive with both lower extremities (Fig. 7.3) [2].

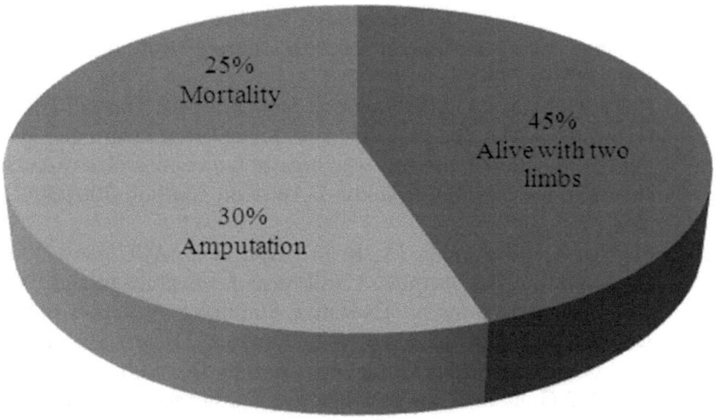

Fig. 7.3 One-year outcomes of patients presenting with critical limb ischemia (Reproduced, with permission, from Elsevier, Hirsch et al. [2])

While a fair amount of data exist regarding the global and technical success following revascularization in patients with CLI, as commonly measured by graft patency, limb salvage, and survival, such traditional outcome measures have been found to be poor predictors of functional and qualitative outcomes. Robust data with regard to the effect of revascularization on overall physical recovery, quality of life, and functional status remains limited. Such outcomes may prompt physicians to consider a more patient-centered approach to the treatment of individuals with CLI, rather than the current lesion-focused approach. This change in paradigm could help identify which groups of patients are unlikely to benefit from interventional procedures and would be better served with primary amputation or medical management only.

Rollins and colleagues [97] performed a review of ten studies examining the functional outcomes of patients following revascularization for CLI. Only three studies noted any improvement in ambulation status, with up to 45 % of patients remaining nonambulatory following vascular intervention. None of the studies found any improvement in residential status as 3–17 % of patients continued to live in a dependent manner after intervention. Preoperative dependent functional status was also noted to be a significant predictor for midterm mortality. Similarly, Crawford et al. [98] examined 30-day outcomes from the NSQIP database and demonstrated dependent functional status as an independent predictor of major complications and death after lower extremity bypass grafting. Dependent functional status combined with dialysis-dependent renal failure, emergency presentation, or age greater than 80 years was associated with a 13-, 38-, and 87-fold increase in the odds of death respectively.

The PREVENT III trial is the largest study to date that prospectively evaluated patient's quality of life after surgical revascularization of the lower extremity [99, 100]. Significant improvements in quality of life were observed based on questionnaires at both 3 and 12 months following revascularization compared to baseline. Diabetes and graft-related events were associated with failure to improve quality of life. Moreover, improvement in health-related quality of life was seen in both the surgery and angioplasty arms of the BASIL trial [36]. A trend toward continued improvement in quality of life was seen in the surgery group with longer follow-up; however, this difference was not statistically significant.

References

1. Norgren L, Hiatt WR, Dormandy JA, Nehler MR, Harris KA, Fowkes FG. Inter-society consensus for the management of peripheral arterial disease (TASC II). J Vasc Surg. 2007;45(Suppl S):S5–67.
2. Hirsch AT, Haskal ZJ, Hertzer NR, et al. ACC/AHA 2005 Practice Guidelines for the Management of Patients with Peripheral Arterial Disease (lower extremity, renal, mesenteric, and abdominal aortic): a collaborative report from the American Association for Vascular Surgery/Society for Vascular Surgery, Society for Cardiovascular Angiography and Interventions, Society for Vascular Medicine and Biology, Society of Interventional Radiology, and the ACC/AHA Task Force on Practice Guidelines (Writing Committee to Develop Guidelines for the Management of Patients With Peripheral Arterial Disease): endorsed by the American Association of Cardiovascular and Pulmonary Rehabilitation; National Heart, Lung, and Blood Institute; Society for Vascular Nursing; TransAtlantic Inter-Society Consensus; and Vascular Disease Foundation. Circulation. 2006;113(11):e463–654.
3. Varu VN, Hogg ME, Kibbe MR. Critical limb ischemia. J Vasc Surg. 2010;51(1):230–41.
4. Suggested standards for reports dealing with lower extremity ischemia. Prepared by the Ad Hoc Committee on Reporting Standards, Society for Vascular Surgery/North American Chapter, International Society for Cardiovascular Surgery. J Vasc Surg. 1986;4(1):80–94.
5. DeWeese JA, Leather R, Porter J. Practice guidelines: lower extremity revascularization. J Vasc Surg. 1993;18(2):280–94.
6. Hirsch AT, Criqui MH, Treat-Jacobson D, et al. Peripheral arterial disease detection, awareness, and treatment in primary care. JAMA. 2001;286(11):1317–24.
7. O'Hare AM, Katz R, Shlipak MG, Cushman M, Newman AB. Mortality and cardiovascular risk across the ankle-arm index spectrum: results from the Cardiovascular Health Study. Circulation. 2006;113(3):388–93.
8. Selvin E, Erlinger TP. Prevalence of and risk factors for peripheral arterial disease in the United States: results from the National Health and Nutrition Examination Survey, 1999–2000. Circulation. 2004;110(6):738–43.
9. Smith Jr SC, Milani RV, Arnett DK, et al. Atherosclerotic vascular disease conference: writing group II: risk factors. Circulation. 2004;109(21):2613–6.
10. Criqui MH, Fronek A, Klauber MR, Barrett-Connor E, Gabriel S. The sensitivity, specificity, and predictive value of traditional clinical evaluation of peripheral arterial disease: results from non-invasive testing in a defined population. Circulation. 1985; 71(3):516–22.
11. Hankey GJ, Norman PE, Eikelboom JW. Medical treatment of peripheral arterial disease. JAMA. 2006;295(5):547–53.
12. Fowkes FG, Housley E, Cawood EH, Macintyre CC, Ruckley CV, Prescott RJ. Edinburgh Artery Study: prevalence of asymptomatic

and symptomatic peripheral arterial disease in the general population. Int J Epidemiol. 1991;20(2):384–92.
13. Mehler PS, Coll JR, Estacio R, Esler A, Schrier RW, Hiatt WR. Intensive blood pressure control reduces the risk of cardiovascular events in patients with peripheral arterial disease and type 2 diabetes. Circulation. 2003;107(5):753–6.
14. Dormandy JA, Murray GD. The fate of the claudicant – a prospective study of 1969 claudicants. Eur J Vasc Surg. 1991;5(2): 131–3.
15. Koelemay MJ, den Hartog D, Prins MH, Kromhout JG, Legemate DA, Jacobs MJ. Diagnosis of arterial disease of the lower extremities with duplex ultrasonography. Br J Surg. 1996;83(3):404–9.
16. Eiberg JP, Gronvall Rasmussen JB, Hansen MA, Schroeder TV. Duplex ultrasound scanning of peripheral arterial disease of the lower limb. Eur J Vasc Endovasc Surg. 2010;40(4):507–12.
17. Sensier Y, Hartshorne T, Thrush A, Nydahl S, Bolia A, London NJ. A prospective comparison of lower limb colour-coded Duplex scanning with arteriography. Eur J Vasc Endovasc Surg. 1996; 11(2):170–5.
18. Larch E, Minar E, Ahmadi R, et al. Value of color duplex sonography for evaluation of tibioperoneal arteries in patients with femoropopliteal obstruction: a prospective comparison with anterograde intraarterial digital subtraction angiography. J Vasc Surg. 1997;25(4):629–36.
19. Katsamouris AN, Giannoukas AD, Tsetis D, Kostas T, Petinarakis I, Gourtsoyiannis N. Can ultrasound replace arteriography in the management of chronic arterial occlusive disease of the lower limb? Eur J Vasc Endovasc Surg. 2001;21(2):155–9.
20. Heijenbrok-Kal MH, Kock MC, Hunink MG. Lower extremity arterial disease: multidetector CT angiography meta-analysis. Radiology. 2007;245(2):433–9.
21. Met R, Bipat S, Legemate DA, Reekers JA, Koelemay MJ. Diagnostic performance of computed tomography angiography in peripheral arterial disease: a systematic review and meta-analysis. JAMA. 2009;301(4):415–24.
22. Fleischmann D, Hallett RL, Rubin GD. CT angiography of peripheral arterial disease. J Vasc Interv Radiol. 2006;17(1):3–26.
23. Swan JS, Carroll TJ, Kennell TW, et al. Time-resolved three-dimensional contrast-enhanced MR angiography of the peripheral vessels. Radiology. 2002;225(1):43–52.
24. Meaney JF, Ridgway JP, Chakraverty S, et al. Stepping-table gadolinium-enhanced digital subtraction MR angiography of the aorta and lower extremity arteries: preliminary experience. Radiology. 1999;211(1):59–67.
25. Willmann JK, Wildermuth S, Pfammatter T, et al. Aortoiliac and renal arteries: prospective intraindividual comparison of contrast-enhanced three-dimensional MR angiography and multi-detector row CT angiography. Radiology. 2003;226(3):798–811.
26. Owen AR, Robertson IR, Annamalai G, et al. Critical lower-limb ischemia: the diagnostic performance of dual-phase injection MR angiography (including high-resolution distal imaging) compared with digital subtraction angiography. J Vasc Interv Radiol. 2009;20(2):165–72.
27. Krous HF, Breisch E, Chadwick AE, Pinckney L, Malicki DM, Benador N. Nephrogenic systemic fibrosis with multiorgan involvement in a teenage male after lymphoma, Ewing's sarcoma, end-stage renal disease, and hemodialysis. Pediatr Dev Pathol. 2007;10(5):395–402.
28. Kucher C, Steere J, Elenitsas R, Siegel DL, Xu X. Nephrogenic fibrosing dermopathy/nephrogenic systemic fibrosis with diaphragmatic involvement in a patient with respiratory failure. J Am Acad Dermatol. 2006;54(2 Suppl):S31–4.
29. Criqui MH, Langer RD, Fronek A, et al. Mortality over a period of 10 years in patients with peripheral arterial disease. N Engl J Med. 1992;326(6):381–6.
30. Wong T, Detsky AS. Preoperative cardiac risk assessment for patients having peripheral vascular surgery. Ann Intern Med. 1992;116(9):743–53.
31. Kelly R, Staines A, MacWalter R, Stonebridge P, Tunstall-Pedoe H, Struthers AD. The prevalence of treatable left ventricular systolic dysfunction in patients who present with noncardiac vascular episodes: a case-control study. J Am Coll Cardiol. 2002;39(2): 219–24.
32. Fleisher LA, Beckman JA, Brown KA, et al. ACC/AHA 2007 Guidelines on Perioperative Cardiovascular Evaluation and Care for Noncardiac Surgery: Executive Summary: A Report of the American College of Cardiology/American Heart Association Task Force on Practice Guidelines (Writing Committee to Revise the 2002 Guidelines on Perioperative Cardiovascular Evaluation for Noncardiac Surgery) Developed in Collaboration With the American Society of Echocardiography, American Society of Nuclear Cardiology, Heart Rhythm Society, Society of Cardiovascular Anesthesiologists, Society for Cardiovascular Angiography and Interventions, Society for Vascular Medicine and Biology, and Society for Vascular Surgery. J Am Coll Cardiol. 2007;50(17):1707–32.
33. Rooke TW, Hirsch AT, Misra S, et al. ACCF/AHA focused update of the guideline for the management of patients with peripheral artery disease (updating the 2005 guideline): a report of the American College of Cardiology Foundation/American Heart Association Task Force on Practice Guidelines: developed in collaboration with the Society for Cardiovascular Angiography and Interventions, Society of Interventional Radiology, Society for Vascular Medicine, and Society for Vascular Surgery. Catheter Cardiovasc Interv. 2011;79(4):501–31.
34. Long-term mortality and its predictors in patients with critical leg ischaemia. The I.C.A.I. Group (Gruppo di Studio dell'Ischemia Cronica Critica degli Arti Inferiori). The Study Group of Critical Chronic Ischemia of the Lower Extremities. Eur J Vasc Endovasc Surg. 1997;14(2):91–5.
35. Adam DJ, Beard JD, Cleveland T, et al. Bypass versus angioplasty in severe ischaemia of the leg (BASIL): multicentre, randomised controlled trial. Lancet. 2005;366(9501):1925–34.
36. Bradbury AW, Adam DJ, Bell J, et al. Bypass versus Angioplasty in Severe Ischaemia of the Leg (BASIL) trial: an intention-to-treat analysis of amputation-free and overall survival in patients randomized to a bypass surgery-first or a balloon angioplasty-first revascularization strategy. J Vasc Surg. 2010;51(5 Suppl):5S–17.
37. Taylor SM, Kalbaugh CA, Gray BH, et al. The LEGS score: a proposed grading system to direct treatment of chronic lower extremity ischemia. Ann Surg. 2003;237(6):812–8; discussion 818–9.
38. Couch NP, Clowes AW, Whittemore AD, Lombara JA, Henderson BA, Mannick JA. The iliac-origin arterial graft: a useful alternative for iliac occlusive disease. Surgery. 1985;97(1):83–7.
39. Brewster DC, Darling RC. Optimal methods of aortoiliac reconstruction. Surgery. 1978;84(6):739–48.
40. Littooy FN, Steffan G, Steinam S, Saletta C, Greisler HP. An 11-year experience with aortofemoral bypass grafting. Cardiovasc Surg. 1993;1(3):232–8.
41. Mingoli A, Sapienza P, Feldhaus RJ, di Marzo L, Burchi C, Cavallaro A. Aortoiliofemoral bypass graft in young adults: long-term results in a series of sixty-eight patients. Surgery. 1997;121(6):646–53.
42. Tiek J, Remy P, Sabbe T, et al. Laparoscopic versus open approach for aortobifemoral bypass for severe aorto-iliac occlusive disease – a multicentre randomised controlled trial. Eur J Vasc Endovasc Surg. 2012;43(6):711–5.
43. Connolly JE, Price T. Aortoiliac endarterectomy: a lost art? Ann Vasc Surg. 2006;20(1):56–62.

44. Carsten 3rd CG, Kalbaugh CA, Langan 3rd EM, et al. Contemporary outcomes of iliofemoral bypass grafting for unilateral aortoiliac occlusive disease: a 10-year experience. Am Surg. 2008;74(6):555–9; discussion 559–60.
45. Schneider JR, McDaniel MD, Walsh DB, Zwolak RM, Cronenwett JL. Axillofemoral bypass: outcome and hemodynamic results in high-risk patients. J Vasc Surg. 1992;15(6):952–62; discussion 962–63.
46. Chiu KW, Davies RS, Nightingale PG, Bradbury AW, Adam DJ. Review of direct anatomical open surgical management of atherosclerotic aorto-iliac occlusive disease. Eur J Vasc Endovasc Surg. 2010;39(4):460–71.
47. Dattilo PB, Casserly IP. Critical limb ischemia: endovascular strategies for limb salvage. Prog Cardiovasc Dis. 2011;54(1):47–60.
48. Jongkind V, Akkersdijk GJ, Yeung KK, Wisselink W. A systematic review of endovascular treatment of extensive aortoiliac occlusive disease. J Vasc Surg. 2010;52(5):1376–83.
49. Kashyap VS, Pavkov ML, Bena JF, et al. The management of severe aortoiliac occlusive disease: endovascular therapy rivals open reconstruction. J Vasc Surg. 2008;48(6):1451–7. 1457. e1451–3.
50. Klinkert P, Schepers A, Burger DH, van Bockel JH, Breslau PJ. Vein versus polytetrafluoroethylene in above-knee femoropopliteal bypass grafting: five-year results of a randomized controlled trial. J Vasc Surg. 2003;37(1):149–55.
51. Klinkert P, Post PN, Breslau PJ, van Bockel JH. Saphenous vein versus PTFE for above-knee femoropopliteal bypass. A review of the literature. Eur J Vasc Endovasc Surg. 2004;27(4):357–62.
52. Faglia E, Dalla Paola L, Clerici G, et al. Peripheral angioplasty as the first-choice revascularization procedure in diabetic patients with critical limb ischemia: prospective study of 993 consecutive patients hospitalized and followed between 1999 and 2003. Eur J Vasc Endovasc Surg. 2005;29(6):620–7.
53. Albers M, Romiti M, Brochado-Neto FC, De Luccia N, Pereira CA. Meta-analysis of popliteal-to-distal vein bypass grafts for critical ischemia. J Vasc Surg. 2006;43(3):498–503.
54. Okazaki J, Guntani A, Homma K, et al. Mid-term clinical outcome of critical limb ischemia after infrapopliteal bypass surgery. Fukuoka Igaku Zasshi. 2011;102(2):31–9.
55. Quinones-Baldrich WJ, Prego AA, Ucelay-Gomez R, et al. Long-term results of infrainguinal revascularization with polytetrafluoroethylene: a ten-year experience. J Vasc Surg. 1992;16(2):209–17.
56. Fichelle JM, Marzelle J, Colacchio G, Gigou F, Cormier F, Cormier JM. Infrapopliteal polytetrafluoroethylene and composite bypass: factors influencing patency. Ann Vasc Surg. 1995;9(2):187–96.
57. Lancaster RT, Conrad MF, Patel VI, Cambria RP, LaMuraglia GM. Predictors of early graft failure after infrainguinal bypass surgery: a risk-adjusted analysis from the NSQIP. Eur J Vasc Endovasc Surg. 2012;43(5):549–55.
58. LaMuraglia GM, Conrad MF, Chung T, Hutter M, Watkins MT, Cambria RP. Significant perioperative morbidity accompanies contemporary infrainguinal bypass surgery: an NSQIP report. J Vasc Surg. 2009;50(2):299–304, 304.e291–4.
59. Conrad MF, Kang J, Cambria RP, et al. Infrapopliteal balloon angioplasty for the treatment of chronic occlusive disease. J Vasc Surg. 2009;50(4):799–805 e4.
60. Bolia A, Brennan J, Bell PR. Recanalisation of femoro-popliteal occlusions: improving success rate by subintimal recanalisation. Clin Radiol. 1989;40(3):325.
61. Nadal LL, Cynamon J, Lipsitz EC, Bolia A. Subintimal angioplasty for chronic arterial occlusions. Tech Vasc Interv Radiol. 2004;7(1):16–22.
62. Yan BP, Moran D, Hynes BG, Kiernan TJ, Yu CM. Advances in endovascular treatment of critical limb ischemia. Circ J. 2011;75(4):756–65.
63. Sidhu R, Pigott J, Pigott M, Comerota A. Subintimal angioplasty for advanced lower extremity ischemia due to TASC II C and D lesions of the superficial femoral artery. Vasc Endovascular Surg. 2010;44(8):633–7.
64. Tartari S, Zattoni L, Rizzati R, et al. Subintimal angioplasty as the first-choice revascularization technique for infrainguinal arterial occlusions in patients with critical limb ischemia. Ann Vasc Surg. 2007;21(6):819–28.
65. Clair DG. Critical limb ischemia: will atherectomy and laser-directed therapy be the answer? Semin Vasc Surg. 2006;19(2):96–101.
66. Collaborative overview of randomised trials of antiplatelet therapy – II: maintenance of vascular graft or arterial patency by antiplatelet therapy. Antiplatelet Trialists' Collaboration. BMJ. 1994;308(6922):159–68.
67. Collaborative meta-analysis of randomised trials of antiplatelet therapy for prevention of death, myocardial infarction, and stroke in high risk patients. BMJ. 2002;324(7329):71–86.
68. A randomised, blinded, trial of clopidogrel versus aspirin in patients at risk of ischaemic events (CAPRIE). CAPRIE Steering Committee. Lancet. 1996;348(9038):1329–39.
69. Bhatt DL, Fox KA, Hacke W, et al. Clopidogrel and aspirin versus aspirin alone for the prevention of atherothrombotic events. N Engl J Med. 2006;354(16):1706–17.
70. Anand S, Yusuf S, Xie C, et al. Oral anticoagulant and antiplatelet therapy and peripheral arterial disease. N Engl J Med. 2007;357(3):217–27.
71. Alonso-Coello P, Bellmunt S, McGorrian C, et al. Antithrombotic therapy in peripheral artery disease: Antithrombotic Therapy and Prevention of Thrombosis, 9th ed: American College of Chest Physicians Evidence-Based Clinical Practice Guidelines. Chest. 2012;141(2 Suppl):e669S–90.
72. Jorneskog G, Brismar K, Fagrell B. Low molecular weight heparin seems to improve local capillary circulation and healing of chronic foot ulcers in diabetic patients. Vasa. 1993;22(2):137–42.
73. Efficacy of oral anticoagulants compared with aspirin after infrainguinal bypass surgery (The Dutch Bypass Oral Anticoagulants or Aspirin Study): a randomised trial. Lancet. 2000;355(9201):346–51.
74. Johnson WC, Williford WO. Benefits, morbidity, and mortality associated with long-term administration of oral anticoagulant therapy to patients with peripheral arterial bypass procedures: a prospective randomized study. J Vasc Surg. 2002;35(3):413–21.
75. Thompson PD, Zimet R, Forbes WP, Zhang P. Meta-analysis of results from eight randomized, placebo-controlled trials on the effect of cilostazol on patients with intermittent claudication. Am J Cardiol. 2002;90(12):1314–9.
76. Enoch S, Grey JE, Harding KG. ABC of wound healing. Non-surgical and drug treatments. BMJ. 2006;332(7546):900–3.
77. Eginton MT, Brown KR, Seabrook GR, Towne JB, Cambria RA. A prospective randomized evaluation of negative-pressure wound dressings for diabetic foot wounds. Ann Vasc Surg. 2003;17(6):645–9.
78. Kranke P, Bennett M, Roeckl-Wiedmann I, Debus S. Hyperbaric oxygen therapy for chronic wounds. Cochrane Database Syst Rev. 2004;(2):CD004123.
79. Cavanagh PR, Bus SA. Off-loading the diabetic foot for ulcer prevention and healing. Plast Reconstr Surg. 2011;127 Suppl 1:248S–56.
80. Frykberg RG, Lavery LA, Pham H, Harvey C, Harkless L, Veves A. Role of neuropathy and high foot pressures in diabetic foot ulceration. Diabetes Care. 1998;21(10):1714–9.

81. Pham H, Armstrong DG, Harvey C, Harkless LB, Giurini JM, Veves A. Screening techniques to identify people at high risk for diabetic foot ulceration: a prospective multicenter trial. Diabetes Care. 2000;23(5):606–11.
82. Sultan S, Esan O, Fahy A. Nonoperative active management of critical limb ischemia: initial experience using a sequential compression biomechanical device for limb salvage. Vascular. 2008;16(3):130–9.
83. Kavros SJ, Delis KT, Turner NS, et al. Improving limb salvage in critical ischemia with intermittent pneumatic compression: a controlled study with 18-month follow-up. J Vasc Surg. 2008;47(3): 543–9.
84. Patel GK. The role of nutrition in the management of lower extremity wounds. Int J Low Extrem Wounds. 2005;4(1):12–22.
85. Pedersen NW, Pedersen D. Nutrition as a prognostic indicator in amputations. A prospective study of 47 cases. Acta Orthop Scand. 1992;63(6):675–8.
86. Isner JM, Pieczek A, Schainfeld R, et al. Clinical evidence of angiogenesis after arterial gene transfer of phVEGF165 in patient with ischaemic limb. Lancet. 1996;348(9024):370–4.
87. Baumgartner I, Pieczek A, Manor O, et al. Constitutive expression of phVEGF165 after intramuscular gene transfer promotes collateral vessel development in patients with critical limb ischemia. Circulation. 1998;97(12):1114–23.
88. Shintani S, Murohara T, Ikeda H, et al. Mobilization of endothelial progenitor cells in patients with acute myocardial infarction. Circulation. 2001;103(23):2776–9.
89. Kamihata H, Matsubara H, Nishiue T, et al. Implantation of bone marrow mononuclear cells into ischemic myocardium enhances collateral perfusion and regional function via side supply of angioblasts, angiogenic ligands, and cytokines. Circulation. 2001;104(9):1046–52.
90. Horsch S, Claeys L. Epidural spinal cord stimulation in the treatment of severe peripheral arterial occlusive disease. Ann Vasc Surg. 1994;8(5):468–74.
91. Klomp HM, Spincemaille GH, Steyerberg EW, Habbema JD, van Urk H. Spinal-cord stimulation in critical limb ischaemia: a randomised trial. ESES Study Group. Lancet. 1999;353(9158): 1040–4.
92. Lundell A, Lindblad B, Bergqvist D, Hansen F. Femoropoplitealcrural graft patency is improved by an intensive surveillance program: a prospective randomized study. J Vasc Surg. 1995;21(1): 26–33; discussion 33–4.
93. Illig KA, Surowiec S, Shortell CK, Davies MG, Rhodes JM, Green RM. Hemodynamics of distal revascularization-interval ligation. Ann Vasc Surg. 2005;19(2):199–207.
94. Ihlberg L, Luther M, Alback A, Kantonen I, Lepantalo M. Does a completely accomplished duplex-based surveillance prevent veingraft failure? Eur J Vasc Endovasc Surg. 1999;18(5):395–400.
95. Ihlberg L, Luther M, Tierala E, Lepantalo M. The utility of duplex scanning in infrainguinal vein graft surveillance: results from a randomised controlled study. Eur J Vasc Endovasc Surg. 1998;16(1):19–27.
96. Arvela E, Dick F. Surveillance after distal revascularization for critical limb ischaemia. Scand J Surg. 2012;101(2):119–24.
97. Rollins KE, Coughlin PA. Functional outcomes following revascularisation for critical limb ischaemia. Eur J Vasc Endovasc Surg. 2012;43(4):420–5.
98. Crawford RS, Cambria RP, Abularrage CJ, et al. Preoperative functional status predicts perioperative outcomes after infrainguinal bypass surgery. J Vasc Surg. 2010;51(2):351–8; discussion 358–9.
99. Nguyen LL, Moneta GL, Conte MS, Bandyk DF, Clowes AW, Seely BL. Prospective multicenter study of quality of life before and after lower extremity vein bypass in 1404 patients with critical limb ischemia. J Vasc Surg. 2006;44(5):977–83; discussion 983–4.
100. Conte MS, Bandyk DF, Clowes AW, et al. Results of PREVENT III: a multicenter, randomized trial of edifoligide for the prevention of vein graft failure in lower extremity bypass surgery. J Vasc Surg. 2006;43(4):742–51; discussion 751.

Lower Extremity Amputations

8

Jason T. Chiriano and Ahmed M. Abou-Zamzam Jr.

Introduction

Although the number of lower extremity amputations has been declining over time, amputation rates vary considerably around the world [1]. Amputations constitute a significant portion of any surgical practice as demonstrated by the fact that over 60,000 major amputations are performed annually in the United States alone [2]. Diabetes and peripheral arterial disease (PAD) are two common comorbidities that increase the risk of limb loss. Individuals with diabetes face up to a 12-fold increase in risk of amputation over their lifetime and comprise 40–45 % of all amputees [1, 3]. A large study of 2,015 diabetic patients found the cumulative risk of amputation to be 11 % 25 years after diagnosis [4]. Other variables associated with increased amputation rates include lower socioeconomic status, ethnicity, and inexperienced physicians caring for patients with critical limb ischemia and diabetes [1–3].

Limb loss has a profound impact on a patient's lifestyle and life expectancy. A study of almost 3,000 patients taken from the National Surgical Quality Improvement Program (NSQIP) found that the 30-day mortality after major amputation was 7 % and complication rates increased with renal insufficiency, cardiac issues, history of sepsis, steroid use, COPD, and advanced age [5]. The Trans-Atlantic Inter-Society Consensus Guidelines (TASC II) reported that patients who undergo major amputation for critical limb ischemia have a 1-year mortality of 25 % and a 30 % incidence of contralateral amputation [6]. Another study found that the 5-year mortality after major amputation ranged between 62.6 and 84.3 % [7].

Amputation survivors frequently face depression not only in the perioperative period, but up to 30 years postamputation [8]. An amputation can disrupt a patient's social function, distort his or her body image, and create new anxieties. These negative social and psychological consequences do not seem to correlate with the level of amputation. In fact, one study found that patients with below knee amputations suffer more depression presumably because they are less disabled overall and tend to compare their activity level to their non-amputee peers more so than above knee amputees [8].

Preventing an amputation starts with the daunting task of controlling complex diseases including critical limb ischemia and diabetes. The challenge becomes more difficult because of patient noncompliance and intransigent social forces, which can sabotage preventive measures and derail limb salvage efforts. Patients can be their own worst enemy by ignoring medical advice or not having the knowledge of or access to healthcare resources. Factors associated with increased amputation rates include sudden rapid progression of disease, limited access to healthcare providers, and poor education [9].

Surgeons who perform amputations should take a holistic approach to patients facing limb loss. Ideally, all possibilities for limb salvage should be exhausted before proceeding with an amputation. Efforts at limb preservation must uncover the etiology of limb threat and explore the potential for correcting it. Factors that determine if an amputation is necessary include the ability to improve perfusion, control infection, and preserve musculoskeletal architecture. If limb salvage is not possible, the optimal level of amputation should be determined with the goal of maximizing limb length and function while minimizing the risk of local complications in the residual limb. An interdisciplinary team consisting of physical therapists, mental health professionals, nutritionists, and physicians can expand the rehabilitation potential following amputation.

This chapter will outline the indications for amputation, discuss exams that help determine the level of the amputation,

J.T. Chiriano, DO, FACS (✉)
Department of Cardiovascular and Thoracic Surgery, Loma Linda University Medical Center, 11175 Campus Street, Suite 21123, Loma Linda, CA 92354, USA
e-mail: jchiriano@msn.com

A.M. Abou-Zamzam Jr., MD, FACS
Division of Vascular Surgery, Loma Linda University School of Medicine, Loma Linda, CA, USA

V. Gahtan and M.J. Costanza (eds.), *Essentials of Vascular Surgery for the General Surgeon*,
DOI 10.1007/978-1-4939-1326-8_8, © Springer Science+Business Media New York 2015

Table 8.1 Indications for foot and lower extremity amputations

Absolute indications for amputation	Relative indications for amputation
Nonsalvageable foot or lower extremity due to extensive tissue loss	Severe Charcot foot deformity limiting functional status
Nonsalvageable foot or lower extremity in the setting of acute limb ischemia	Failed prior revascularization with continued tissue loss or infection
Severe life-threatening foot/limb infection	Poor surgical candidate with critical limb ischemia
Nonambulatory patients with nonhealing wounds or infection including patients with severe lower extremity contractures	No revascularization targets in patients with critical limb ischemia and ongoing tissue loss or severe rest pain
	Chronic osteomyelitis and nonhealing wounds

and describe the surgical technique of major amputations. The goal of this chapter is to give the reader an understanding of the workup and treatment for patients who require an amputation of the toe, foot, or lower extremity.

Indications for Amputation

Indications for a lower extremity amputation include life-threatening infection, failure of prior revascularization, poor functional status with an unsalvageable leg or foot, and fixed joint contractures with recurrent lower extremity wounds (Table 8.1). Challenging decisions about whether to proceed with an amputation can be clarified with a stepwise evaluation of the ability to salvage the lower extremity, the etiology of the wounds, and the functional status of the patient.

The first decision point along the path to amputation determines whether the lower extremity is worth saving. Nonsalvageable lower extremities suffer from extensive tissue loss that would be impossible to heal or would require massive debridement ultimately compromising the architecture and function of the foot. Other factors favoring a lower extremity amputation include extensive heel gangrene particularly with underlying osteomyelitis, widespread soft tissue infection, and severe Charcot deformity of the foot with loss of function. Any of these clinical scenarios represents a clear indication for lower extremity amputation.

If the patient does not have an obvious indication for amputation because of the factors described above, the next step involves determining the etiology of the lower extremity wounds. Patients may present with ischemic, neuroischemic, neuropathic, pressure-induced, or venous wounds. The investigation begins with a complete pulse exam to evaluate the vascular supply to the lower extremity. Absence of palpable lower extremity pulses frequently indicates underlying peripheral arterial disease (PAD). An ankle-brachial index (ABI) provides an objective, bedside exam to detect PAD defined as an ABI less than 0.9. A systolic ankle pressure less than 70 mmHg identifies patients with severe ischemia of the foot who are unlikely to heal their wounds without a revascularization procedure [6]. Falsely elevated ABIs (greater than 1.3) usually indicate tibial vessel calcification. In this situation, toe pressures measured by the noninvasive vascular lab provide a more accurate assessment of perfusion with values less than 50 mmHg indicating significant foot ischemia. Transcutaneous pressures may also help predict wound healing after an amputation. Several studies have shown that a threshold level of 30 mmHg correlates with improved wound healing. Ballard et al. reported a 73 % healing rate at this level, while Chiriano et al. found that 67 % of patients with PAD and underlying wounds healed with a TcpO2 level above 30 mmHg [10–12].

If ischemia caused the lower extremity wounds, the next step involves determining which patients will benefit from revascularization. Although revascularization is the treatment of choice for patients with underlying arterial disease and tissue loss, it is not universally successful. Lower extremity wounds can recur after failed surgical bypasses or endovascular interventions. Abou-Zamzam et al. found that over 50 % of patients undergoing an amputation had either a prior attempt at revascularization or no revascularization options based on anatomy [13]. In patients with limb-threatening ischemia, the surgeon must determine the feasibility and benefit of revascularization.

Imaging studies such as computed tomography angiography (CTA) or magnetic resonance angiography (MRA) can map the arterial anatomy to help determine revascularization options. Although CTA and MRA can detect iliac, femoral, and popliteal artery lesions, their accuracy diminishes in the tibial vessels. Catheter-directed angiography may be indicated if noninvasive imaging does not identify target vessels for revascularization. Patient factors that make angiography unreasonable include severe renal insufficiency in a highly debilitated patient or progression of wounds that would make the limb unsalvageable. Angiography should include images of the foot to evaluate for distal revascularization targets. While axial flow to the foot has traditionally been preferred for healing pedal wounds, a peroneal artery bypass can be successful if adequate collaterals to the pedal vessels are present at the ankle [14].

Patients who have no revascularization targets usually require an amputation. Some patients have distal arterial targets but lack an autogenous conduit to function as a bypass. Although distal bypasses with prosthetic grafts are feasible, they have inferior patency rates and increased infection risk [15].

Debilitated, nonambulatory patients with extensive ischemic tissue loss and no autogenous conduit are better served with an amputation instead of repeat revascularization.

Patients without underlying peripheral arterial disease who present with nonhealing lower extremity wounds most often suffer from diabetes. Several studies cite diabetes as the most common risk factor for amputation because of its association with infection, neuropathy, and architectural deformity of the foot. Malone ranked the indications for amputation starting with complications of diabetes (60–80 %), infections without diabetes (15–25 %), ischemia without infection (5–10 %), chronic osteomyelitis (3–5 %), trauma (2–5 %), and miscellaneous (5–10 %) [2, 16]. Diabetic patients can present with overwhelming infections which require urgent amputation as a matter of life over limb. Elective amputations may be necessary for loss of function after multiple wound debridements for underlying osteomyelitis or severe Charcot deformity. Preventing amputations in patients with foot deformities or neuropathic ulcers requires orthotics to off load pressure on the foot, advanced wound care, and surgical correction of architectural deformities whenever possible. Fortunately, most patients who undergo an amputation for the indications described above maintain an acceptable quality of life.

Functional status represents the final component to evaluate in patients being considered for amputation. Invasive limb salvage procedures have no role in the management of extremely debilitated patients. Nonambulatory patients with extensive lower extremity wounds and patients with fixed joint contractures and pressure-induced tissue necrosis should undergo primary amputation. Patients with limited survival including patients with malignancy, severe CHF, and severe dementia and elderly patients on dialysis should be considered for primary amputation [17–19].

Determining the Level of Amputation

Although an amputation is often perceived as a failure of limb salvage, it still requires preoperative planning and sound surgical judgment. Choosing the appropriate level of amputation plays a critical role in achieving a successful outcome. Amputations that fail to heal delay rehabilitation and frequently require further surgery with its associated risks. While the amputation level should be tailored to each patient's anatomic and functional needs, any amputation must adhere to three general principles. Firstly, it should ensure the removal of all nonviable tissue and infection. Secondly, the level of amputation should be chosen to maximize the chances of uncomplicated wound healing. Finally, it should give the patient the best opportunity for future prosthetic use.

Successful healing after amputation depends on multiple factors including hemodynamic status, infection, glucose level, and the patients' underlying comorbidities (Table 8.2). It should be noted that although wound healing is the easiest outcome variable to observe, it is not the only measure of success after an amputation. Other important outcome measures for amputations include successful rehabilitation, functional status, and overall survival.

Table 8.2 Factors that influence healing at amputation site

SPP	>30 mmHg
TcPO2	>30 mmHg
Ankle pressures	>70 mmHg
Toe pressure	>50 mmHg
Physical exam	Palpable popliteal pulse
Level of amputation	Below the ankle < above the ankle
Presence of comorbidities	CAD, cerebrovascular disease, ESRD, diabetes, COPD, increased age

SPP skin perfusion pressure, *TcPO2* transcutaneous pressure of oxygen, *CAD* coronary artery disease, *ESRD* end-stage renal disease, *COPD* chronic obstructive pulmonary disease

While there is no consensus on which noninvasive tests can determine the optimal level of amputation, it is clear that physical exam alone and presence of bleeding during debridement are poor predictors of successful wound healing. Although the presence of a palpable pulse immediately proximal to the amputation site nearly always predicts healing, the absence of a pulse does not consistently lead to wound failure [2]. Using the pulse exam alone to determine amputation level would therefore unnecessarily preclude some patients from having more distal amputations. Several studies have documented toe pressures and TcPO2 levels as predictors of wound healing particularly in forefoot procedures such as digit, ray, and transmetatarsal amputations. Vitti et al. retrospectively studied 136 men undergoing forefoot amputations and found universal failure of healing in diabetic patients with toe pressures less than 38 mmHg and universal success with toe pressures greater than 68 mmHg. This threshold did not predict outcome in nondiabetic patients [20].

Several studies have explored alternatives to the "clinical judgment" method of determining amputation level which has proven to be notoriously inaccurate. Poredos et al. attempted to establish a minimal TcPO2 level necessary for amputation healing by studying 71 limbs of which 55 were below knee amputations. In all patients, the level of amputation was based solely on clinical factors. Sixteen patients (22.5 %) required conversion to above knee amputation due to failure of healing. The patients that failed to heal had significantly lower TcPO2 levels versus those that healed (18 mmHg vs. 37 mmHg, $p<0.01$) [21]. Holstein found that only one failed below knee amputation out of 15 exhibited clinical signs of ischemia prior to amputation, whereas all of the failures had skin perfusion pressures (SPP) less than 30 mmHg. Only 3 % of the amputations in this series with an SPP greater than 30 mmHg failed to heal [22].

These studies and others like them highlight the inaccuracy of clinical judgment alone in deciding on the level of amputation. Skin perfusion pressure seems to correlate well with below knee amputation healing; however, other factors also contribute to successful outcomes following major amputation.

Ankle and toe pressures should be measured as surrogates for local perfusion at the site of the surgical procedure. A study of 44 consecutive major lower extremity amputations (38 for severe limb ischemia) revealed that all patients with ankle pressures greater than 70 mmHg achieved successful wound healing. In contrast only 50 % of those with ankle pressures less than 70 mmHg healed their wounds. Notably, these findings were only significant for amputations proximal to the ankle; foot amputations had worse outcomes overall. The authors found no significant outcome differences with respect to skin temperature, gender, age, blood chemistry, or duration of diabetes [23]. Data from large series suggest that TcPO2 and skin perfusion pressures are also less significant predictors of wound healing in forefoot amputations compared to more proximal amputations [24]. Toe pressures may offer a more accurate predictor of healing after forefoot amputations. The TASC II document cites toe pressures less than 50 mmHg as a sign of severe ischemia at the level of the forefoot suggesting that this may increase the risk of failed healing in forefoot amputations [6].

Although hemodynamic factors play an important role in selecting the level of amputation, other more global variables such as prior ambulatory status and presence of comorbidities may also help the surgeon select which amputation to perform. A retrospective review of 80 patients undergoing 91 transmetatarsal amputations found that initial healing of the amputation negatively correlated with the presence of end-stage renal disease and infection [25]. In a different series of patients, the authors found no correlation between healing transmetatarsal amputations and preoperative demographic factors such as CAD, DM, and renal insufficiency. In this cohort, a history of MI and the presence of COPD were associated with mortality after BKA, while ESRD and COPD were the strongest predictors of mortality after AKA [24]. These comorbid conditions seem to correlate better with amputations proximal to the ankle and lose some degree of predictability for foot and toe amputations.

One of the largest outcome studies of lower extremity amputations used the NSQIP database including 4,250 patients from 121 hospitals nationally. In this study, wound complication risk increased with an elevated INR, age 50–59 as compared with older patients, high BMI, and current tobacco use. Thirty-day mortality was 7.6 and 12 % after BKA and AKA, respectively, and predictors of mortality corroborated previous study results with history of MI and presence of COPD associated with mortality after BKA and ESRD and COPD predicting mortality after AKA [26]. Although predicting outcomes based on preoperative risk factors is not always reliable, it is clear that wound complications increase with uncontrolled diabetes, presence of renal disease, COPD, and CAD. These results highlight the importance of pursuing medical optimization prior to performing an elective amputation.

While preoperative planning focuses on achieving local wound healing, a healed stump does not completely define a successful amputation. The amputation level selected should also maximize the functional capacity of the patient. Achieving this goal requires integrating multiple factors that influence the amputation level including extremity perfusion, comorbid conditions, pre-amputation ambulatory status, and life expectancy. Taylor and associates reported on a comprehensive definition of amputation success in 3,000 patients undergoing major lower extremity amputations (309 BKAs) from 1998 to 2004. They defined success as wound healing without need for revision to a higher level, maintenance of ambulatory status for 1 year, and survival for at least 6 months. Only 51 % of patients met this definition of success and the overall mortality was 3.2 %. Preoperative factors associated with poor outcomes included CAD, cerebrovascular disease, COPD, diabetes, impaired ambulatory status, and increased age. Independent predictors of clinical failure included presence of coronary artery disease, cerebrovascular disease, and impaired preoperative ambulatory status. If any two of these factors were present, the probability of success was only 23 %, and if all were present, the success rate dropped to 10.4 %. The probability of success was 67.5 % if none of the factors were present [27].

Return to ambulation should be a primary consideration when determining amputation level. Ambulating with a prosthetic requires more energy, and the energy expenditure increases as the level of amputation moves proximally. Tang et al. found that below knee amputations, knee disarticulation, above knee amputation, and hip disarticulation have energy requirements above baseline of 10–40 %, 71.5 %, 63 %, and 82 %, respectively [28]. Approximately 80 % of patients return to ambulation after a below knee amputation and up to 50 % after an above knee amputation, and less than 10 % of patients walk after a hip disarticulation.

In summary, determining the level of amputation remains challenging and has a significant clinical impact. Although forefoot and below knee amputations have acceptable functional outcomes, they carry an increased risk of wound complication and need for proximal revision. The overall mortality for amputations ranges from 6 to 17 % and peaks among patients with renal failure, prior coronary revascularization, advanced age, and transfemoral versus transtibial amputation [26, 27, 29–32]. In general, transmetatarsal amputations have a significantly lower healing potential than amputations proximal to the ankle and should be reserved for patients with high functional status who have few if any hemodynamic risk factors for wound failure. Most patients

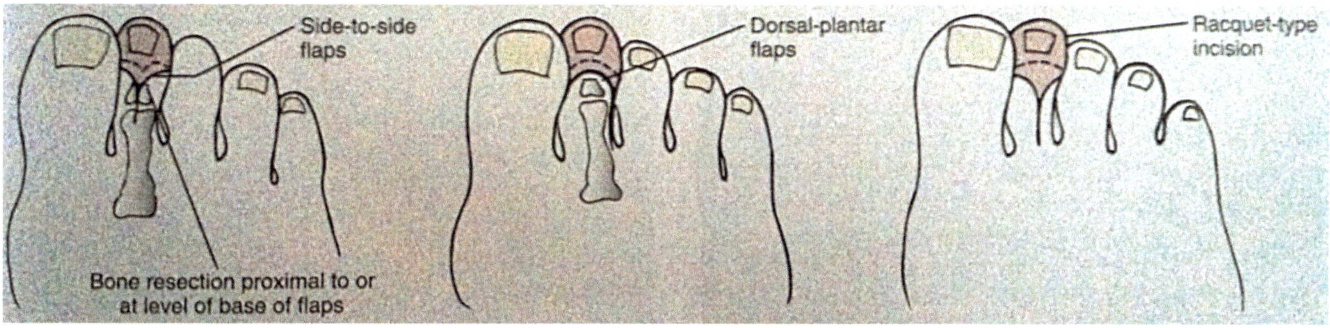

Fig. 8.1 Digital amputation (Adapted from Brodsky [33])

who have failed prior revascularization for critical limb ischemia will not be candidates for amputations below the ankle because of impaired preoperative ambulatory status or severe comorbid conditions including renal dysfunction.

Below knee amputation is a reasonable option for ambulatory patients with hemodynamic factors that predict postoperative wound healing including adequate skin perfusion pressures (generally above 30 mmHg). The presence of a palpable popliteal pulse has also been consistently associated with successful wound healing [2]. An overall successful wound healing rate of 85 % should be expected from patients undergoing below knee amputations. Above knee amputations are indicated for nonambulatory or minimally ambulatory patients and for patients who have a low likelihood of healing any distal amputation. These criteria apply even when the wound is completely confined to the forefoot.

Procedures

Digital Amputation

While digital amputations can be performed at several levels, this section will focus on metatarsophalangeal amputations. Planning the skin incision should allow for adequate skin coverage after bony amputation. Usually an elliptical incision oriented in the vertical direction minimizes the space between the digits after wound healing. The incision should begin at the level of the proximal phalanx providing there is viable skin at that level. Dissection should then proceed circumferential through the soft tissue to expose the bone of the proximal phalanx and the metatarsophalangeal joint space. Any bleeding from the digital arteries can usually be controlled with electrocautery. The metatarsophalangeal joint should then be disarticulated. If this is not possible, the proximal phalanx can be transected with a bone cutter and the bone can be removed back to the joint space using a rongeur. We prefer to rongeur the cartilage off of the head of the metatarsal bone because its relative avascularity can complicate wound healing. After achieving hemostasis, closure involves interrupted subcutaneous absorbable sutures followed by interrupted simple nylon sutures for the skin (Fig. 8.1). Amputations performed for acute infection should be left open and packed.

Ray Amputation

Ray amputation refers to removal of the toe with a part of its corresponding metatarsal bone. The skin incisions vary depending on which toe is being amputated, but all incisions attempt to preserve as much skin as possible for closure. Flap coverage of the remaining bone segment can be achieved with a subperiosteal resection of the metatarsal proximal to the soft tissue incision. For the first and fifth toe resections, the incision is similar to a digital amputation with a proximal extension along the medial (first toe) or lateral (fifth toe) foot to obtain access to the metatarsal bone. The incision is closed along its length after resection of the bone. For central ray resections, the incision again is similar to that of a digital amputation with extension proximally along the dorsal aspect of the foot. Preserving the plantar skin whenever possible plays a critical role in recovery as it will allow for early weight bearing [33] (Fig. 8.2).

Transmetatarsal Amputation (TMA)

Patients being considered for a transmetatarsal amputation should have adequate plantar skin to create a flap that will heal and provide soft tissue support for any forefoot prosthesis. If the plantar skin is compromised, a TMA can be performed in a guillotine fashion with subsequent skin grafting. The incision begins transversely across the dorsum of the foot at the level of the midmetatarsal. It then extends distally on the medial and lateral side of the foot and before crossing on the plantar aspect of the foot at the level of the metatarsophalangeal joint to create a posterior flap. Dissection is performed through the subcutaneous tissue along the incision line. After exposing the metatarsal bones, a periosteal elevator is used to

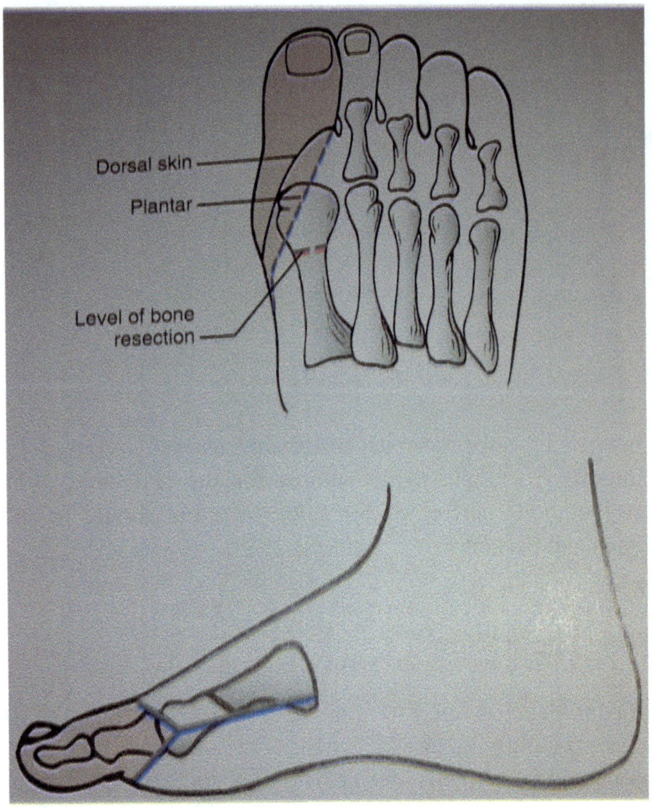

Fig. 8.2 Ray amputation (Adapted from Brodsky [33])

create a cephalad flap on the dorsal surface. The skin should be retracted cephalad and the metatarsal bones should be transected at the level of the midshaft or proximal third. In order to preserve the plantar fat pad, a periosteal elevator is used to separate the plantar surface of the metatarsal bones from the soft tissue. The digital arteries can either be suture ligated or cauterized to obtain hemostasis. Starting with the transected shafts of the metatarsal bones, the fat pad is then dissected away and the forefoot is removed. A tension-free closure is then performed by approximating the fascia of the dorsum of the foot with the soft tissue of the plantar fat pad with interrupted absorbable sutures. The skin can either be stapled or closed with interrupted 3–0 nylon sutures. There is no need for a drain in the subcutaneous tissue; however, a local pump that functions to slowly infuse local anesthetic may help reduce the need for narcotics postoperatively. The foot is wrapped with moderate compression to minimize the risks of postoperative hematoma or edema (Fig. 8.3).

Outcomes of transmetatarsal amputations vary depending on the presence of infection and critical limb ischemia. Hosch and associates found that healing rates were significantly better if the amputation was performed for infection in the absence of critical limb ischemia. The need for revision to a more proximal amputation was appeared to be greater in patients with hypoalbuminemia and in patients who were not prescribed an adequate postoperative prosthetic [34]. Another study reported that 27 % of patients undergoing transmetatarsal amputation required revision to a below knee amputation [35]. Although TMA healing rates can be poor, this amputation should be offered to suitable candidates as it provides an opportunity for limb preservation particularly in the diabetic population without critical limb ischemia [36]. Patients with severe peripheral arterial disease being considered for TMA usually require revascularization prior to the amputation to insure wound healing.

Below Knee Amputation

Below knee amputations require meticulous surgical technique to minimize the risk of postoperative complications and subsequent conversion to an above knee amputation. Several factors play a role in the planning and execution of a below knee amputation. Firstly, the surgeon must decide on the location and type of incision to use. Young patients with an injury to the foot itself who have normal perfusion and good skin quality may benefit from a slightly longer stump, whereas older patients with severe peripheral vascular disease may have a better chance of healing with a shorter stump. Secondly, the skin quality may prohibit a long posterior flap, and the surgeon may opt for a fishmouth incision to construct medial and lateral flaps (Fig. 8.4a, b). Thirdly, below knee amputations demand meticulous hemostasis as postoperative hematoma creates a nidus for infection that ultimately requires reoperation and conversion to an above knee amputation. Patients who are on antiplatelet therapy or Coumadin may benefit from closed suction drainage which can give an early warning of postoperative bleeding within the stump. Finally, all nonviable tissue should be removed intraoperatively to maximize wound healing. With appropriate patient selection and surgical technique, 85 % of below knee amputations should achieve initial wound healing.

Patients undergoing below knee amputation often have open wounds below the ankle. To minimize contamination and the risk of perioperative infection, the foot should be isolated from the surgical field by wrapping it with adherent drapes and placing it in a stockinet. The leg is then prepped and draped in a sterile fashion from the foot to the midthigh.

When planning a below knee amputation with a long posterior flap, the incision should follow the 2/3–1/3 rule. The level of the transverse anterior skin incision depends on the desired length of the stump, but it is usually placed 5–10 cm distal to the tibial tuberosity. The circumference of the calf is measured at this level, and the transverse anterior incision extends for 2/3 the circumference. The incision should then transition to medial and lateral longitudinal incisions which extend distally for a distance of at least 1/3 the calf circumference (Fig. 8.5). Electrocautery dissection then deepens the incision to the crural fascia along the length of the incision.

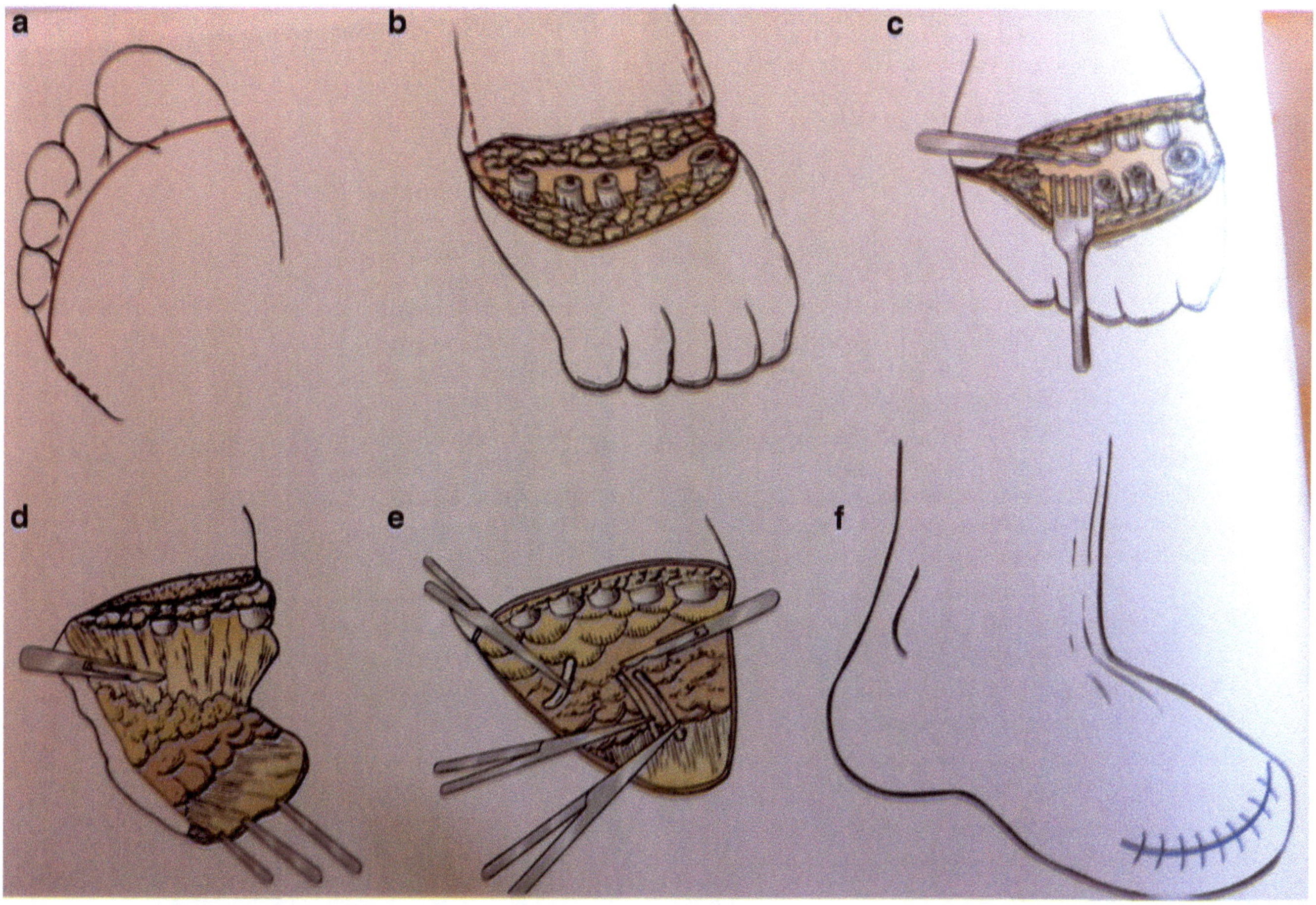

Fig. 8.3 Transmetatarsal amputation. (**a**) Incision on plantar aspect of foot at level of metatarsophalangeal joint. (**b**) Transection of metatarsal bones. (**c**) Dissection of fat pad while retracting forefoot. (**d**) Creation of plantar flap. (**e**) Ligation of digital arteries (**f**) Skin closure

The authors prefer an anatomic dissection in which each compartment is methodically dissected in order to minimize blood loss and tissue trauma. The fascia of the anterior compartment is incised to allow transection of the muscles and visualization of the anterior tibial artery, deep peroneal nerve, and tibial vein which travel anterior to the interosseous membrane near the tibia (Fig. 8.6). This neurovascular bundle is ligated and divided. Next, the lateral compartment is entered by incising the crural fascia. The muscles are transected and the fibula is exposed at this level. There are no named vessels that require division in the lateral compartment. Medially, the posterior compartments are entered by incising the overlying crural fascia. The saphenous vein should be ligated and divided if it has not already been harvested for a revascularization procedure. The gastrocnemius muscle is reflected posteriorly and the soleus muscle is separated from the tibia to create a window into the lateral portion of the leg.

A large clamp is then placed directly behind the tibia to bring a laparotomy pad through the back of the calf as protection for the popliteal vessels during transection of the tibia. A periosteal elevator is then used to mobilize and anterior skin flap that should be retracted cephalad with rakes during tibial transection. At this point the soft tissue should be cleared off of the fibula with electrocautery and periosteal elevators. The tibia is then transected with a mechanical or power saw 1–2 cm proximal to the skin incision anteriorly taking care not to injure the posterior vasculature. The fibula is transected in a similar fashion 1 cm proximal to the level of the tibial transection. A bone hook is then placed into the marrow cavity of the distal tibia to elevate it away from the popliteal neurovascular bundle (Fig. 8.7).

The popliteal artery/vein and tibial nerve are then identified and separately suture ligated and divided. If not already performed, the distal posterior incision should be completed at this time and deepened through the crural fascia. An amputation knife is then used to dissect the deep compartment musculature posteriorly from the tibia and fibula, this is performed to the distal posterior incision, and the soft tissue is transected at this level to remove the lower leg. There is often hemorrhage from the transected peroneal and posterior tibial arteries and veins, which are easily clamped and suture ligated. All bleeding vessels and soft tissue are then meticulously controlled with

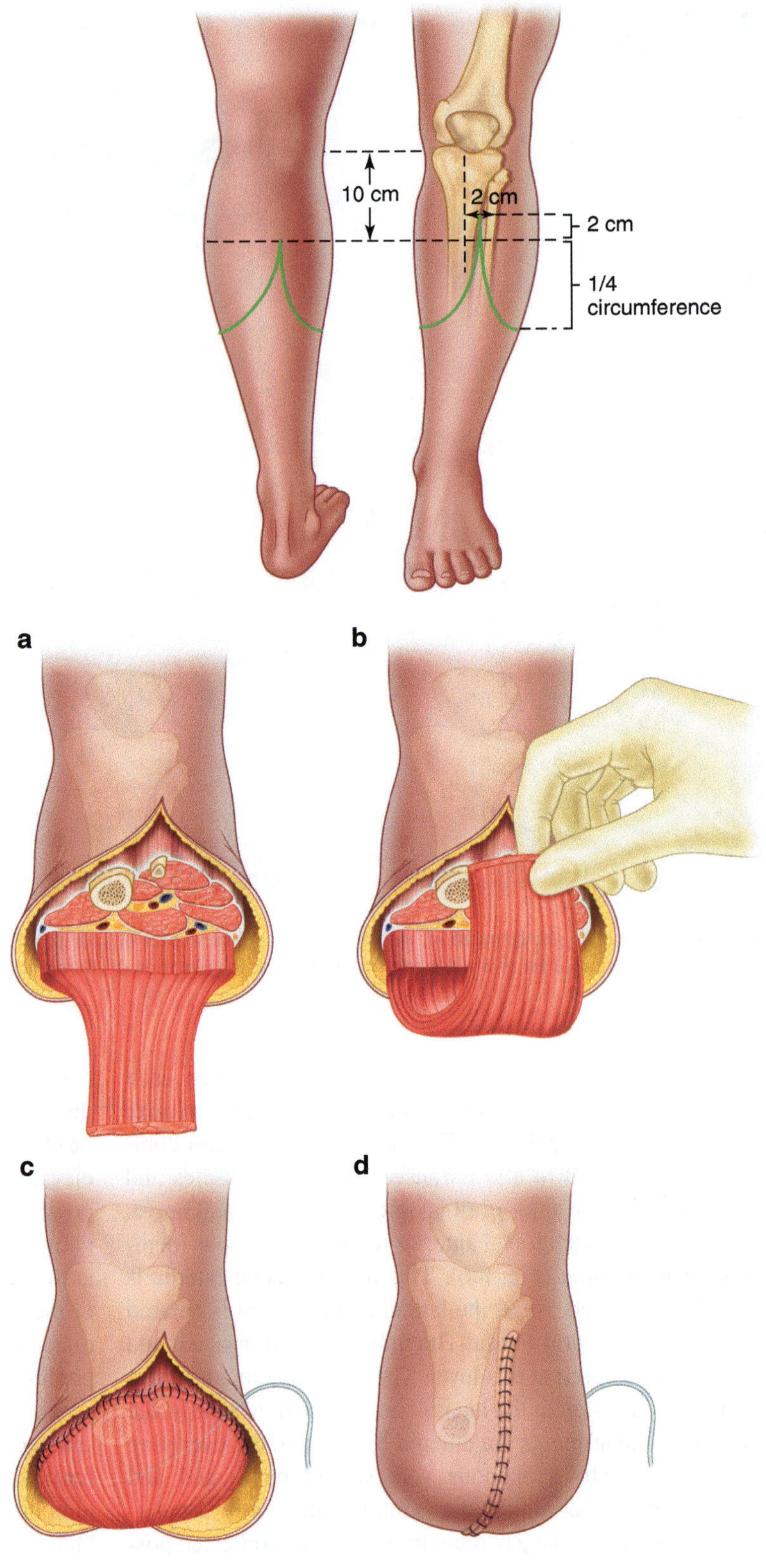

Fig. 8.4 Skew flaps for below knee amputation using fishmouth incision. (**a**) and (**b**) development of gastrocnemius muscle flap. (**c**) and (**d**) closure of wound with drain in place

electrocautery and suture ligation. After obtaining hemostasis, copious irrigation removes any devitalized tissue and bone fragments from the amputation site.

At this point, the surgeon must decide if the soleus muscle must be excised in order to facilitate a tension-free closure. If the flap is bulky such as is found in muscular patients, one can separate the soleus from the gastrocnemius muscle in an avascular plane and partially or totally excise it leaving the gastrocnemius as the main pad of the posterior flap (Fig. 8.8). Additionally, the tibia may need to be shortened in order to

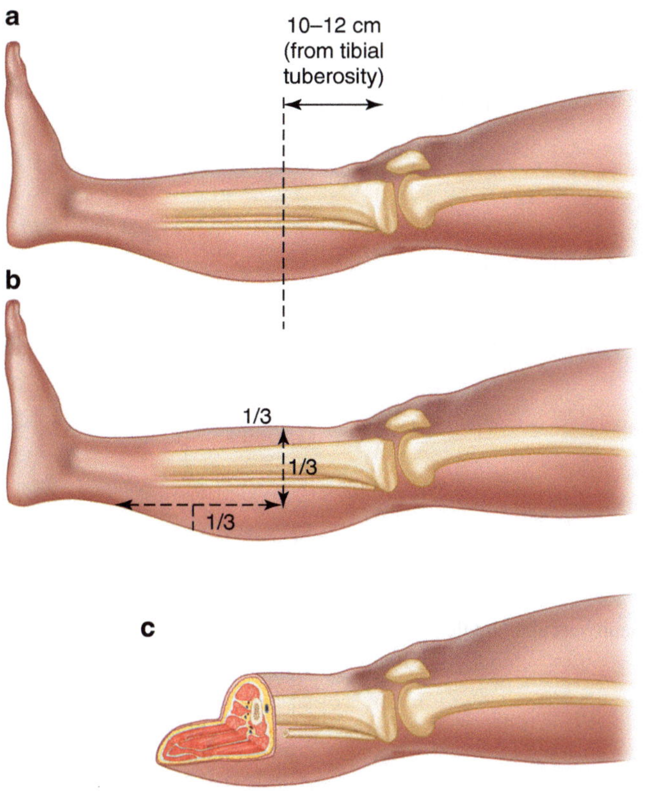

Fig. 8.5 (**a**) Transverse skin incision located 10-12 cm distal to tibial tuberosity. (**b**) Anterior inicison is 2/3rd circumference of the calf (1/3rd on each side of midline), while the posterior flap length is 1/3rd the circumference. (**c**) Below knee amputation with posterior flap before wound closure

prevent protrusion into the posterior flap. Once the tibia is at the proper length, the authors prefer to bevel its anterior surface to create a smoother edge of the bone in order to minimize pressure while wearing a prosthetic.

Closure of the amputation starts by approximating the anterior and posterior fascia with interrupted 2-0 braided absorbable sutures. There should be no gaps through which a digit or an instrument can pass. The authors prefer to place a local anesthetic pain pump catheter deep to the fascial closure near the transected nerves and exiting through the skin medially or laterally. By achieving localized pain relief, the pain pump can minimize the need for narcotic medications postoperatively. The skin should be closed with either staples or interrupted nylon sutures (Fig. 8.9). The stump is then wrapped with gauze and an ACE bandage and placed into a knee immobilizer brace to decrease the risk of a flexion contracture at the knee.

Above Knee Amputation (AKA)

Above knee amputations boast the highest initial healing rates; however, fewer patients return to ambulation after this procedure compared to below knee amputations. A longer AKA stump length can improve the ability to ambulate. Therefore, the length of the amputation should be maximized for patients that have promising rehabilitation potential and in whom there is a possibility for prosthetic use. The incision should be made on the distal thigh just above the knee joint whenever possible. The commonly used fishmouth incision can be outlined dividing the circumference of the site of amputation by two and creating a cephalad bevel in the incision on each side of the thigh. This facilitates closure with no dog-ears and keeps the incision line more anterior in order to avoid undue pressure while the patient is supine (Fig. 8.10).

After carrying the incision through the subcutaneous tissue with electrocautery, the fascia and muscles of the anterior compartment of the thigh are transected to expose the femur. Incising the subcutaneous tissue and fascia of the medial and lateral thigh and transecting the lateral and medial thigh muscles provide more exposure of the femur. A periosteal elevator is then used to mobilize an anterior musculocutaneous flap to be used during closure. The femoral/popliteal vessels are then isolated posterior to the distal femur and dissected free of the surrounding soft tissue (Fig. 8.11). The artery and vein are individually double ligated with heavy silk suture and transected. The sciatic nerve which is located lateral and posterior to the vessels should be mobilized as far proximally as possible, ligated, and divided, thereby allowing it to retract deep into the proximal musculature. Handling the sciatic nerve in this way will keep it well back from the skin incision and may prevent it from forming a neuroma which leads to chronic pain in the stump. The posterior portion of the amputation is then completed by incising the skin and posterior fascia followed by division of the posterior muscles with electrocautery. Large rakes are then used to retract the anterior skin and muscles, and the femur is transected with a power saw 2 cm proximal to the level of the incision. Meticulous hemostasis is carried out with electrocautery and suture ligation of any small bleeding vessels. The amputation site is then thoroughly irrigated before approximating the anterior and posterior fascia with interrupted 2-0 braided absorbable sutures. The authors insert a small pain pump to infuse local anesthetic for 48–72 h postoperatively in an attempt to minimize narcotic use. The skin can either be sutured closed with interrupted nylon sutures or stapled. The site is then wrapped with Kerlix gauze and a compressive ACE bandage.

Technical errors for an above knee amputation often involve inadequate shortening of the femur. In these cases, the distal muscle provides inadequate padding and the stump is vulnerable to pressure sores and skin breakdown if the patient uses a prosthetic for ambulation. Creating a tension-free closure with an appropriate proximal resection of the femur can facilitate perioperative healing and prevent future wound complications.

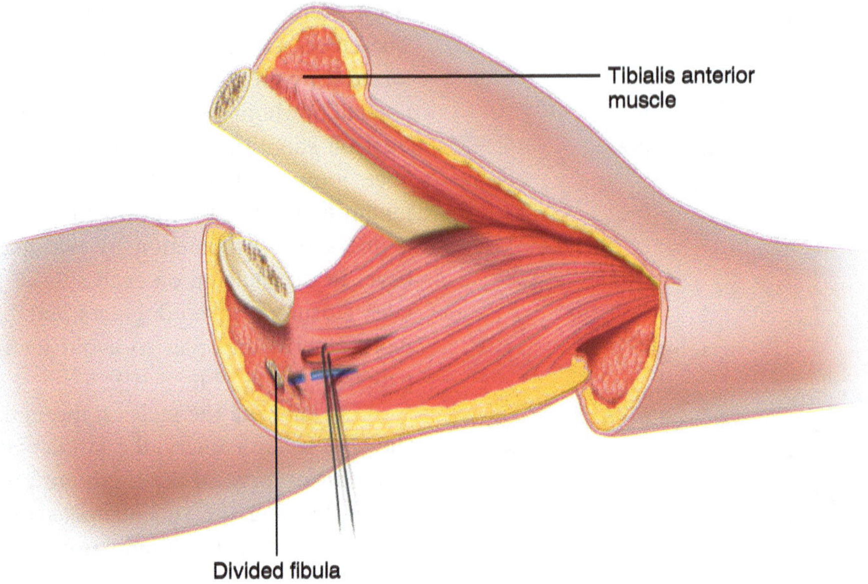

Fig. 8.6 Division and superior retraction of the tibia exposes the popliteal neurovascular bundle

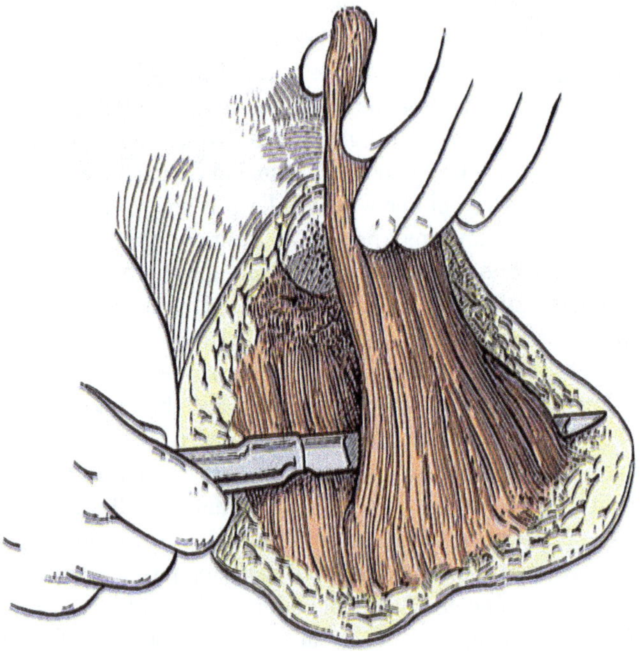

Fig. 8.7 Excision of the soleus muscle to facilitate posterior flap closure

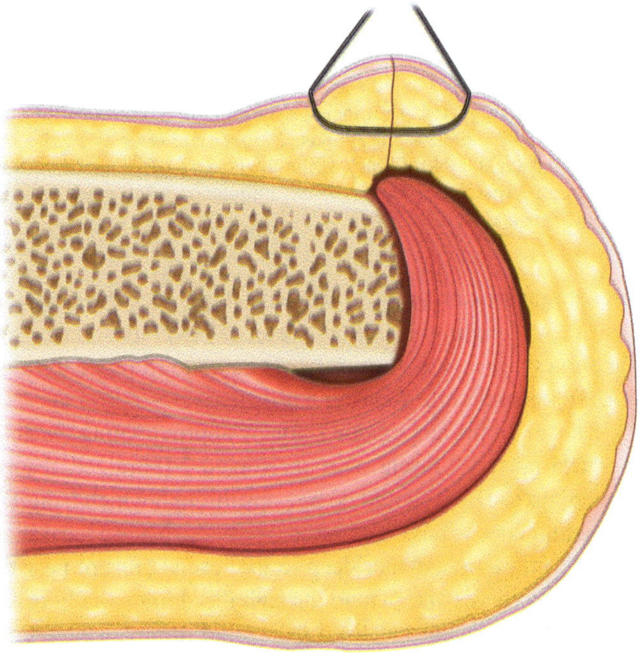

Fig. 8.8 Closure of posterior flap over distal end of the tibia

Alternative Lower Extremity Amputations

Less commonly performed amputations of the foot and ankle include Chopart, Lisfranc, and Syme's procedures. Although these foot amputations have the attraction of salvaging the limb, their healing rates are not as robust as the more commonly performed amputations, and the procedures themselves tend to be more technically demanding.

Chopart's amputation implies a disarticulation of the talonavicular and calcaneocuboid joints combined. This amputation is thought to be easier to perform than the Syme's amputation. The patient can wear a shoe after this procedure if fitted with a proper orthotic. This is in contrast to the knee high prosthesis that is needed after a below knee amputation and a Syme's amputation. Proponents of the Chopart's amputation cite the fact that the weight bearing surface includes the relatively resilient plantar skin which can toler-

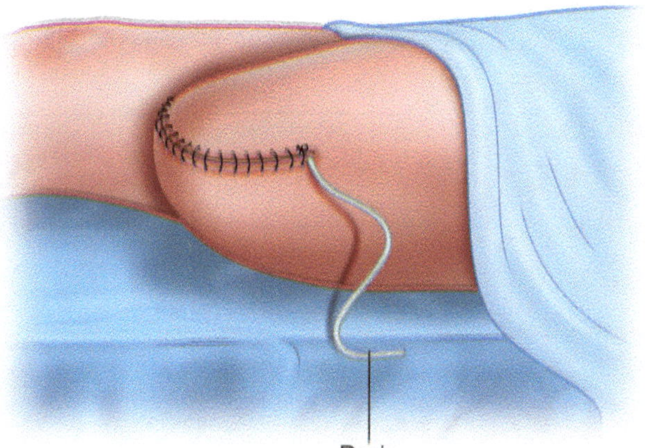

Fig. 8.9 Fishmouth incision for above knee amputation

ate the pressure load and stress incurred during ambulation. Patients with this amputation may be prone to tendon imbalance due to foot deformities and the unopposed pull of the Achilles tendon. Subsequent procedures to divide or lengthen Achilles tendon may be necessary to achieve an acceptable functional outcome. In contrast, a below knee amputation has relatively straightforward fitting process for a knee high prosthesis [2, 33].

Lisfranc's amputation is a tarsometatarsal disarticulation which creates a shorter, more proximal version of the transmetatarsal amputation. Although it is considered a limb salvage procedure, Lisfranc's amputation requires a comprehensive orthotic to be functional. Similar to a transmetatarsal amputation, this procedure carries the risk of poor healing, especially in patients with critical limb ischemia. Counterbalancing this risk is the promise of limb salvage and higher ambulation rates compared to below knee amputation. To be successful, Lisfranc's amputations require viable plantar skin and should allow for removal of all nonviable tissue. Patients who had deep foot abscesses and associated plantar incisions for drainage may be better served with a below knee amputation, as operative stump corrections are necessary in 20–30 % of patients following Lisfranc's amputation [33, 37, 38].

Syme's amputation is an ankle disarticulation which was initially described during an era when below knee amputations carried a 20–25 % mortality rate. This less extensive procedure with a smaller wound had a survival advantage and offered a good functional alternative to below knee amputation. Proponents of the Syme's amputation argue that the increased leg length makes ambulation easier compared to more proximal amputations [39]. Enthusiasm for the Syme's amputation has waned with the advent of more technologically advanced below knee prostheses. Prosthetic options for the distal leg are limited and often fail to reproduce the propulsion created at the ankle joint during ambulation compared to below knee prostheses. Healing this level of amputation can be tenuous and appears to depend on the status of the posterior tibial artery. Laughlin and associates found a 90 % healing rate in patients with a palpable pulse or triphasic Doppler signal over the posterior tibial artery, as compared with a 57 % healing rate in patients with a monophasic Doppler signal. In their study, 90 % of patients that healed were fitted for prosthesis and achieved functional ambulation [39]. Frykberg and associates found a 50 % healing rate 1 year after a Syme's amputation in high-risk patients in whom a more proximal amputation had been initially recommended. They could not identify predictors of success or failure due to the small sample size. All of the patients in this study had diabetes or severe peripheral arterial disease, and 65 % of those that healed went on to ambulate with a prosthetic [40]. The authors favor a below knee amputation in patients with underlying severe peripheral arterial disease, reserving a Syme's amputation for diabetic patients with normal arterial perfusion.

Other more proximal lower extremity amputations include disarticulation procedures such as a through-knee amputation and hip disarticulation. Hip disarticulations are rarely performed and comprise only 0.5 % of all lower extremity amputations in the United States [41]. They are usually indicated in the setting of uncontrolled infection or a failed high above knee amputation with severe osteomyelitis of the proximal femur. Mortality rates range from 30 to 44 % and increase in patients requiring an urgent operation for severe infection [41–43]. The high mortality rate coupled with its technical complexity makes hip disarticulation an amputation of last resort for most surgeons. The functional outcome after hip disarticulation also varies in the literature. Energy needed for ambulation after this procedure is even greater than an above knee amputation which usually requires 100 % more energy than normal ambulation [43]. Conversely, these patients have lower skin and wound complications most likely because they wear their prostheses less than other amputees. Although Yari and associates found significant functional limitations in patients that undergo hip disarticulation, technological advances may overcome these challenges [44]. Prosthetics now incorporate microprocessors to control the knee joint which decrease the energy required for ambulation and improve mobility [45].

Finally, a knee disarticulation or through-knee amputation has several potential advantages over the traditional above knee amputation. The through-knee amputation may improve mobility by creating a longer stump with a more bulbous end that can easily fit into a prosthesis. Only the vessels, nerves, and tendons are transected during the procedure. Preserving the thigh muscles and femur maximizes the mechanical advantage of the stump and decreases the energy required for ambulation. Patients with properly performed bilateral through-knee amputee can full weight bear on the stumps without prosthesis. Weight bearing is made possible

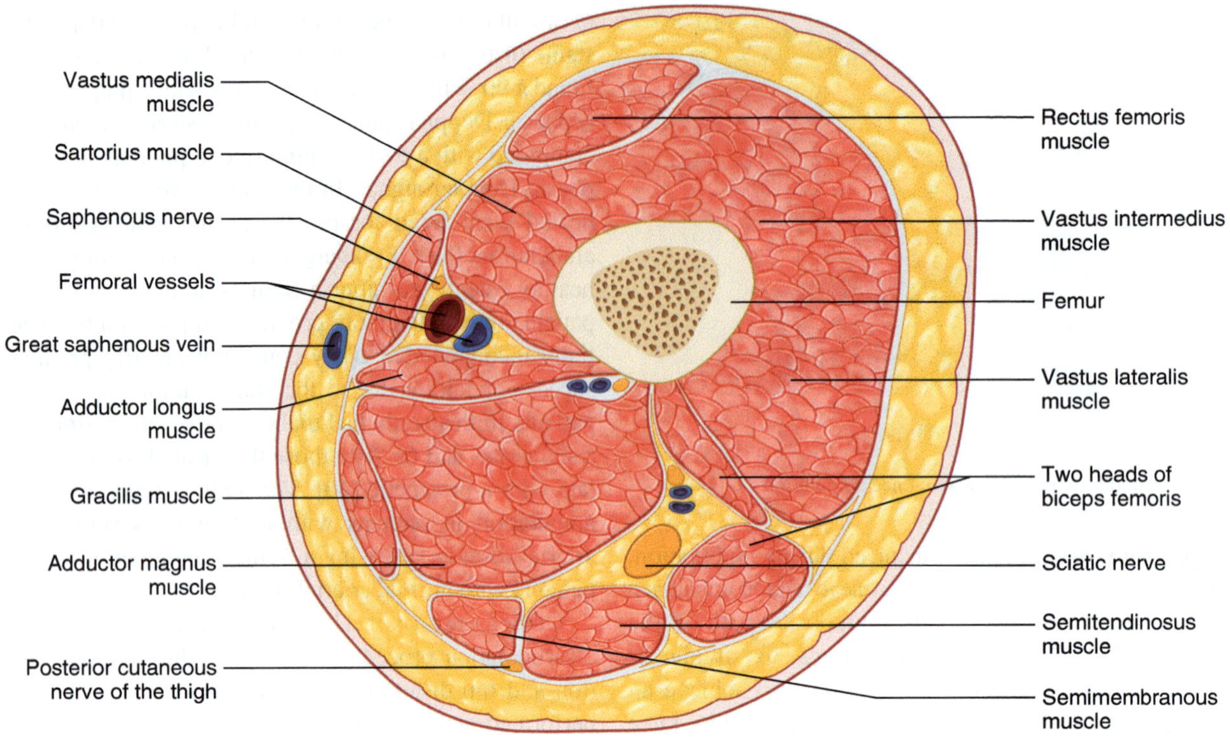

Fig. 8.10 Cross section showing location of the neurovascular structures within the muscle compartments of the leg

by leaving the meniscal cartilage on the femoral condyles to function as a shock absorber. If there is not enough soft tissue for closure, the femoral condyles may be partially or totally excised. These amputations are particularly prone to decubitus ulcers and require appropriate postoperative bandaging and leg elevation to facilitate healing. Prosthetic fitting is usually possible 3–6 weeks after a through-knee amputation [46].

Amputations for Infection

Patients with diabetes or critical limb ischemia and tissue loss are at high risk for developing severe foot infections that ultimately require major amputation. Foot infection is the most common reason for hospitalization and subsequent lower extremity amputation in patients with diabetes [47]. The clinical spectrum ranges from superficial cellulitis to a deep plantar abscess and necrotizing infection. Additionally, osteomyelitis may lead to wounds that will not heal without debridement and bony resection. Treatment for foot infections may require drainage and debridement for source control with revascularization to allow for healing. In severe infections with advanced tissue destruction and systemic signs of sepsis, the only option for control may be a major amputation. These cases fall into the category of "life over limb."

An open guillotine amputation above the ankle or ankle disarticulation can control life-threatening sepsis in patients with severe infection and an unsalvageable foot. After sepsis resolves, a definitive amputation with a concomitant vascular reconstruction if necessary can be planned. One group found that staging amputations in the setting of pedal sepsis resulted in a higher healing rate for below knee amputations. They reported that 25 % of patients required conversion to an above knee amputation when the below knee amputation was performed in the setting of pedal sepsis. In contrast, patients treated with an ankle guillotine amputation first followed by a definitive below knee amputation had an AKA conversion rate of only 6.7 % [48]. Likewise, Altindas et al. found that only one of 62 patients treated with a staged below knee amputation required conversion to an above knee amputation. Nearly two-thirds of these patients healed completely without wound complications. According to this study, an initial tibiotalar disarticulation reduces the risk of failure for secondary below knee amputation in patients with advanced foot infections [49].

Results have been mixed in comparison with staged versus initial closed amputation in patients who present with osteomyelitis or a foot infection with a salvageable foot. A study of 46 patients with infected diabetic foot ulcers and osteomyelitis found faster healing rates, decreased exudation, edema, and reinfection in patients undergoing primary surgical closure. In contrast, a study of 204 patients with forefoot osteomyelitis or infected gangrene found that patients treated with staged amputations had limb salvage rates approaching those of patients with less invasive infections in whom a primary closure was performed. Drawbacks of the staged approach included prolonged wound healing and the need for repeat interventions.

All patients who require a forefoot amputation for infection face the possibility of early limb loss [50, 51]. Limb salvage efforts should focus on restoring perfusion to the foot and optimizing medical management for the patient's infection and underlying comorbidities. Foot infections in patients with critical limb ischemia require prompt diagnosis and imaging with the intention of early revascularization. Initial broad-spectrum antibiotic coverage should be tailored to cover the specific pathogens identified from cultures of the bone or deep tissue. Tight glycemic control and local wound care can achieve durable healing and limb preservation. In a study of 330 patients with osteomyelitis who were treated with a combination of optimal surgical and medical therapy, the local wound recurrence rate was only 12.1 % over a 1-year period following forefoot amputation [52].

In summary, a patient with life-threatening sepsis from a severe foot infection requires an immediate guillotine amputation above the ankle or an ankle disarticulation to gain control of the infection. The timing of the definitive below or above knee amputation is controversial, but is usually safe when the patient has recovered from systemic sepsis and the wound has stabilized. If the foot appears to be salvageable, all nonviable tissue and bone should be removed, and revascularization should be planned. Clinical judgment based on the extent of the initial infection determines whether an initial closed amputation is feasible. The operating surgeon should have a low threshold to perform an open, partial foot amputation or debridement with later wound closure as this has been found to have acceptable limb salvage rates, at a cost of more frequent secondary procedures and prolonged wound healing.

Summary

Limb loss poses a serious threat to all patients with diabetes and peripheral arterial disease. Few surgical procedures rival the profound social and lifestyle changes caused by a lower extremity amputation. Although its overall incidence has decreased, amputation continues to have a significant economic impact on the healthcare system [53]. The surgeon taking care of this patient population must be well versed in strategies to maximize limb salvage including optimal medical management of comorbidities, arterial reconstruction when necessary, and local wound care. When these strategies fail, an amputation that is appropriately planned and skillfully performed can maximize a patient's recovery and functional outcome. The overall goals of a lower extremity amputation should focus on achieving initial wound healing, avoiding long-term stump complications, and to returning the patient to ambulatory status whenever possible.

References

1. Moxey PW, Gogalniceanu P, Hinchliffe RJ, et al. Lower extremity amputations-a review of global variability in incidence. Diabet Med. 2011;28:1144–53.
2. Zhang W, Abou-Zamzam Jr AM. Lower extremity amputation: general considerations. In: Rutherford textbook of vascular surgery. 8th ed. Saunders, Philadelphia, Pennsylvania, USA
3. Dormandy J, Heeck L, Vig S. Major amputations: clinical patterns and predictors. Semin Vasc Surg. 1999;12(2):154–61.
4. Humphrey LL, Palumbo PJ, Butters MA, et al. The contribution of non-insulin dependent diabetes to lower-extremity amputation in the community. Arch Intern Med. 1994;154(8):885–92.
5. Belmont Philip J, Davey S, Orr J, et al. Risk factors for 30-day postoperative complications and mortality after below-knee amputation: a study of 2,911 patients from the National Surgical Quality Improvement Program. J Am Coll Surg. 2011;213:370–8.
6. Norgren L, Hiatt WR, Dormandy MR. Inter-society consensus for the management of peripheral arterial disease (TASC II). Eur J Vasc Endovasc Surg. 2007;33(Suppl):S1–75.
7. Corey M, Julien J, Miller C. Patient education level affects functionality and long term mortality after major lower extremity amputation. Am J Surg. 2012;204(5):626–30.
8. Horgan O, Malcolm M. Psychological adjustment to lower-limb amputation: a review. Disabil Rehabil. 2004;26(14–15):837–50.
9. Feinglass J, Shively V, Martin G, et al. How 'preventable' are lower extremity amputations? A qualitative study of patient perceptions of precipitating factors. Disabil Rehabil. 2012;34(25):2158–65.
10. Chiriano J, Bianchi C, Teurya TH, et al. Management of lower extremity wounds in patients with peripheral arterial disease: a stratified conservative approach. Ann Vasc Surg. 2010;24(8):1110–6.
11. Ballard JL, Eke C, Bunt TJ, et al. Prospective evaluation of transcutaneous oxygen measurement in the management of diabetic foot problems. J Vasc Surg. 1995;22:485–92.
12. DeGraaf JC, Ubbinck DT, Legemate DA, et al. Evaluation of toe pressure and transcutaneous oxygen measurements in management of chronic critical leg ischemia: a diagnostic randomized clinical trial. J Vasc Surg. 2003;38:528–34.
13. Abou-zamzam AM, Teruya TH, Killeen JD, Ballard JL. Major Lower extremity amputation in an academic vascular center. Ann Vasc Surg. 2003;17:86–90.
14. Abou-Zamzam Jr AM, Moneta GL, Lee RW, et al. Peroneal bypass is equivalent to inframalleolar bypass for ischemic pedal gangrene. Arch Surg. 1996;131(8):894–8.
15. Veith F, Gupta K, Ascer E, et al. Six-year prospective multicenter randomized comparison of autologous saphenous vein and expanded polytetrafluoroethylene grafts in infrainguinal arterial constructions. J Vasc Surg. 1996;3(1):104–14.
16. Malone JM. Lower extremity amputations. In: Moore WS, editor. Vascular surgery: a comprehensive review. Philadelphia: WB Saunders; 2002. p. 875–917.
17. Nehler MR, Hiatt WR, Taylor LM. Is revascularization and limb salvage always the best treatment for critical limb ischemia? J Vasc Surg. 2003;37:704.
18. Nehler MR, Coll JR, Hiatt WR, et al. Functional outcome in a contemporary series of major lower extremity amputations. J Vasc Surg. 2003;38:7–14.
19. Taylor SM, Kalbaugh CA, Blackhurst SW, et al. Preoperative clinical factors predict postoperative functional outcomes after major

lower extremity amputation: an analysis of 553 consecutive patients. J Vasc Surg. 2005;42:227.
20. Vitti MJ, Robinson DV, Hauer-Jensen M. Wound healing in forefoot amputations: the predictive value of toe pressure. Ann Vasc Surg. 1994;8(1):99–106.
21. Poredos P, Rakovec S, Guzic- Salobir B. Determination of amputation level in ischaemic limbs using TcPO2 measurement. Vasa. 2005;34(2):108–12.
22. Holstein P. Level selection in leg amputation for arterial occlusive disease: a comparison of clinical evaluation and skin perfusion pressure. Acta Orthop Scand. 1982;53(5):821–31.
23. Wang CL, Wang M, Liu TK. Predictors for wound healing in ischemic lower limb amputation. J Formos Med Assoc. 1994;93(10):849–54.
24. Landry G, Silverman D, Liem T, Mitchell E, Moneta G. Predictors of healing and functional outcome following transmetatarsal amputations. Arch Surg. 2011;146(9):1005–9.
25. Salonga B, Garbalosa J, Pierre-Paul D, et al. Predictors for the healing of transmetatarsal amputations: retrospective study of 91 amputations. Vascular. 2007;15(3):126–33.
26. Hasanadka R, McLafferty R, Moore C. Predictors of wound complications following major amputation for critical limb ischemia. J Vasc Surg. 2011;54:1374–82.
27. Taylor S, Corey K, Cass A. 'Successful outcome' after below-knee amputation: an objective definition and influence of clinical variables. Am Surg. 2008;74:607–13.
28. Tang P, Ravji K, Key JJ, et al. Let them walk! Current prosthesis options for leg and foot amputees. J Am Coll Surg. 2008;206:548.
29. Stone PA, Flaherty SK, AbuRahma AF. Factors affecting perioperative mortality and wound related complications following major lower extremity amputations. Ann Vasc Surg. 2006;20:209–16.
30. Bates B, Stineman MG, Reker DM, et al. Risk factors associated with mortality in veteran population following transtibial or transfemoral amputation. J Rehabil Res Dev. 2006;43:917–28.
31. Cruz CP, Eidt JF, Capps C, et al. Major lower extremity amputations at a Veterans Affairs Hospital. Am J Surg. 2003;186:449–54.
32. Aulivola B, Hile CN, Hamdan AD. Major lower extremity amputation: outcome of a modern series. Arch Surg. 2004;139:395–9.
33. Brodsky J. Amputations of the foot and ankle. In: Coughlin MJ, editor. Surgery of the foot and ankle. St. Louis: Mosby; 2007. p. 1369–98.
34. Hosch J, Quiroga C, Bosma J, et al. Outcomes of transmetatarsal amputations in patients with diabetes mellitus. J Foot Ankle Surg. 1997;36(6):430–4.
35. Elsharawy MA. Outcomes of midfoot amputations in diabetic gangrene. Ann Vasc Surg. 2011;25(6):778–82.
36. Stone PA, Back MR, Armstrong PA, et al. Midfoot amputations expand limb salvage rates for diabetic foot infections. Ann Vasc Surg. 2005;19(6):805–11.
37. Baumgartner R. Forefoot and midfoot amputations. Oper Orthop Traumatol. 2011;23(4):254–64.
38. DeCotiis MA. Lisfranc and Chopart amputations. Clin Podiatr Med Surg. 2005;22(3):385–93.
39. Laughlin RT, Chambers RB. Syme amputation in patients with severe diabetes mellitus. Foot Ankle. 1993;14(2):65–70.
40. Frykberg RG, Abraham S, Tierney E. Syme amputation for limb salvage:early experience with 26 cases. J Foot Ankle Surg. 2007;46(2):93–100.
41. Zalavaras CG, Rigopoulos N, Ahlmann E, Patzakis M. Hip disarticulation for severe lower extremity infections. Clin Orthop Relat Res. 2009;467:1721–6.
42. Unruh T, Fisher Jr DF, Unruh TA, et al. Hip disarticulation. An 11-year experience. Arch Surg. 1990;125:791–3.
43. Endean ED, Schwarcz TH, Barker DE, Munfakh NA. Hip disarticulation: factors affecting outcome. J Vasc Surg. 1991;14:398–404.
44. Yari P, Dijkstra P, Geertzen J. Functional outcome of hip disarticulation and hemipelvectomy : a cross-sectional national descriptive study in the Netherlands. Clin Rehabil. 2008;22:1127–33.
45. Chin T, Sawamura S, Shiba R, et al. Energy expenditure during walking in amputees after disarticulation of the hip. A microprocessor- controlled swing- phase control knee versus a mechanical-controlled stance-phase control knee. J Bone Joint Surg Br. 2005;87(1):117–9.
46. Baumgartner R. Knee disarticulation and through-knee amputation. Oper Orthop Traumatol. 2011;23(4):289–95.
47. Zgonis T, Roukis T. A systematic approach to diabetic foot infections. Adv Ther. 2005;22(3):244–61.
48. Desai Y, Robbs JV, Keenan JP. Staged below-knee amputations for septic peripheral lesions due to ischaemia. Br J Surg. 1986;73:392–4.
49. Altindas M, Klic A, Cinar C. A reliable surgical approach for the two-staged amputation in unsalvageable limb and life threatening acute progressive diabetic foot infections: tibiotalar disarticulation with vertical crural incisions and secondary transtibial amputation. Foot Ankle Surg. 2011;17(1):13–8.
50. Garcia-Morales E, Lazaro-Martinez JL, Aragon-Sanchez J, et.al. Surgical complications associated with primary closure in patients with diabetic foot osteomyelitis. Diabet Foot Ankle. 2012;3. Epub Sept 2012;1–5.
51. Berceli S, Brown J, Irwin P, et al. Clinical outcomes after closed, staged, and open forefoot amputations. J Vasc Surg. 2006;44:347–51.
52. Widatalla AH, Mahadi SE, Shawer MA, et al. Diabetic foot infections with osteomyelitis: efficacy of combined surgical and medical treatment. Diabet Foot Ankle. 2012;3. Epub Oct 1 2012;1–6.
53. Jindeel A, Narahara KA. Nontraumatic amputation: incidence and cost analysis. Int J Low Extrem Wounds. 2012;11(3):177–9. Epub Aug 2 2012;1–6.

Part IV

Venous Disease

Deep Venous Thrombosis

9

Anthony J. Comerota and Hussein Barayan

Introduction

Deep venous thrombosis (DVT) is a common global health problem affecting the populations of both developed and developing countries. Studies show that acute venous thrombosis resulting in pulmonary embolism (PE) kills more people than acute myocardial infarction or acute stroke [1]. Over one million people per year will suffer an acute venous thromboembolic event in the United States alone. The postthrombotic morbidity that follows is substantial and is proportional to the extent of venous thrombosis [2–4].

The goal of treating DVT is to prevent PE and death from PE, reduce the risk of recurrence, and avoid postthrombotic morbidity. Choosing the appropriate treatment depends upon the anatomic distribution, extent of thrombus, and degree of luminal obstruction. Patients with extensive thrombus involving the iliofemoral veins represent a clinically relevant subset of DVT patients who have acute obstruction of the single venous outflow pathway of the lower extremity. These patients develop high muscle compartment pressures and venous hypertension which, if undertreated, can result in debilitating symptoms of postthrombotic syndrome.

Although anticoagulation remains the mainstay of treatment for acute DVT, many patients are not adequately anticoagulated both early in their course of therapy and over the long term. This failure in anticoagulation therapy can result in more severe postthrombotic morbidity and an increased risk of recurrent venous thromboembolism. Moreover, patients with iliofemoral DVT benefit from a strategy of early thrombus removal in addition to therapeutic anticoagulation, as the severity of postthrombotic venous disease correlates directly with the extent and persistence of venous thrombus. Thrombus removal techniques include surgical venous thrombectomy, catheter-directed thrombolysis, and pharmacomechanical thrombectomy, all of which have been shown in randomized trials and observational studies to minimize postthrombotic morbidity and decrease DVT recurrence [5–13].

Several factors contribute to the increasing incidence of venous thromboembolic complications. The aging population puts more patients at risk and more operative procedures are being performed on higher risk patients. In addition, the greater awareness of venous thromboembolic complications coupled with more sensitive diagnostic imaging likely factors into the higher reported incidence.

Risk Factors

Most risk factors for DVT relate to one or more elements of the classic triad described by Rudolf Ludwig Karl Virchow [14]. Over 150 years ago Virchow recognized that changes in blood elements (hypercoagulability), reduced blood flow velocity (stasis), and vein wall injury (endothelial damage) combined to create an environment promoting thrombus formation. Hypercoagulability can take the form of genetic or acquired risk factors as listed in Table 9.1. Although stasis alone does not cause DVT, stasis can be an important predisposing or permissive factor in the presence of other more potent pro-thrombotic risks. The precise role that endothelial damage plays in DVT formation remains unclear. While few would argue that direct injury to a vein wall leads to the thrombus formation, most postoperative DVTs begin in the calf veins which are usually distant from the surgical site and undamaged by operative trauma.

A.J. Comerota, MD, FACS, FACC (✉)
Jobst Vascular Institute, ProMedica Toledo Hospital, 2109 Hughes Dr, Suite 400, Toledo, OH 43606, USA

Section of Vascular Surgery, Cardiovascular Center, University of Michigan Medical Center, Ann Arbor, MI 48109, USA
e-mail: anthony.comerotamd@promedica.org; marilyn.gravett@promedica.org

H. Barayan, MD
Jobst Vascular Institute, ProMedica Toledo Hospital, 2109 Hughes Dr, Suite 400, Toledo, OH 43606, USA

V. Gahtan and M.J. Costanza (eds.), *Essentials of Vascular Surgery for the General Surgeon*,
DOI 10.1007/978-1-4939-1326-8_9,

Table 9.1 Congenital and acquired risk factors for DVT

Acquired	Congenital
Age	Antithrombin deficiencies
Malignancy	Proteins C & S deficiencies
Surgery/trauma	Factor V Leiden
Immobilization	Prothrombin 20210A
Oral contraceptives	Blood group non-O
Hormone replacement therapy	Hyperhomocysteinemia
Pregnancy	Factor XI, IX, VII, VIII, X, and II excess
Obesity	Dysfibrinogenemia
Neurological disease	Dysplasminogenemia
Cardiac disease	Plasminogen activator inhibitor-1
Antiphospholipid antibodies	Reduced activity of heparin cofactor II

When a DVT occurs in a patient with no known risk factors, the diagnosis is considered an idiopathic DVT presumably provoked by a transient risk factor such as surgery or trauma. In a prospective, multicenter registry of 2,119 patients with venous thromboembolism (VTE), 43 % were deemed to have idiopathic DVT [15]. Approximately 42 % of the patients with idiopathic DVT had temporary risk factors with immobilization (15 %), surgery (14.4 %), and severe medical illness (8.2 %) occurring most frequently.

Most patients have more than one thrombotic risk factor at the time of their presentation. Fifty percent of thrombotic events in patients with inherited thrombophilia occur in the presence of an additional acquired risk factor (e.g., surgery, prolonged bed rest, pregnancy, oral contraceptives). Some patients have more than one form of inherited thrombophilia or more than one form of acquired thrombophilia and appear to carry an even greater risk for thrombosis. In a population-based study, 53 % of patients with VTE had three or more of the following risk factors: >48 h of immobility in the preceding month, hospital admission, surgery, malignancy, infection in the past 3 months, or current hospitalization [16].

Genetic Risk Factors

The most frequent causes of an inherited (primary) hypercoagulable state are factor V Leiden mutation, prothrombin gene mutation, protein S deficiency, protein C deficiency, antithrombin deficiency, and dysfibrinogenemia. The pathophysiology and genetics of each of those disorders are beyond the scope of this chapter; however, their associated thrombotic risk has been assessed in two ways: evaluation of patients with DVT and evaluation of families with thrombophilia [17]. In a Spanish study of 2,132 consecutive unselected patients with VTE, 12.9 % had an anticoagulant protein deficiency (7.3 % with protein S deficiency, 3.2 % with protein C deficiency, and 0.5 % with antithrombin deficiency) [18].

Acquired Risk Factors

According to the previously cited population-based study, many patients with an episode of VTE have more than one acquired risk factor for thrombosis [16]. The most prevalent preexisting medical characteristics include the following: greater than 48 h of immobility in the preceding month (45 %), hospital admission (39 %), surgery (34 %), malignancy (34 %), infection in the past 3 months (34 %), and current hospitalization (26 %). Of the 587 episodes of VTE, only 11 % had no preexisting medical characteristics present, while 36 and 53 % had one to two and three or more risk factors, respectively.

Malignancy

Patients with cancer often harbor a hypercoagulable state due to the production of substances with procoagulant activity (e.g., tissue factor and cancer procoagulant). The risk of VTE in such patients peaks during the initial hospitalization and onset of chemotherapy, as well as at the time of disease progression [19]. Approximately 20 % of patients with symptomatic DVT have a known active malignancy. In a retrospective study of over 63,000 patients admitted to Danish nonpsychiatric hospitals from 1977 to 1992 for a diagnosis of VTE, 18 % had received a diagnosis of cancer (other than non-melanoma skin cancer) prior to the thromboembolic event [20]. The majority of cancers associated with thromboembolic events are clinically evident and have been previously diagnosed at the time of the event. In the Danish study, 78 % of the cancers were diagnosed before the event with the most common sites being lung (17 %), pancreas (10 %), colon and rectum (8 %), kidney (8 %), and prostate (7 %) [20].

Surgery

Thrombotic risk increases during surgery, particularly orthopedic, neurologic, and cancer surgery [21–23]. The 2012 American College of Chest Physicians (ACCP) guidelines estimate that patients undergoing orthopedic surgery have a 2.80 % risk of having a symptomatic thrombotic event if untreated with initial thromboprophylaxis during the first 2 weeks following surgery, with a cumulative 35-day risk of 4.3 % if untreated during the entire perioperative period [24].

The ACCP guidelines for nonorthopedic surgery stratify patients into categories based on their estimated untreated VTE risk [25]. Outpatient or same-day surgery patients make up the very low-risk category (<0.5 % VTE risk in the absence of thromboprophylaxis). The low-risk category (1.5 % VTE risk) applies to patients having spinal surgery for nonmalignant disease. Patients undergoing gynecologic (noncancer), cardiothoracic surgery, and those having spinal surgery for malignant disease fall into the medium-risk category.

The high-risk category (6 % VTE risk) includes patients having bariatric surgery, surgery for gynecologic cancer, a craniotomy, and major trauma surgery.

Trauma

The risk of thrombosis increases after all forms of major trauma [26–29]. A study of 716 patients admitted to a regional trauma unit found lower extremity DVT in 58 % of patients with adequate venographic studies, 18 % of whom had proximal vein thrombosis [27]. Venous thrombi were detected in 54 % of patients with a major head injury, 61 % of patients with a pelvic fracture, 77 % of patients with a tibial fracture, and 80 % of those with a femoral fracture. The sequence of events that trigger activation of the coagulation system following surgery or trauma remains unclear. Conditions which favor venous thrombosis include decreased venous blood flow in the lower extremities, diminished fibrinolysis, immobilization, release or exposure of tissue factor, and depletion of endogenous anticoagulants such as antithrombin [30]. A large population-based study investigated the VTE risk following a minor injury defined as one not requiring surgery, a plaster cast, hospitalization, or extended bed rest at home for at least 4 days [31]. A minor injury occurring in the preceding 3–4 weeks increased the DVT risk three- to fivefold overall and 50-fold in carriers of factor V Leiden.

Pregnancy

Pregnancy increases the risk of thrombosis due in part to obstruction of venous return by the enlarged uterus and the hypercoagulable state associated with pregnancy. Estimates of the age-adjusted incidence of VTE range from 5 to 50 times higher in pregnant versus nonpregnant women with an absolute incidence of 1 in 500–2,000 pregnancies (0.025–0.10 %) [32, 33].

Drugs

While several drugs increase the risk of venous thrombosis, oral contraceptives have the greatest impact because of their widespread use. Among young women, oral contraceptive use represents the most important cause of thrombosis [34]. Observational studies, the HERS trials, and a meta-analysis published before the Women's Health Initiative, identified an association between hormone replacement therapy (HRT) and venous thromboembolism (VTE). These studies reported that HRT caused an approximately twofold increase in VTE risk, which appeared to be greatest in the first year of treatment [35–38]. Other medications associated with increased risk of VTE include tamoxifen and bevacizumab.

Immobilization

Immobilization favors venous stasis which increases the risk of DVT and subsequent PE. Warlow et al. evaluated the effect of immobilization by using radiolabeled fibrinogen to study patients with unilateral lower extremity paralysis [39]. They found that DVT developed in 60 % of the paralyzed limbs compared with a DVT rate of only 7 % in the contralateral normal leg which acted as an internal control. Prolonged immobilization during air travel may increase the risk of DVT; however, its clinical impact remains unclear. A meta-analysis reported a slightly increased rate of asymptomatic DVT after long haul air travel defined as flight duration greater than 7 h. None of the reviewed studies reported any symptomatic DVTs, deaths, or pulmonary emboli [40].

Prior Episode of VTE

In an outpatient prospective cohort study, the risk of recurrence after an acute episode of venous thrombosis was 18, 25, and 30 % at 2, 5, and 8 years, respectively [42]. In a community epidemiologic study, a history of VTE conferred a relative risk (RR) of 7.9 for VTE recurrence [43]. The association between lower extremity superficial venous thrombophlebitis (SVTP) and DVT risk is less clear. A retrospective study showed a DVT rate of 2.7 % following an episode of SVTP compared to 0.2 % in control patients (OR 10.2). This relationship became less robust and lost statistical significance when the authors controlled for a previous history of VTE [41].

Antiphospholipid Antibodies

The presence of antibodies directed against phospholipid-bound plasma proteins characterizes the antiphospholipid syndrome. Patients can present clinically with venous or arterial thrombosis, recurrent fetal loss, and occasional thrombocytopenia. The disorder may be classified as primary or associated with systemic lupus erythematosus and other connective tissue diseases. In one large series, antiphospholipid antibodies were present in 4.1 % of 2,132 consecutive patients presenting with DVT [18].

Anatomic Factors Associated with Increased Risk of DVT

May-Thurner syndrome involves hemodynamically significant compression of the left common iliac vein between the overlying right common iliac artery and the underlying vertebral body. Although this anatomic pattern is common in asymptomatic subjects, May-Thurner syndrome has been implicated in patients with unprovoked left iliofemoral DVT or chronic venous insufficiency [44]. The incidence of May-Thurner syndrome peaks in women between the ages of 20 and 50, and it may be more common in those with reduced left common iliac vein diameters and/or severe degrees of iliac vein compression. Recurrent episodes of DVT may respond poorly to treatment with anticoagulation alone requiring catheter-directed thrombolysis and balloon angioplasty with intravascular stenting, especially in those with limb-threatening thrombosis.

Paget-Schroetter syndrome, also referred to as spontaneous upper extremity venous thrombosis, usually results from an underlying compressive anomaly at the thoracic outlet. Compression of the subclavian vein usually occurs between the first rib and a hypertrophied scalene or subclavius tendon or between the tendons themselves.

Diagnosis

The clinical diagnosis of DVT is unreliable because the nonspecific signs and symptoms of venous thrombosis can be easily confused with other disease processes. Lower extremity swelling, the most common physical sign of DVT, has several nonvenous causes including inflammation from infection and soft tissue injury. Furthermore, nonocclusive venous thrombus can remain asymptomatic until it embolizes or completely occludes the vein. Despite these diagnostic challenges, a thorough history and physical examination can help correctly identify DVT when it is present and rule it out when it is absent. Venous duplex ultrasound provides a noninvasive, objective tool for detecting DVT and guiding treatment.

Clinical Assessment

Wells et al. developed a clinical model to determine the probability of DVT prior to definitive diagnostic testing in symptomatic outpatients [45]. Patients were stratified into high-, moderate-, or low-probability groups based on a score derived from their clinical characteristics (Table 9.2). Applying this scoring system to 529 patients, they reported that a DVT was detected in 85 % of patients in the high pretest probability category, 33 % in the moderate, and 5 % in the low category. They also demonstrated that using a clinical model in conjunction with ultrasound would decrease the number of false-positive and false-negative diagnoses if ascending phlebography was used when the ultrasound result and pretest probability disagreed. These investigators subsequently integrated D-dimer testing with clinical probability to conserve vascular laboratory resources [46].

In a prospective multicenter management study, Elf et al. theorized that if a patient was categorized as low pretest probability and a moderate sensitivity D-dimer test was negative, DVT could be ruled out without further diagnostic testing [47]. In a study of 110 patients, only one patient who had both low pretest probability and negative D-dimer developed an episode of venous thromboembolism within the next 3 months. Others have reported similar results in outpatients with low pretest probability score and negative D-dimer results [48]. A negative D-dimer, however, cannot be used to exclude DVT in patients with a high pretest probability score, as up to 20 % of these patients have a DVT confirmed subsequent to test results [48].

Table 9.2 Pretest clinical probability (Wells' score) [45]

Characteristic	Score
Active cancer	1
Paresis, paralysis, or recent immobilization of lower limb	1
Bedridden >3 days or major surgery <4 weeks	1
Localized tenderness	1
Entire leg swollen	1
Calf swelling >3 cm (compared with asymptomatic limb)	1
Pitting edema	1
Collateral superficial veins	1
Alternative diagnosis as likely or greater than DVT	−2

High risk: ≥3
Moderate risk: 1–2
Low risk: 0

Table 9.3 Venous duplex diagnosis of acute DVT: criteria

Component	Criteria
B-mode imaging	Noncompressibility of vein
	Visible intraluminal thrombus
	Dilated veins
	Enlarged branch veins (collaterals)
Doppler	Loss of respiratory phasicity
	Loss of spontaneous venous signal
	Abnormal augmentation
	Elevated flow velocity (wind tunnel sound) in main vein
	Elevated flow velocity in branch veins (collaterals)

Venous Duplex Ultrasound

Venous duplex ultrasound is the diagnostic method of choice for most patients being evaluated for acute DVT. Table 9.3 lists the duplex criteria used to detect a DVT, the most important of which is compressibility of the vein being examined. Duplex ultrasound examination of a normal, patent vein demonstrates a black lumen that can be completely compressed by exerting pressure on the ultrasound probe. Acute thrombus has the same density as blood and therefore the lumen of a thrombosed vein also appears black (anechoic) by ultrasound examination. The distinguishing characteristic of an acute DVT is the inability to completely compress the vein under the probe. In the setting of an iliofemoral thrombosis, the more distal lower extremity veins may be patent but non-compressible because of the high venous pressures caused by the proximal occlusion. The sensitivity and specificity reported in any single study of venous duplex ultrasound depend on the number of isolated iliac and calf vein thromboses included in the patient sample, as these are more difficult to diagnose.

Additional sonographic signs of acute DVT include dilated veins and enlarged venous collaterals. As thrombus ages, the density increases, making it more echogenic and visible by ultrasound. A negative venous duplex examination reliably excludes DVT, and withholding anticoagulation on the basis of one or more negative ultrasound evaluations is a safe and well-established practice [49–51]. The most reliable physical sign of acute DVT is unilateral leg edema which warrants a definitive ultrasound examination. In most cases, the patient should receive empiric anticoagulation therapy if the ultrasound examination will be significantly delayed.

In the past, venous duplex ultrasound exams focused on compression of the common femoral and popliteal veins assuming that the diagnosis of calf vein DVT was unreliable and clinically inconsequential. More recent studies demonstrate that DVT frequently begins in the calf veins [52, 53] and that isolated calf DVT progresses into the popliteal vein in 25–30 % of cases [53–56]. Moreover, pulmonary emboli have been reported in 8–34 % of patients with isolated calf vein thrombosis [57]. Although the accuracy of venous duplex for detecting calf vein thrombosis varies, some reports cite sensitivity and specificity rates of 90 and 100 %, respectively [58, 59].

The diagnostic sensitivity of venous ultrasound may vary between symptomatic and high-risk asymptomatic patients. In a study of postoperative orthopedic patients, 24 % of symptomatic and 88 % of asymptomatic patients had isolated calf vein thrombosis [60]. In the symptomatic group, venous duplex ultrasound had 85 % sensitivity and 86 % specificity, but in the asymptomatic group, the sensitivity dropped to 16 % although the specificity was 99 %.

Ultrasound diagnosis of an isolated iliac vein thrombosis can be challenging. The physical finding of unilateral lower extremity edema extending distally from the inguinal ligament should raise clinical suspicion for an isolated iliac vein thrombosis. In contrast, patients with internal iliac vein thrombosis or nonocclusive thrombus of the common iliac or proximal external iliac veins often remain asymptomatic. Compressibility, the most accurate ultrasound test for DVT, cannot be used to evaluate the iliac veins or inferior vena cava because of their location in the pelvis and retroperitoneum. Diagnosing an iliac vein or caval thrombosis therefore depends on indirect ultrasound findings including color flow imaging and venous velocity profiles, in addition to the grayscale image itself. Unfortunately, patients with abdominal obesity or extensive bowel gas present technical challenges to imaging the iliac veins and cava, and up to 24 % of these patients have a nondiagnostic exam [61].

Phlebography and Venography

In the past, ascending phlebography had widespread use as a diagnostic tool for detecting lower extremity DVT. Although it required venous access in the foot and could cumbersome to perform, ascending phlebography proved to be an accurate test with high sensitivity and specificity. Weinmann and Salzman reported a 2–3 % risk of contrast-induced thrombosis following phlebography; however, the use of nonionic contrast, elevation of the leg, and flushing with heparinized saline reduces this risk considerably [62]. Ascending phlebography now plays a very limited role in diagnosing DVT having been replaced by other noninvasive imaging modalities, most notably venous duplex ultrasound.

Computerized tomographic (CT) and magnetic resonance (MR) venography have several advantages, particularly in imaging patients with a suspected pelvic DVT. Both types of cross-sectional imaging can detect abdominal, pelvic, and chest pathology (pelvic masses, abdominal or thoracic malignancies) that may be etiologically associated with the development of venous thrombosis. CT and MR venography can also show iliac vein compression resulting from the overlying iliac artery (May-Thurner syndrome). Disadvantages of CT and MR venography include radiation exposure (CT), high cost, and limited availability.

D-Dimer Tests

After factor XIII stabilizes cross-linked fibrin during clot formation, autogenous plasmin breaks down the fibrin, releasing the fragments into the blood stream. D-dimer represents one type of fragment which can be detected with a blood test [63]. A positive D-dimer test indicates the presence of thrombus; however, it cannot determine the thrombus location or its clinical significance. In practice, the D-dimer test acts as a sensitive but nonspecific diagnostic tool which has clinical utility in excluding the diagnosis of DVT in patients with low thrombotic risk. A negative D-dimer test in a patient with a low clinical suspicion results in a 99 % negative predictive value for DVT [45, 47, 64]. In this clinical situation, no further testing is required and anticoagulation can be safely withheld. Other conditions can elevate D-dimer levels including inflammation, recent surgery, infection, and pregnancy, making the D-dimer test more accurate in the outpatient setting.

The evaluation of patients with suspected venous thrombosis begins with a thorough clinical assessment to gauge the pretest probability of DVT. The D-dimer blood test along with venous duplex ultrasound provide adjunctive diagnostic tools that can help exclude or confirm the presence of DVT.

Treatment Strategies

Appropriate treatment of acute DVT can significantly improve short- and long-term patient outcomes. Several studies highlight the short-term benefit of early and sustained therapeutic anticoagulation for acute DVT. Other studies focusing on the duration of anticoagulation show that longer treatment times lower the risk of recurrent DVT. A new generation of oral anticoagulants promises greater ease of use and may eliminate some of the logistic barriers to outpatient anticoagulation therapy. The key to making sound treatment decisions is recognizing that not all venous thromboses are the same. Some patients do well with anticoagulation alone (e.g., isolated calf vein thrombosis), whereas patients with extensive iliofemoral DVT often benefit from a strategy of thrombus removal followed by effective anticoagulation. The treatment strategies outlined in the following sections are based on the level and extent of venous thrombosis, the known natural history of acute DVT, and the recognized benefits of therapy.

Importance of Anticoagulation

The goal of immediate anticoagulation with heparin is to interrupt ongoing thrombosis while long-term oral anticoagulation with warfarin attempts to prevent recurrent DVT. Brandjes et al. demonstrated the importance of initial therapeutic anticoagulation by randomizing patients to either prompt anticoagulation with heparin followed by vitamin K antagonists (VKA) or VKAs alone [65]. Patients receiving a VKA alone had recurrent thrombotic events three times more frequently than those who received heparin immediately. The authors associated this finding with the fact that patients treated with warfarin alone had a delay of several days before they reached therapeutic anticoagulation. Hull et al. confirmed the need for early therapeutic anticoagulation [66]. They reported a 24.5 % rate of recurrence in patients whose treatment with heparin failed to achieve therapeutic levels within the first 24 h, compared with a 1.6 % recurrence rate in those reaching an early therapeutic level. Current guidelines favor low-molecular-weight heparin (LMWH) over unfractionated heparin (UFH) in the initial period and advise that heparin overlap a VKA for a minimum of 5 days to ensure therapeutic anticoagulation. Studies on the duration of suggest that the longer anticoagulation is continued, the lower the risk of recurrence. Decisions on the length of treatment must always strike a balance between the risk of recurrent thrombosis and the risk of bleeding.

The emergence of new oral anticoagulants may change the paradigm of care for acute DVT. Randomized clinical trials on direct inhibitors of factor Xa (rivaroxaban, apixaban) or factor IIa-thrombin (dabigatran) show that these compounds are effective and safe in the management of patients with venous thromboembolic disease [67, 68]. The new oral anticoagulants have several advantages including the fact that they are rapidly absorbed, require no monitoring, have fewer drug and food interactions than VKAs, and do not require parenteral heparin. The enhanced safety profile and ease of use associated with the new oral agents may ultimately shift the risk-benefit analysis in favor of prolonged anticoagulation to prevent DVT recurrence [68–71].

Determining Treatment by Type of DVT

Calf Vein Thrombosis

Although patients with isolated calf vein thrombosis have the lowest thrombotic burden and the best overall prognosis, they still carry a risk of thrombus extension or thromboembolic sequelae. A randomized trial of idiopathic calf DVT compared 3 months of therapeutic anticoagulation with 5 days of anticoagulation followed by placebo. Thrombus propagated or recurred in 19 % of patients who received only 5 days of anticoagulation compared to no major thromboembolic complications observed in patients anticoagulated for 3 months [54]. Current guidelines recommend 3 months of anticoagulation for symptomatic calf DVT. For asymptomatic calf DVT, 2 weeks of serial ultrasound Doppler examinations should be performed and anticoagulation should be initiated if thrombus extension occurs [72]. We recommend treating isolated calf DVT with anticoagulation and compression stockings unless the patient is at high risk for bleeding. In patients with a high bleeding risk, we recommend compression and ambulation with serial ultrasound surveillance.

Femoral Vein Thrombosis

Patients with isolated femoral vein thrombus, particularly in the mid or upper thigh, typically do well with anticoagulation alone due to collateral venous drainage from the popliteal and profunda femoral veins to the common femoral vein. Often, functional valves exist above and below the vein segment involved with thrombus. Recanalization of the thrombus does not play a critical role as long as the popliteal and common femoral veins remain free of obstructive thrombus.

Popliteal Vein Thrombosis

Patients with occlusive femoropopliteal vein thrombosis extending into the popliteal vein "trifurcation" frequently have severe acute symptoms. Occlusion of the axial venous drainage of the calf causes distal venous hypertension and significant postthrombotic morbidity. We consider active patients with symptomatic femoropopliteal DVT to be candidates for catheter-directed thrombolysis followed by compression and 3–6 months of anticoagulation.

Iliofemoral DVT

Although a DVT in any location can result in postthrombotic complications, an iliofemoral DVT poses the threat of debilitating PTS symptoms especially when patients are treated with anticoagulation alone [4, 73]. Anatomically, the common femoral, external iliac, and common iliac veins make up the single outflow venous channel for the entire lower extremity. Thrombotic obliteration of this lone outflow channel therefore results in the highest venous pressures and the most severe postthrombotic morbidity.

Labropoulos et al. studied arm-foot pressure differentials at rest and during postocclusive reactive hyperemia in post-thrombotic patients who were treated with anticoagulation alone at the time of their acute DVT [74]. They found that iliofemoral DVT patients had the highest resting and hyperemic venous pressures. Qvarfordt and Eklof et al. provided objective evidence that immediate thrombus removal reduced venous pressure in patients with iliofemoral DVT [75]. They recorded lower extremity compartment pressures (a surrogate for venous pressures) in patients with acute iliofemoral DVT before and after venous thrombectomy and found very high compartment pressures preoperatively which normalized postoperatively.

Another important but generally overlooked observation in patients with iliofemoral DVT is the risk of recurrence. Douketis and colleagues found that patients with iliofemoral DVT had a greater than twofold risk of recurrent venous thromboembolism compared to patients with infrainguinal DVT (11.8 % vs. 5.2 %) [76]. Several clinical outcome studies show that recurrent DVT increases the frequency and severity of postthrombotic syndrome.

Treatment with a Strategy of Thrombus Removal

Thrombus removal attempts to minimize the clinical impact of acute DVT by reducing the risk of PTS and recurrent thrombosis. The rationale behind thrombus removal can be traced to natural history studies of acute DVT treated with anticoagulation alone. Efficient endogenous fibrinolysis, which resolved thrombus within 60–90 days, restored venous patency and preserved valve function [77]. Extended follow-up in the same patient cohort showed that patients whose thrombus did not resolve had a much higher rate of recurrent DVT [78–80].

PTS occurs in 25–46 % of patients following acute DVT and represents a major source of morbidity which significantly reduces patients' quality of life [4, 42, 73, 81–83]. Factors that increase the risk of PTS include iliofemoral DVT, residual thrombus, and recurrent thrombosis. Thrombus removal attempts to counteract the risk factors for PTS by restoring venous patency, preserving valve function, and reducing the rate of DVT recurrence. Aziz et al. [12] reported that recurrent DVT following catheter-directed thrombolysis for iliofemoral DVT correlated with the quantity of residual thrombus remaining after treatment. Patients experiencing successful thrombolysis had significantly less recurrence than patients with >50 % of their initial thrombus burden remaining after thrombolysis.

Treatment strategies designed to eliminate thrombus from the deep veins include operative venous thrombectomy, catheter-directed thrombolysis, and percutaneous pharmacomechanical thrombolysis. An algorithm that illustrates our suggested strategy of thrombus removal is shown in Fig. 9.1.

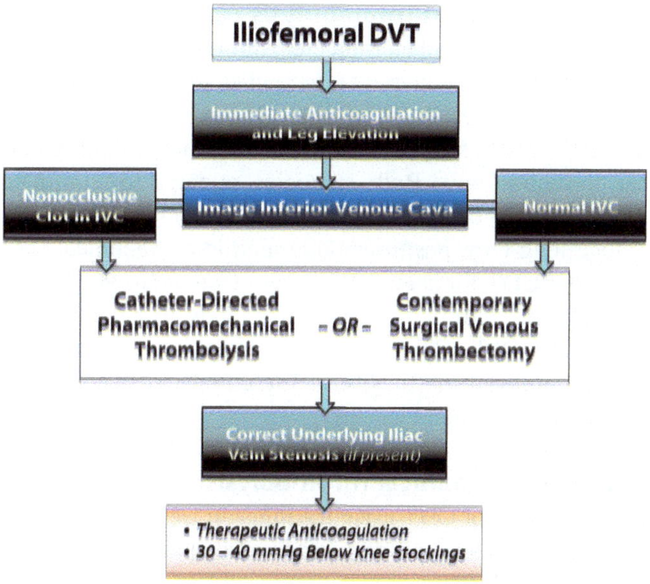

Fig. 9.1 Algorithm illustrates suggested strategy of thrombus removal for patients with iliofemoral DVT

Surgical Venous Thrombectomy

Surgical venous thrombectomy represents the first technique developed for eliminating venous thrombus. Although it is an invasive procedure, surgical venous thrombectomy is effective in removing thrombus and decreasing the risk of PTS. Plate et al. randomized patients to surgical venous thrombectomy plus anticoagulation versus anticoagulation alone [6, 84, 85]. They found that patients randomized to thrombectomy had higher venous patency rates, improved venous hemodynamics, and a reduced risk for developing PTS. More recent studies confirm that venous thrombectomy significantly reduces early morbidity in patients with iliofemoral DVT who present with severe symptoms including phlegmasia cerulea dolens. Comerota and Gale described the basic principles and operative techniques of contemporary surgical venous thrombectomy [86]. Technical improvements include the use of venous thrombectomy catheters, infrainguinal thrombectomy, fluoroscopic-guided iliocaval thrombectomy with completion intraoperative phlebography, correction of underlying venous outflow stenoses, construction of an arteriovenous fistula, and immediate and prolonged therapeutic anticoagulation in the postoperative period with catheter-directed heparin infusion into the thrombectomized venous system. The long-term benefits of venous thrombectomy stem from its ability to restore proximal venous patency and preserve the competence of venous valves. Both of these benefits depend upon the initial technical success of the procedure and the avoidance of recurrent thrombosis.

Catheter-Directed Thrombolysis

In recent years, catheter-directed thrombolyis (CDT) has emerged as a less-invasive alternative to surgical venous thrombectomy. CDT targets patients with extensive iliofemoral DVT and shares the same treatment objectives as surgical thrombectomy. Both strategies attempt to eliminate thrombus in order to relieve acute pain and suffering and reduce long-term postthrombotic morbidity. Technical success after CDT for acute DVT ranges from 80 to 90 % [87]. In a cohort-controlled observational study of patients with iliofemoral DVT, Comerota et al. showed that CDT significantly improved the quality of life compared to treatment with anticoagulation alone [83].

Pharmacomechanical Thrombolysis

One drawback of CDT using the infusion technique involves the long treatment times required to adequately clear the clot. Sillesen et al. [88] reported the results of standard CDT using drip technique in a young patient cohort (mean age of 31 years) with iliofemoral DVT who had a short duration of symptoms (less than 6 days). At hospital discharge and 1-year follow-up, 93 % of their patients had patent veins and normal venous valve function. These results required a mean treatment time of 71 h, which may exceed the capacity of many health systems and the patience of many physicians. Integrating percutaneous mechanical thrombectomy into the treatment regimen can accelerate thrombolysis while reducing the dose of lytic agent and shortening overall treatment time. Pharmacomechanical thrombolysis, the combination of lytic infusion and mechanical thrombectomy, has gained popularity as an alternative to the standard drip method of CDT.

A number of studies compared percutaneous mechanical thrombectomy alone with treatment regimens that combine mechanical clot removal with enzymatic thrombolysis [89, 90]. While percutaneous mechanical thrombectomy alone achieved limited success, significant benefit was observed when plasminogen activators were incorporated into the mechanical clot disruption.

Parikh et al. evaluated the technique of ultrasound-accelerated thrombolysis in 53 patients with acute DVT (60 % lower extremity) [91]. After a median infusion time of 22 h, 70 % of the patients had greater than 90 % lysis, 91 % had complete or partial lysis, and only 4 % of patients developed a major complication. When compared to historical controls, there was a significant advantage of ultrasound-accelerated lysis in reducing the lytic dose and shortening treatment times.

Baker et al. reported different results in a single-center retrospective analysis of CDT ($N=19$) versus ultrasound-accelerated thrombolysis ($N=64$) in patients with iliofemoral DVT [92]. The baseline parameters, extent of DVT, and time since onset of symptoms did not differ between groups. Both treatment groups had a similar and substantial resolution of thrombus load (CDT = 89 %, ultrasound = 82 %; $P=0.560$). There were no significant differences in the lytic drug infusion rate, dose of plasminogen activator, infusion time, or use of adjunctive procedures between groups. Major and minor bleeding complications were observed in 8.4 and 4.8 % of patients and were not statistically different between groups. Resolving the conflicting data regarding ultrasound-accelerated thrombolysis will require an appropriately designed randomized trial.

The technique of isolated segmental pharmacomechanical thrombolysis (ISPMT) employs a double-balloon catheter known as the Trellis catheter (Covidien, Mansfield, MA). After inflating the two balloons, thrombolytic agent is directly infused into the isolated venous segment. A dispersion wire is then advanced into the catheter, causing the catheter to assume a spiral configuration between the two balloons. The catheter is activated to spin at 3,500 rpm for 20 min and is then aspirated to remove the macerated and dissolved thrombus. After deflating the balloons repeat venography assesses venous patency. If the results are satisfactory, the catheter can be repositioned to treat additional vein segments. If thrombolysis is inadequate, treatment can be repeated. Although some physicians use up to 10 mg of recombinant tissue plasminogen activator (rtPA) per segment, the authors feel that this represents an unnecessarily excessive dose. Using 2–3 mg of rtPA in the infusate should yield the same efficacy without exposing the patient to the potential risk of a systemic lytic effect if multiple runs were required. This is supported by personal observation and the evolution of catheter-directed thrombolysis during the past 10–12 years. Overall, the interventional community has started to recognize the success of lower doses of rtPA delivered in higher volumes of infusion (50–100 cc/h). Future studies may show that even 2–3 mg of rtPA is overdosing if smaller doses prove to be equally effective.

Martinez et al. evaluated the benefit of ISPMT in a study of 43 consecutive patients treated at the Jobst Vascular Institute [10]. Twenty-one patients were treated with CDT using the drip technique and 22 patients were treated with ISPMT plus CDT when necessary. All patients had venoplasty and stenting to correct an underlying stenosis when it was present, and all patients had subsequent therapeutic anticoagulation. After evaluating the quantity of thrombus pre- and posttreatment, the investigators found that patients undergoing ISPMT had better overall lysis than those treated with the catheter-directed drip technique. Significantly, more patients in the ISMPT group had complete (>95 %) thrombolysis with a shorter treatment time (23.4 versus 54.4 h; $P=0.001$) and lower dose of rtPA (33.4 versus 59.3 mg; $P=0.007$). There was no difference in ICU or hospital length of stay due to the patient's underlying comorbidity, and there was no difference in bleeding complications or transfusions.

Randomized Trials

Only two randomized trials comparing CDT to anticoagulation alone have been reported. Elsharawy et al. randomized 35 patients with iliofemoral DVT to CDT or anticoagulation alone [7]. Patency was restored in 72 % of the CDT group versus 12 % in the anticoagulation group ($P<0.001$). Although CDT preserved normal valve function in more patients (89 % vs. 59 % at 6 months), the true difference in valve function may not have been underestimated by this study. Evaluating valve function requires a patent vein and most of the veins in the anticoagulation group remained obstructed. Longer follow-up allowing recanalization may have yielded a higher percentage of abnormal valves in the anticoagulation group and further emphasized the advantage of CDT.

Enden et al. examined the clinical outcomes of patients with a first-time, acute iliofemoral DVT [5]. In their multicenter randomized trial, patients with symptoms for up to 21 days received either CDT or standard anticoagulation alone with 30 mmHg gradient compression stockings. The primary clinical endpoint was the frequency of the postthrombotic syndrome at 24 months and iliofemoral patency at 6 months. After a mean treatment duration of 2.4 days, 43 % of patients in the CDT group had complete lysis, 37 % had partial, and 10 % were deemed unsuccessful. Major bleeding complications occurred in 3 % of patients receiving CDT versus none randomized to anticoagulation alone. At 6 months, 66 % of CDT patients and 47 % of anticoagulation patients had a patent iliofemoral system. At 24 months, fewer patients in the CDT group had postthrombotic syndrome compared with the anticoagulation cohort (41 % vs 56 %, $P=0.047$).

A National Institutes of Health-sponsored trial, the ATTRACT study [93] is currently underway with over 390 patients randomized. It is anticipated that this study will offer definitive data regarding the benefit of thrombus removal versus anticoagulation alone for iliofemoral DVT. Patients with acute proximal DVT will be stratified by DVT distribution (iliofemoral or femoropopliteal) and results evaluated according to the procedural strategy (pharmacomechanical vs. CDT drip) compared to anticoagulation alone.

Phlegmasia Cerulea Dolens

Phlegmasia cerulea dolens (PCD) represents a limb-threatening condition that results from an extensive DVT most commonly involving the iliofemoral segment (Fig. 9.2). Patients with PCD have a painful, edematous, and cyanotic extremity due to multilevel venous occlusion. Cyanosis occurs because of the inability of the dermal venous plexus to drain blood containing increased levels of carboxyhemoglobin. In contrast, phlegmasia alba dolens occurs in patients with less-extensive venous occlusion and is characterized by a pale, painfully swollen extremity. PCD occurs more frequently than is generally thought and is associated with severe postthrombotic morbidity and high recurrence rates if treated with anticoagulation alone [4, 73, 81]. Although the left lower extremity is the most commonly affected, up to 5 % of PCD cases occur in the upper extremity [94, 95].

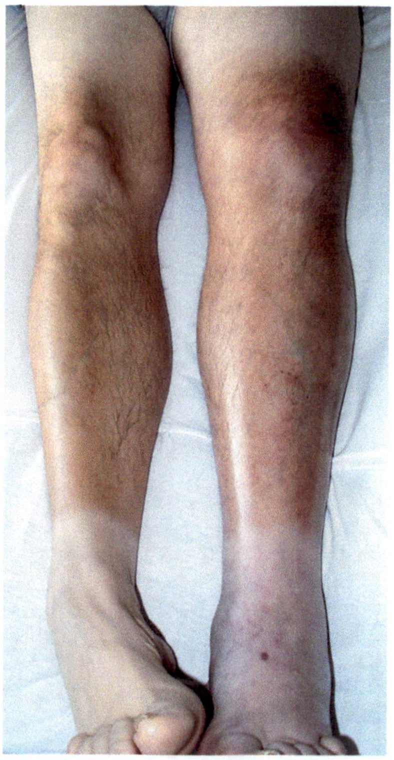

Fig. 9.2 Phlegmasia cerulea dolens of the left lower extremity. Photo illustrates swelling and cyanosis. The patient experienced continuous discomfort

PCD symptoms include pain, cyanosis, and edema which often starts distally and progresses proximally over a period of a few hours to several days. Pain occurs from the associated venous hypertension and elevated muscle compartment pressures. Skin blistering indicates high tissue pressures which can result in partial-thickness necrosis if the venous outflow patency is not rapidly reestablished. Irreversible tissue loss due to full-thickness skin necrosis represents venous gangrene.

Most patients with PCD have palpable pedal pulses or audible Doppler signals in the feet. Arterial compromise is unusual, but when it occurs, the lower extremity pain changes in character and becomes unremitting. Sensory or motor deficits indicate impending venous gangrene and predict a poor prognosis for limb viability. Skin blistering and arterial or neural compromise warrants immediate intervention to remove the thrombus, restore venous outflow, and salvage the limb.

Doppler ultrasonography should be used to confirm the diagnosis of PCD. It is important to assess the inferior vena cava (IVC) for thrombus as it may alter treatment options.

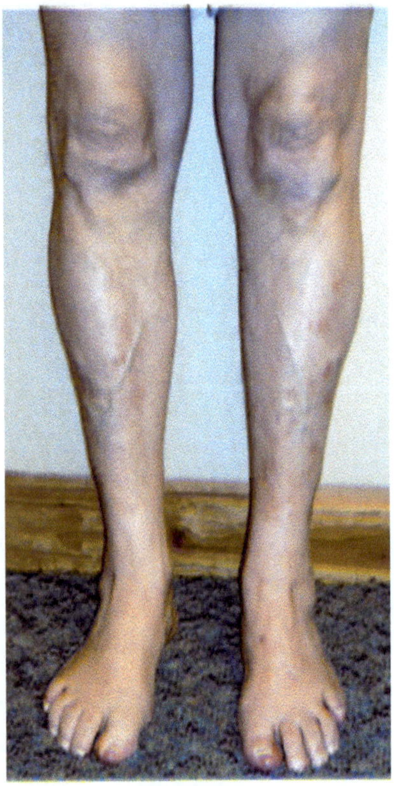

Fig. 9.3 Photograph of patient's leg 16 months following treatment with a strategy of thrombus removal. The patient was asymptomatic; the veins were patent and had normal valve function

Computed tomography angiography (CTA), magnetic resonance venography (MRV), and standard venography offer diagnostic imaging alternatives. While an MRV takes more time than CTA, it eliminates radiation and avoids the use of nephrotoxic iodinated agents that can cause complications in the setting of severe volume depletion. If catheter-based techniques will be used for thrombus removal, direct study of the IVC can be performed at the time of intervention.

Testing for hypercoagulability or thrombophilia is often performed in patients presenting with PCD. These investigations do not usually affect patient management decisions either acutely or over the long term. However, in patients with PCD from an idiopathic DVT, a thrombophilia evaluation should be performed on first-degree female relatives of childbearing age as the results may impact their care during future pregnancies.

PCD should be treated with a strategy of thrombus removal to avoid postthrombotic morbidity and reduce the risk of recurrence (Fig. 9.3) [8, 9, 12, 96]. Initial management should incorporate therapeutic anticoagulation, elevation of the affected limb, snug compression bandaging of the limb from toes to upper thigh, appropriate fluid resuscitation, and ambulation. Although surgical venous thrombectomy with or without an arteriovenous fistula is effective, catheter-based strategies are now more commonly performed [97].

Catheter-directed thrombolysis for patients with PCD has a success rate of 85–95 % [11, 98, 99]. When CDT is combined with percutaneous mechanical thrombectomy techniques, the amount of clot removed is greater over a short period of time using a lower dose of lytic agent [10, 100]. All patients should wear 30–40 mmHg compression stockings from awakening until returning to bed, and long-term oral anticoagulation with warfarin should target an international normalized ratio (INR) of 2.0–3.0. Although some practitioners believe that fasciotomy should be universally performed, it is often unnecessary if venous drainage is quickly restored. Restoring iliofemoral venous drainage should be considered the top treatment priority.

Long-Term Sequelae of DVT

Mortality

Not surprisingly, mortality after acute DVT is increased compared to age-matched controls. The in-hospital case fatality rate for acute DVT is approximately 5 %, and subsequent 1-, 3-, and 5-year mortality rates of 22, 30, and 39 %, respectively, have been reported [3, 101, 102]. Cancer is the most common cause of early death in patients with acute DVT, especially in patients over 44 years of age [101, 103]. The 1-month mortality rate among cancer patients with DVT is as high as 25 %, while the 1-year mortality rate is 63 % compared to 12.6 % in patients without cancer [101, 104]. The duration of increased mortality risk for patients with DVT and cancer persists for at least 3 years after diagnosis, whereas the mortality risk following secondary DVT (due to a transient risk) returns to that of the general population after 6 months [101].

DVT has also been linked to arterial thrombotic events, specifically cardiovascular death. Acute thrombosis is the common denominator for both DVT and myocardial infarction. Therefore, it is not surprising that the presence of residual venous thrombus at the time anticoagulants are stopped after treating a DVT may be a marker for a cardiovascular event [105, 106]. There appears to be a definite association between idiopathic venous thromboembolic events (VTE) and clinical cardiovascular disease. Patients with idiopathic VTE have more atherosclerotic risk factors and a higher 10-year risk of a symptomatic cardiovascular event compared to patients with secondary VTE (25.4 % vs. 12.9 %) [107, 108].

Pathophysiology of Postthrombotic Morbidity

Venous valvular dysfunction and outflow obstruction lead to ambulatory venous hypertension and are the underlying cause of chronic venous disease and the postthrombotic syndrome [109, 110]. While venous valvular function can be easily identified and precisely quantified, venous obstruction often remains undiagnosed. Current invasive and noninvasive imaging studies often fail to detect venous obstruction, and venous obstruction cannot be quantified. Therefore, the importance of venous obstruction as a contributor to postthrombotic morbidity has been largely underappreciated. Patients with venous obstruction generally have significant postthrombotic symptoms, and when obstruction and valve incompetence occur in the same patient, postthrombotic morbidity can be severe [109, 111].

A well-recognized risk factor for postthrombotic morbidity is ipsilateral recurrent venous thrombosis. DVT recurs in up to 24 % of patients at 5 years and 30 % of patients at 8 years following initial diagnosis [80, 106, 112]. Patients with idiopathic DVT or thrombophilia have a 2.5- to 3-fold increased risk of recurrence compared to patients with transient thrombotic risk factors. The risk of recurrent DVT appears to correlate with the adequacy of anticoagulation throughout the course of treatment for acute DVT. Subtherapeutic anticoagulation early in the treatment of acute DVT is associated with a 15-fold increased risk of recurrence. Over the long term, the risk of new thrombotic events increases 1.4 fold for each 20 % reduction in the time of therapeutic anticoagulation [66, 113].

Persistent luminal obstruction and ongoing thrombus activity also increase the risk of recurrent thrombosis. Following termination of anticoagulation, failure of complete recanalization manifested by persistent luminal obstruction on duplex ultrasound was associated with a significantly higher risk of recurrence compared to patients with a normal duplex examination [80, 112, 114]. Furthermore, ongoing thrombus activity detected as an elevated D-dimer level 1 month after stopping anticoagulation is associated with a 310 % increased risk for recurrent thrombosis [115, 116].

Complications of Anticoagulation

Bleeding Complications

Although it is commonly believed that the risk of bleeding from heparin increases as the dose increases, this observation may only apply to patients with comorbid risk factors such as recent surgery or trauma [117]. In this subset of patients, monitoring heparin activity with vitro tests of coagulation such as the activated partial thromboplastin time (aPTT) can help identify patients at risk for bleeding. However, in the vast majority of patients without concomitant risk factors, an association between supratherapeutic aPTT response and the risk of bleeding remains unproven and aPTT levels provide minimal guidance in predicting bleeding [118].

Bleeding can also complicate anticoagulation therapy with oral agents. When vitamin K antagonists (VKA) are used, the bleeding risk correlates with prolongation of the prothrombin time and elevation of the international normalized ratio (INR) [119]. Bleeding risk accelerates once the INR exceeds 4.0. Warfarin-induced skin necrosis represents a nonhemorrhagic complication that can occur if VKAs are given without overlapping heparin therapy. VKAs inhibit the naturally occurring anticoagulants Protein C and S faster than they inhibit the vitamin K-dependent procoagulants. Patients with underlying protein C or S deficiency and some patients with cancer may develop skin necrosis because the initial dosing of warfarin makes them hypercoagulable [120–123]. This situation can often be avoided by extending anticoagulation with heparin until achieving a therapeutic INR with warfarin.

Warfarin compounds cross the placenta and cause teratogenic effects when given during the first trimester of pregnancy [124, 125]. Because of similar risks during the second trimester, as well as the threat of fetal bleeding during and after delivery, warfarin compounds should be avoided during pregnancy. All women of childbearing potential who are taking warfarin must avoid becoming pregnant. Long-term adjusted dose subcutaneous heparin is recommended for pregnant patients who require anticoagulation [126].

Heparin-Induced Thrombocytopenia

Heparin-induced thrombocytopenia is a potentially life- and limb-threatening complication associated with the use of unfractionated heparin (UFH) and, to a lesser extent, low-molecular-weight heparin (LMWH) [127]. HIT should be suspected when a patient receiving UFH or LMWH has a drop in their platelet count of 50 % or more. HIT affects patients receiving UFH ten times more commonly than those being treated with LMWH. In patients that have not been previously sensitized to heparin, HIT typically occurs 5–14 days after starting heparin [128]. Patients with recent prior heparin exposure may have already developed heparin antibodies which can accelerate the onset of HIT, causing a rapid, precipitous thrombocytopenia and acute thrombosis. Thrombotic complications occur in up to 50 % of HIT patients and are most commonly venous [129]. Potential complications include deep venous thrombosis (DVT) of the arms and legs, pulmonary embolism (PE), cerebral vein thrombosis, adrenal vein thrombosis, and venous gangrene. Acute limb ischemia, stroke, myocardial infarction, cardiac thrombus or embolus, and mesenteric, renal, spinal, or arterial thrombosis have also been reported [127–129]. Heparin-induced thrombocytopenia can cause acute graft thrombosis following lower extremity bypass as a result of platelet deposition at the sites of vascular injury.

Heparin-dependent IgG antibodies mediate the pathophysiology of HIT [130, 131]. Normally, heparin binds to platelet factor 4 (PF-4) which is released from the alpha granules within activated platelets. Some patients recognize PF-4 bound heparin as a target antigen and generate IgG (HIT) antibodies. The PF-4 bound heparin and IgG antibodies form immune complexes which attach to the Fc receptor on platelets resulting in platelet activation [132]. Unchecked platelet activation not only consumes platelets (resulting in thrombocytopenia), it also generates large quantities of platelet microparticles. These procoagulant-rich microparticles are thought to be responsible for the venous and arterial thrombosis associated with HIT. The diagnosis of HIT requires the appropriate clinical setting of thrombocytopenia in a patient with current or recent exposure to heparin and the detection of heparin-dependent antibodies.

Based on clinical presentation, HIT is divided into two types. Type I HIT is associated with a mild thrombocytopenia that usually occurs within 4 days of starting heparin. It is nonimmune mediated and appears to be caused by the direct agglutinating effect of heparin on platelets. Type I is not associated with thrombosis and resolves spontaneously despite continuing anticoagulation with heparin. Type II HIT is associated with severe thrombocytopenia or a significant decrease (greater than 50 %) in the platelet count that occurs between 5 and 14 days after starting heparin. Type II is immune mediated and may be associated with both arterial and venous thrombosis.

Management Recommendations

Platelet counts should be checked every 2–3 days in patients receiving heparin who are thought to have greater than 1 % risk for developing HIT. Monitoring should continue from days 4–14 of heparin therapy or until heparin is discontinued, whichever occurs first. The first step in treating HIT involves immediate cessation of all heparin-related compounds. A direct thrombin inhibitor such as lepirudin, argatroban, or danaparoid should be started to maintain anticoagulation. Oral anticoagulation with VKAs should not be started until the platelet count returns to normal or near normal. At that point, the VKA can be initiated and should be overlapped with the parenteral nonheparin anticoagulant for a minimum of 5 days. Patients with HIT rarely require platelet transfusions. In patients with severe thrombocytopenia, platelet transfusions should only be given if bleeding occurs or the patient requires an invasive procedure that is associated with a high risk of bleeding.

Summary

The sheer number of invasive procedures performed on patients with thrombotic risk factors ensures that nearly all surgeons will encounter patients with DVT. The choice of treatment for acute DVT depends on the extent and location of the thrombus as well as the patient's clinical situation. All patients without a significant bleeding risk should receive immediate anticoagulation to achieve therapeutic levels quickly. Anticoagulation therapy requires monitoring and awareness of potential complications including bleeding and heparin-induced thrombocytopenia. Catheter-directed thrombolysis and pharmacomechanical thrombectomy have emerged as minimally invasive techniques that effectively restore venous patency. Convincing evidence shows that early thrombus removal improves functional outcomes and minimizes the risk of postthrombotic syndrome. Active patients who have an acute iliofemoral DVT and a low risk of bleeding stand to gain the greatest benefit from percutaneous thrombolytic procedures. Extensive venous thrombosis leading to phlegmasia cerulea dolens or venous gangrene can threaten a patient's life and limb. These patients cannot afford to wait for thrombolytic therapy to take effect and require an emergent surgical venous thrombectomy for limb salvage. This chapter has outlined treatment strategies to help practicing surgeons effectively manage acute DVT and prevent its potentially fatal and disabling consequences.

References

1. Heit JA, Kobbervig CE, James AH, Petterson TM, Bailey KR, Melton III LJ. Trends in the incidence of venous thromboembolism during pregnancy or postpartum: a 30-year population-based study. Ann Intern Med. 2005;143:697–706.
2. Strandness Jr DE, Langlois Y, Cramer M, Randlett A, Thiele BL. Long-term sequelae of acute venous thrombosis. JAMA. 1983;250:1289–92.
3. Beyth RJ, Cohen AM, Landefeld CS. Long-term outcomes of deep-vein thrombosis. Arch Intern Med. 1995;155:1031–7.
4. Delis KT, Bountouroglou D, Mansfield AO. Venous claudication in iliofemoral thrombosis: long-term effects on venous hemodynamics, clinical status, and quality of life. Ann Surg. 2004;239:118–26.
5. Enden T, Haig Y, Klow NE, et al. Long-term outcome after additional catheter-directed thrombolysis versus standard treatment for acute iliofemoral deep vein thrombosis (the CaVenT study): a randomised controlled trial. Lancet. 2012;379:31–8.
6. Plate G, Einarsson E, Ohlin P, Jensen R, Qvarfordt P, Eklof B. Thrombectomy with temporary arteriovenous fistula: the treatment of choice in acute iliofemoral venous thrombosis. J Vasc Surg. 1984;1:867–76.
7. Elsharawy M, Elzayat E. Early results of thrombolysis vs anticoagulation in iliofemoral venous thrombosis. A randomised clinical trial. Eur J Vasc Endovasc Surg. 2002;24:209–14.
8. Comerota AJ, Grewal N, Martinez JT, et al. Postthrombotic morbidity correlates with residual thrombus following catheter-directed thrombolysis for iliofemoral deep vein thrombosis. J Vasc Surg. 2012;55:768–73.
9. Grewal N, Martinez J, Andrews L, Comerota AJ. Quantity of clot lysed after catheter-directed thrombolysis for iliofemoral deep venous thrombosis correlates with post-thrombotic morbidity. J Vasc Surg. 2010;51:1209–14.
10. Martinez Trabal JL, Comerota AJ, LaPorte FB, Kazanjian S, DiSalle R, Sepanski DM. The quantitative benefit of isolated, segmental, pharmacomechanical thrombolysis (ISPMT) for iliofemoral venous thrombosis. J Vasc Surg. 2008;48:1532–7.

11. Mewissen MW, Seabrook GR, Meissner MH, Cynamon J, Labropoulos N, Haughton SH. Catheter-directed thrombolysis for lower extremity deep venous thrombosis: report of a national multicenter registry. Radiology. 1999;211:39–49.
12. Aziz F, Comerota AJ. Quantity of residual thrombus after successful catheter-directed thrombolysis for iliofemoral deep venous thrombosis correlates with recurrence. Eur J Vasc Endovasc Surg. 2012;44:210–3.
13. Le Gal G, Carrier M, Kovacs MJ, et al. Residual vein obstruction as a predictor for recurrent thromboembolic events after a first unprovoked episode: data from the REVERSE cohort study. J Thromb Haemost. 2011;9:1126–32.
14. Virchow R. Neuer Fall von todlicher Emboli er Lungenarterie. Arch Pathol Anat. 1856;10:225.
15. Agnelli G, Verso M, Ageno W, et al. The MASTER registry on venous thromboembolism: description of the study cohort. Thromb Res. 2008;121:605–10.
16. Spencer FA, Emery C, Lessard D, et al. The Worcester Venous Thromboembolism study: a population-based study of the clinical epidemiology of venous thromboembolism. J Gen Intern Med. 2006;21:722–7.
17. Koster T, Rosendaal FR, de Ronde H, Briet E, Vandenbroucke JP, Bertina RM. Venous thrombosis due to poor anticoagulant response to activated protein C: Leiden Thrombophilia Study. Lancet. 1993;342:1503–6.
18. Mateo J, Oliver A, Borrell M, Sala N, Fontcuberta J. Laboratory evaluation and clinical characteristics of 2,132 consecutive unselected patients with venous thromboembolism–results of the Spanish Multicentric Study on Thrombophilia (EMET-Study). Thromb Haemost. 1997;77:444–51.
19. Lyman GH. Venous thromboembolism in the patient with cancer: focus on burden of disease and benefits of thromboprophylaxis. Cancer. 2011;117:1334–49.
20. Sorensen HT, Mellemkjaer L, Olsen JH, Baron JA. Prognosis of cancers associated with venous thromboembolism. N Engl J Med. 2000;343:1846–50.
21. White RH, Zhou H, Romano PS. Incidence of symptomatic venous thromboembolism after different elective or urgent surgical procedures. Thromb Haemost. 2003;90:446–55.
22. Lee AY, Gent M, Julian JA, et al. Bilateral vs. ipsilateral venography as the primary efficacy outcome measure in thromboprophylaxis clinical trials: a systematic review. J Thromb Haemost. 2004; 2:1752–9.
23. Maxwell GL, Synan I, Dodge R, Carroll B, Clarke-Pearson DL. Pneumatic compression versus low molecular weight heparin in gynecologic oncology surgery: a randomized trial. Obstet Gynecol. 2001;98:989–95.
24. Falck-Ytter Y, Francis CW, Johanson NA, et al. Prevention of VTE in orthopedic surgery patients: Antithrombotic Therapy and Prevention of Thrombosis, 9th ed: American College of Chest Physicians Evidence-Based Clinical Practice Guidelines. Chest. 2012;141:e278S–325.
25. Gould MK, Garcia DA, Wren SM, et al. Prevention of VTE in nonorthopedic surgical patients: Antithrombotic Therapy and Prevention of Thrombosis, 9th ed: American College of Chest Physicians Evidence-Based Clinical Practice Guidelines. Chest. 2012;141:e227S–77.
26. Geerts WH, Code KI, Jay RM, Chen E, Szalai JP. A prospective study of venous thromboembolism after major trauma. N Engl J Med. 1994;331:1601–6.
27. Geerts WH, Jay RM, Code KI, et al. A comparison of low-dose heparin with low-molecular-weight heparin as prophylaxis against venous thromboembolism after major trauma. N Engl J Med. 1996;335:701–7.
28. Montgomery KD, Geerts WH, Potter HG, Helfet DL. Thromboembolic complications in patients with pelvic trauma. Clin Orthop Relat Res. 1996;(329):68–87.
29. McLaughlin DF, Wade CE, Champion HR, Salinas J, Holcomb JB. Thromboembolic complications following trauma. Transfusion. 2009;49 Suppl 5:256S–63.
30. Owings JT, Gosselin R. Acquired antithrombin deficiency following severe traumatic injury: rationale for study of antithrombin supplementation. Semin Thromb Hemost. 1997;23 Suppl 1:17–24.
31. Van Stralen KJ, Rosendaal FR, Doggen CJ. Minor injuries as a risk factor for venous thrombosis. Arch Intern Med. 2008;168:21–6.
32. Marik PE, Plante LA. Venous thromboembolic disease and pregnancy. N Engl J Med. 2008;359:2025–33.
33. Greer IA. Thrombosis in pregnancy: maternal and fetal issues. Lancet. 1999;353:1258–65.
34. Kujovich JL. Hormones and pregnancy: thromboembolic risks for women. Br J Haematol. 2004;126:443–54.
35. Miller J, Chan BK, Nelson HD. Postmenopausal estrogen replacement and risk for venous thromboembolism: a systematic review and meta-analysis for the U.S. Preventive Services Task Force. Ann Intern Med. 2002;136:680–90.
36. Grodstein F, Stampfer MJ, Goldhaber SZ, et al. Prospective study of exogenous hormones and risk of pulmonary embolism in women. Lancet. 1996;348:983–7.
37. Perez GS, Garcia Rodriguez LA, Castellsague J, Duque OA. Hormone replacement therapy and risk of venous thromboembolism: population based case-control study. BMJ. 1997;314: 796–800.
38. Hulley S, Furberg C, Barrett-Connor E, et al. Noncardiovascular disease outcomes during 6.8 years of hormone therapy: Heart and Estrogen/progestin Replacement Study follow-up (HERS II). JAMA. 2002;288:58–66.
39. Warlow C, Ogston D, Douglas AS. Venous thrombosis following strokes. Lancet. 1972;1:1305–6.
40. Clarke M, Hopewell S, Juszczak E, Eisinga A, Kjeldstrøm M. Compression stockings for preventing deep vein thrombosis in airline passengers. Cochrane Database Syst Rev. 2006;(2): CD004002.
41. van Weert H, Dolan G, Wichers I, de Vries C, ter Riet G, Buller H. Spontaneous superficial venous thrombophlebitis: does it increase risk for thromboembolism? A historic follow-up study in primary care. J Fam Pract. 2006;55:52–7.
42. Prandoni P, Lensing AW, Cogo A, et al. The long-term clinical course of acute deep venous thrombosis. Ann Intern Med. 1996; 125:1–7.
43. Samama MM. An epidemiologic study of risk factors for deep vein thrombosis in medical outpatients: the Sirius study. Arch Intern Med. 2000;160:3415–20.
44. Kibbe MR, Ujiki M, Goodwin AL, Eskandari M, Yao J, Matsumura J. Iliac vein compression in an asymptomatic patient population. J Vasc Surg. 2004;39:937–43.
45. Wells PS, Hirsh J, Anderson DR, et al. Accuracy of clinical assessment of deep-vein thrombosis. Lancet. 1995;345:1326–30.
46. Wells PS, Anderson DR, Rodger M, et al. Evaluation of D-dimer in the diagnosis of suspected deep-vein thrombosis. N Engl J Med. 2003;349:1227–35.
47. Elf JL, Strandberg K, Nilsson C, Svensson PJ. Clinical probability assessment and D-dimer determination in patients with suspected deep vein thrombosis, a prospective multicenter management study. Thromb Res. 2009;123:612–6.
48. Kelly J, Hunt BJ. Role of D-dimers in diagnosis of venous thromboembolism. Lancet. 2002;359:456–8.
49. Noren A, Lindmarker P, Rosfors S. A retrospective follow-up study of patients with suspected deep vein thrombosis and negative results of colour duplex ultrasound. Phlebography. 1997; 12:56–9.
50. Schellong SM, Schwarz T, Halbritter K, et al. Complete compression ultrasonography of the leg veins as a single test for the diagnosis of deep vein thrombosis. Thromb Haemost. 2003;89: 228–34.

51. Elias A, Mallard L, Elias M, et al. A single complete ultrasound investigation of the venous network for the diagnostic management of patients with a clinically suspected first episode of deep venous thrombosis of the lower limbs. Thromb Haemost. 2003; 89:221–7.
52. Cogo A, Lensing AW, Prandoni P, Hirsh J. Distribution of thrombosis in patients with symptomatic deep vein thrombosis. Implications for simplifying the diagnostic process with compression ultrasound. Arch Intern Med. 1993;153:2777–80.
53. Philbrick JT, Becker DM. Calf deep venous thrombosis. A wolf in sheep's clothing? Arch Intern Med. 1988;148:2131–8.
54. Lagerstedt CI, Olsson CG, Fagher BO, Oqvist BW, Albrechtsson U. Need for long-term anticoagulant treatment in symptomatic calf-vein thrombosis. Lancet. 1985;2:515–8.
55. Huisman MV, Buller HR, ten Cate JW, Vreeken J. Serial impedance plethysmography for suspected deep venous thrombosis in outpatients. The Amsterdam General Practitioner Study. N Engl J Med. 1986;314:823–8.
56. Lohr JM, James KV, Deshmukh RM, Hasselfeld KA, Allastair B. Karmody Award. Calf vein thrombi are not a benign finding. Am J Surg. 1995;170:86–90.
57. Moreno-Cabral R, Kistner RL, Nordyke RA. Importance of calf vein thrombophlebitis. Surgery. 1976;80:735–42.
58. Fraser JD, Anderson DR. Deep venous thrombosis: recent advances and optimal investigation with US. Radiology. 1999; 211:9–24.
59. Elias A, Le CG, Bouvier JL, Benichou M, Serradimigni A. Value of real time B mode ultrasound imaging in the diagnosis of deep vein thrombosis of the lower limbs. Int Angiol. 1987;6:175–82.
60. Sumner DS. Diagnosis of deep vein thrombosis with real-time color and duplex scanning. In: Bernstein EF, editor. Vascular diagnosis. 4th ed. St. Louis: Mosby; 1993. p. 794–5.
61. Messina LM, Sarpa MS, Smith MA, Greenfield LJ. Clinical significance of routine imaging of iliac and calf veins by color flow duplex scanning in patients suspected of having acute lower extremity deep venous thrombosis. Surgery. 1993;114: 921–7.
62. Weinmann EE, Salzman EW. Deep-vein thrombosis. N Engl J Med. 1994;331:1630–41.
63. Bauer KA. Laboratory markers of coagulation and fibrinolysis. In: Colman RW, Marder VJ, Clowes A, Genge JN, Goldhaber SZ, editors. Hemostasis and thrombosis. 5th ed. Philadelphia: Lippincott, Williams, and Wilkins; 2006. p. 835–50.
64. Wells PS. Integrated strategies for the diagnosis of venous thromboembolism. J Thromb Haemost. 2007;5 Suppl 1:41–50.
65. Brandjes DP, Heijboer H, Buller HR, de Rijk M, Jagt H, ten Cate JW. Acenocoumarol and heparin compared with acenocoumarol alone in the initial treatment of proximal-vein thrombosis. N Engl J Med. 1992;327:1485–9.
66. Hull RD, Raskob GE, Hirsh J, et al. Continuous intravenous heparin compared with intermittent subcutaneous heparin in the initial treatment of proximal-vein thrombosis. N Engl J Med. 1986; 315:1109–14.
67. Schulman S, Kearon C, Kakkar AK, et al. Dabigatran versus warfarin in the treatment of acute venous thromboembolism. N Engl J Med. 2009;361:2342–52.
68. Bauersachs R, Berkowitz SD, Brenner B, et al. Oral rivaroxaban for symptomatic venous thromboembolism. N Engl J Med. 2010; 363:2499–510.
69. Schulman S, Eriksson H, Goldhaber SZ. Dabigatran or warfarin for extended maintenance therapy of venous thromboembolism [Abstract]. J Thromb Haemost. 2011;9:731–2.
70. Schulman S, Baanstra D, Eriksson H. Dabigatran vs. placebo for extended maintenance therapy of venous thromboembolism [Abstract]. J Thromb Haemost. 2011;9:22.
71. Agnelli G, Buller HR, Cohen A, et al. Apixaban for extended treatment of venous thromboembolism. N Engl J Med. 2013; 368:699–708.
72. Kearon C, Akl EA, Comerota AJ, et al. Antithrombotic therapy for VTE disease: Antithrombotic Therapy and Prevention of Thrombosis, 9th ed: American College of Chest Physicians Evidence-Based Clinical Practice Guidelines. Chest. 2012;141: e419S–94.
73. Akesson H, Brudin L, Dahlstrom JA, Eklof B, Ohlin P, Plate G. Venous function assessed during a 5 year period after acute ilio-femoral venous thrombosis treated with anticoagulation. Eur J Vasc Surg. 1990;4:43–8.
74. Labropoulos N, Volteas N, Leon M, et al. The role of venous outflow obstruction in patients with chronic venous dysfunction. Arch Surg. 1997;132:46–51.
75. Qvarfordt P, Eklof B, Ohlin P. Intramuscular pressure in the lower leg in deep vein thrombosis and phlegmasia cerulae dolens. Ann Surg. 1983;197:450–3.
76. Douketis JD, Crowther MA, Foster GA, Ginsberg JS. Does the location of thrombosis determine the risk of disease recurrence in patients with proximal deep vein thrombosis? Am J Med. 2001; 110:515–9.
77. Meissner MH, Manzo RA, Bergelin RO, Markel A, Strandness Jr DE. Deep venous insufficiency: the relationship between lysis and subsequent reflux. J Vasc Surg. 1993;18:596–605.
78. Meissner MH, Caps MT, Bergelin RO, Manzo RA, Strandness Jr DE. Propagation, rethrombosis and new thrombus formation after acute deep venous thrombosis. J Vasc Surg. 1995;22:558–67.
79. Roumen-Klappe EM, Den HM, Janssen MC, van der Vleuten C, Thien T, Wollersheim H. The post-thrombotic syndrome: incidence and prognostic value of non-invasive venous examinations in a six-year follow-up study. Thromb Haemost. 2005;94:825–30.
80. Prandoni P, Lensing AW, Prins MH, et al. Residual venous thrombosis as a predictive factor of recurrent venous thromboembolism. Ann Intern Med. 2002;137:955–60.
81. Kahn SR, Ginsberg JS. Relationship between deep venous thrombosis and the postthrombotic syndrome. Arch Intern Med. 2004; 164:17–26.
82. O'Donnell TF, Browse NL, Burnand KG, Thomas ML. The socioeconomic effects of an iliofemoral venous thrombosis. J Surg Res. 1977;22:483–8.
83. Comerota AJ, Throm RC, Mathias SD, Haughton S, Mewissen M. Catheter-directed thrombolysis for iliofemoral deep venous thrombosis improves health-related quality of life. J Vasc Surg. 2000;32:130–7.
84. Plate G, Akesson H, Einarsson E, Ohlin P, Eklof B. Long-term results of venous thrombectomy combined with a temporary arterio-venous fistula. Eur J Vasc Surg. 1990;4:483–9.
85. Plate G, Eklof B, Norgren L, Ohlin P, Dahlstrom JA. Venous thrombectomy for iliofemoral vein thrombosis–10-year results of a prospective randomised study. Eur J Vasc Endovasc Surg. 1997;14:367–74.
86. Comerota AJ, Gale SS. Technique of contemporary iliofemoral and infrainguinal venous thrombectomy. J Vasc Surg. 2006;43: 185–91.
87. Comerota AJ. Thrombolysis for deep venous thrombosis. J Vasc Surg. 2012;55:607–11.
88. Sillesen H, Just S, Jorgensen M, Baekgaard N. Catheter-directed thrombolysis for treatment of ilio-femoral deep venous thrombosis is durable, preserves venous valve function and may prevent chronic venous insufficiency. Eur J Vasc Endovasc Surg. 2005; 30:556–62.
89. Kasirajan K, Gray B, Ouriel K. Percutaneous AngioJet thrombectomy in the management of extensive deep venous thrombosis. J Vasc Interv Radiol. 2001;12:179–85.

90. Vedantham S, Vesely TM, Parti N, Darcy M, Hovsepian DM, Picus D. Lower extremity venous thrombolysis with adjunctive mechanical thrombectomy. J Vasc Interv Radiol. 2002;13:1001–8.
91. Parikh S, Motarjeme A, McNamara T, et al. Ultrasound-accelerated thrombolysis for the treatment of deep vein thrombosis: initial clinical experience. J Vasc Interv Radiol. 2008;19:521–8.
92. Baker R, Samuels S, Benenati JF, Powell A, Uthoff H. Ultrasound-accelerated vs standard catheter-directed thrombolysis-a comparative study in patients with iliofemoral deep vein thrombosis. J Vasc Interv Radiol. 2012;23:1460–6.
93. Comerota AJ. The ATTRACT trial: rationale for early intervention for iliofemoral DVT. Perspect Vasc Surg Endovasc Ther. 2009;21:221–4.
94. Perkins JM, Magee TR, Galland RB. Phlegmasia caerulea dolens and venous gangrene. Br J Surg. 1996;83:19–23.
95. Mousa A, Henderson P, Dayal R, Bernheim J, Kent KC, Faries PL. Endoluminal recanalization in a patient with phlegmasia cerulea dolens using a multimodality approach. Vascular. 2005;13:313–7.
96. Baekgaard N, Broholm R, Just S, Jorgensen M, Jensen LP. Long-term results using catheter-directed thrombolysis in 103 lower limbs with acute iliofemoral venous thrombosis. Eur J Vasc Endovasc Surg. 2010;39:112–7.
97. Sarwar S, Narra S, Munir A. Phlegmasia cerulea dolens. Tex Heart Inst J. 2009;36:76–7.
98. Bjarnason H, Kruse JR, Asinger DA, et al. Iliofemoral deep venous thrombosis: safety and efficacy outcome during 5 years of catheter-directed thrombolytic therapy. J Vasc Interv Radiol. 1997;8:405–18.
99. Comerota AJ, Kagan SA. Catheter-directed thrombolysis for the treatment of acute iliofemoral deep venous thrombosis. Phlebology. 2000;15:149–55.
100. Lin PH, Zhou W, Dardik A, et al. Catheter-direct thrombolysis versus pharmacomechanical thrombectomy for treatment of symptomatic lower extremity deep venous thrombosis. Am J Surg. 2006;192:782–8.
101. Naess IA, Christiansen SC, Romundstad P, Cannegieter SC, Rosendaal FR, Hammerstrom J. Incidence and mortality of venous thrombosis: a population-based study. J Thromb Haemost. 2007; 5:692–9.
102. Anderson Jr FA, Wheeler HB, Goldberg RJ, et al. A population-based perspective of the hospital incidence and case-fatality rates of deep vein thrombosis and pulmonary embolism. The Worcester DVT Study. Arch Intern Med. 1991;151:933–8.
103. Cushman M, Tsai AW, White RH, et al. Deep vein thrombosis and pulmonary embolism in two cohorts: the longitudinal investigation of thromboembolism etiology. Am J Med. 2004;117:19–25.
104. White RH. The epidemiology of venous thromboembolism. Circulation. 2003;107:I4–8.
105. Savory L, Harper P, Ockelford P. Posttreatment ultrasound-detected residual venous thrombosis: a risk factor for recurrent venous thromboembolism and mortality. Curr Opin Pulm Med. 2007;13:403–8.
106. Young L, Ockelford P, Milne D, Rolfe-Vyson V, Mckelvie S, Harper P. Post-treatment residual thrombus increases the risk of recurrent deep vein thrombosis and mortality. J Thromb Haemost. 2006;4:1919–24.
107. Hong C, Zhu F, Du D, Pilgram TK, Sicard GA, Bae KT. Coronary artery calcification and risk factors for atherosclerosis in patients with venous thromboembolism. Atherosclerosis. 2005;183:169–74.
108. Prandoni P, Ghirarduzzi A, Prins MH, et al. Venous thromboembolism and the risk of subsequent symptomatic atherosclerosis. J Thromb Haemost. 2006;4:1891–6.
109. Shull KC, Nicolaides AN, Fernandes e Fernandes J, et al. Significance of popliteal reflux in relation to ambulatory venous pressure and ulceration. Arch Surg. 1979;114:1304–6.
110. Nicolaides AN, Schull K, Fernandes E. Ambulatory venous pressure: new information. In: Nicolaides AN, Yao JS, editors. Investigation of vascular disorders. New York: Churchill Livingstone; 1981. p. 488–94.
111. Johnson BF, Manzo RA, Bergelin RO, Strandness Jr DE. Relationship between changes in the deep venous system and the development of the postthrombotic syndrome after an acute episode of lower limb deep vein thrombosis: a one- to six-year follow-up. J Vasc Surg. 1995;21:307–12.
112. Lindmarker P, Schulman S. The risk of ipsilateral versus contralateral recurrent deep vein thrombosis in the leg. The DURAC Trial Study Group. J Intern Med. 2000;247:601–6.
113. Caps MT, Meissner MH, Tullis MJ, et al. Venous thrombus stability during acute phase of therapy. Vasc Med. 1999;4:9–14.
114. Prandoni P, Prins MH, Lensing AW, et al. Residual thrombosis on ultrasonography to guide the duration of anticoagulation in patients with deep venous thrombosis: a randomized trial. Ann Intern Med. 2009;150:577–85.
115. Eichinger S, Minar E, Bialonczyk C, et al. D-dimer levels and risk of recurrent venous thromboembolism. JAMA. 2003;290:1071–4.
116. Palareti G, Cosmi B, Legnani C, et al. D-dimer testing to determine the duration of anticoagulation therapy. N Engl J Med. 2006;355:1780–9.
117. Landefeld CS, Cook EF, Flatley M, Weisberg M, Goldman L. Identification and preliminary validation of predictors of major bleeding in hospitalized patients starting anticoagulant therapy. Am J Med. 1987;82:703–13.
118. Conti S, Daschbach M, Blaisdell FW. A comparison of high-dose versus conventional-dose heparin therapy for deep vein thrombosis. Surgery. 1982;92:972–80.
119. Turpie AG, Gunstensen J, Hirsh J, Nelson H, Gent M. Randomised comparison of two intensities of oral anticoagulant therapy after tissue heart valve replacement. Lancet. 1988;1:1242–5.
120. McGehee WG, Klotz TA, Epstein DJ, Rapaport SI. Coumarin necrosis associated with hereditary protein C deficiency. Ann Intern Med. 1984;101:59–60.
121. Kazmier FJ. Thromboembolism, coumarin necrosis, and protein C. Mayo Clin Proc. 1985;60:673–4.
122. Martin BF, Phillips JD. Gangrene of the female breast with anticoagulant therapy: report of two cases. Am J Clin Pathol. 1970; 53:622–6.
123. Everett RN, Jones Jr FL. Warfarin-induced skin necrosis. A cutaneous sign of malignancy? Postgrad Med. 1986;79:97–103.
124. Hall JG, Pauli RM, Wilson KM. Maternal and fetal sequelae of anticoagulation during pregnancy. Am J Med. 1980;68:122–40.
125. Stevenson RE, Burton OM, Ferlauto GJ, Taylor HA. Hazards of oral anticoagulants during pregnancy. JAMA. 1980;243: 1549–51.
126. Comerota AJ. Thrombophlebitis in obstetrics and gynecology. In: Rakel RE, editor. Conn's current therapy. Philadelphia: WB Saunders; 1985. p. 903–7.
127. Arepally GM, Ortel TL. Clinical practice. Heparin-induced thrombocytopenia. N Engl J Med. 2006;355:809–17.
128. Warkentin TE, Greinacher A, Koster A, Lincoff AM. Treatment and prevention of heparin-induced thrombocytopenia: American College of Chest Physicians Evidence-Based Clinical Practice Guidelines (8th Edition). Chest. 2008;133:340S–80.
129. Warkentin TE, Levine MN, Hirsh J, et al. Heparin-induced thrombocytopenia in patients treated with low-molecular-weight heparin or unfractionated heparin. N Engl J Med. 1995;332:1330–5.
130. Kelton JG, Sheridan D, Santos A, et al. Heparin-induced thrombocytopenia: laboratory studies. Blood. 1988;72:925–30.
131. Chong BH, Fawaz I, Chesterman CN, Berndt MC. Heparin-induced thrombocytopenia: mechanism of interaction of the heparin-dependent antibody with platelets. Br J Haematol. 1989; 73:235–40.
132. Amiral J, Bridey F, Dreyfus M, et al. Platelet factor 4 complexed to heparin is the target for antibodies generated in heparin-induced thrombocytopenia. Thromb Haemost. 1992;68:95–6.

Superficial Thrombophlebitis

10

Anil Hingorani and Enrico Ascher

Introduction

Superficial venous thrombophlebitis (SVT) is a common disorder that carries the risk of thrombus progression, embolization, and recurrence. Despite these potentially serious consequences, SVT has always been the stepchild of deep venous thrombosis (DVT) and received limited attention in the literature. Previous studies estimate that SVT occurs in 125,000 patients per year; however, the actual incidence is probably higher as many cases of SVT are unreported [1]. Traditional teaching classified SVT as a self-limited process that posed little if any risk. This inaccurate but widely held perception prompted physicians to dismiss patients with the clinical diagnosis of SVT believing that the best treatment was "benign neglect." In an attempt to dispel this and other misconceptions, this chapter will examine current data regarding SVT and its management.

Clinical Presentation

Approximately 54–65 % of patients diagnosed with SVT are women with an average age of 58, while the average age for men is about 54 [2, 3]. Varicose veins represent the most common predisposing risk factor for SVT occurring in 62 % of patients. Others factors associated with SVT include age older than 60, obesity, tobacco use, and previous history of DVT or SVT. Factors associated with progression of SVT include age older than 60, male sex, and history of DVT.

The physical diagnosis of SVT is based on the presence of erythema and tenderness in the distribution of the superficial veins. Thrombus can often be appreciated as a palpable cord following the course of a superficial vein. Pain and warmth are clinically evident, and significant extremity swelling can be present despite the absence of a DVT. Some patients present with erythema, pain, and tenderness as a streak along the arm or leg. If a duplex ultrasound does not detect a DVT or SVT in these patients, the diagnosis of cellulitis or lymphangitis should be considered.

Etiology

Over 100 years ago, Virchow identified stasis, endothelial damage, and hypercoagulability as the primary risk factors for thrombosis. Although stasis and endothelial trauma have direct links to SVT, the relationship between hypercoagulability and SVT remains unclear. When a DVT occurs in the presence of an SVT, the two thrombotic segments are often not contiguous. The fact that the DVT rarely represents a direct extension of the SVT provides circumstantial evidence that systemic factors such as hypercoagulability could play a role in the pathophysiology of SVT.

In order to determine whether a hypercoagulable state contributes to the development of SVT, Hanson et al. measured anticoagulant levels in 29 patients with acute SVT [4]. All patients had duplex ultrasound scans performed on both the superficial and deep venous systems. Patients with SVT were treated with nonsteroidal anti-inflammatory drugs, while those with both SVT and a concomitant DVT were treated with heparin and warfarin. All patients had a coagulation profile performed including (1) protein C antigen and activity, (2) activated protein C (APC) resistance, (3) protein S antigen and activity, (4) antithrombin (AT), and (5) lupus-type anticoagulant. Twelve patients (41 %) had abnormal results consistent with a hypercoagulable state. Five of the

A. Hingorani, MD (✉)
Vascular Institute of New York, Lutheran Medical Center, 960 50th Street, Brooklyn, NY 11219, USA

Division of Vascular Surgery, Department of Surgery, Lutheran Medical Center, Brooklyn, NY, USA
e-mail: ahingorani@lmcmc.com

E. Ascher, MD
Division of Vascular Surgery, Department of Surgery, Lutheran Medical Center, Brooklyn, NY, USA

V. Gahtan and M.J. Costanza (eds.), *Essentials of Vascular Surgery for the General Surgeon*,
DOI 10.1007/978-1-4939-1326-8_10, © Springer Science+Business Media New York 2015

patients (38 %) with combined SVT and DVT and seven of the patients (44 %) with SVT alone were found to be hypercoagulable. Four patients had decreased levels of AT only, and four patients had APC resistance. One patient had decreased protein C and protein S, and three patients had deficiencies of AT, protein C, and protein S. The most prevalent hypercoagulable condition was AT deficiency. In a subsequent separate data set of patients, anticardiolipin antibodies were detected in 33 % of patients with recurrent SVT [5]. These observations suggest that patients with SVT have a higher prevalence of underlying hypercoagulability disorders.

Pathology

The cellular mechanics involved in DVT formation and resolution have been thoroughly investigated. An extensive amount of literature has focused on the contribution of cytokines and chemokines and the importance of the leukocyte/vessel wall interaction in the pathophysiology of DVT. Whether these processes also apply to SVT is a matter of speculation. Although it is intuitively appealing to believe that the underlying pathology of SVT is analogous to DVT, this hypothesis remains unsupported.

SVT: Other Topics

SVT can occur in any superficial vein due to a variety of inciting causes. The most common clinical scenario for SVT involves the great saphenous vein (GSV) in a patient with underlying varicose veins. Several other locations and etiologies for SVT are briefly discussed in this section.

Trauma

An intravenous (IV) cannula represents the most common source of venous trauma leading to SVT. Erythema, warmth, and tenderness along the course of the cannulated vein usually indicate the presence of SVT. Treatment starts with removal of the cannula and warm compresses. After the acute inflammation resolves, a lump may persist for months afterward.

Suppurative

Suppurative SVT (SSVT) is a rare form of SVT characterized by pus and intense pain at an IV site that is often associated with systemic signs of infection such as fever and leukocytosis [6]. Although both SVT and SSVT can be triggered by an IV cannula, the more common clinical scenario for SSVT is a patient with a history of IV drug abuse. In contrast to uncomplicated SVT which typically resolves on its own, SSVT can be fatal if it deteriorates into septicemia. Treatment for SSVT begins with prompt removal of the foreign body and IV antibiotics. Excision of the vein is rarely needed to clear infection; however, it should be considered in a patient with purulence at an IV site who fails to improve with noninterventional management.

Migratory

In 1845, Jadioux first described migratory thrombophlebitis as repeated superficial venous thrombosis at varying sites, most commonly in the lower extremity [7]. Migratory thrombophlebitis has been associated with underlying malignancy and may be present several years before the cancer is diagnosed. Consequently, the diagnosis of migratory thrombophlebitis often warrants an evaluation for occult malignancy.

Mondor's Disease

Mondor's disease is defined as thrombophlebitis of the thoracoepigastric vein of the breast and chest wall. This diagnosis has been associated with breast carcinoma or a hypercoagulable state; however, cases with no identifiable cause have also been reported [8]. Recently, the term "penile Mondor's disease" has been used to describe SVT of the dorsal vein of the penis [9]. Treatment consists of noninterventional measures including warm compresses and nonsteroidal anti-inflammatory drugs.

Small Saphenous Vein SVT

Although it does not receive as much attention as SVT of the GSV, small saphenous vein (SSV) SVT can have significant clinical consequences. SSV SVT can extend proximally and become a popliteal DVT. In a group of 56 patients with SSV SVT, 16 % suffered from PE or DVT [2]. Therefore, patients with SSV SVT should be managed using a similar approach to those diagnosed with GSV SVT. Treatment includes a thorough duplex ultrasound examination, vigilant follow-up, and anticoagulation or ligation of the SSV if the thrombus approaches the popliteal vein.

SVT with Varicose Vein Disease

Patients with SVT and varicose veins may have a different underlying pathophysiology compared to those without varicose veins. In several studies, only 3–20 % of SVT patients with varicose veins developed a DVT, compared to 44–60 % of patients without varicose veins [10, 11, 12]. In contrast, a more recent study showed no difference in the incidence of DVT or PE among 186 SVT patients with and without varicose veins [2]. Therefore, it remains unclear if SVT patients with and without associated varicose veins should be classified as belonging to different patient subsets.

SVT involving varicose veins may remain localized to a cluster of tributary varicosities or extend into the GSV [2]. SVT of varicose vein tributaries can occur without antecedent trauma and is frequently found in varicosities surrounding venous stasis ulcers. The diagnosis should be confirmed by duplex ultrasound scan as the clinical exam often underestimates the true extent of SVT. Treatment consists of noninterventional therapy including warm compresses and nonsteroidal anti-inflammatory drugs.

Upper Extremity SVT

Upper extremity SVT often results from intravenous cannulation and infusion of caustic substances that damage the endothelium. In contrast to lower extremity SVT, upper extremity SVT does not have a tendency to progresses into a DVT and rarely becomes the source of a PE [13]. Initial treatment of symptomatic upper extremity SVT associated with a catheter requires catheter removal followed by warm compresses and nonsteroidal anti-inflammatory medications.

Peripheral inserted central catheters (PICCs) have become nearly ubiquitous in modern medical practice. Their accessibility, cost-effectiveness, and perceived safety profile have led to widespread use of PICCs across all specialties in both the inpatient and outpatient setting. The proliferation of PICCs has focused attention on their potential complications, the most common of which are infection and venous thrombosis. The exact incidence and relative risk of PICC-associated thrombotic episodes remains unclear because some studies have reported on only symptomatic patients, while others have included asymptomatic patients diagnosed by ultrasound screening. Periard et al. prospectively compared PICCs to peripheral IV cannulas in patients requiring IV therapy for at least 5 days [14]. Ultrasound screening of all 60 patients demonstrated a high but similar rate of upper extremity SVT in both the PICC and peripheral IV groups (29 % vs. 34 %). In a review of symptomatic upper extremity venous thrombosis, Liem et al. found a much lower incidence of PICC-associated SVT: 1.9 % for basilic PICCs and 7.2 % for cephalic PICCs [15]. Despite the low incidence, the large number of PICCs placed per year makes PICC-associated venous thrombosis an important and commonly encountered clinical problem. According to Liem et al. PICCs were associated with 20 % of all upper extremity SVTs diagnosed by their vascular lab in 1 year. PICC-associated DVT had an even greater clinical impact accounting for over 35 % of all upper extremity DVTs diagnosed in 1 year.

PICC-associated SVT usually results from catheter-induced trauma to the venous endothelium. Any patient with a current or recent PICC who has upper extremity edema, pain, or a palpable cord warrants a complete ultrasound exam to evaluate for thrombus and determine its extent. The presence of the catheter often impairs sonographic evaluation of the veins and may obscure direct visualization of the thrombus. Obtaining multiple views, changing the angle of insonation, and using a combination of gray imaging, spectral wave analysis and color flow imaging can usually overcome these technical challenges. As the previously cited studies show, clinical symptoms occur in only a minority of patients with PICC-associated SVT. Screening ultrasonography has not been widely adopted since the clinical significance of detecting SVT in an asymptomatic patient remains unclear.

If a symptomatic PICC-associated SVT is diagnosed, we do not suggest removing the catheter as long as the PICC is functional and is not associated with systemic or local infection. If the patient needs to continue receiving IV therapy, we recommend using the PICC rather than removing it and placing a new PICC at a different location. The rationale for this recommendation comes in part from the findings of Jones et al. in their study of catheter-associated upper extremity DVT [16]. They found an 86 % incidence of new site DVT when a catheter was removed and immediately replaced in the other extremity. Although their study focused on upper extremity DVT, we believe that underlying thrombotic risk factors may also apply to catheter-associated SVT. If a PICC is maintained in a patient with an SVT, we usually repeat the duplex ultrasound scan in 3–7 days to assess for progression to DVT.

Diagnosis

In the past, clinically apparent SVT was thought to follow a benign, self-limited course that required no further evaluation unless symptoms failed to resolve quickly on their own [17]. This guideline now appears to be antiquated and flawed as it ignores evidence showing that DVT associated with SVT may be clinically silent [2]. Failure to completely evaluate SVT could therefore overlook a coexisting DVT which requires active treatment.

Since it first description in 1982, duplex ultrasonography has become the diagnostic test of choice for venous thrombosis in the upper and lower extremities [18]. Duplex ultrasound is a readily available and sensitive method of evaluating the deep and superficial venous systems. Compared to the standard clinical exam, ultrasound scanning provides a more complete assessment of the location, extent, and severity of thrombosis. Duplex ultrasound also has the advantage of being inexpensive and noninvasive making it ideal for follow-up imaging surveillance. The success and reliability of duplex ultrasound has nearly eliminated the need for contrast venography as a diagnostic exam. Not only is venography less accurate, it is also an invasive test that can trigger phlebitis.

Duplex imaging detects a concomitant DVT in 5–40 % of patients with SVT [2, 19, 20, 21]. Interestingly, up to 25 % of these DVTs are not contiguous with the SVT and may even be in the contralateral extremity [2]. This finding suggests that some patients have an underlying hypercoagulability state contributing to the etiology of thrombosis.

Treatment

The location of the SVT determines the most appropriate treatment. Treatment strategies differ depending on whether the SVT involves the venous tributaries of the GSV, the GSV in the distal thigh, or the GSV in the proximal thigh. Likewise, treatment for SVT in the distal calf SSV differs from treatment for SVT approaching the confluence with the popliteal vein. Conservative treatment for SVT localized in tributaries of the GSV and the GSV in the distal thigh consists of ambulation, warm soaks or compresses, and nonsteroidal anti-inflammatory drugs [1, 22, 23]. Surgical excision of the GSV has a more limited role and is usually reserved for patients with recurrent thrombophlebitis despite of adequate medical management.

Symptomatic treatment for distal SVT does not address the possibility of clot progression or the development of a DVT. Chengelis et al. studied the progression of isolated lower extremity SVT to DVT with follow-up duplex ultrasonography on 263 patients [12]. Duplex scans performed on an average of 6.3 days after the initial diagnosis showed that 30 patients (11 %) had progression of their SVT to deep venous involvement. The most common site of deep vein involvement was the progression of disease from the GSV in the thigh into the common femoral vein (21 patients), with 18 of these extensions noted to be nonocclusive and 12 having a free-floating component. In three patients above-knee saphenous vein thrombi extended through thigh vein perforators to occlude the femoral vein. Below-knee small saphenous vein SVT extended into the popliteal vein in three patients, and three additional patients had SVT extend through calf perforators into the tibioperoneal veins. None of the 30 patients with SVT progression to DVT were being treated with anticoagulants at the time of diagnosis. The results of this study support a protocol for obtaining follow-up imaging for patients diagnosed with lower extremity SVT. We recommend a repeat duplex ultrasound after 48 h to assess for thrombus progression and DVT [21].

SVT within 1 cm of the saphenofemoral junction has a well-recognized potential for extending into the deep venous system and embolizing [24–28]. High ligation of the GSV with or without saphenous vein stripping may prevent this complication by physically interrupting the primary connection between the superficial and deep venous system. Lohr et al. studied the outcome of 43 patients treated with ligation of the saphenofemoral junction with or without local common femoral vein thrombectomy and stripping of the GSV [3]. Approximately 86 % of the patients were discharged within 3 days; two patients had postoperative contralateral DVT, one of whom had a PE. Four patients developed wound cellulitis requiring antibiotics, and one patient had wound hematoma treated nonoperatively. Although this study reported satisfactory results, it also raised several unanswered questions regarding GSV ligation. Whether or not to strip the GSV in addition to high ligation remains unclear. Proponents of stripping the GSV argue that patients experience less pain after the SVT is removed. Despite GSV ligation and removal, however, some patients still developed noncontiguous, post-ligation DVT and PE. This observation suggests that ligation alone may not provide adequate therapy for SVT encroaching on the saphenofemoral junction. Systemic anticoagulation could be necessary to counteract the thrombotic risk factors present in at least a subset of patients with lower extremity SVT.

Husni and Williams conducted a prospective nonrandomized study on using systemic anticoagulation alone to manage saphenofemoral junction thrombophlebitis (SFJT) [12]. Over a 2-year period, 20 consecutive patients with SFJT were hospitalized and systemically anticoagulated with heparin. Duplex ultrasonography before admission and 2–4 days later was performed to establish the diagnosis, evaluate the deep venous system, and assess resolution of SFJT. Patients with SFJT which resolved were maintained on warfarin for 6 weeks, while patients with SFJT and DVT received warfarin for 6 months. The efficacy of anticoagulation therapy was evaluated by measuring SFJT resolution, recurrent episodes of SFJT, and occurrence of PE.

In this study, the incidence of concurrent DVT was 40 % (8 of 20 patients). Of these eight patients, DVT was contiguous with SFJT in five patients and noncontiguous in three patients. Repeat imaging studies showed that only one patient failed to have complete or partial resolution of SFJT. At a maximum follow-up of 14 months, there were no episodes of PE, thrombotic recurrences, or anticoagulation complications. Despite including a small number of patients, this study suggests that anticoagulation alone is a feasible strategy for SFJT. The surprisingly high incidence of DVT associated with SFJT underscores the value of ultrasonography to evaluate the deep venous system in patients with lower extremity SVT [29]. Studies that focus on preventing SVT progression in the short term and the effect of anticoagulation on local recurrence of SVT have not been conducted yet.

Proponents of surgical intervention for SFJT have suggested that high ligation of the GSV is more cost effective than 6 months of systemic anticoagulation [3]. This argument fails to consider several areas of potential cost saving. The duration of anticoagulation for patients with SVT remains an unresolved issue and could be shortened. For the last 10 years, we have treated patients with SFJT with 6 weeks of anticoagulation and had no episodes of PE or complications of anticoagulation. Significant cost savings can also be realized if low-molecular-weight heparin or the newer oral agents are used in an outpatient setting instead of unfractionated intravenous heparin. The fact that surgical ligation does not address the hypercoagulable state of these patients and may create injury to the endothelium at the saphenofemoral junction makes it a less appealing treatment option compared to anticoagulation.

Belcaro et al. attempted to clarify the issue of anticoagulation versus surgical therapy in a prospective study consisting of 444 patients with SVT randomized to six different treatment plans (compression only, early surgery [with and without stripping], low-dose subcutaneous heparin, low-molecular-weight heparin (LMWH), and oral anticoagulant treatment) [30]. Patients presenting with SVT and large varicose veins without any systemic disorder were included in this study. Inclusion criteria were venous incompetence (by duplex); a tender, indurated cord along a superficial vein; and redness and heat in the affected area. Exclusion criteria were obesity, cardiovascular or neoplastic diseases, nonambulatory status, bone/joint disease, problems requiring immobilization, age >70 years, and patients with SVT without varicose veins. Color duplex ultrasound scans at 3 and 6 months were used to detect concomitant DVT and to evaluate the extension or reduction of SVT.

After 3 and 6 months, the incidence of SVT extension was significantly higher in the elastic compression and saphenous ligation groups and lowest in the group of patients treated with vein stripping. There was no significant difference in the incidence of DVT among the treatment groups. While treatment with compression stockings costs the least, it had the highest overall social cost which factored in lost workdays and inactivity. Anticoagulation with LMWH was the most expensive form of therapy.

Although this study provides some insight into the different treatment options for SVT, it has limited value as a practical guide to managing SVT. The details of the treatment protocols were not specifically identified, and the exclusion criteria applied in the study would eliminate many patients diagnosed with SVT in a real-world clinical practice. The study also suffered from a nonuniform patient population by including any patient with an SVT regardless of its anatomic location.

Lower extremity SVT that approaches the femoral or popliteal vein threatens to become a DVT or a potentially fatal venous thromboembolism. The ideal treatment for this condition should weigh the thromboembolic risk of an SVT versus its tendency to resolve without progression. Sullivan et al. attempted to perform a meta-analysis of surgical versus medical therapy for isolated above-knee SVT [31]. Although a paucity of comparable data precluded a formal meta-analysis, their review made several useful observations. Medical management with anticoagulants was found to be slightly superior for minimizing complications and preventing subsequent DVT and PE, while surgical ligation with stripping provided superior pain relief. Based on the available, albeit scarce, evidence, we recommend systemic anticoagulation for patients with SVT involving the proximal GSV or SSV. Future studies focusing on the natural history and pathophysiology of SVT will help evaluate and refine the treatment options.

Conclusion

Superficial venous thrombophlebitis (SVT) is a common and important clinical problem that surgeons encounter on a regular basis. Contrary to popular belief, SVT is not a universally benign condition that always resolves on its own. In addition to causing localized discomfort, SVT poses significant risks including thrombus progression, embolization, and recurrence. Patients with SVT may require treatment with conservative measures, systemic anticoagulation, or surgical intervention depending on the clinical scenario. This chapter has provided an up-to-date review of SVT so that surgeons can make rational, informed decisions regarding its diagnosis and treatment.

References

1. DeWeese MS. Nonoperative treatment of acute superficial thrombophlebitis and deep femoral venous thrombosis. In: Ernst CB, Stanley JC, editors. Current therapy in vascular surgery. Philadelphia: BC Decker Inc; 1991. p. 952–60.
2. Lutter KS, Kerr TM, Roedersheimer LR, Lohr JM, Sampson MG, Cranley JJ. Superficial thrombophlebitis diagnosed by duplex scanning. Surgery. 1991;110:42–6.
3. Lohr JM, McDevitt DT, Lutter KS, Roedersheimer LR, Sampson MG. Operative management of greater saphenous thrombophlebitis involving the saphenofemoral junction. Am J Surg. 1992;164: 269–75.
4. Hanson JN, Ascher E, DePippo P, Lorensen E, Scheinman M, Yorkovich W, Hingorani A. Saphenous vein thrombophlebitis (SVT): a deceptively benign disease. J Vasc Surg. 1998;27:677–80.
5. de Godoy JM, Batigalia F, Braile DM. Superficial thrombophlebitis and anticardiolipin antibodies–report of association. Angiology. 2001;52:127–9.
6. Hammond JS, Varas R, Ward CG. Suppurative thrombophlebitis: a new look at a continuing problem. South Med J. 1988;81:969–71.
7. Glasser ST. Principles of peripheral vascular surgery. Philadelphia: FA Davis; 1959.

8. Mayor M, Buron I, de Mora JC, Lazaro TE, Hernandez-Cano N, Rubio FA, Casado M. Mondor's disease. Int J Dermatol. 2000;39: 922–5.
9. Sasso F, Gulino G, Basar M, Carbone A, Torricelli P, Alcini E. Penile Mondors' disease: an underestimated pathology. Br J Urol. 1996;77:729–32.
10. Bergqvist D, Jaroszewski H. Deep vein thrombosis in patients with superficial thrombophlebitis of the leg. Br Med J. 1986;292:658–9.
11. Prountjos P, Bastounis E, Hadjinikolaou L, Felekuras E, Balas P. Superficial venous thrombosis of the lower extremities co-existing with deep venous thrombosis. A phlebographic study on 57 cases. Int Angiol. 1991;10:263–5.
12. Chengelis DL, Bendick PJ, Glover JL, Brown OW, Ranval TJ. Progression of superficial venous thrombosis to deep vein thrombosis. J Vasc Surg. 1996;24:745–9.
13. Sassu GP, Chisholm CD, Howell JM, Huang E. A rare etiology for pulmonary embolism: basilic vein thrombosis. J Emerg Med. 1990;8:45–9.
14. Periard D, Monney P, Waeber G, Zurkinden C, Mazzolai L, Hayoz D, Doenz F, Zanetti G, Wasserfallen J-B, Denys A. Randomized controlled trial of peripherally inserted central catheters vs. peripheral catheters for middle duration in-hospital intravenous therapy. J Thromb Haemost. 2008;6:1281–8.
15. Liem TK, Yanit KE, Moseley SE, Landry GJ, DeLoughery TG, Rumwell CA, Mitchell EL, Moneta GL. Peripherally inserted central catheter usage patterns and associated symptomatic upper extremity venous thrombosis. J Vasc Surg. 2012;55:761–7.
16. Jones MA, Lee DY, Segall JA, Landry GJ, Liem TK, Mitchell EL, Moneta GL. Characterizing resolution of catheter-associated upper extremity deep venous thrombosis. J Vasc Surg. 2010;51:108–13.
17. Section XIII. Medical and surgical complication in pregnancy. In: Williams Obstetrics. Ed. McGraw-Hill F. Cunningham. 22nd ed. Sanford: Appleton & Lange. p. 1084.
18. Talbot SR. Use of real-time imaging in identifying deep venous obstruction: a preliminary report. Bruit. 1982;6:41–2.
19. Skillman JJ, Kent KC, Porter DH, Kim D. Simultaneous occurrence of superficial and deep thrombophlebitis in the lower extremity. J Vasc Surg. 1990;11:818–23.
20. Jorgensen JO, Hanel KC, Morgan AM, Hunt JM. The incidence of deep venous thrombosis in patients with superficial thrombophlebitis of the lower limbs. J Vasc Surg. 1993;18:70–3.
21. Blumenberg RM, Barton E, Gelfand ML, Skudder P, Brennan J. Occult deep venous thrombosis complicating superficial thrombophlebitis. J Vasc Surg. 1998;27:338–43.
22. Ludbrook J, Jamieson GG. Disorders of veins. In: Sabiston Jr DC, editor. Textbook of surgery. 12th ed. Philadelphia: WB Saunders; 1981. p. 1808–27.
23. Hobbs JT. Superficial thrombophlebitis. In: Hobbs JT, editor. The treatment of venous disorders. Philadelphia: JB Lippincott; 1977. p. 414–27.
24. Husni EA, Williams WA. Superficial thrombophlebitis of lower limbs. Surgery. 1982;91:70–3.
25. Lofgren EP, Lofgren KA. The surgical treatment of superficial thrombophlebitis. Surgery. 1981;90:49–54.
26. Gjores JE. Surgical therapy of ascending thrombophlebitis in the saphenous system. Angiology. 1962;13:241–3.
27. Plate G, Eklof B, Jensen R, Ohlin P. Deep venous thrombosis, pulmonary embolism and acute surgery in thrombophlebitis of the log saphenous vein. Acta Chir Scand. 1985;151:241–4.
28. Decousus H, Quéré I, Presles E, Becker F, Barrellier MT, Chanut M, Gillet JL, Guenneguez H, Leandri C, Mismetti P, Pichot O, Leizorovicz A, POST (Prospective Observational Superficial Thrombophlebitis) Study Group. Superficial venous thrombosis and venous thromboembolism: a large, prospective epidemiologic study. Ann Intern Med. 2010;152(4):1–48.
29. Ascer E, Lorensen E, Pollina RM, Gennaro M. Preliminary results of a nonoperative approach to saphenofemoral junction thrombophlebitis. J Vasc Surg. 1995;22:616–21.
30. Belcaro G, Nicolaides AN, Errichi BM, Cesarone MR, De Sanctis MT, Incandela L, Venniker R. Superficial thrombophlebitis of the legs: a randomized, controlled, follow-up study. Angiology. 1999; 50:523–9.
31. Sullivan V, Denk PM, Sonnad SS, Eagleton MJ, Wakefield TW. Ligation versus anticoagulation: treatment of above-knee superficial thrombophlebitis not involving the deep venous system. J Am Coll Surg. 2001;193:556–62.

Chronic Venous Insufficiency

11

Kathleen J. Ozsvath

Introduction

Venous disease is a global health problem which affects hundreds of millions of people and accounts for over five billion dollars of annual healthcare spending [1]. In the United States, one third of the adult population has chronic venous insufficiency (CVI), and 1 % of adults have a venous ulcer, the most severe manifestation of CVI. The annual risk of developing CVI is 2.6 % in women and 1.9 % in men [2]. Deep venous thrombosis (DVT), another form of venous disease, occurs in 250,000 people per year in the United States alone [3]. Pulmonary embolism (PE) and DVT cause over a half a million hospitalizations and 200,000 deaths per year [4]. Approximately 90 % of patients with an iliofemoral DVT go on to have persistent lower extremity swelling and pain which is collectively known as post-thrombotic syndrome (PTS) [5–7].

Chronic venous disease has an economic and social impact which extends beyond its clinical symptoms. CVI and PTS cause disability resulting in the loss of more than two million workdays per year. Patients with severe symptoms of venous disease become socially isolated and often develop psychosocial adjustment problems. Effective management strategies for venous disease can improve the symptoms and restore productivity and quality of life to patients affected by this chronic and often demoralizing disease. Surgeons who encounter patients with chronic edema and skin breakdown should be able to recognize venous disease and initiate an appropriate treatment plan. This chapter will outline the pathophysiology, clinical diagnosis, and management options for patients with CVI and PTS.

K.J. Ozsvath, MD (✉)
The Vascular Group, Albany Medical College,
Albany Medical Center Hospital, 43 New Scotland Avenue
MC157, Albany, NY 12208, USA
e-mail: ozsvathk@albanyvascular.com

Venous Anatomy and Physiology

The earliest description of a patient with symptoms of venous disease dates back to 1550 B.C. [8]. Since the disease only occurs in humans, CVI may have its origin in our upright posture and ambulation. Lower extremity veins are conduits allowing blood to return from the periphery to the central circulation. Normally, almost all of the blood volume returns through the deep venous system with minimal contribution from the superficial system. Deep veins form a complex system within the muscular compartments of the leg, while superficial veins course through the subcutaneous tissue above the muscle fascia. The muscles of the leg act as a mechanical pump that squeeze the veins, propelling blood toward the central venous circulation. All veins contain bicuspid, one-way valves which act as checkpoints designed to counter gravity and keep blood from pooling in the extremities.

The deep veins of the calf join together behind the knee to form the popliteal vein. In the thigh, the popliteal vein continues as the femoral vein which becomes confluent with the profunda femoral vein to form the common femoral vein in the proximal thigh. The leg veins and pelvic veins then drain into the iliac veins which in turn drain into the inferior vena cava (IVC). The IVC usually lies to the right of the vertebral column, while the aorta is on the left. This anatomic configuration can cause external compression of the left common iliac vein between the overlying right common iliac artery and the vertebral column. In some patients, this obstructive condition can lead to May-Thurner syndrome which is characterized by left iliac vein thrombosis and leg swelling. A similar anatomic problem occurs in patients with subclavian-axillary vein thrombosis, which is also known as effort thrombosis or Paget-Schroetter syndrome. In this condition, the thoracic outlet compresses the subclavian vein leading to vein thrombosis and arm swelling.

The small and great saphenous veins make up the superficial venous system of the lower extremity. The small saphenous vein begins posterior to the lateral malleolus and courses

V. Gahtan and M.J. Costanza (eds.), *Essentials of Vascular Surgery for the General Surgeon*,
DOI 10.1007/978-1-4939-1326-8_11, © Springer Science+Business Media New York 2015

cephalad in the posterior calf before joining the popliteal vein at the saphenopopliteal junction behind the knee. The great saphenous vein originates anterior to the medial malleolus and travels up the medial calf and thigh before joining the common femoral vein at the saphenofemoral junction near the inguinal crease. Perforating veins form connections between the deep and superficial venous systems throughout the leg and thigh. Venous tributaries in the subcutaneous tissue of the lower extremity originate from the superficial veins. If these superficial venous tributaries become engorged and protrude visibly under the skin, they are known as varicose veins.

Chronic Venous Insufficiency

Venous disease encompasses a wide spectrum of clinical conditions including acute thrombosis, varicose veins, and chronic venous insufficiency. Chapters 9 and 12 focus on venous thrombosis and varicose veins, respectively. This chapter will address CVI which causes circulatory dysfunction on the macro- and microvascular level leading to a variety of clinical manifestations. Risk factors for CVI include obesity, ambulatory jobs, history of pregnancy, female gender, and previous thrombophlebitis [9].

Pathophysiology

In the most general terms, blood travels in arteries from the heart to the periphery and returns from the periphery to the heart via veins. Unlike arteries, veins do not have a centrally located pump to drive blood flow. Veins in the lower extremities rely on several mechanisms to overcome gravity and return venous blood flow to the central circulation. During ambulation, the muscles of the foot, calf, and thigh externally compress the deep veins which propel blood flow cephalad. Bicuspid valves located throughout all veins act as checkpoints to prevent the blood column from refluxing backward down the leg. This system of segmental venous compression and check valves can overcome gravity and move blood from the distal lower extremity to the central circulation even in the upright position.

Normally, venous pressure in the lower extremity decreases after ambulation. Muscle contraction increases pressure within the fascial compartments which forces blood up the deep venous system. Bicuspid valves in the deep veins prevent blood from traveling retrograde, while valves in perforating veins prevent reflux through to the superficial venous system. The combination of muscle pumps and competent valves maintains low venous pressure and keeps venous blood flowing from distal to cephalad and superficial to deep. With prolonged standing, the veins slowly refill and become distended which opens the venous valves and increases venous pressure. Contraction of the muscle pump then empties the veins and reduces the pressure.

Patients with CVI have persistently high venous pressure as the lower extremity venous system fails to conduct blood from the periphery back to the central circulation. The underlying pathophysiology can involve venous obstruction, valvular incompetence, muscle pump weakness, or a combination of problems. Venous thrombosis is one of the most prominent conditions causing venous obstruction. An acute DVT triggers a cellular and humoral response in the affected vein. Although the influx of inflammatory cells, chemokines, and enzymes helps resolve the acute thrombus, it can also cause permanent changes to the vein wall and venous endothelium. In many patients, the sequelae of an acute DVT cause the vein to become chronically occluded or severely stenotic. This obstructive process known as post-thrombotic syndrome will be discussed in more detail in the next section. Extrinsic compression can also cause venous obstruction. In May-Thurner syndrome, the left common iliac vein is compressed between the overlying right common iliac artery and the underlying vertebral column.

Valvular incompetence can affect the deep, superficial, and perforating venous systems. Deep venous valves usually fail because of damage inflicted by previous acute thrombotic events. Dysfunctional deep valves allow venous blood that has just been ejected by the muscular pump to reflux retrograde down the leg, quickly refilling and repressurizing the distal venous segments. Valvular incompetence in the superficial veins most commonly occurs because of intrinsic weakness in the vein wall due to an unclear etiology. Less rigid or "floppy" vein walls prevent the cusps of the venous valves from coapting leading to an incompetent valve which allows retrograde venous flow. Venous reflux down the great and small saphenous veins can transmit elevated venous pressure into the superficial venous tributaries causing dilation and varicose vein formation. Superficial valve dysfunction can also result from valvular damage caused by phlebitis or excessive vein dilation due to hormonal effects or high pressure. Valvular incompetence in the perforator veins allows blood to reflux from the deep to the superficial veins. In severe cases, perforator incompetence can cause secondary failure of the superficial venous valves. Clinical manifestations can include a localized cluster of dilated superficial veins which ascends up the leg.

Failure of the muscle pump eliminates the driving force that empties veins and maintains a low venous pressure in the distal lower extremity. Instead of decreasing after ambulation, venous pressure increases to levels nearly as high as the pressure reached after prolonged standing. An ineffective muscle pump can be the primary etiology of CVI in some cases such as neuromuscular disorders and muscle wasting. More commonly, failure of the muscle pump occurs in the setting of severe venous reflux or obstruction.

Regardless of its underlying etiology, CVI stagnates lower extremity blood flow and increases venous pressure. The deep venous system transmits these hemodynamic changes though the perforating and superficial veins and ultimately into the microcirculation of the subcutaneous tissue and skin. The ensuing microangiopathy has several consequences including fluid accumulation from increased capillary permeability and lymphatic damage, hyperpigmentation from extravasated red blood cells, and nerve dysfunction causing altered vasoregulation. Theories to explain the pathophysiology of CVI have incorporated histologic findings such as fibrin cuff formation in the pericapillary space and trapping of growth factors and white blood cells which could inhibit healing and prolong inflammation [10].

Table 11.1 CEAP classification of venous disease

C0 – No signs of visible or palpable venous disease
C1 – Telangectasias or reticular veins
C2 – Varicose veins
C3 – Edema
C4a – Pigmentation, eczema
C4b – Lipodermatosclerosis or atrophie blanche
C5 – Healed venous ulcer
C6 – Open venous ulcer
S – Symptomatic, ache, pain, tightness, skin irritation, heaviness, muscle cramps
A – Asymptomatic

Adapted from Vasquez et al. [11]

Clinical Presentation

Patients with CVI usually have lower extremity edema, pain, dilated veins, and skin changes. Edema occurs as fluid accumulates in the dependent lower leg usually beginning near the medial malleolus or gaiter region. Pain described as leg heaviness and aching may result from increased pressure and volume within the compartments and subcutaneous tissue. Superficial venous tributaries develop into varicose veins when they enlarge and become tortuous. Skin changes include hyperpigmentation from hemosiderin deposits, eczematous dermatitis, and lipodermatosclerosis which denotes fibrosis of the skin and subcutaneous tissue.

Compromised skin and poor wound healing predispose patients with CVI to recurrent episodes of cellulitis and skin ulceration. Venous ulcers are the most severe manifestation of CVI and seem to occur more frequently in elderly men with long-standing CVI. Although venous ulcers can be painful and carry a risk of infection, the impact of venous ulcers extends beyond their localized symptoms. Patients with venous ulcers often feel ashamed of their condition which leads them to withdraw from family and friends. Work hours are lost in patients who would otherwise be productive in the labor force. Wound care for venous ulcers requires a significant investment of time, resources, and healthcare spending to secure the necessary supplies and nursing care.

An international consensus conference developed the Clinical-Etiology-Anatomy-Pathophysiology (CEAP) classification to standardize the classification of patients with CVI [11] (Table 11.1). The clinical variable has seven categories and is further categorized by the presence or absence of symptoms. Etiology depends on whether the underlying cause of CVI was congenital, primary, or secondary. Congenital causes of CVI such as Klippel Trenauay and Parkes Webber syndrome are present at birth but may not manifest until later in life. Primary causes of CVI have an unclear origin, while secondary causes are linked to an acquired condition such as a previous DVT. The involvement of the deep, superficial, or perforating veins determines the anatomic classification. Pathophysiology, the final variable, describes the underlying mechanism of CVI as obstruction, valvular incompetence, or a combination of both conditions. The venous severity score (VSS) provides a more detailed assessment of CVI by assigning a numeric score to three components: clinical severity, anatomic segment, and disability [12]. VSS can complement the CEAP classification and provide a more accurate tool for assessing a patient's response to treatment.

Diagnosis

The diagnosis of CVI derives from the history and physical exam along with adjunctive information from noninvasive testing. The history should characterize the presence, duration, and severity of symptoms including edema, pain, fluid drainage, and skin breakdown. Patients should be questioned about previous thrombotic episodes and evaluated for the presence of thrombotic risk factors such as family history, personal traits, and medication use. Documenting previous treatments for CVI that have succeeded or failed can help in the making of decisions regarding future therapy.

Physical examination begins with visual inspection and palpation of the lower extremity skin. Dilated, tortuous varicose veins may be obvious at first glance, or they have a more subtle appearance as localized, palpable skin bulges. The upright posture will maximally distend the veins making them easier to detect and characterize. Cutaneous changes associated with CVI range from hyperpigmentation to fibrosis to frank ulceration (Fig. 11.1). Sites of healed venous ulceration referred to as "atrophie blanche" appear as a localized area of white scarring with an absence of capillaries. Edema usually gives way to palpation and is described

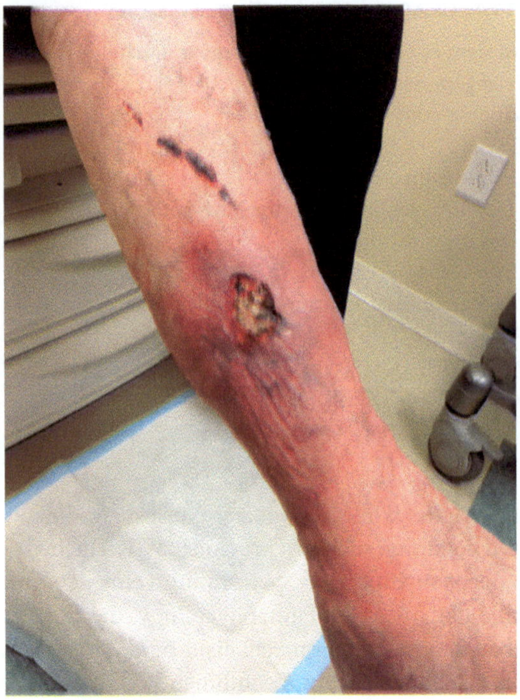

Fig. 11.1 Chronic venous ulcer of the lower extremity

as "pitting edema." Patients with long-standing CVI and underlying fibrosis often develop brawny edema that does not indent with palpation.

Simple bedside maneuvers can help detect the presence and nature of venous reflux. In the Trendelenburg or tourniquet test, the veins of leg are first emptied by elevating the lower extremity with the patient supine [13]. The patient then assumes an upright position with a tourniquet or manual pressure applied to various levels. In the presence of superficial venous reflux, the varicose veins distal to the tourniquet will remain collapsed until the tourniquet is released. With deep venous reflux, varicose veins immediately reappear upon standing despite the presence of a tourniquet or manual compression. More detailed information regarding venous reflux can now be gained from duplex ultrasound examination making bedside maneuvers a less important component of the physical exam.

Before making a definitive diagnosis of CVI, other conditions should be considered in the differential. The most serious cause of limb edema is acute DVT which can be detected with a duplex ultrasound exam. Systemic causes of lower extremity edema include congestive heart failure, renal insufficiency, liver disease, endocrine disorders, and medication side effects. Localized conditions such as a ruptured popliteal cyst, hematoma, exertional compartment syndrome, gastrocnemius muscle tear, and lymphedema can also cause lower extremity edema. A carefully performed history and physical exam and appropriately selected noninvasive tests can usually clarify the diagnosis.

Noninvasive Testing

Lower extremity venous duplex ultrasound exams first evaluate for acute thrombosis by checking the patency of the deep and superficial venous systems. Sonographic evidence of a previous thrombotic event can take the form of intraluminal echoes, thickened vein walls, and prominent venous collaterals. These chronic venous changes would support an obstructive etiology for CVI. Diagnosing venous reflux involves measuring the duration of reversed blood flow at various locations. The standard venous reflux exam involves inflation and rapid deflation of cuffs on the lower extremity with the patient standing. The duration of reversed flow after cuff deflation corresponds to the valve closure time [14]. In the deep venous system, abnormal reflux is defined as reversed flow longer than 1.0 s, while the threshold for reflux is 0.5 s in the superficial venous system. Reflux can also be elicited using the Valsalva maneuver with the patient supine in 30° reversed Trendelenburg position. Patients with persistent stasis dermatitis or recalcitrant venous ulcers, especially those who have already been treated for axial (great and/or small saphenous vein) reflux, should be evaluated for perforator reflux. Reversed flow going from deep to superficial veins lasting longer than 0.3 s indicates reflux in the perforating venous system.

Although duplex ultrasonography can detect venous reflux, the results of the exam do not correlate with the clinical manifestations or severity of CVI [15]. Other less widely used noninvasive exams provide a more complete assessment of the venous hemodynamics in the lower extremity. Air plethysmography (APG) uses pressure cuffs and physical maneuvers to measure the variables that contribute to CVI: obstruction, reflux, and muscle pump dysfunction. During an APG exam, changes in the volume of air displaced in air-filled cuffs quantifies the venous outflow fraction, refilling index, and ejection fraction. A low venous outflow fraction correlates with obstruction; a high refilling index detects reflux; and a poor ejection fraction indicates muscle pump dysfunction [16]. APG can determine how much each variable contributes to CVI making APG a valuable tool in planning interventions and assessing the response to treatment. Photoplethysmography is a more convenient but less quantitative method for detecting venous reflux and assessing overall venous function.

Invasive Testing

Invasive testing rarely plays a role in the diagnosis of CVI. Contrast venography involves a lower extremity venipuncture and the injection of radiopaque contrast. Descending venography using femoral vein access usually employs a tilt table to evaluate for reflux in the femoral and great saphenous veins. Ascending venography injects contrast through a vein on the dorsum of the foot to assess venous anatomy and patency. Once considered the diagnostic standard, venography has been almost completely replaced by noninvasive exams. Venograms are now most commonly performed in conjunction with venous thrombolytic procedures. In the rare patient being considered for venous reconstruction, venography may be helpful in planning surgery or clarifying inconclusive ultrasound images.

Lower extremity venous cannulation can also be used to measure ambulatory venous pressure (AVP). After placing a catheter in a vein on the dorsum of the foot, the venous pressure is measured in various positions and before and after walking and toe raises. These exercises yield several physiologic parameters including mean ambulatory pressure and refill time. Previous studies suggest that AVP and the results generated correlate with CVI severity, risk of ulceration, and response to treatment [17]. Other studies have questioned the value of AVP especially in light of noninvasive exams which have reasonable accuracy in evaluating overall venous competence [18]. The performance of this study is not commonplace.

Treatment

Treatment for CVI ranges from conservative measures to invasive procedures depending on disease severity. All patients with CVI should adopt behavioral modifications designed to minimize lower extremity edema including leg elevation, avoidance of prolonged standing, and weight loss (if indicated) to reduce intra-abdominal pressure. Conservative therapy consisting of external compression usually suffices for patients with mild venous disease. Patients with more severe manifestations of CVI (CEAP class 4 to 6) may warrant referral to a vein specialist to consider interventional therapy. Even patients with CEAP class 3 and extensive edema may benefit from more aggressive treatment to reduce the risk of recurrent skin breakdown and nonhealing venous ulcers.

Noninterventional Therapy

Compression stockings exert an external force on the leg to oppose the hydrostatic pressure caused by venous hypertension. Graded compression stockings exert the most force at the ankle and decrease in pressure as they go up the leg. By keeping blood from pooling in the lower leg, compression stockings usually improve symptoms related to venous congestion such as edema, leg fatigue, and aching discomfort. In addition to symptomatic relief, compression stockings may also have physiologic benefit by improving muscle pump function and reducing venous reflux.

Prescriptions for compression stockings should specify the tension and length. Tension varies with clinical severity starting with 20–30 mmHg for patients with mild edema, 30–40 mmHg for CEAP class 4–6, and 50 mmHg for patients with recurrent venous ulcers. Knee-high stockings are the easiest to use and usually provide symptomatic relief. Although thigh-high and waist-high stockings may be indicated for patients with extensive edema, they are cumbersome and usually generate patient complaints and noncompliance. Measuring leg diameter at the ankle, calf, and thigh improves the fit of compression stockings and can be performed in the office or at the medical supply facility.

Patients should be instructed to apply the stockings as soon as they get up in the morning when the lower extremities have the least edema. The stockings should be worn throughout the day and taken off in the evening before bed. Education about stockings should emphasize the importance of daily use as patient compliance has a significant impact on treatment success. With regular use, compression stockings lose their elasticity in 6–9 months and should be replaced accordingly.

Used regularly, compression stockings can relieve the symptoms of CVI even to the point of healing venous ulcers. Unfortunately, noncompliance often prevents patients from achieving the full benefit of compression therapy. Barriers that keep patients from regularly wearing compression stockings include lack of physical strength, arthritis, inconvenience, and ulceration or drainage requiring frequent dressing changes. Pain can also be a factor in noncompliance as some patients have too much lower extremity discomfort to tolerate any external compression. Other medical devices have been designed to address lower extremity edema. Although twice daily use of external compression pumps can be effective, compression stockings are often necessary to prevent edema from returning between treatment sessions.

Dry skin associated with CVI requires moisturizers, while topical steroids may be necessary to treat stasis dermatitis. Left unchecked, compromised skin can break down to form a venous ulcer, the most severe and difficult to heal manifestation of CVI. Treatment of the ulcer begins by controlling edema and infection. Nonviable tissue must be debrided to healthy tissue with either pharmacologic agents or sharp debridement. The formation of granulation tissue and neovascularization in the wound bed allows for epithelialization and healing. Silver-impregnated dressings can help manage wounds affected by infection or bacterial overgrowth.

Although wound care promotes healing, venous ulcers do not usually resolve without compression to control edema. The Unna boot has been used for over a century to apply external compression to patients with lower extremity wounds. Medicated dressings form the first layer of an Unna boot followed by a noncompliant wrap to exert compression. Unna boots have the advantage of being able to stay in place for up to a week at a time; however, the wraps tend to loosen and exert less pressure as time passes. Four-layer wraps maintain their strength longer and have been shown to promote ulcer healing [19]. Blair et al. found that 82 % of patients using four-layer wraps had healed their ulcers within 20 weeks.

Used in conjunction with external compression, bioengineered skin substitutes can accelerate ulcer healing rates compared to control. Split-thickness skin grafting can also be considered in selected patients.

Medical therapy offers a potentially promising treatment for CVI. Coumarins, flavonoids, saponosides, and other plant extracts have venoactive properties that may improve venous tone and decrease capillary permeability. Although these medications are used in Europe, they have not been approved for use in the United States. Pentoxifyllene which is normally used in the treatment of claudication may improve venous ulcer healing rates. The magnitude of this effect appears to be small and pentoxifyllene does not currently have a well-defined role in the treatment of CVI [20]. Exercise programs also have an unclear role in the management of CVI. Directed rehabilitation programs improve muscle pump function, but they do not decrease the amount of venous reflux [21].

Interventional Therapy

Healing for venous ulcers often proves to be fleeting. Severe ulcers can become completely refractory to conservative measures, and recurrence after healing is as high as 80 % in the first year [22]. Patients who have nonhealing ulcers or persistent disability and ulcer recurrence despite maximal noninvasive therapy should be considered for surgical or endovascular interventions. Interventional techniques attempt to correct the underlying pathophysiology of CVI by minimizing venous reflux and relieving venous obstruction.

Superficial venous reflux increases lower extremity edema, promotes varicose vein formation, and exacerbates deep venous reflux. Eliminating superficial reflux improves venous hemodynamics which provides symptomatic relief and may assist in ulcer healing. In a randomized study of patients with venous ulcers, surgery to eliminate superficial venous reflux reduced the rate of ulcer recurrence by more than half compared to compression therapy alone. Interventions for superficial venous reflux including saphenous vein stripping, endovenous ablation, and sclerotherapy can be applied to all CEAP clinical classes 2–6. Chapter 12 has a full description of these techniques.

Unlike superficial venous reflux, reflux in the deep veins cannot be eliminated by surgical stripping or endovenous ablation procedures. A small number of vascular specialists perform surgery to restore deep vein valvular competency in highly selected patients with recurrent venous ulcers and severe reflux. Surgical techniques for valvular reconstruction include external valvuloplasty, brachial/axillary valve transfer, and vein transpositions [23, 24].

Reflux in the perforating veins may be the primary underlying problem in patients with persistent ulcers despite external compression and treatment of axial reflux. Interventional treatment for perforator reflux has evolved over time. Open perforator ligation caused significant morbidity as incisions were performed in diseased, ulcerated skin. Subfascial endoscopic perforator surgery (SEPS) offered the ability to ligate perforators using access from a remote site away from the diseased skin. In practice, opening the subfascial space was a limiting factor and SEPS had difficulty treating veins near the ankle due to scarring. The use of SEPS has decreased in favor of endovenous techniques for eliminating perforator reflux. Sclerotherapy attempts to obliterate the incompetent perforator by injecting sclerosant directly into the vein using ultrasound guidance [25]. Risks include skin hyperpigmentation, ulceration, DVT, and allergic reaction to the sclerosant. Other techniques use an ablation catheter inserted directly into the perforator vein to deliver radio frequency or laser energy.

Approximately 10–30 % of patients with severe CVI have occlusion or stenosis of the iliac veins causing chronic venous outflow obstruction. Palma described transposing the great saphenous vein to the contralateral femoral vein to create a cross-femoral venous bypass [26]. The other surgical option involves directly bypassing the occluded iliac veins with a prosthetic conduit. Endovascular therapy has emerged as a less invasive alternative to surgery for chronic venous obstruction. Wire recanalization, balloon angioplasty, and venous stent placement can often restore patency to chronically occluded iliofemoral veins. In a large single-center series, 55 % of patients completely healed their venous ulcer after iliac vein stenting [27]. More recently, Alhabouni et al. reported that over half of their patients presenting with venous ulcers had venous outflow obstruction. After treatment with venous stent placement, 58 % of the open ulcers healed [28]. Optimizing the long-term patency for venous stents requires close follow-up and early intervention if in-stent restenosis occurs. In the future, stents designed specifically for the venous system may improve the technical success and long-term durability of endovascular therapy for CVI.

Post-thrombotic Syndrome (PTS)

PTS refers to symptoms of CVI such as leg pain, edema, and skin ulcers that develop and persist after an acute DVT. Venous thrombosis can cause permanent obstruction and valvular damage which leads to PTS in 15–50 % of patients within 1–2 years of an acute DVT [29].

Approximately 10 % of these patients develop severe symptoms, and 170,000 new cases of venous ulceration per year in the United States are attributable to PTS [30].

Pathophysiology

The pathophysiology of PTS centers around chronic venous hypertension caused by obstruction, valvular incompetence, or a combination of both. Incomplete recanalization after an acute DVT causes venous outflow obstruction which reroutes blood flow into collateral and superficial veins leading to progressive dilation and incompetence. At the same time, acute thrombosis and the process of recanalization damage venous valves rendering them incapable of stopping retrograde venous flow. The end result of these two conditions is venous hypertension, which can cause edema from capillary leakage, tissue hypoxia, and skin breakdown in severe cases. Patients with PTS have signs and symptoms which mirror those of CVI including leg pain, heaviness, edema, varicose veins, hyperpigmentation, lipodermatosclerosis, and ulceration (healed or active).

In some patients with PTS, venous obstructive symptoms outweigh all other clinical findings. These patients usually have complete venous outflow occlusion as a result of a previous iliofemoral DVT. Walking usually triggers lower extremity pain, which is often described as a bursting sensation. Venous claudication is a term coined to describe clinical symptoms of walking discomfort brought on by venous occlusion. Interventional treatment options for severe venous claudication include endovenous balloon angioplasty and stenting or surgical bypass. Preventing complete venous occlusion may be one of the benefits of treating acute iliofemoral DVT with immediate thrombolysis. In a study by Criqui et al., 44 % of patients treated for acute iliofemoral DVT with anticoagulation alone developed venous claudication [31].

Diagnosis

PTS should be considered in patients with a history of DVT who present with the characteristic signs and symptoms discussed above. Since the pain, edema, and inflammation caused by an acute DVT takes 3–6 months to resolve, the diagnosis of PTS is usually deferred until after this time period has passed. Patients without a history of DVT should be questioned about prior orthopedic surgery, prolonged immobilization, and any episode of acute leg edema that resolved on its own. Documenting a previous DVT and the hemodynamic consequences can help confirm the diagnosis of PTS. Sonographic findings which suggest a previous DVT include thickened vein walls, hyperechoic intraluminal thrombus, and prominent venous collaterals. Venous reflux demonstrated by duplex ultrasound or air/photoplethysmography also supports the diagnosis of PTS. Note that asymptomatic patients do not have PTS even if they have objective evidence of venous reflux after a DVT.

Distinguishing between PTS and recurrent venous thrombosis can be challenging. A recurrent, acute DVT usually causes an abrupt increase in edema and pain which persists rather than improves over 24 h. Objective imaging exams often fail to provide a definitive diagnosis in this clinical scenario. Duplex ultrasound exams remain abnormal in 80 % of patients 3 months after and 50 % of patients 1 year after a proximal DVT [32]. Non-compressibility of a venous segment therefore does not necessarily represent a recurrent DVT. In some cases, comparing the results of the duplex exam to previous studies can be helpful. A previously normal segment of the vein that becomes non-compressible or an increase in the diameter of the femoral or popliteal vein during compression by 4 mm or more correlates with recurrent DVT. Unfortunately, not all patients have a previous duplex exam available, and comparing studies can be time consuming [33]. D-dimer offers limited diagnostic value in patients suspected of having a recurrent DVT. Although a normal D-dimer test excludes an acute DVT, a positive D-dimer is nondiagnostic.

Prevention

Despite studies on a wide range of patient characteristics, the only clear risk factor for PTS is a recurrent, ipsilateral DVT [34]. Efforts to minimize the impact of PTS must therefore focus on preventing DVT. Thromboprophylaxis for selected patients in high-risk settings can minimize the risk of DVT, and several evidence-based guidelines have been established [35]. To reduce the risk of recurrent DVT, patients should receive adequate intensity and full duration anticoagulation for their initial thrombotic episode. Risk factors for recurrent DVT should be identified including idiopathic or unprovoked DVT, proximal DVT, cancer, and hypercoagulable states. Patients with previous DVT who no longer take anticoagulants should receive situation-specific thromboprophylaxis.

Graduated compression stockings can improve the symptoms of PTS by reducing lower extremity edema, improving tissue microcirculation, and assisting the calf muscle pump. In unblinded studies, the use of compression stockings after an acute proximal DVT was associated with a lower incidence of PTS [36]. In contrast, a randomized study using sham stockings failed to show a significant benefit for daily use of compression stocking in preventing or treating PTS [37]. Likewise, a crossover trial of compression stockings during exercise did not show a benefit for exercise-induced symptoms and edema [38]. Although compression stockings carry little if any risk of harm, they are expensive and difficult to apply. Patient compliance can be challenging as the stockings are hot, itchy, constraining, and generally uncomfortable to wear. Selective use of compression stockings after an acute DVT seems to be a reasonable approach. Patients with residual leg pain and edema after a DVT should be prescribed compression stockings, and they should be used for as long as the patient achieves symptomatic relief.

Catheter-directed thrombolysis (CDT) has shown promise as an endovascular intervention for patients with an acute, proximal DVT [39]. By dissolving the thrombus, CDT can immediately restore venous patency while protecting the venous valves and endothelium from damage associated with recanalization. In the long term, successful CDT may preserve valvular competence while reducing the risk of chronic venous obstruction. A recent meta-analysis concluded that the symptomatic benefits of CDT appeared to translate into a lower incidence of PTS [40]. A more detailed discussion of CDT and its role in the treatment of acute DVT can be found in Chap. 9.

Treatment

PTS represents a chronic condition that lacks a single, definitive treatment. The management of patients with PTS should therefore focus on DVT prevention and symptomatic relief. As previously discussed, recurrent, ipsilateral DVT poses the highest risk of PTS, and patients with PTS have an increased thrombotic risk given their history of DVT. Adhering to the established guidelines for anticoagulation and thromboprophylaxis can help minimize the risk of recurrent DVT. Graduated compression stockings remain the first-line therapy for chronic lower extremity edema and discomfort. Although practitioners unfamiliar with venous disease often prescribe diuretics, these medications do not decrease PTS-related edema. In severe cases of PTS, skin breakdown and venous ulcers often recur despite treatment with topical dressings, external compression, and leg elevation. Although valve reconstruction and venous bypass procedures have been described, they are rarely performed and have a limited role in the management of PTS [40]. Evidence on the benefit of surgery for PTS is confined to small patient series from single, specialized centers.

PTS is a common, chronic condition that can develop months or years after an acute DVT. Since the incidence of venous thrombosis has remained constant over time, the prevalence of PTS may increase. Ongoing research efforts may help identify at-risk patients who can benefit from thrombolysis and other interventions aimed at preventing and minimizing the impact of PTS.

Conclusion

Chronic venous disease undermines a patient's quality of life by causing persistent edema, pain, and ulcers in severe cases. The economic impact of CVI and PTS encompasses the direct medical costs for prolonged treatment and the indirect costs from lost productivity at work and in the home. Despite the high prevalence and significant morbidity of chronic venous disease, many clinicians are not familiar with the underlying pathophysiology. This chapter will empower general surgeons to recognize patients with chronic venous disease and initiate appropriate management strategies.

References

1. Cullum N, Nelson E, Fletcher A, Sheldon T. Compression for venous leg ulcers (review). Cochrane Database Syst Rev. 2001;(2):CD000254.
2. Brand FN, Dannenberg AL, Abbott RD, Kannel WB. The epidemiology of varicose veins: the Framingham Study. Am J Prev Med. 1988;4:96–101.
3. Wakefield TW, Downing LJ, Strieter RM. Pathophysiology of venous thrombosis. In: Ernst CB, Stanley JC, editors. Current therapy in vascular surgery. 4th ed. St. Louis: Mosby; 2001. p. 817–20.
4. Anderson Jr FA, Wheeler HB, Goldberg RJ, et al. A population based perspective of hospital incidence and case fatality rates of deep vein thrombosis and pulmonary embolism: the Worcester DVT study. Arch Intern Med. 1991;151:933–8.
5. Stewart GJ. Neutrophils and deep venous thrombosis. Haemostasis. 1993;23 Suppl 1:27–140.
6. Akesson H, Brudin L, Dahlstrom JA, Eklof B, Ohlin P, Plate G. Venous function assessed during a 5 year period after acute ilio-femoral venous thrombosis treated with anticoagulation. Eur J Vasc Surg. 1990;4:43–8.
7. O'Donnell Jr TF, Browse NL, Burnand KG, Thomas ML. The socioeconomic effects of an iliofemoral venous thrombosis. J Surg Res. 1977;22:483–8.
8. Majno G. The healing hand: man and wound in the ancient world. Cambridge, MA: First Harvard University Press; 1975.
9. Criqui MH, Denenberg JO, Bergan J, Langer RD, Fronek A. Risk factors for chronic venous disease: the San Diego population study. J Vasc Surg. 2007;46:331–7.
10. Pappas PJ, Duran WN, Hobson RW. Pathology and cellular physiology of chronic venous insufficiency. In: Goviczki P, Yao JS, editors. Handbook of venous disorders. 2nd ed. New York: Arnold; 2001. p. 58–67.
11. Vasquez MA, Rabe E, McLafferty RB, Shortell CK, Marston WA, Gillespie D, Meissner MH, Rutherford RB, American Venous Forum Ad Hoc Outcomes Working Group. Revision of the venous clinical severity score: venous outcomes consensus statement: special communication of the American Venous Forum Ad Hoc Outcomes Working Group. J Vasc Surg. 2010;52(5):1387–96.
12. Rutherford RB, Padberg FT, Comerota AJ, Kistner RL, Meissner MH, Moneta GL. Venous severity scoring: an adjunct to venous outcome assessment. J Vasc Surg. 2001;31:1307–12.
13. Bradbury A, Ruckley CV. Clinical assessment of patients with venous disease. In: Goviczki P, Yao JS, editors. Handbook of venous disorders. 2nd ed. New York: Arnold; 2001. p. 58–67.

14. Labropoulos N, Tiongson J, Pryor L, Toassiopoulos AK, Kang SS, Ashraf Mansour M, Baker WH. Definition of venous reflux in the lower-extremity veins. J Vasc Surg. 2003;38:793–8.
15. Eberhardt RT, Raffetto JD. Chronic venous insufficiency. Circulation. 2005;111:2398–409.
16. Criado E, Farber MA, Marston WA, Daneil PF, Burnham CB, Keagy BA. The role of air plethysmography in the diagnosis of chronic venous insufficiency. J Vasc Surg. 1998;27:660–70.
17. Nicolaides AN, Hussein MK, Szendro G, Christopoulos D, Vasdekis S, Clarke H. The relation of venous ulceration with ambulatory venous pressure measurements. J Vasc Surg. 1993;17:414–19.
18. Neglen P, Raju S. Ambulatory venous pressure revisited. J Vasc Surg. 2000;31:1206–13.
19. Blair SD, Wright DDI, Backhouse CM, Riddle E, McCollum CN. Sustained compression and healing of chronic venous ulcers. Br Med J. 1988;297:1159–61.
20. Dale JJ, Ruckley CV, Harper DR, Gibson B, Nelson EA, Prescott RJ. A randomised double-blind placebo controlled trial of oxpentifylline in the treatment of venous leg ulcers. Phlebology. 1995;Suppl 1:917–18.
21. Padberg FT, Johnston MV, Sisto SA. Structured exercise improves calf muscle pump function in chronic venous insufficiency: a randomized trial. J Vasc Surg. 2004;39:79–87.
22. Mayberry JC, Moneta GL, Taylor Jr LM, et al. Fifteen-year results of ambulatory compression therapy for chronic venous ulcers. Surgery. 1991;109(5):575–81.
23. Sottiurai V. Technique in direct venous valvuloplasty. J Vasc Surg. 1988;8:646–8.
24. Sottiurai VS. Incompetence transplanted arm vein valves: surgical correction and result. Phlebologie. 1991;6:41–6.
25. Breu FX, Guggenbichler S. European consensus meeting on foam sclerotherapy, April 4–6, 2003, Tegernsee, Germany. Dermatol Surg. 2004;30:709–17.
26. Palma EC, Esperon R. Vein Transplants and grafts in the surgical treatment of the post-phlebitic syndrome. J Cardiovasc Surg (Torino). 1960;1:94–107.
27. Neglen P, Raju S. Intravascular ultrasound scan evaluation of the obstructed vein. J Vasc Surg. 2002;35:694–700.
28. Alhalbouni S, Hingorani A, Shiferson A, Gopal K, Jung D, Novak D, Marks N, Ascher E. Iliac-femoral venous stenting for lower extremity venous stasis symptoms. Ann Vasc Surg. 2012;26(2):185–9.
29. Schulman S, Lindmarker P, Holmstrom M, Larfars G, Carlsson A, Nicol P, Svensson E, Ljunberg B, Viering S, Nordlander S, Leijd B, Jahed K, Hjorth M, Linder O, Beckman M. Post-thrombotic syndrome, recurrence, and death 10 years after the first episode of venous thromboembolism treated with warfarin for 6 weeks or 6 months. J Thromb Haemost. 2006;4:734–42.
30. Heit JA, Rooke TW, Silverstein MD, et al. Trends in the incidence of venous stasis syndrome and venous ulcer: a 25 year population-based study. J Vasc Surg. 2001;33:1022–7.
31. Delis KT, Bountouroglou D, Mansfield AO. Venous claudication in iliofemoral thrombosis: long-term effects on venous hemodynamics, clinical status, and quality of life. Ann Surg. 2004;239:118–26.
32. Prandoni P, Cogo A, Bernardi E, et al. A simple ultrasound approach for detection of recurrent proximal-vein thrombosis. Circulation. 1993;88:1730–5.
33. Kahn SR, Ginsberg JS. The post-thrombotic syndrome: current knowledge, controversies, and directions for future research. Blood Rev. 2002;16:155–65.
34. Prandoni P, Villala S, Bagatella P, et al. The clinical course of deep vein thrombosis. Prospective long-term follow-up of 528 symptomatic patients. Haematologica. 1997;82:423–8.
35. Geerts WH, Pineo GF, Heit JA, Bergqvis D, Lassen MR, Colwell CW, Ray JG. Prevention of venous thromboembolism: the seventh ACCP conference on antithrombotic and thrombolytic therapy. Chest. 2004;126:338S–400.
36. Brandjes DPM, Buller JR, Heijboer H, et al. Randomized trial of effect of compression stockings in patients with symptomatic proximal vein thrombosis. Lancet. 1997;349:759–62.
37. Ginsberg JS, Hirsh J, Julian J, et al. Prevention and treatment of postphlebitic syndrome: results of a 3 part study. Arch Intern Med. 2001;161:2105–9.
38. Kahn S, Hirsch A, Shrier I, Stulovitch C, Azoulay L, Haber M. The impact of elastic compression socks worn during exercise after deep venous thrombosis. Blood. 2001;98:Abstract#1125.
39. Watson L, Broderick C, Armon MP. Thrombolysis for acute deep vein thrombosis. Cochrane Database Syst Rev. 2014;(23):CD002783.
40. Eklof BG, Kistner RL, Masuda EM. Venous bypass and valve reconstruction: long term efficacy. Vasc Med. 1998;3:157–64.

Varicose Veins

12

Jennifer A. Heller

Introduction

Venous disease affects a large segment of the United States population with approximately 20 % of American adults having varicose veins and over two million people suffering from disabling complications of advanced chronic venous insufficiency. The economic burden associated with venous disease is measured in hundreds of millions of dollars for healthcare costs and lost work days. As the population ages, the prevalence of venous disorders will increase which highlights the need for practitioners who can diagnose and effectively manage patients with venous insufficiency. This chapter will review the basic pathophysiology and clinical presentation of superficial venous insufficiency and varicose veins with specific attention to diagnosis using duplex ultrasonography, indications for treatment, and interventional treatment techniques.

Pathophysiology

The precise sequence of events leading to varicose veins remains unclear. Rather than being mutually exclusive, many theories regarding the pathophysiology of varicose veins and venous insufficiency represent interrelated parts of the larger puzzle. Valve dysfunction has traditionally been identified as the primary trigger for venous hypertension and subsequent varicose vein formation. According to this hypothesis, varicose veins develop from a single incompetent valve, usually at the saphenofemoral junction. Valvular dysfunction at this proximal "entrance point" creates venous reflux by allowing retrograde venous flow into the distal lower extremity. Venous reflux generates venous hypertension, which ultimately causes venous tributaries in the thigh and leg to sequentially dilate into varicose veins. Despite its anatomic support and intuitive appeal, this theory alone cannot completely explain the pathophysiology of varicose veins. Increasing evidence suggests that varicose veins do not always follow a "proximal to distal" pattern of progression. Varicose veins can develop in any location on the lower extremity as the result of factors other than valvular incompetence. Over the past decade, research has identified key roles for inflammation and hormone activation in the pathogenesis of varicose veins and venous insufficiency [1]. On a molecular level, patients with varicose veins and venous insufficiency share unique characteristics including increased levels of TGF-beta and matrix metalloproteinases (MMPs) and changes in the extracellular matrix which forms a perivascular cuff. Researchers now focus their attention on how these molecular changes interact with and contribute to valvular incompetence to create varicose veins [2].

Clinical Evaluation

Patients with varicose veins typically report aching, throbbing, and heaviness in the lower extremity. Prolonged sitting or standing exacerbates these complaints because having the extremity in a dependent position increases venous hypertension and engorgement of branch varicosities. Patients often intuitively elevate the affected extremity to relieve discomfort. Progression of venous disease gives rise to more advanced symptoms such as a burning sensation, warmth within varicosities, and pruritus. Intense pain is not a characteristic of venous disease or varicose veins and should prompt an investigation for another etiology.

The physical exam of a patient with varicose veins should begin with a thorough evaluation of both the arterial and venous systems. Assessment of the bilateral femoral, popliteal, dorsal pedal, and posterior tibial pulses can be performed with the patient supine. Asking the patient to stand will allow filling of the venous circulation making branch varicosities more prominent and easy to recognize.

J.A. Heller, MD, FACS (✉)
Department of Surgery, Johns Hopkins Vein Centers,
Johns Hopkins University, 4940 Eastern Avenue, Baltimore,
MD 21212, USA
e-mail: jheller6@jhmi.edu

V. Gahtan and M.J. Costanza (eds.), *Essentials of Vascular Surgery for the General Surgeon*,
DOI 10.1007/978-1-4939-1326-8_12, © Springer Science+Business Media New York 2015

The anatomic paths of the superficial axial veins should be inspected to determine if they are easily palpable. Varicose vein tributaries can then be examined for communication with a specific axial system. Edema of the extremities, particularly asymmetric swelling, is also most apparent with the patient standing.

Findings consistent with advanced venous insufficiency should be recorded including: venous stasis dermatitis, lipodermatosclerosis (LPD), atrophie blanche, and healed or active ulcers. Venous stasis dermatitis can masquerade as a generalized dermatitis, which appears in the gaiter distribution of the distal medial calf and is commonly clustered within or adjacent to hemosiderin deposition or varicosities. LPD is a manifestation of long-standing venous hypertension and chronic inflammation. Affected extremities have a woody fibrosis of the distal calf with contracted skin whose texture is similar to a tree trunk. Over time, the distal calf becomes so contracted that the leg resembles an upside down champagne bottle. Severe fibrosis from prolonged venous hypertension can involve the Achilles tendon and limit the ankle joint range of motion. Atrophie blanche appears as a shiny, whitish patch of skin around the medial malleolus. Although it can look like an ulcer or a healed ulcer, atrophie blanche is actually a harbinger of an active venous stasis ulcer.

Occasionally, patients have a clinical presentation suggesting both arterial occlusive disease and venous insufficiency. Physical findings may include decreased pulses with hemosiderin deposition and LPD. In this situation, ankle brachial indices and a venous reflux exam must be performed. In the presence of both arterial occlusive disease and advanced venous changes, efforts to improve arterial perfusion should precede any venous intervention.

In women, proximal venous obstruction can cause pelvic congestion syndrome which is characterized by pelvic pain and dyspareunia. Physical clues to pelvic congestion include vaginal or labial varicosities and clusters of varicose veins at the inguinal crease and medial upper thigh. Recognizing pelvic congestion syndrome can be challenging, and the condition is often a diagnosis of exclusion. Although clinical presentations vary, pelvic congestion syndrome usually affects premenopausal, multiparous women who report symptoms of pelvic fullness or heaviness, postcoital pain, and exacerbation of these issues during the menstrual cycle. Diagnostic imaging modalities can involve transabdominal/transvaginal ultrasound, magnetic resonance venography (MRV) of the abdomen and pelvis, and pelvic venography with concomitant embolization as a therapeutic intervention. Findings consistent with the diagnosis include dilated periuterine varices on MRV and ovarian vein reflux during venography. Over the past several years, surgical ligation of the ovarian vein via a retroperitoneal or laparoscopic approach has been replaced with percutaneous embolization of the incompetent pelvic veins using a combination of sclerosants, plugs, and coils. The management of pelvic congestion syndrome continues to evolve, and further investigation is required to establish standards of care for both diagnosis and treatment.

Table 12.1 CEAP classification

Clinical classification	
C0	No disease
C1	Telangiectasia
C2	Varicose veins
C3	Edema
C4a	Hemosiderin deposition, venous stasis dermatitis
C4b	Lipodermatosclerosis
C5	Healed venous ulcer
C6	Active/open venous ulcer
Etiologic classification	
Ec	Congenital
Ep	Primary; idiopathic
Es	Secondary
Anatomic classification	
As	Superficial
Ad	Deep
Ap	Perforator
Pathophysiologic classification	
Pr	Reflux
Po	Obstruction
Pr,o	Reflux and obstruction in combination

Both men and women can have other physical signs suggestive of proximal venous obstruction including abdominal varicosities and severe unilateral lower extremity edema. In some patients with no obvious physical signs, the clinical history may offer the only clue to presence of proximal venous obstruction. These patients may complain of a bursting pain in the leg that occurs with walking and requires leg elevation for relief. The term "venous claudication" has been coined to describe symptoms attributable to proximal venous obstruction. Most cases require further imaging exams to confirm the diagnosis such as an MRV of the abdomen and pelvis with contrast. Up to 30 % of patients with advanced chronic venous insufficiency, particularly venous ulcer disease, may harbor pelvic venous pathology. In patients with chronic venous ulcers that are refractory to superficial venous intervention, the pelvic venous anatomy should be interrogated [3].

In 1994, the American Venous Forum devised the CEAP system to uniformly classify venous disease (Table 12.1) [4]. Figures 12.1, 12.2, 12.3, 12.4, 12.5, and 12.6 show examples of the different clinical grades using the CEAP classification system. Although the CEAP system can reliably define the severity of venous disease, this classification is a static instrument that cannot measure clinical outcome. The Venous Clinical Severity Scoring (VCSS) system incorporates subjective criteria which give the scoring system a dynamic element allowing researchers to measure clinical outcomes by calculating the VCSS score before and after venous interventions (Table 12.2). Although venous disease

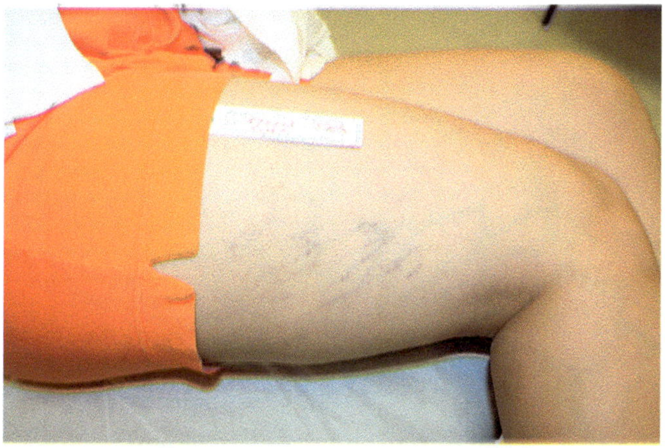

Fig. 12.1 Right leg showing telangiectasia, C1

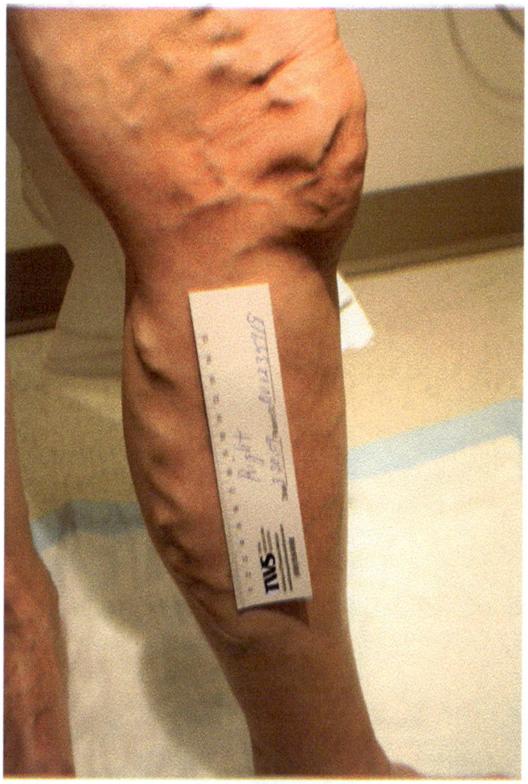

Fig. 12.2 Left leg varicose veins, C2

encompasses a wide spectrum of conditions, this chapter will primarily focus on varicose vein disease management.

Diagnostic Evaluation: The Duplex Ultrasound Examination

Venous reflux refers to flow in the veins away from the heart and toward the periphery which is the opposite direction of the normal venous blood flow. This retrograde venous flow generates venous hypertension which can distend branch

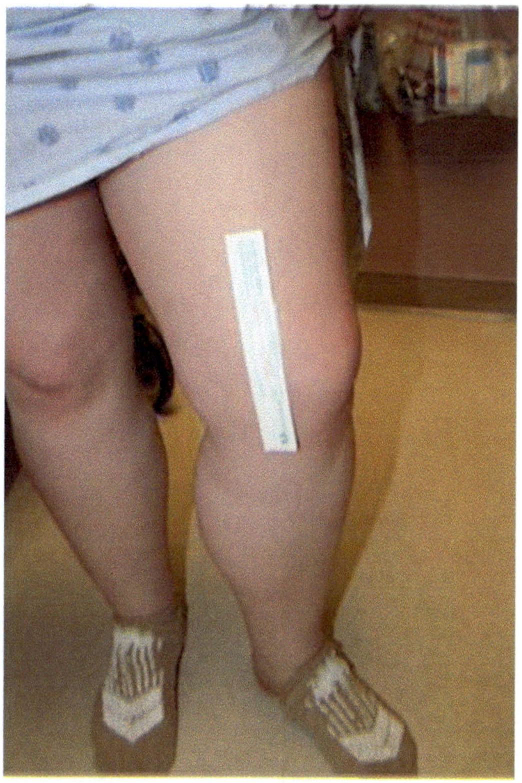

Fig. 12.3 Left leg edema, C3

varicosities, trigger inflammation, and produce clinical symptoms such as leg fatigue, discomfort, and edema. Although this description oversimplifies the pathophysiology, there is little doubt that venous reflux plays an important role in varicose veins. All varicose vein treatment strategies attempt to eliminate or minimize the impact of venous reflux. The success of any therapy, therefore, requires a sensitive and practical test for detecting and characterizing venous reflux. Duplex ultrasonography meets these requirements and has become the gold standard imaging modality for evaluation of venous disease. It is a noninvasive test that can accurately assess all of the variables relevant to patients being evaluated for varicose veins including:

1. Evidence of GSV and SSV reflux
2. Severity and extent of superficial, perforator, and deep venous reflux
3. Presence of variant tributaries of the superficial venous system
4. Diameter of proximal, mid-, and distal GSV and SSV
5. Patency of the deep venous system

Limitations of venous duplex ultrasound include its reliance on the sonographer's technical skills and the inability to visualize veins in patients with extensive bandages, severe edema, and extremely obese body habitus.

Evaluating for reflux in the femoral veins and at the saphenofemoral junction should ideally be done with the patient standing for two reasons. First, standing dilates the

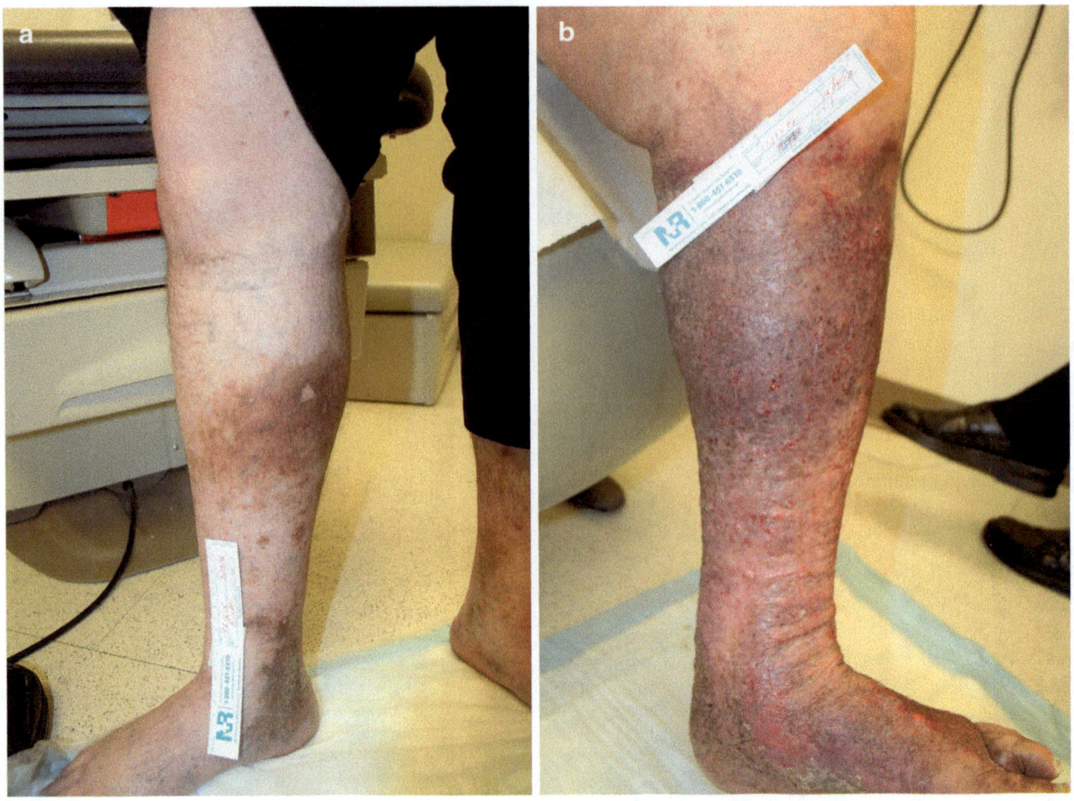

Fig. 12.4 (**a**) Right leg with hemosiderin deposits, C4a. (**b**) Left leg with lipodermatosclerosis, C4b

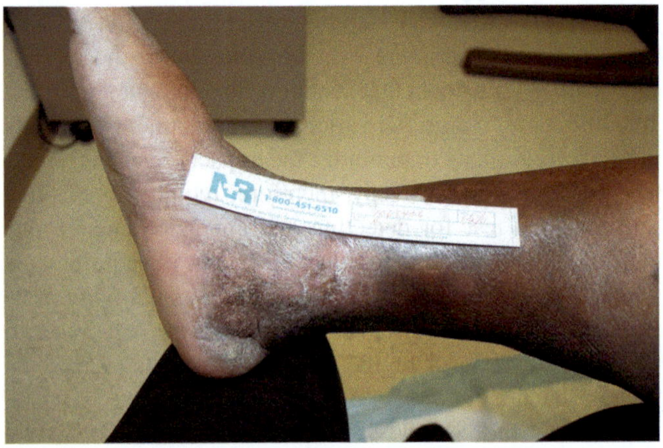

Fig. 12.5 Right leg with healed venous stasis ulcer, C5

lower extremity veins making them easier to identify and follow. Second, the upright position provokes reflux by increasing the hydrostatic pressure on the venous valves. Overall, the physiologic consequences of standing upright improve the sensitivity and specificity for detecting venous reflux. Conducting a duplex exam with the patient standing requires some safety precautions. A walker or fixed support bar allows patients to brace themselves in order to take weight off of the leg being examined. Keeping the knee in a

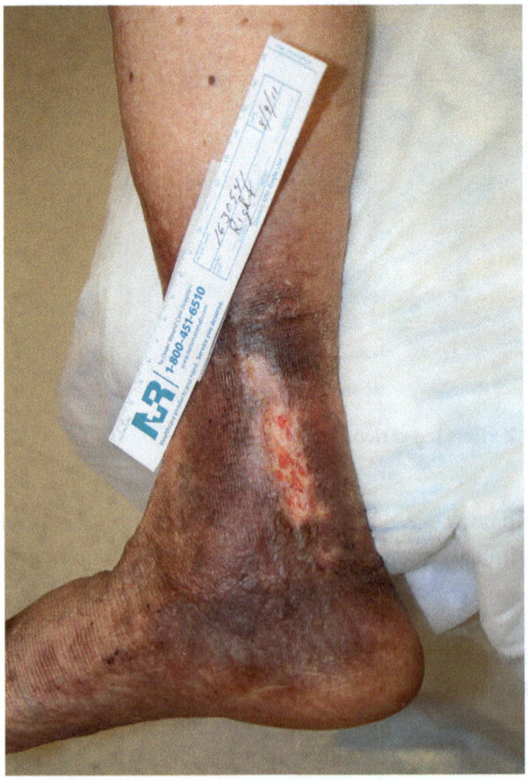

Fig. 12.6 Right leg with active venous stasis ulcer, C6

Table 12.2 Venous Clinical Severity Scoring (VCSS)

NAME:

	LEFT						RIGHT					
	Initial	Pre-Op	3-4 Days	3-4 Weeks	3-4 Months	1 Year	Initial	Pre-Op	3-4 Days	3-4 Weeks	3-4 Months	1 Year
DATE:												
CEAP (0-6)												
Fatigue: (Y/N)												
VCSS **(0-3 Each)**												
Pain												
Varicose Vein												
Venous Edema												
Pigmentation												
Inflammation												
Induration												
Active Ulcers												
Ulceration Duration												
Active Ulcer Size												
Compressive Therapy												
Total												
Complications: Blank (none) to 3 (severe)												
Hyperpigmentation												
Phlebitis												
Paresthesia												
Erythema												
Ecchymosis												
Infection												
Thermal Injury												
Other												
Patient Satisfaction: (None/Partly/Very)												
Varicose Veins:(None/ Residual/New/Recur)												
Outcome:(Not successful/ Successful/N/A)												

slightly flexed position helps facilitate a complete exam. Before beginning, the patient should be instructed to communicate any feelings of dizziness that arise during the exam. In some patients, the overall atmosphere of the room coupled with the audible Doppler signals can elicit a fainting response. These symptoms tend to occur less frequently when the exam is performed silently. Patients who cannot tolerate standing during the exam can be evaluated on a stretcher placed in reverse Trendelenburg position.

The superficial axial veins, that is, the GSV and SSV, should be mapped and interrogated with sequential compression throughout their course. The GSV resides in a fascial sheath with sonographically distinct anterior and posterior borders. When compressed the normal GSV appears as a winking eye within the sheath [5]. Incomplete compression indicates acute thrombus or chronic phlebitis if the image is associated with thickened walls or intraluminal septae. Vein segments visualized outside of the saphenous sheath are accessory vein branches, not the axial vein, and anomalous venous anatomy or branching should be noted. The SSV appears in a triangular sheath created by the two heads of the gastrocnemius and the surrounding fascia.

Reflux testing employs provocative maneuvers designed to elicit retrograde venous flow. The Valsalva maneuver generates retrograde venous flow in the proximal GSV. With the transducer positioned to visualize the saphenofemoral junction, the patient takes a deep breath and bears down with a closed epiglottis. Color flow imaging demonstrates reversed flow in the proximal GSV. The exact duration of retrograde flow can then be determined by reviewing the spectral analysis of the venous waveform recorded during the Valsalva maneuver. Venous reflux is defined as prolonged retrograde flow lasting longer than 0.5 s (500 ms). The Valsalva test for reflux can only be used to evaluate the saphenofemoral junction since a competent valve will interrupt the transmission of pressure distally [6].

Evaluating for reflux in the more distal veins of the lower extremity employs a series of compression and release maneuvers. After distal compression and rapid release, venous flow reverses until contact with a competent venous

Table 12.3 Criteria for reflux

Vein	Criteria
Femoral, popliteal tibial	Greater than 1,000 ms
Great and small saphenous (GSV, SSV)	Greater than 500 ms
Perforating veins	Greater than 350 ms (diameter greater than 3.5 mm)

valve. In perforator veins, a cutoff time of 350 ms is used to define venous reflux, while 1,000 ms is used for the femoral and popliteal veins (Table 12.3). To be effective, the compression and release of the thigh and calf should be done quickly and sharply. Automated pressure cuffs can substitute for manual compression and offer a more standardized, albeit more cumbersome, exam [6].

In addition to evaluating for reflux, duplex examination also provides essential information regarding superficial venous anatomy, patency, and diameter. Duplicated veins and accessory tributaries occur relatively frequently in the lower extremity. More than 18 % of patients have duplicated saphenous systems, and other veins may be hypoplastic or aplastic. The diagnostic duplex study should actively search for and characterize duplicated and accessory veins. In some cases, reflux may occur only in an accessory venous tributary, while the GSV remains uninvolved. Knowledge of these anatomic variants allows practitioners to direct venous interventions at only those segments which demonstrate venous reflux [7].

The duplex ultrasound exam should also assess the patency of the superficial and deep veins because the presence of venous thrombosis or obstruction can limit interventional treatment options. Complete venous wall apposition during compression confirms patency. A dilated vein that fails to compress indicates acute thrombosis, while thickened vein walls and altered inhomogeneous color flow suggest chronic thrombosis or partial recanalization. Acute or chronic obstruction of the GSV or SSV may prevent advancement of the venous stripper or ablation catheter precluding surgical vein stripping or endovenous ablation, respectively. Likewise, obstruction of the deep venous system represents a relative contraindication to interventions on the superficial venous system. In these cases, the superficial axial veins should be preserved because they may be acting as important venous collaterals providing venous outflow for the lower extremity.

The diameter of the GSV helps determine the presence of venous reflux. Diameters larger than 7.3 mm at the saphenofemoral junction, 6 mm in the midthigh, and 4 mm in the midcalf are predictive of an incompetent GSV. In contrast, diameters smaller than 5.5 mm, 3 mm, and 2 mm at the same respective levels are associated with GSV competence. Vein diameter and distance from the skin also play a role in planning for endovenous ablation procedures. These variables help determine what energy level will ablate the vein without risking thermal injury to the skin. Ultrasound diameter measurements of the saphenous and accessory veins should be conducted with the patient supine since ablation procedures are performed in that position. The GSV 3–4 cm below the knee deserves particular attention because it is the most common entry point for percutaneous access and it must be of adequate caliber to accept the therapeutic catheters.

Noninterventional Management

The initial management of varicose veins usually involves noninterventional therapy consisting of compression stockings, lower extremity elevation, exercise, and anti-inflammatory medication as needed. Compression stockings exert graduated pressure on the lower extremity which keeps varicose veins from becoming distended during prolonged standing, walking, and sitting with the legs in a dependent position. This extrinsic compression may provide symptomatic relief by minimizing the inflammatory response triggered by varicose vein engorgement and lower extremity edema. Compression stockings come in a variety of lengths (knee high, thigh high, pantyhose) and various pressure ranges: 8–15 mmHg, 15–20 mmHg, 20–30 mmHg, 30–40 mmHg, and greater than 40 mmHg. An adequate trial of noninterventional therapy requires use of compression stockings with a minimum pressure of 20–30 mmHg.

Although compression stockings effectively control the symptoms of varicose veins, they cannot work if they are not worn regularly. Patients should be instructed to put the stockings on as soon as they get out of bed in the morning when leg edema and varicose vein distention are least prominent. They should wear the stockings all day while performing their activities of daily living and remove them in the evening prior to bed. Some patients lack the physical strength or manual dexterity to pull on their stockings. Advanced age, severe musculoskeletal disease, and high body mass index can render stocking use nearly impossible. In addition, patients who have concomitant arterial occlusive disease (ABI less than 0.5) should not wear compression stockings to avoid compromising the tenuous arterial perfusion. Physicians can improve patient compliance by emphasizing the advantages of compression stockings including their noninvasive nature, excellent safety profile, and ability to improve symptoms with use. Below-knee stockings are the easiest to wear and should be prescribed regularly unless patients have varicosities around the popliteal fossa. Patients must be measured by a certified stocking fitter who can act as a useful resource to help patients understand proper stocking application. Compliance generally improves with stocking education.

Lower extremity elevation allows passive emptying of the axial and tributary veins and provides relief of symptoms associated with ambulatory venous hypertension. Patients are instructed to keep their "toes above the nose" for 15 min twice a day. Despite being brief in duration, these intervals of lower extremity venous decompression can alleviate some of the symptoms associated with varicose veins.

Exercise plays an essential role in noninterventional management of varicose veins and superficial venous insufficiency. The specific type of exercise is not important as long as it involves activation of the gastrocnemius and soleus muscles. Calf muscle contraction pumps venous blood from the GSV and SSV of the superficial system into the femoral and popliteal veins of the deep system. The lower extremity venous pump also augments venous blood flow from the distal leg into the proximal thigh and ultimately increases venous outflow into the iliac veins and inferior vena cava. Overall, exercise decreases lower extremity venous pressure [8]. Although not required, some patients report that wearing compression stockings during exercise provides additional symptomatic relief.

Medical therapy for venous disease primarily involves anti-inflammatory medications to relieve symptoms associated with varicose veins and superficial phlebitis. Outside of the United States, venoactive agents are used more regularly to treat symptomatic venous insufficiency. Studies involving horse chestnut extract, gamma-benzopyrenes, flavinoids, and pine bark extract have reported a decrease in leg edema. Although these small studies had promising results, a recent Cochrane review concluded that there was insufficient evidence to support widespread use of venoactive agents. In patients with advanced chronic venous insufficiency, flavinoids (MPFF) or pentoxifylline may accelerate ulcer healing, and the Society of Vascular Surgery/American Venous Forum (SVS/AVF) Guidelines Committee recommends using one of these agents as adjuvant therapy to compression (Grade 2B) [9].

Treatment

Indications for Intervention

The initial management of symptomatic varicose veins consists of a trial of conservative measures including compression stockings, anti-inflammatory medication, and leg elevation. After 3 months, patients should be reevaluated to determine the success of noninterventional therapy. If the patient's symptoms persist despite adequate compliance, interventional treatment options should be considered. Patients who present with complications related to varicose veins such as superficial thrombophlebitis or bleeding can often forego a trial of conservative treatment and be considered for immediate intervention.

All interventions for varicose veins share the same treatment objective: to remove branch varicosities and eliminate superficial venous reflux. Various forms of phlebectomy and sclerotherapy physically remove or close off branch varicosities, thereby abolishing the source of symptoms and the most obvious physical manifestation of the disease. Procedures directed at superficial venous reflux focus on the unseen source of venous hypertension and varicose veins. Surgical stripping and percutaneous ablation of the GSV are techniques designed to reduce venous hypertension by eliminating superficial venous reflux. In addition to providing symptomatic relief, successful vein stripping or ablation procedures also decrease the rate of recurrent varicose veins.

Surgical Vein Stripping

Surgical techniques for eliminating superficial venous reflux started to develop over 100 years ago. Keller introduced saphenous vein invagination and stripping, while Mayo pioneered the use of an external stripper to remove the saphenous vein. Babcock described stripping the saphenous vein intraluminally from the ankle to groin. High ligation of the GSV briefly gained popularity as a method for treating venous reflux without removing the GSV. Unfortunately, ligation usually fails to eliminate venous reflux, and it has been largely abandoned as an isolated treatment for superficial venous incompetence. Modern surgical treatment for superficial venous reflux involves high ligation and stripping of the GSV from the knee to the groin. This method of GSV removal minimizes the risk of nerve injury compared to stripping that extends to the ankle.

High ligation and vein stripping usually requires general or spinal anesthesia. A transverse or oblique groin incision is made just medial to the femoral artery pulse and inferior to the inguinal crease. Sharp dissection allows identification of the proximal GSV and other venous tributaries which can be ligated and divided. A brief exploration to identify the presence of a duplicate saphenous system should be performed. The GSV can then be brought up into the surgical field with gentle traction on the saphenofemoral junction. This maneuver affords further visualization of any missed tributaries that require ligation. The GSV should be ligated with a nonabsorbable suture and transected near its confluence with the femoral vein.

Attention is then directed to the below-knee segment of the GSV by making a small transverse incision on the proximal, medial calf. The GSV is identified, ligated distally, and transected. The Codman stripper is advanced proximally through the GSV to exit out the transected vein in the groin incision. The bulb is then attached to the end of the Codman stripper that exits the groin incision, and a handle is attached to the other end (exiting the calf incision). The saphenous vein should be secured to the bulb of the stripper and inverted onto itself. Forcefully pulling on the handle of the Codman stripper removes the GSV from the groin to the knee. Prior to stripping, the lower extremity should be wrapped circumferentially to aid in hemostasis and prevent postoperative edema and permanent hyperpigmentation due to blood extravasation. An additional method to decrease hyperpigmentation involves soaking gauze in 1 % lidocaine with epinephrine solution and attaching it to the end of the stripper. The gauze will pass through the vein tract and can be briefly left in place after stripping to encourage hemostasis.

SSV stripping requires placing the patient in the prone position to optimize surgical exposure. The procedure starts with a proximal dissection involving the saphenopopliteal junction and follows the same techniques used in stripping the GSV. Stripping of the small saphenous should only be done to the level of the midcalf to avoid injury to the closely aligned sural nerve [10].

Complications

Neovascularization refers to the development of new venous tributaries and varicose veins around the previously ligated and divided saphenofemoral junction. The incidence of neovascularization after high ligation and stripping of the GSV exceeds 30 % according to some reports. Interestingly, neovascularization does not occur after endovenous ablation procedures which obviate the need for a groin dissection or venous tributary ligation. This observation challenges the long-held tenet of varicose vein surgery which stressed the importance of a meticulous groin dissection with ligation of all visible venous tributaries. Rather than being beneficial, surgical dissection and tributary ligation may actually trigger neovascularization and varicose vein recurrence. Monitoring for this complication usually involves periodic duplex ultrasound examination.

Saphenous nerve injury is a well-documented complication that occurs more frequently when the GSV is stripped all the way to the ankle. Anatomically, the saphenous nerve runs in closer proximity to the GSV in the calf compared to the thigh where the nerve and vein have more separation. This anatomic detail may explain why stripping only from the knee to the thigh reduces the risk of nerve injury.

Percutaneous Vein Ablation

Percutaneous endovenous ablation of the superficial axial veins revolutionized the treatment for superficial venous insufficiency. As a minimally invasive alternative to surgical vein stripping, percutaneous endovenous ablation can be performed on an outpatient basis with local anesthesia. Advantages of this technique include less patient discomfort and a more rapid recovery. Patients now actively seek treatment for varicose veins prompting the proliferation of outpatient vein treatment centers. There are three types of endovenous therapy for the superficial axial veins: radiofrequency ablation, laser ablation, and ultrasound-guided sclerotherapy (UGS). The first two therapies will be described in this section, and the sclerotherapy section will include a review of UGS.

Table 12.4 Patient characteristics that warrant consideration of LMWH prophylaxis

Body mass index (BMI) >30
Use of oral contraceptives
Tobacco use
History of thrombotic episode
Documented thrombophilia

Endovenous ablation requires minimal pre-procedure preparation. Healthy patients with no medical history do not require lab work, while standard lab evaluation is usually obtained for patients with significant medical comorbidities. Patients who are on anticoagulation should remain on their standard regimen. The risk of bridging therapy is greater than the risk of keeping patients on their baseline anticoagulation as long as the INR is 3 or less. Guidelines for periprocedural DVT prophylaxis have yet to be widely accepted. The author gives a single pre-procedure dose of low-molecular heparin to patients with two or more risk factors for DVT listed in Table 12.4. All antiplatelet medications can be continued throughout the procedural course. Although the author does not routinely administer prophylactic antibiotics, patients with advanced chronic venous insufficiency and skin changes usually receive a pre-procedure dose of cefazolin.

Anesthesia for endovenous ablation procedures can range from local injections to moderate sedation. Many patients tolerate the procedure with minimal anesthesia consisting only of tumescent infusion of dilute lidocaine around the GSV. Ideally, these patients can be treated in an office setting. Moderate sedation requires hemodynamic monitoring equipment and is more suited for an outpatient surgical center. The choice of anesthesia ultimately depends on the preferences of the patient and physician as well as the available resources and practice environments.

As previously described, the venous duplex ultrasound plays an essential role in planning endovenous ablation procedures. The ultrasound exam should provide the treating physician with the following information: patency of the deep venous system, location of normal and refluxing axial veins, areas of communication between the varicosities and the axial vein, and the presence of duplicate or accessory refluxing vein segments.

An acute occlusive DVT is an absolute contraindication to endovenous ablation while a chronically recanalized deep

Table 12.5 Ultrasonographic findings that contraindicate intervention

Acute occlusive deep venous thrombus
Poor recanalization of chronic deep veins
Acute thrombus (partial or long segment) of GSV or SSV

venous system is a relative contraindication. In patients who have secondary venous insufficiency, the superficial veins play a more important role in venous drainage compared to patients with a pristine deep venous system and primary venous insufficiency. Care must be taken to ensure that superficial venous ablation will not compromise the venous outflow of the postthrombotic limb (Table 12.5).

The site of percutaneous access depends on the patient's symptoms and the location of their varicose vein tributaries. If endovenous ablation of the GSV is planned in a patient with painful varicosities on the proximal calf, it is helpful to evaluate these branches with ultrasound. Percutaneous access on the distal calf just inferior to the varicose veins will ensure that maximum resolution of the tributary branches is achieved with endovenous therapy.

Radiofrequency ablation and laser energy deliver two different types of energy to the vein lumen. Radiofrequency heat is delivered at a temperature of 120 °C. The radiofrequency directly injures the vein wall endothelium, resulting in collagen contraction and thrombosis of the treated vein. As the vein becomes fibrotic, new collagen matrix further constricts the vein lumen resulting in long-term occlusion of the vein. Laser energy delivers energy to the blood itself. Steam bubbles are generated with the laser energy, and coagulation occurs after completion of laser energy is delivered. Radiofrequency catheters vary in length but not in temperature delivered. In contrast, laser energy catheters come in different wavelengths ranging from 810 to 1,470 nm. Investigators have demonstrated that the higher wavelength fibers appear to be associated with less post-procedural discomfort.

Technique

In most cases, the extremity should be placed in a position of external rotation with the knee slightly flexed. A sheet "bump" may help the patient maintain this position. Placing the patient in reverse Trendelenburg can help dilate the vein to be accessed. After the standard sterile prep and draping, the ultrasound probe is brought onto the field in a sterile transducer cover. The author reexamines the vein to be treated along its entire course noting areas of aneurysmal dilation or tortuosity that may affect catheter placement (Table 12.6). Ideally, the puncture site should be distal to the lowest level of truncal reflux and provide unobstructed access to the refluxing vein segment.

At the chosen site of percutaneous access, the ultrasound probe is positioned to obtain a stable gray-scale image of the vein in either the transverse or sagittal plane. After puncturing the skin, limited, small movements of the 21 gauge needle help identify its tip on the ultrasound image. Using real-time imaging, the needle is guided into the vein lumen and exchanged over a wire for a 6 or 7 French sheath using the modified Seldinger technique. With ultrasound guidance, the RF catheter or laser catheter is then advanced through the sheath, and the ultrasound probe is positioned in the groin to visualize the catheter tip, saphenofemoral junction, and the deep system. Using ultrasound guidance, the tip of the ablation catheter is placed 2–3 cm distal to the saphenofemoral junction in order to minimize the chance of heat transmission into the femoral vein. Ideally, the probe should be placed just distal to ostium of the superficial epigastric vein. Definitive positioning of the therapeutic catheter must be completed at this point, prior to the administration of local anesthesia during the next stage of the procedure. Imaging artifacts from the tumescent anesthesia tend to impede visualization of the catheter tip making it difficult to adjust its position.

Table 12.6 Ultrasonographic findings that affect the endovenous procedure

Venous dilatation or aneurysmal segment of superficial axial vein
Webbing, septae of GSV, SSV
Attenuated infrapopliteal GSV
Variable endpoint of the SSV (no communication with the popliteal system)
Duplicate system
Accessory branches

Before beginning tumescent anesthesia, the patient should be placed in the Trendelenburg position to help empty the vein. Tumescent anesthesia is the infusion of a large volume of dilute local anesthetic. Although there are many recipes for tumescent solution, the main components are lidocaine, epinephrine, and sodium bicarbonate diluted with Ringer's lactate or normal saline. During laser treatment and radiofrequency ablation procedures, tumescent anesthesia performs three functions: (1) anesthesia provided over a large area, (2) vein compression around the therapeutic catheter, and (3) creation of a protective barrier to prevent heating of nontarget tissues including skin, nerves, arteries, and the deep veins.

For GSV procedures, the target of tumescent anesthesia is the saphenous canal which consists of the deep and superficial fascial layer surrounding the GSV. When viewed in the transverse plane, the saphenous canal resembles an eye, and the ultrasound image is often referred to as the "saphenous eye." Administration of tumescent anesthesia starts distally on the lower extremity and progresses proximally. Real-time ultrasound imaging guides a 21–25 gauge needle into the saphenous canal to deliver the tumescent anesthesia. When injected into the proper perivenous tissue plane, the tumescent anesthesia will track up and around the target vein. A long-axis ultrasound view gives the best image of fluid spreading

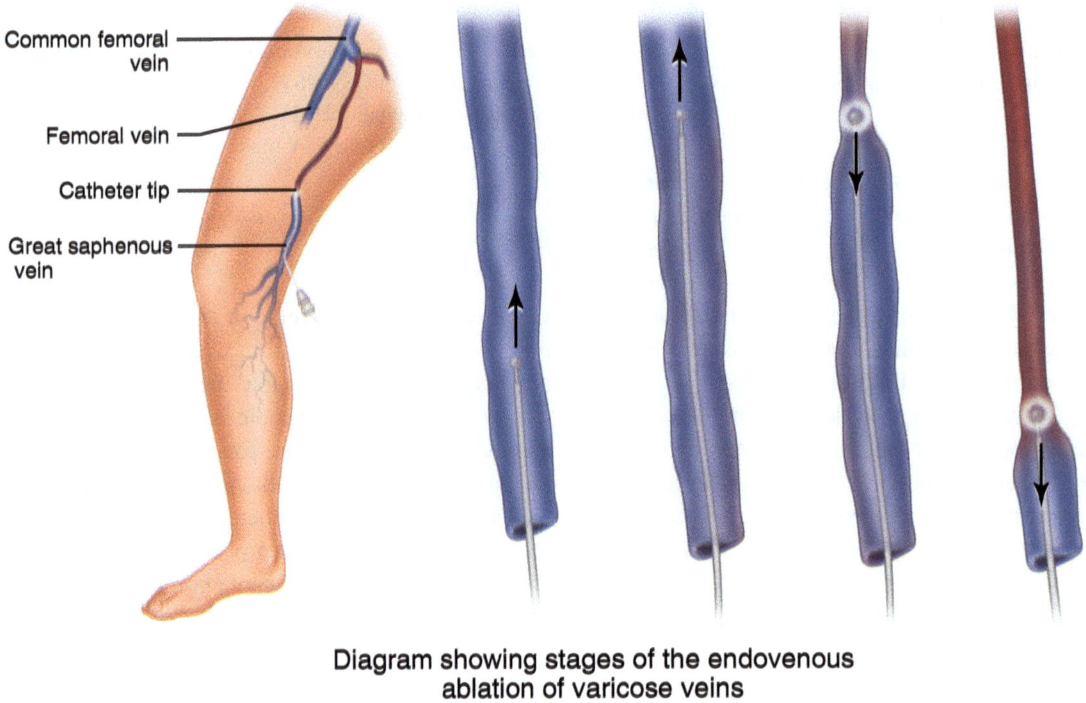

Fig. 12.7 Endovenous ablation. Top common femoral vein (line ends at blue vessel). Next label leave off, third is femoral vein, fourth catheter tip for vein ablation, fifth great saphenous vein

up the saphenous canal. Multiple skin punctures and injections are performed until the vein has a 10 mm halo of tumescent anesthesia along its entire course. The targeted vein segment is then reinspected by ultrasound to ensure that the vein is compressed around the therapeutic catheter and adequately separated from the overlying skin.

Radiofrequency energy or laser energy is then applied to the vein segment by activating and slowly withdrawing the therapeutic catheter (Fig. 12.7). The specifics of retrograde pullback depend on the type of catheter. Radiofrequency energy involves a segmental pullback governed by hash marks on the catheter and a timed activation on the accompanying generator. Laser energy catheters are variable: some have a slow continuous pullback, while others require a segmental pullback. Gray-scale ultrasound images can often detect steam bubbles generated by the laser fiber. For some practitioners, this ultrasound finding serves as proof that the laser fiber is functioning properly.

Regardless of the type of energy delivered, once the vein has been completely treated, the sheath and accompanying catheter are removed. Ultrasound imaging should confirm the patency of the femoral vein as well as successful occlusion of the GSV. Color Doppler is often the only way to assess patency at this point because of the distortion caused by the ablation and the surrounding tumescent anesthesia. The author also routinely evaluates venous flow in the epigastric vein. Retrograde flow from the epigastric vein into the proximal GSV may help prevent the post-procedural development of endovenous heat-induced thrombus.

Post-procedural instructions vary. Usually, the patient's extremity is wrapped in a layered compression dressing, or a 20–30 mmHg compression stocking is applied. The patient is instructed to walk every hour until bed. Regular activity except for vigorous cardiovascular exercise can be resumed the following day. After a satisfactory post-procedural duplex, all activity restrictions are lifted.

All follow-up protocols should include a duplex ultrasound exam 2–5 days after the procedure. The duplex ultrasound ensures that the deep venous system remains patent and confirms that the GSV has been ablated. Reported rates of DVT following endovenous procedures range from 0 to 16 % after radiofrequency ablation and 0–7.7 % after laser ablation. Although the incidence of a post-ablation DVT is extremely low, duplex ultrasound can detect thrombus in the proximal GSV which can extend into the common femoral vein. Kabnick coined the term endovenous heat-induced thrombus (EHIT) to describe this ultrasound finding. He classified EHIT into four different levels based on the size of the thrombus and its extension into the deep venous system (Fig. 12.8 and Table 12.7).

The mechanism of EHIT formation remains unclear. General consensus assumes that heat-triggered thrombus in the GSV propagates into the saphenofemoral junction and encroaches on the deep venous system. EHIT and acute DVT

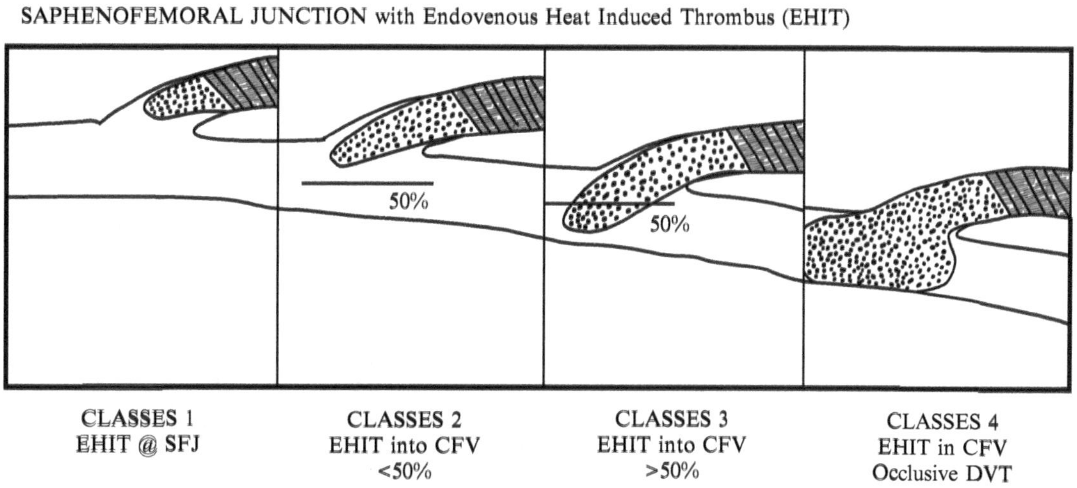

Fig. 12.8 Endovenous heat-induced thrombus classification

Table 12.7 Classification of endovenous heat-induced thrombus

	Location of and extent of thrombus
Class 1	Flush with saphenofemoral junction
Class 2	Proximal extension of saphenofemoral junction with cross-sectional diameter of <50 %
Class 3	Proximal extension of the saphenofemoral junction with cross-sectional diameter of >50 %
Class 4	Occlusive deep venous thrombosis

differ in their sonographic characteristics and natural history. EHIT becomes sonographically echogenic very quickly (less than 24 h), while acute DVT usually remains hypoechoic for several days after its initial detection. Although EHIT appears to have a low propensity to propagate or embolize, pulmonary embolism has been reported after venous ablation procedures. Follow-up ultrasound exams usually demonstrate retraction or complete resolution of EHIT within 7–10 days. Given this benign natural history, most practitioners do not treat Class 1 and Class 2 EHIT. Class 3 EHIT which involves partial, nonocclusive extension into the deep venous system usually warrants anticoagulation therapy, the duration of which can vary based on physician discretion. Since Class 4 EHIT represents occlusive DVT, it requires a 3-month course of anticoagulation [11].

RFA or Laser?

The choice of whether to use RFA or laser as the energy source for venous ablation procedures remains a matter of physician preference. Randomized prospective studies comparing the two techniques have detected very few differences. Patients treated with laser ablation tended to have more discomfort in the very early post-procedural period; however, all other outcome variables were similar [12, 13].

Phlebectomy

Preoperative Considerations

Patients who are on anticoagulation do not require reversal or bridging as the risk of bleeding is less than the risk associated with altering a stable anticoagulation regimen. The author considers an INR of 3 or less to be safe. Patients can also continue using aspirin.

Preoperatively the varicose vein tributaries should be marked with the patient standing to allow adequate venous distension. Occasionally, the patient may need to ambulate to facilitate vein filling. The varicosities are marked directly with a permanent pen, and pre-procedural photographs are taken. Varicose vein phlebectomy qualifies as a clean case that does not require prophylactic perioperative antibiotics. Any type of anesthesia can be used, and the appropriate choice depends on the clinical setting and patient factors. Ambulatory phlebectomy can be performed under local anesthesia by instilling lidocaine adjacent to the marked varicose vein segments. Patients with extensive varicosities, multiple comorbidities, or a high level of anxiety may be more comfortable with moderate sedation.

Technique

Surgical phlebectomy employs several small incisions (1 mm) made along Langer's skin lines. The author uses an 11 blade scalpel to make the incisions adjacent to the previously marked varicose veins. A hook device inserted into the subcutaneous plane is swept in a circular fashion to locate the vein. The tactile sensation of rubbery counter tension indicates that the hook has entered the vein. Once the vein is hooked, the vein is brought up through the skin incision and grasped with a pediatric mosquito hemostat. Executing a

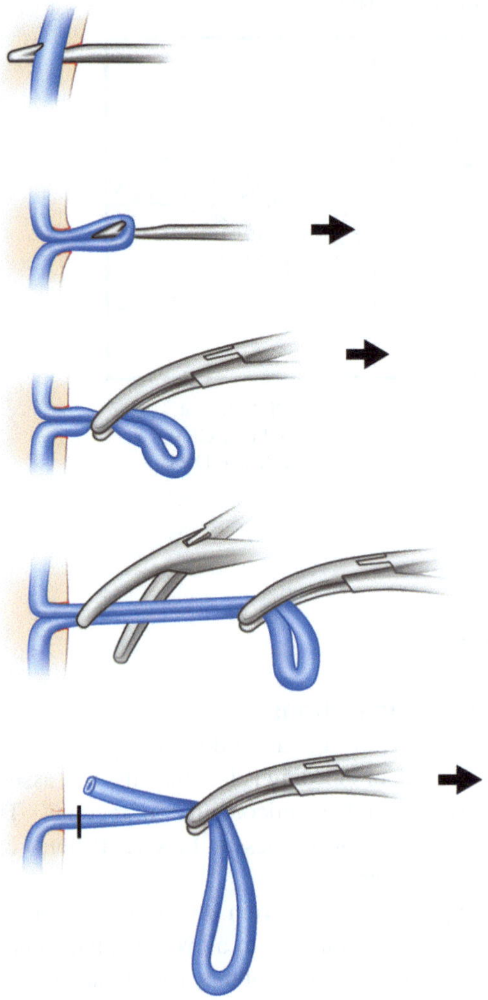

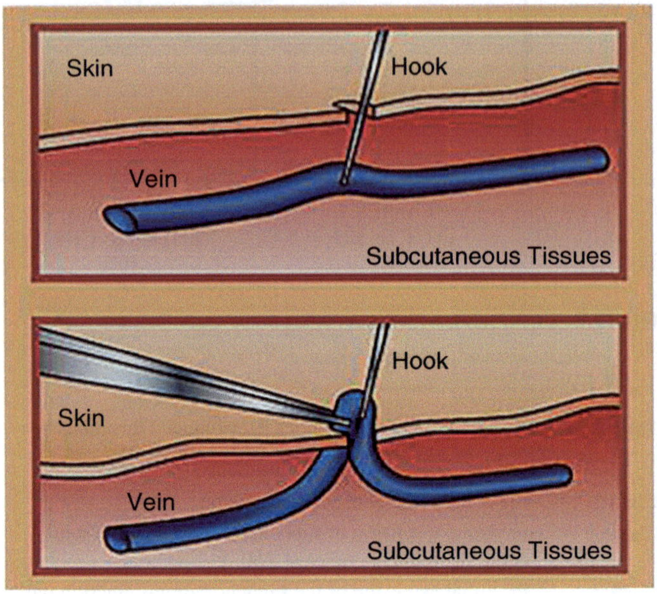

Figs. 12.9 and 12.10 Illustration of technique for stab phlebectomy

series of gentle pronation and supination movements while holding tension on the mosquito clamp will deliver an appreciable length of the vein. As this occurs, another mosquito hemostat is applied to the vein as close to the skin as possible. This process continues, removing as much of the vein as possible until the vein avulses (Figs. 12.9 and 12.10). Applying gentle finger pressure will quickly achieve hemostasis. Placement of the next incision depends on the length of the vein obtained from the preceding avulsion. Keeping the incisions small allows them to reapproximate with an excellent cosmetic result. A steri strip or simple suture in rare cases can close larger incisions. Patients with multiple, large varicosities may require a multilayer compression dressing. For focal small- and moderate-sized varicosities, the incisions can be closed with steri strips and padded with a small piece of gauze. A compression stocking can then be placed directly over the dressings. This method is most commonly used for ambulatory phlebectomy performed under local anesthesia.

Precautions/Additional Considerations

Redundant skin, particularly around the popliteal fossa, can cause small incisions to elongate dramatically. Care must be taken to avoid hooking the subcutaneous tissue aggressively or multiple times through a single incision site. Removing varicosities from the pretibial region has been associated with higher rates of paresthesias. Pedal edema can occur with overzealous phlebectomy of the foot, and this possibility should be discussed with the patient prior to the procedure.

Complications

Complications of surgical phlebectomy include sensory paresthesias which are usually temporary. Nerve injury resulting in a motor deficit has been rarely reported. More limited phlebectomy attempts around the ankle, foot, and popliteal fossa may decrease the risk of this complication. DVT and pulmonary embolism are rare but reported events. Perioperative DVT prophylaxis is recommended for patients who have multiple thrombotic risk factors.

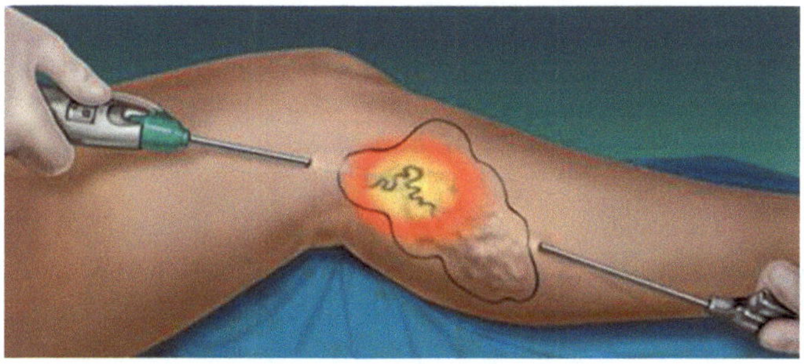

Fig. 12.11 Transilluminated powered phlebectomy

Transilluminated Powered Phlebectomy

Spitz and colleagues developed a minimally invasive vein extracting device in the early 1990s. With the transilluminated powered phlebectomy technique, one hand holds a device that delivers tumescence and provides transillumination, while the other hand operates the motorized resector (Fig. 12.11). Most practitioners administer moderate sedation when performing the powered phlebectomy; however, some investigators reported promising preliminary outcomes with using only local anesthesia [14].

Preoperatively the clusters of varicosities to be resected should be identified with the patient standing and marked circumferentially. After adequate anesthesia is administered, a small incision is made outside the marking to allow entry of the transilluminator into the subcutaneous plane. Administration of tumescence hydrodissects the tissue around the varicose veins. The resector is then placed across from the transilluminator, and the varicosities are resected under direct vision and expelled through the resector device. Applying counter traction on the skin can help facilitate vein removal. Punch holes (1.5 or 2 mm) are placed within the phlebectomy field to provide drainage during the procedure. Multilayer compression dressings are applied to the extremity. Most patients experience drainage due to effluence of the tumescent solution through the punch hole sites. A post-procedural follow-up visit is required to change the dressings and assess the incisions.

Precautions/Additional Considerations

In experienced hands, powered phlebectomy is an excellent device. Transillumination provides direct visualization enabling practitioners to remove branch vein tributaries rapidly with fewer incisions than surgical phlebectomy. This technique is particularly advantageous in patients with extensive neovascularization. Effective use of powered phlebectomy is associated with a steep learning curve. Hematomas, retained vein segments, and extensive ecchymoses are common complications. The resector device is disposable, so the cost of equipment needs to be weighed against faster procedure times. The post-procedural visit required to manage the bulky dressings also adds to the overall cost.

Complications

Most of the complications associated with powered phlebectomy involve inadequate drainage of the surgical site which can result in a hematoma, ecchymosis, and skin staining. Retained vein segments can lead to localized phlebitis. Temporary and permanent paresthesias have been reported and are likely due to apparatus manipulation in the subcutaneous space.

Sclerotherapy

Sclerotherapy consists of injecting a sclerosant or detergent directly into the targeted vein. The sclerosant damages the vein endothelium eventually causing fibrosis, contraction, and, in smaller veins, reabsorption (Fig. 12.12). A wide range of veins can be treated with sclerotherapy including telangiectasias, small varicose veins (1–3 mm), and residual veins that persist after axial ablation procedures.

Sclerotherapy performed on small telangiectasias or "spider veins" is a cosmetic procedure. Therefore, an explicit discussion with the patient regarding expected outcomes, aesthetic results, and potential complications is extremely important. Photographs are recommended both for documentation and for assessment of post-procedure outcome. A variety of sclerosants and concentrations are available. The two main FDA approved agents used in the United States are polidocanol and sodium tetradecyl sulfate.

Sclerotherapy should be performed by injecting small regions at a time. It is better to be too superficial than too deep with the injection. The needle caliber should be as small as the operator can use and still be able to appreciate its tip. Wearing magnification loupes may be helpful. The bevel of the needle should be positioned up, and some practitioners prefer to gently bend the needle to aid in vein entry. Blood should be aspirated prior to injecting the sclerosant to ensure that the needle is in the vein lumen. Caution must be exercised when contemplating sclerotherapy for veins at the ankle and foot. These areas have a small amount of subcutaneous tissue which increases the risk of nerve injury, hyperpigmentation, and necrotic ulceration.

The treated leg can be wrapped in a layered dressing, or the compression stocking can be placed over the extremity. Patients are instructed to ambulate for 20 min before driving home. Low-grade compression stocking use for 2 weeks following the procedure has been shown to improve the final aesthetic result. Patients should avoid exposing the extremity to direct sunlight for the first 7 days following the injection.

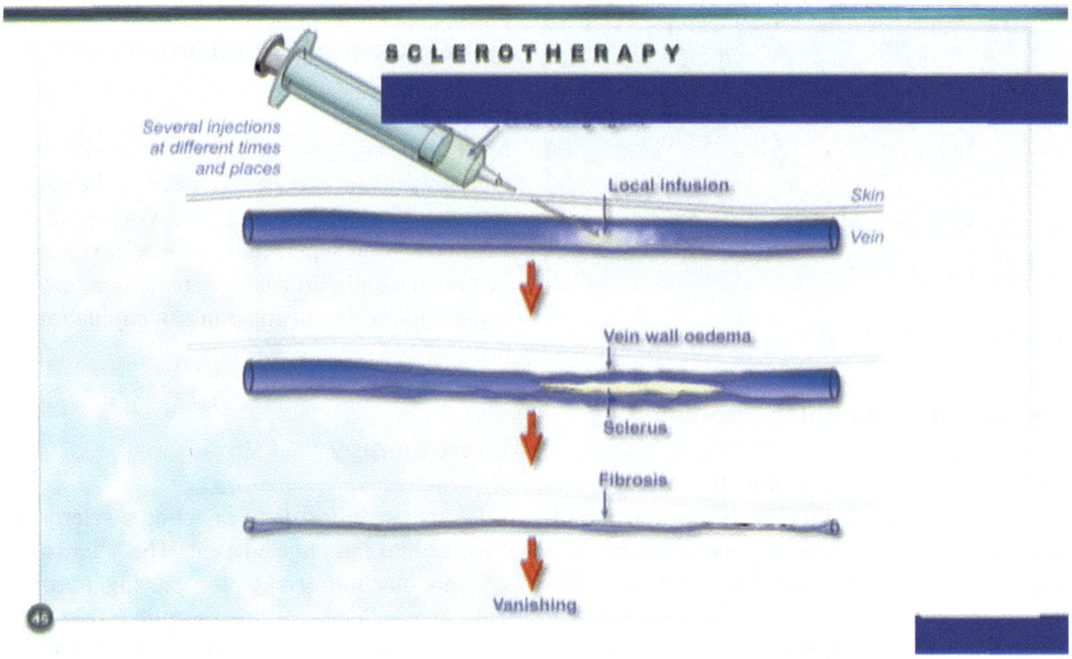

Fig. 12.12 Illustration of sclerotherapy

Complications

Complications associated with sclerotherapy for telangiectasias include hyperpigmentation, matting, and trapped blood filling small venules. Patients are instructed to return for follow-up evaluation 7–10 days following the procedure. If necessary, trapped blood can be aspirated or punctured and expressed with a small needle during the follow-up visit. Telangiectatic matting can resolve with time or further sclerotherapy sessions [15].

Ultrasound-Guided Sclerotherapy

Ultrasound-guided sclerotherapy (UGS) gained popularity as a simple, minimally invasive technique that allows patients to rapidly return to their baseline activity level. Since its first description in 1989, the use of UGS has expanded to treating incompetent perforator branches and large venous tributaries caused by neovascularization. Preparation for UGS requires a comprehensive duplex examination.

The closed needle technique is the most common method for performing UGS. A 25 gauge needle is used as this is the smallest caliber needle that can be visualized with gray-scale ultrasound. The needle is attached to a syringe containing the sclerosant. The vein can be sonographically visualized in a transverse or longitudinal plane depending on the operator's preference. The frequency of the transducer is dependent on the depth of the vein to be treated. High-frequency transducers visualize superficial veins better, while deeper veins require lower frequency transducers. The needle tip must be visualized immediately as it penetrates the dermis. After entering the vein, the needle should be aspirated to confirm its position within the vein lumen. Injecting a small test dose of sclerosant provides further confirmation of the needle position. An alternative method of UGS uses a butterfly needle instead of the needle attached to a syringe.

Volumes and concentrations of sclerosant are dependent on the size and length of vein to be treated. In general UGS requires high concentrations of sclerosant due to the large caliber of the targeted veins. Specific details regarding sclerosant preparation are outside the scope of this chapter. Additional training is recommended with this technique before attempting to perform UGS independently.

Anatomically, perforator veins have a direct connection with the deep venous system. Treating these veins with UGS requires caution to prevent sclerosant from entering the deep vein. The deep vein should be visualized sonographically throughout the procedure. Applying pressure on ultrasound transducer compresses the vein providing some degree of protection. Foam sclerosant tends to rise, and placing the patient in Trendelenburg position provides another level of protection from proximal embolization [16].

Immediately following UGS, patients should ambulate for approximately 30 min. They are instructed to continue daily ambulation and wear 20–30 mmHg compression hose for 2 weeks. Post-procedure follow-up consists of ultrasound evaluation to assess the treated vein and associated deep venous tributaries.

Complications

Minor complications of UGS include hyperpigmentation, superficial phlebitis, pain, swelling, and allergic reaction. Transient visual disturbances and headache have also been reported. Major complications include DVT, pulmonary embolus, and intra-arterial injection. Paradoxical embolism and stroke after UGS have been reported in patients with a patent foramen ovale (PFO). Due to the very low prevalence of PFO, it is not considered cost effective to perform an echocardiogram on every patient scheduled for UGS.

Conclusion

As awareness of venous disease increases among the general public and healthcare practitioners, more people will seek treatment for their varicose veins and superficial venous reflux. Achieving successful outcomes in these patients requires knowledge of the underlying pathophysiology, technical skill in performing endovenous procedures, and sound judgment to avoid pitfalls and complications. A stepwise approach to the patient with varicose veins and superficial venous reflux begins with a thorough physical exam and accurate ultrasound interpretation to determine the optimal treatment regimen. With this mindset, both the surgeon and patient will be satisfied and benefit from these minimally invasive techniques.

References

1. Bergan JJ, Schmid-Schoenbein GW, Smith PD, et al. Chronic venous disease. N Engl J Med. 2006;355:488.
2. Woodside KJ, Hu M, Burke A, et al. Morphologic characteristics of varicose veins: possible role of metalloproteinases. J Vasc Surg. 2003;38:162.
3. Neglen P, Raju S. Proximal lower extremity venous outflow obstruction: recognition and treatment. Semin Vasc Surg. 2002; 15:57.
4. Eklof B, Rutherford RB, Bergan JJ, American Venous Forum International Ad Hoc Committee for Revision of the CEAP Classification, et al. Revision of the CEAP classification for chronic venous disorders: consensus statement. J Vasc Surg. 2004;40:1248.
5. Caggiati A. Fascial relationships of the long saphenous vein. Circulation. 1999;100:2547–9.
6. Labropoulos N, Tiongson J, Landon P, et al. Definition of venous reflux in lower extremity veins. J Vasc Surg. 2003;38:793–8.
7. Caggiati A, Ricci S. The caliber of the human long saphenous vein and its congenital variations. Anat Anz. 2000;182:195–201.
8. Padberg Jr F, Johnson MV, Sisto SA. Structured exercise improves calf muscle pump function in chronic venous insufficiency: a randomized trial. J Vasc Surg. 2004;39:79.
9. Gloviczki P, Comerota AJ, Dalsing MC, et al. The care of patients with varicose veins and associated chronic venous diseases and clinical practice guidelines of the Society for Vascular Surgery and the American Venous Forum. J Vasc Surg. 2011;53(5 Suppl):2S–48.
10. Bergan JJ. Surgical procedures for varicose veins: axial stripping and stab avulsion. In: Bergan JJ, Kistner RL, editors. Atlas of venous surgery. Philadelphia: WB Saunders; 1992.
11. Marsh P, Proce BA, Holdstock J, et al. Deep venous thrombosis (DVT) after venous thermal ablation techniques: rates of endovenous heat induced thrombus and classical DVT after radiofrequency and endovenous laser ablation in a single centre. Eur J Vasc Endovasc Surg. 2010;40(4):521–7.
12. Lurie F, Creton D, Eklof B, et al. Prospective randomized study of endovenous radiofrequency obliteration (closure) versus ligation and vein stripping (EVolVeS): two year follow up. Eur J Vasc Endovasc Surg. 2005;29:67.
13. Rasmussen LH, Lawaetz M, Bjoern L, et al. Randomized controlled trial comparing endovenous laser ablation, radiofrequency ablation, foam sclerotherapy and surgical stripping for great saphenous veins. Br J Surg. 2011;98(8):1079–87.
14. Spitz GA, Braxton JM, Bergan JJ. Outpatient varicose vein surgery with transilluminated powered phlebectomy. Vasc Surg. 2000; 34:547–55.
15. Guex JJ. Foam sclerotherapy; an overview of use for primary venous insufficiency. Semin Vasc Surg. 2005;18:25.
16. Masuda EM, Kessler DM, Lurie F, et al. The effect of ultrasound-guided sclerotherapy of incompetent perforator veins on clinical severity and disability scores. J Vasc Surg. 2006;43:551–6.

Inferior Vena Cava Filters

13

Misaki M. Kiguchi and Ellen D. Dillavou

History and Introduction

Despite heightened public awareness and advances in chemoprophylaxis, venous thromboembolism (VTE) remains a significant source of morbidity and mortality. Defined as any clot within the deep or pulmonary veins, VTE affects 1 per 1,000 people in the United States resulting in 600,000 cases of clinically significant pulmonary embolism (PE) and approximately 200,000 deaths [1]. Anticoagulation is the standard treatment for VTE with proven safety and efficacy. Patients with a contraindication to anticoagulation usually require temporary or permanent caval interruption with an inferior vena cava (IVC) filter. IVC filter placement in the United States has grown exponentially over the past three decades, from approximately 2,000 device deployments in 1979 to 167,000 filters placed in 2007 [2–4]. The widespread use of IVC filters means that all clinicians will regularly encounter patients who either already have a filter or have a potential indication for IVC filter placement. Making rational treatment decisions for this growing patient population requires an evidence-based analysis of the benefits and potential risks involved in IVC filter deployment and maintenance.

The concept of caval interruption began in the eighteenth century when physicians realized that lower extremity deep vein thrombosis (DVT) could fragment and travel through the IVC into the lungs. In 1784, John Hunter ligated the femoral veins in an attempt to mechanically prevent venous thromboembolism. Morbidity from lower extremity venous stasis prompted efforts to ligate the infrarenal IVC, suggested by Trouseeau in 1868, and performed by Bottini in 1893 [5]. This procedure offered little improvement in patient outcomes with mortality rates as high as 39 % and a significant morbidity including lower extremity edema, disabling venous claudication, ulceration, and varicose veins [6, 7].

Techniques aimed at trapping large venous thromboemboli while maintaining the patency of the IVC started to appear in the 1960s. These early attempts at preventing a PE involved externally plicating the IVC with sutures, staples, or external clips all of which required general anesthesia and a laparotomy for placement. These procedures proved no better than caval ligation as they usually resulted in thrombosis of the IVC with high rates of associated morbidity and mortality [8–10].

The earliest precursor to the modern IVC filter was the Mobin-Uddin device which consisted of a silicone membrane with perforations to allow blood flow (Fig. 13.1). Instead of requiring a laparotomy for placement, the Mobin-Uddin filter could be placed transvenously without altering the anatomy of the IVC. Although it proved to be effective in preventing recurrent PE (3 % incidence), the Mobin-Uddin filter was subsequently removed from the market due to a high incidence of IVC thrombosis (>50 %) and device migration [12, 13].

The modern era of IVC filters began in 1973 with the introduction of the transvenous Greenfield filter (Boston Scientific/Meditech, Natick, MA), a stainless steel umbrella made of six legs radiating from the apex. The Greenfield filter was the earliest device to effectively trap venous emboli while maintaining caval patency. Its funnel-shaped design forces trapped thrombi into the center while preserving circumferential blood flow which allows the Greenfield filter to minimize the risk of IVC thrombosis. Twenty years of long-term follow-up demonstrated a 4 % rate of recurrent PE and a filter patency rate of 98 % [14, 15]. The durability and safety of the Greenfield continue to be the standard benchmarks for modern IVC filters.

Early versions of the Greenfield filter used large introducer sheaths for placement and usually required a surgical venous cutdown. This part of the procedure increased the

M.M. Kiguchi, MD, MBA • E.D. Dillavou, MD, FACS, RPVI (✉)
Department of Surgery/Vascular Surgery, University of Pittsburgh Medical Center, Suite 307 MOB, Shadyside Hospital, 5200 Centre Avenue, Pittsburgh, PA 15232, USA
e-mail: dillavoued@upmc.edu

V. Gahtan and M.J. Costanza (eds.), *Essentials of Vascular Surgery for the General Surgeon*,
DOI 10.1007/978-1-4939-1326-8_13, © Springer Science+Business Media New York 2015

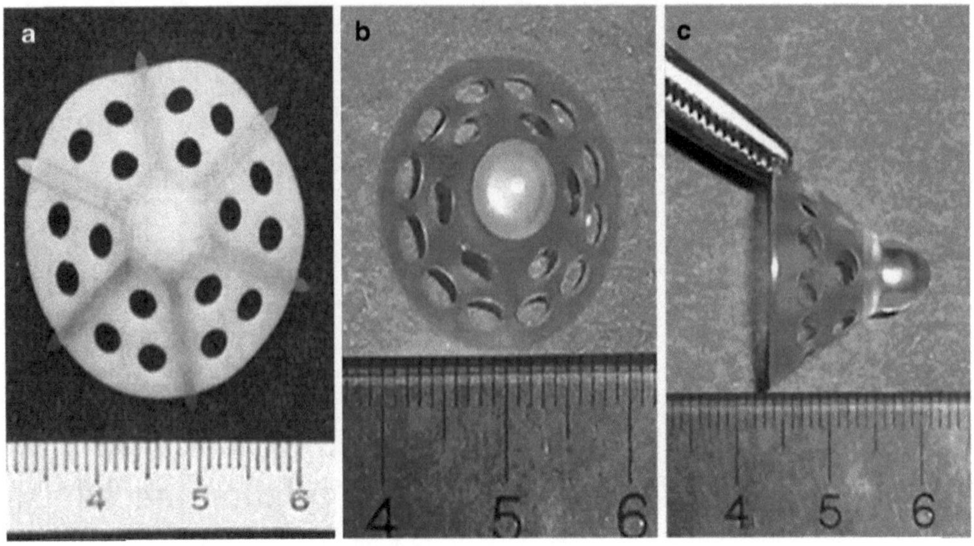

Fig. 13.1 (**a**) Top view of the 28 mm diameter Mobin-Uddin filter, scaled in centimeters (**b**) top view of the 20 mm diameter Mobin-Uddin filter (**c**) Side view of the 20 mm diameter Mobin-Uddin filter (Reprinted with permission from Elsevier Harlal et al. [11])

morbidity and introduced the risk of DVT at the surgical insertion site. Advances in technology then allowed for percutaneous insertion using smaller introducer sheaths. The Greenfield filter was first placed percutaneously in 1984 marking the advent of a new generation of devices with improved ease of deployment, flexibility, clot-trapping effectiveness, and, in recent years, retrievability [16].

Indications

While therapeutic anticoagulation remains the first-line treatment for DVT and PE, patients with proximal DVT who have a contraindication to or proven failure of anticoagulation require an IVC filter [17, 18]. For this group of patients, IVC filter placement provides an effective method of PE prophylaxis that is well supported by level 1 evidence and recent consensus guidelines [18]. Appropriate patient selection that strictly adheres to well-defined insertion criteria will ensure that IVC filters are used responsibly with a favorable risk-benefit ratio [19–21] (Tables 13.1, 13.2, 13.3, 13.4, and 13.5).

The ease of use and retrievability of modern IVC filters have blurred the indications for treatment and lowered the threshold for IVC filter insertion. In response to the dramatic rise in the use of IVC filters, the American College of Chest Physicians (AACP) and the Society of Interventional Radiology (SIR) published indication guidelines specific to retrievable IVC filters [20, 21]. These retrievable filters can be removed when the risk of VTE is reduced and/or anticoagulation therapy is no longer contraindicated.

Table 13.1 Absolute indications for inferior vena cava filters

• Contraindication to anticoagulation with documented PE, IVC, iliofemoral, femoral, or popliteal DVT
• Recurrent PE on therapeutic anticoagulation
• Hemorrhage on anticoagulation for PE/DVT

Table 13.2 Relative indications for inferior vena cava filters

• Free-floating IVC/iliac thrombus
• Septic pulmonary embolism
• Extension of DVT despite adequate anticoagulation
• High risk for complications from anticoagulation for DVT/PE: syncope, unsteady gait, poor compliance
• Massive PE with residual DVT with limited reserve for further insult (pulmonary hypertension or cor pulmonale)
• Occlusion of >50 % of the pulmonary vascular bed without reserve
• Recurrent PE with IVC filter
• DVT with severe cardiopulmonary disease and limited reserve for further insult
• Recent DVT undergoing major surgery
• Pregnancy with proximal DVT
• During DVT thrombolysis

Table 13.3 Expanded indications for retrievable cava filters

• Prophylaxis
o Need for major surgery with acute DVT (<6 months)
o Need for major surgery with significant thromboembolism risk (hypercoagulable state, history of DVT/PE, venous reconstructions)
o Documented VTE in cancer patient, burn patient, or pregnancy
o Prophylaxis for VTE in "high-risk" surgical, medical, and trauma patients

Table 13.4 Absolute contraindications for IVC filter insertion

• Thrombosis of the IVC without PE
• Complete thrombosis of access vessels (venous obstruction)

Table 13.5 Relative contraindications for IVC filter insertion

• Uncorrectable severe coagulopathy
• Bacteremia/untreated infection
• Pediatric population
• Congenital IVC abnormalities
• Upper extremity DVT

Debate continues on expanding the use of IVC filters to a wider population of patients outside the absolute indications described above (Tables 13.2 and 13.3). Clinicians in favor of placing IVC filters for relative and prophylactic indications cite the fatal consequences of a potentially preventable PE and the low morbidity of filter placement. Despite its intuitive appeal, the argument for lowering the threshold for IVC filter placement relies on nonrandomized data and observational studies. Ingber et al. reviewed the current clinical evidence and concluded that the only inarguable indication for IVC filter use is in patients with proximal DVT and a contraindication to anticoagulation [22]. In this specific context, a retrievable IVC filter should be placed and then removed as soon as therapeutic anticoagulation is reestablished. According to Ingebar et al., major complication rates for IVC filters equaled or exceeded the incidence of PE in patients without an IVC filter. Objective clinical evidence therefore does not support the liberal use of IVC filters for relative or prophylactic indications.

Absolute contraindications for IVC filter placement involve clinical conditions which preclude safe deployment of the device at its intended position. Examples of absolute contraindications include chronic IVC occlusion, IVC anomalies, inability to access the IVC, and IVC compression. Relative contraindications include a variety of clinical situations which increase the risk for IVC filter-associated morbidity. A large diameter IVC which approaches or exceeds the maximum diameter of the filter constitutes a relative contraindication because of the risk of device migration or dislodgement. IVC filters should also not be used in patients for whom placement of the filter is unlikely to improve their clinical course. A noteworthy example of this contraindication is the placement of a filter in the superior vena cava (SVC). The rationale for placing a filter in the SVC is to prevent PE in a patient with upper extremity DVT and a contraindication to anticoagulation. Not only does SVC filter placement have an unacceptably high periprocedural morbidity rate, patients who receive SVC filters also have limited survival due to the severity of their underlying disease [23]. Although IVC filters have been used in the SVC, no commercially available filter is specifically designed for this location [24]. Reported complications of IVC filters placed in the SVC include SVC perforation, cardiac tamponade, SVC thrombosis, and pneumothorax [25].

Evidence of Efficacy

Despite the exponential rise in IVC filter use for an expanding list of indications, data on device efficacy remain limited [4]. Even the core principle and absolute indication for IVC placement has not been critically evaluated. To date, no randomized trial or prospective observational study has been performed to evaluate IVC filters as PE prophylaxis in patients with DVT who cannot receive anticoagulation.

The best available data come from a single, large, randomized controlled European trial examining the use of anticoagulation with or without IVC filters as the initial treatment of DVT. The PREPIC (Prevention du Risque d'Embolie Pulmonaire par Interruption Cave) study has been influential in shaping the current recommendations for IVC filter use. PREPIC randomized patients with a DVT to receive permanent IVC filters and anticoagulation vs. anticoagulation alone for at least 3 months. Patients were discharged on oral anticoagulation if not contraindicated. Pulmonary angiograms performed on day 12 showed a new PE in only 1.1 % of filtered patients compared to 4.8 % of anticoagulated patients who did not have a filter ($P=0.03$). This difference in PE rate did not translate into a decrease in mortality as survival curves were identical for the two groups of patients. Although 2-year data showed no difference in the incidences of symptomatic PE, major bleeding, and overall mortality between the two treatment arms, PE-related death was 10 times higher (0.6 vs. 6.3 %) in the unfiltered group. Patients who received an IVC filter had an increased rate of recurrent DVT (21 %) compared to patients in the no IVC filter group (11.6 %, $P=0.02$) [26]. Of the patients with recurrent DVT in the IVC filter group, 16 patients (9 %) had symptomatic IVC thrombosis.

At 8 years follow-up, less than 50 % of patients in the PREPIC study had received anticoagulation for more than 1 year. There were lower rates of symptomatic PE in the IVC filter group compared to the no filter group (6.2 % vs. 15.1 %, $P=0.008$), and a lower rate of fatal PE with a filter ($P=0.014$). Despite these differences in PE incidence, mortality was the same for both groups, and a filter was not protective relatively to long-term survival according to multivariate analysis. The long-term clinical cost of an IVC filter was a higher incidence of symptomatic DVT (35.7 % vs. 27.5 %, $P=0.042$). Overall IVC filter placement with anticoagulation reduced the risk of PE, but increased the risk of DVT without improving long-term survival. The authors concluded that IVC filter placement should be reserved for patients at high risk of recurrent PE [27].

Although PREPIC stands alone as the only randomized, prospective study on IVC filters, it had several limitations. The study included different types of permanent filters and randomly assigned patients to anticoagulation with unfractionated or low-molecular weight heparin. Long-term anticoagulation was not standardized in terms of drug, dosage, or duration of therapy. Statistical adjustments for multiple comparisons were not performed making the PREPIC data underpowered for subgroup analyses. Although it failed to show long-term survival benefit for IVC filters, PREPIC did show that IVC filters significantly decrease PE. These data provide the best evidence supporting the comparative efficacy of filters while providing an objective analysis of filter complications. Smaller studies have corroborated IVC filter efficacy for PE prophylaxis, as another review also reported a 1.3 % incidence of symptomatic PE after IVC filter placement [28].

Prophylactic Indications in Specific Patient Populations Without Documented DVT

Prophylactic indications for IVC filter placement apply to patients who pose a high risk for VTE and cannot receive standard DVT chemoprophylaxis or anticoagulation. Preemptively placing an IVC filter is an attempt to reduce the PE risk among patients who have no other form of protection from VTE. In theory, a prophylactically placed retrievable IVC filter could be removed when the patient's VTE risk decreased or when the patient could safely receive chemoprophylaxis for DVT. The practice of prophylactic IVC filter placement has gained popularity for several patient populations with varying amounts of supporting evidence.

Trauma Patients

VTE is the third most common cause of death in multiple-injury trauma patients who survive for at least 24 h [29]. Risk factors for VTE in the trauma population include advanced age, severity of injury, head injury, spinal cord injury, pelvic and long-bone fractures, multiple blood transfusions, and prolonged immobility [30–32]. Shackford et al. reported a 7 % incidence of VTE in multi-trauma patients despite thromboprophylaxis compared to a VTE rate of 58 % in comparable trauma patients without prophylactic anticoagulation. Geerts et al. confirmed these high rates of VTE in a similar study [30, 33]. These studies provide solid evidence supporting the recommendation that all trauma patients receive some form of thromboprophylaxis, preferably anticoagulation [34].

Many patients with traumatic injuries cannot receive adequate thromboprophylaxis because of the risk of bleeding. Prophylactic placement of a retrievable IVC filter offers an alternative method of reducing PE risk for this subgroup of trauma patients [35–37]. Clinical studies examining the effectiveness of prophylactic IVC filters have reported mixed results. In one study, 244 IVC filter placements were analyzed in a group of 4,936 trauma patients. Approximately 93 % of retrievable filters were placed for prophylactic indications, while only 59 % were eventually retrieved. Two fractures, two migrations, and one filter tilt were documented. The PE rate was 1.6 % in patients who had IVC filters placed; however, the 0.4 % overall rate of clinically significant PE was not significantly different from the historical rate of 0.7 % (P=NS) [38]. Additional studies failed to detect a significant decrease in the incidence of clinical PE in trauma patients treated with temporary IVC filtration [39–41].

Some guidelines for the treatment of trauma patients cite levels II and III data which suggest a possible benefit of prophylactic IVC filter placement in appropriately selected patients at high risk for VTE [42–44]. Rodriguez et al. studied a cohort of critically injured patients who received IVC filters and found that PE occurred in 3 % of those with IVC filters vs. 18 % in historical controls [45]. Carlin et al. compared trauma patients receiving therapeutic IVC filters for documented PE to those receiving prophylactic IVC filters. Mortality rates were 11 % in the PE group vs. 3 % in the prophylaxis group [44]. Both of these studies compared dissimilar patient populations which undermines the strength of their conclusions. Instead of relying on these flawed studies, clinicians who treat trauma patients should use more sound clinical evidence in deciding on the use of IVC filters. As previously discussed, current evidence argues against prophylactic IVC filter placement.

The cost of the procedure and device along with the potential morbidity of IVC filter placement also contribute to the controversy regarding prophylactic filter use. Cost analysis and modeling in high-risk trauma patients demonstrated that the minimal effectiveness of prophylactic IVC filters had an estimated cost exceeding $380,000 per gained quality of life year. In terms of both in the initial hospitalization and long-term projection, prophylactically placing an IVC filter for the prevention of PE is not a cost-effective intervention [46].

Although there is no level 1 evidence showing that prophylactic IVC filters in trauma patients is superior to other VTE prevention measures, adherence to VTE prophylaxis has a wide regional variation possibly due to conflicting guidelines from different consensus panels (the Eastern Association of Trauma (EAST) vs. the American College of Chest Physicians (ACCP)) [18, 47]. Some institutions place more than 90 % of trauma filters for prophylactic indications [4], while retrieval rates rarely exceed 50 %. Over time, the cost of prophylactic IVC filter placement along with its potential morbidity should temper the excessive enthusiasm for IVC filter placement in trauma patients especially if high-quality, supporting evidence fails to materialize [4]. The authors believe that IVC filters are primarily indicated in trauma patients who fall under the absolute indication for filter use (a proven DVT/PE with a contraindication to therapeutic anticoagulation). Based on limited evidence and in agreement with Geerts et al., prophylactic IVC filter placement should be reserved for trauma patients with high predictive risk factors for VTE who cannot receive pharmacologic thromboprophylaxis for more than 4 days [48]. In the absence of convincing evidence, the use of IVC filters in trauma patients will continue to generate debate, and the ultimate clinical decision remains individualized.

Major Orthopedic Surgery

Major orthopedic surgery poses a high risk for developing VTE. Fortunately, routine perioperative thromboprophylaxis has significantly decreased the incidence of DVT/PE. Although several studies suggest that retrievable filters enhance protection against PE in selected orthopedic patients during the period of highest risk, the lack of level 1 evidence from randomized studies should continue to limit IVC filter use in this patient population [49, 50].

Cancer

Cancer increases the risk for VTE, and IVC filters have a well-defined role in the treatment of VTE in patients with malignancy [51]. In contrast, limited evidence supports the prophylactic use of IVC filters in cancer patients who do not have a documented proximal DVT or PE. Increased rates of venous thrombotic events (e.g., PE, recurrent DVT, and vena caval thrombosis) have been reported in cancer patients with IVC filters [52–54]. Although these complications are not usually fatal, they can significantly diminish comfort and quality of life. Therefore, except in carefully selected patients, prophylactic IVC filter use is generally not indicated in cancer patients. Therapeutic treatment with low-molecular weight heparin is the first-line treatment for cancer patients with DVT/PE. If recurrent DVT/PE occurs despite therapeutic anticoagulation in patients with malignancy, the intensity of anticoagulation is often adjusted instead of automatically proceeding to IVC filter placement [55]. Permanent rather than retrievable IVC filters should be used in appropriately selected cancer patients as the increased risk for PE is likely to be lifelong [56].

Major General Surgery

In patients undergoing major general surgery, the type and duration of surgery and the patient's medical risk factors influence the risk of VTE. Numerous randomized clinical trials recommend routine pharmacologic thromboprophylaxis for patients after major surgical procedures [18, 34]. Preoperative, prophylactic anticoagulation is also safe and effective and may benefit patients at high risk for VTE [57]. The optimal duration of thromboprophylaxis following major surgery remains unclear. Shorter hospital stays raise concerns about prematurely terminating thromboprophylaxis during the postoperative period at highest risk for VTE. Although prophylactic IVC filters could extend PE protection during the postoperative period following discharge home, no solid evidence supporting IVC filter use in this setting exists. Therefore, IVC filter use in patients following major general surgery should be limited to the standard indications that apply to the general population.

Pregnancy

Pregnancy increases the risk of VTE and anticoagulation with low-molecular weight heparin is the first-line therapy for DVT during pregnancy [58]. Indications for IVC filters during pregnancy do not differ from standard guidelines and apply specifically to pregnant patients with a proximal DVT and a contraindication to anticoagulation. There is no evidence to support prophylactic IVC filter placement in pregnant patients based on high-risk status alone. Compression of the infrarenal IVC by the gravid uterus mandates suprarenal positioning of the IVC filter via transjugular access. In most cases, a permanent filter is required as the diameter of the suprarenal cava generally exceeds 28 mm which is the approved size for all retrievable filters. Results from small case series suggest that IVC filters provide safe and effective PE protection for pregnant women with VTE [59, 60].

Bariatric Surgery

Obesity is a strong risk factor for VTE, with an adjusted relative risk of 2.9 in a recent study. Hamad et al. identified BMI greater than 60, truncal obesity, and hypoventilation syndrome in bariatric surgery patients as risk factors for VTE [61, 62]. In addition, appropriate dosing of both therapeutic and prophylactic anticoagulation is difficult in obese patients due to their metabolic variability. Despite using standardized heparin protocols or two thromboprophylactic measures simultaneously, the rate of PE is still 1–3 % in bariatric surgical patients and increases to as high as 17 % in super obese patients (BMI >55 kg/m^2) [63–65].

Due to the difficulties and challenges of prophylactic anticoagulation in this high-risk, morbidly obese population, IVC filter placement for PE prophylaxis has become increasingly common despite an absence of supporting level 1 evidence [66–69]. According to a 2010 study by Birkmeyer et al., IVC filters not only failed to protect bariatric surgery patients from PE, placement of an IVC filter also proved to be a major source of morbidity and mortality in this population. No subgroup of patients benefited from IVC filter placement, and more importantly, half of the complications resulting in death or disability among IVC filter patients were related to the device itself. This study, based on a Michigan statewide registry, was the first to demonstrate that IVC filter use may not be as beneficial as previous data from single centers had suggested [66]. This large prospective cohort study supports the current consensus opinion that prophylactic filters are not beneficial in the morbidly obese patients undergoing bariatric surgery.

Technical Details of Filter Placement

IVC filters are placed most often with the aid of fluoroscopy. Many patients, especially in the trauma population, have a recent CT scan of the abdomen and pelvis available for preprocedural review of renal vein landmarks and anomalies. Contrast venography performed as part of the procedure provides visualization of anatomic landmarks and accurate, real-time positioning of the IVC filter. Venous access usually involves a femoral or internal jugular approach using a vein uninvolved with clot. Previous studies suggest an increased risk of subsequent femoral vein thrombosis related to femoral vein access, particularly in patients receiving prophylactic filters [70, 71]. The use of an ultrasound guidance to evaluate for clot, rule out abnormal anatomy, and assist in venous cannulation can minimize access-related complications. A micropuncture kit is typically used to cannulate the vein. If there is any suspicion for clot between the puncture site and the infrarenal cava, a venogram should be obtained before proceeding any further to decrease the risk of embolizing clot. Once patency has been confirmed, the micropuncture catheter is exchanged over a wire for a larger sheath, and a long starter wire is advanced into the IVC under fluoroscopy (Fig. 13.2a). For a femoral approach, a catheter is positioned near the L4 level under fluoroscopy. An inferior cavagram is obtained with the patient in Valsalva to maximize visualization of the renal veins and to obtain an accurate diameter measurement of the IVC at this level (Fig. 13.2b). In some cases, an adequate venocavogram requires a power injection of contrast (20 cc/s rate; 40 cc total volume). A marker wire or catheter should be used as a reference to measure caval diameter immediately below the renal veins. Caval diameter smaller than 18 mm [72] should preclude filter placement unless the SafeFlo IVC filter designed for smaller vena cavas is used (16–19 mm). In this clinical scenario, the indications for filter placement should be compelling, if not lifesaving, as the radial force of the filter in a small cava can lead to perforation of the struts. Caval diameter >28 mm precludes the use of most standard retrievable filters and mandates the use of the permanent Bird's Nest filter (Cook Medical, Bloomington, IN) if filter placement is essential.

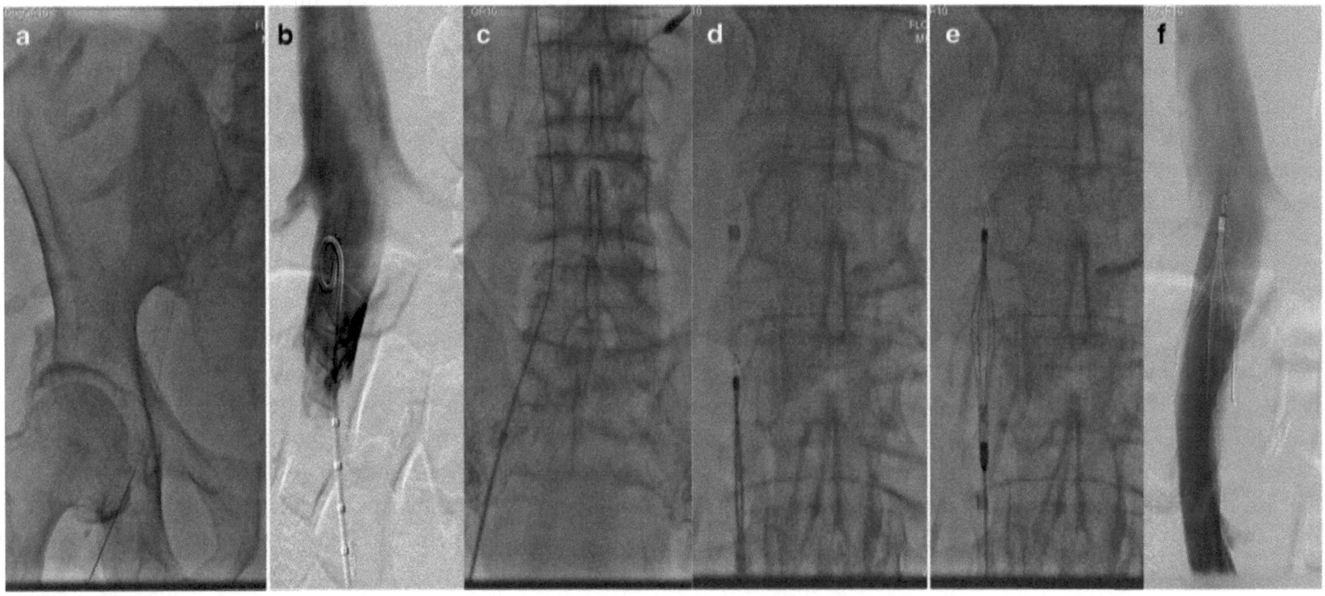

Fig. 13.2 Sequential fluoroscopic images taken during various steps of IVC filter placement. (**a**) A micropuncture wire is advanced though the right common femoral vein; (**b**) inferior venacavogram showing the renal veins; (**c**) the delivery sheath is advanced over the wire; (**d**) the filter is advanced through the delivery sheath; (**e**) the sheath is withdrawn to expose and release the filter; (**f**) completion venacavogram showing the deployed IVC filter

Renal vein anomalies, IVC transposition, IVC duplication, and IVC agenesis are anatomic variants important to identify before IVC filter placement. Empiric placement of IVC filters by bony landmarks alone should be discouraged due to the relatively high prevalence of venous anomalies. Contrast venography performed during filter placement provides a roadmap of venous anatomy and helps identify the renal veins to guide placement of the device. The IVC filter is inserted into the sheath and positioned with the superior tip of its cone between the renal veins. Under direct fluoroscopic guidance, the sheath is slowly withdrawn to release and deploy the IVC filter (Fig. 13.2c, d). A completion venogram is performed to ensure proper placement, confirm IVC patency, and evaluate for significant filter tilt (Fig. 13.2f). The clinical scenarios which warrant suprarenal filter placement are listed in Table 13.6. As previously discussed, the larger diameter of the suprarenal cava usually precludes the use of standard retrievable IVC filters.

Troubleshooting

Occasionally, the nonselective venocavogram fails to demonstrate the location of the renal veins. In these cases, selective cannulation of the renal veins with a curved catheter (Cobra C-2, Terumo Medical Corporation, Somerset, NJ) can determine the level of each renal vein and guide filter placement. If venous anomalies are suspected, selective venography provides more detailed anatomic information which changes the intended location of IVC filter placement in a significant number of patients compared to nonselective venography [73]. In the authors' opinion, the increased cost, time, contrast, and radiation loads to the patient do not justify selective renal vein cannulation in routine cases.

Table 13.6 Indications for suprarenal IVC filter placement

• Thrombus in IVC
• Malpositioned infrarenal filter
• Duplicate IVC
• Gonadal vein thrombosis
• Pregnancy

Filter tilt is common with the traditional triangular, cone-shaped filters especially when deployed from femoral vein access. Internal jugular vein access involves less torque on the filter resulting in a lower tendency to tilt. Retrievable filters placed through the internal jugular vein can also be easily retrieved and redeployed if filter tilt is severe. If a filter is tilted after deployment through the femoral vein, it can be gently manipulated with a J-wire or pigtail catheter to reposition the filter. Attempted manipulation of the filter should be done with caution to avoid dragging the filter inferiorly or causing the cone to tilt into one of the renal veins. If this does occur, the interventionalist should establish access through the internal jugular vein in order to retrieve and reposition the filter.

Rarely, the filter fails to completely deploy because the struts stick together and do not expand to fill the lumen of the IVC (Fig. 13.3). This technical problem can be corrected with gentle manipulation using a pigtail catheter, being careful not to embolize the filter as it is not yet anchored to the caval wall [74]. IVC diameter varies depending on the patient's volume status. All currently available filters can be safely deployed in cavas up to 30 mm in diameter, depending on the specifics of each manufacturer's indications for use. An excessively large diameter IVC or so-called megacava

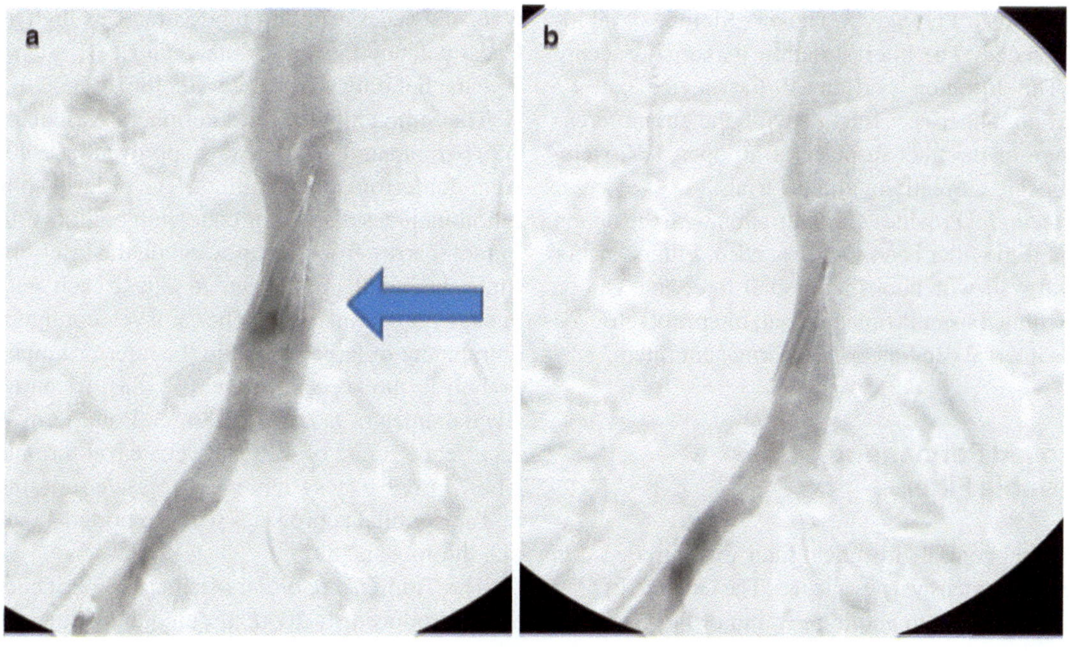

Fig. 13.3 (**a**) Filter is deployed and fails to fully expand (*arrow*). (**b**) After gentle manipulation with a pigtail catheter, the struts expand

may require a Bird's Nest filter which has been approved for the use in caval diameters of up to 40 mm. Alternatively, standard diameter filters can be placed in both the common iliac vein to provide PE protection [75].

Bedside Filter Placement Using Transabdominal or Intravascular Ultrasound

In patients who are too unstable to transfer to the operating room or interventional suite, ultrasound-guided IVC filter placement is safe and cost-effective [76]. Although large body habitus, recent abdominal surgery, and excessive bowel gas make adequate sonographic visualization less predictable, a single-center study reported a 97.7 % technical success rate for IVC filter placement with transabdominal ultrasound. If transabdominal ultrasound was not adequate, intravascular ultrasound was used to place the filter with a technical success rate of 96.2 % [77–79].

Filter Selection

No randomized controlled trials between different IVC filter models have been performed, and comparative observational studies failed to show superiority of one filter over another. The interventionalist placing the filter should consider the features unique to each type of filter as well as the specific clinical scenario in deciding which type of filter to use. IVC filters are designed in the following categories:

- *Permanent filters*: Provides permanent, lifelong caval filtration. The design of these filters maximizes secure fixation to the IVC wall.
- *Convertible filters*: Provides permanent, lifelong caval filtration if needed. The filter structure maximizes secure fixation. The filtration portion of the device can be removed if no longer necessary, leaving the circumferential structure of the filter in place as an open IVC stent. These filters are currently in clinical trials.
- *Retrievable filters*: Provides caval filtration with the option of retrieval if the filter is no longer needed. Filters anchor to the caval wall with hooks and radial force, but can be retrieved within a specific time interval; filters not retrieved within this interval can function as permanent filters.

FDA-Approved Permanent and Retrievable Filters

The stainless steel conical Greenfield filter was introduced in 1973 and has been extensively evaluated. The Greenfield filter spans a diameter of 30 mm and traps 3 mm or larger emboli [2, 14, 15, 80]. Initially, there was a high rate of venous access site thrombosis (up to 41 %), due to the 24 Fr delivery system [81]. In 1989, Greenfield filters were constructed out of titanium alloy (nonthrombogenic, nonferromagnetic, resistant to fatigue and corrosion) and delivered via a 12 Fr sheath. Subsequent modifications have minimized technical complications including tilt (<5 %), migration (1 %), recurrent PE (2 %), and access site thrombosis (4 %). Caval patency after Greenfield filter placement is approximately 98 % [15].

The Bird's Nest filter was introduced in 1982. This permanent filter is delivered by a 12 Fr system. At deployment, two struts are released to attach to the caval wall, and four wires extend in a random "Bird's Nest" configuration. The unique feature of the Bird's Nest filter is the struts which span a diameter of up to 60 mm allowing the filter to accommodate large caliber cavas. Unlike other filters, the Bird's Nest filters rarely perforate the IVC because the devices do not have radially oriented struts [82]. The tighter configuration of the Bird's Nest filter traps smaller emboli resulting in a low recurrent PE rate of 1–7 %. The downside of the Bird's Nest geometry is a higher rate vena caval thrombosis (3–19 %) [2, 83, 84].

The Vena Tech LGM (B Braun, Bethlehem, PA) permanent IVC filter is made from biocompatible and nonferromagnetic Phynox (cobalt, chromium, iron, nickel, molybdenum). It maintains a conical shape with a central apex and six radiating struts containing flat side rails with hooks. The Vena Tech LGM accommodates caval diameters as large as 28 mm and is deployed through a 10 Fr delivery from either a jugular or femoral approach. The Vena Tech Low-Profile (LP) (B Braun, Bethlehem, PA) IVC filter is similar to the LGM but uses a 7 Fr delivery system. An experience with both Vena Tech LGM and LP IVC filters has exposed technical problems and complications including incomplete opening of the filter, recurrent PE rates as high as 6 %, and access site thrombosis rates as high as 23 % [85]. Caval patency rates for Vena Tech LGM filters are 92 % at 2 years, but only 67 % at 9 years [86].

The Simon nitinol (Bard Peripheral Vascular Inc., Tempe, AZ) permanent IVC filter was approved in 1990 and is made from nonferromagnetic nitinol. The bi-level conical configuration includes a superior cone with eight overlapping loops in radial array from the apex, while the inferior cone has six limbs in radial array from its apex, each with a hook to engage the caval wall. The bi-level configuration allows entrapment of large emboli in the inferior limbs and of small emboli in the superior dome [87, 88]. It can accommodate caval diameters as large as 28 mm. Long-term studies report recurrent PE rate of 4 % and vena caval thrombosis of 4 %. The 7 Fr delivery system is appropriate for femoral, jugular, and antecubital approaches with a reported 4 % rate of access site thrombosis [89].

The TrapEase (Cordis, Miami, FL) permanent IVC filter was introduced in 2000. Its unique symmetric trapezoidal double-basket designs connects a cephalic conical basket to its mirror image pointing caudally through six side struts, each with hooks providing filter attachment to the caval wall. A 6 Fr delivery system deploys this 50 mm long and 35 mm wide IVC filter through antecubital, jugular, and femoral approaches. The OptEase (Cordis, Miami, FL) IVC filter is similar to the TrapEase design with the addition of a hook placed on the caudal apex and unidirectional anchoring barbs to allow retrievability. Based on initial safety and efficacy data on retrievals, the FDA approved OptEase IVC filter retrieval up to 14 days after placement [90].

TrapEase and OptEase have high technical success rates with limited filter migration, insertion site thrombosis, and filter fracture rates. In a large single-center experience, symptoms of PE developed in 8 % of patients with TrapEase filters, but only 0.1 % developed into fatal PEs. The double-basket filter design has generated concern that TrapEase and OptEase filters have a higher risk of vena cava occlusion. In animal models, trapped emboli in the TrapEase filter slow blood flow between the inferior basket of the filter and the caval wall. This stagnant blood flow promotes further thrombosis. Schutzer et al. reported symptomatic vena caval thrombosis of 1.5 %, and Corriere et al. reported TrapEase filters had an increased risk for vena caval thrombosis compared to other filter designs [91, 92]. In a large study, venography before retrieval confirmed intrafilter thrombus in 22 % of TrapEase filters; however, the study failed to make a clear distinction between captured emboli and thrombus formation [93].

The Recovery G-2 (Bard Peripheral Vascular Inc., Tempe, AZ) permanent IVC filter was modified from the original Recovery nitinol IVC filter. Approved in 2006, the 41 mm length filter is conical in design with six radiating stabilizing arms and six separate radiating fixation legs with hooks for anchoring. In 2008, the Recovery G-2 IVC filter and G-2 Express filter incorporated a hook at the apex of the conical filter to allow for retrievability. These filters are delivered through a 7 Fr low-profile system and can accommodate caval diameters up to 28 mm. Early reports cite PE rates of 2.8 % and no cases of caval thrombosis [94]. The EVEREST trial recorded a 95 % successful retrieval rate of Recovery G-2 filters with a mean indwelling time of 140 days and a maximum of 300 days [95]. In 2010, the FDA approved the Eclipse, an electropolished finish version of the G-2 Recovery IVC filter (Bard Peripheral Vascular Inc., Tempe, AZ). The electropolish creates an ultrasmooth finish to prevent micro-imperfections.

The nonferromagnetic Gunther Tulip (Cook Medical, Bloomington, IN) IVC filter was approved in 2000 for permanent use and in 2003 for retrieval. The conichrome filter is conical with four filters legs with barbed anchoring hooks radiating from the apex and four additional wires wrapped around these legs. The Gunther Tulip filter is 50 mm long and 30 mm wide and delivered with an 8.5 Fr system from the femoral approach and a 7 Fr system from the jugular approach. A hook at the apex allows removal even after long dwell times of greater than 180 days [96]. Rates of recurrent PE rates are 1–2 %, filter tilt 4–11 %, IVC penetration 2–4 %, and caval thrombosis 5–7 % [97–101].

An updated model of the Tulip IVC filter is the Celect (Cook Medical, Bloomington, IN), approved in 2007 for permanent use and in 2008 for retrievable use. Changes to the tulip structure included eight secondary legs to improve stabilization and centering and a wider base for use in caval diameters up to 30 mm. Although the Celect IVC filter provides PE protection and retrievability (symptomatic PE rate of 2.8 %; successful retrieval 89 % at 52 weeks), it also demonstrated a high incidence of caval penetration by a filter leg [102, 103].

Recently, approved IVC filters include ALN (ALN Implants Chirurgicaux Ghisonaccia, France), SafeFlo (Rafael Medical Technologies, Caesarea, Israel), Crux (Crux Biomedical, Menlo Park, CA), and Option (Rex Medical/Argon Medical Devices, Athens, TX). The ALN filter is designed from nonferromagnetic stainless steel in a conical shape with three additional long curved legs radiating from the apex to facilitate self-centering. After a median follow-up of 21 months in a small group of patients receiving the ALN filter, no recurrent PE or vena caval thrombosis rates were reported [104]. Successful ALN filter retrieval rates dramatically decrease after 3 months; only 50 % of IVC filters were retrieved with failures due to adherence to the wall and filter tilt [105]. SafeFlo IVC filter has a non-tilt spiral shape oversized to a double-ring platform. The available filter sizes correlate with the caval diameter: small, 16–19 mm; medium, 19–22 mm; and large, 22–25 mm. Data on the long-term safety and efficacy of the SafeFlo filter remains limited. The novel design of the Crux filter includes two nitinol spiral parts crimped at the ends to form a double-looped helical structure. A filter mesh is attached to one loop, while three fixation anchors are attached to the opposite loop. Delivered through a 6 Fr system, two sizes are available: one for small cavas (17–22 mm) and one for large cavas (22–28 mm). The symmetric design of the Crux filter allows retrieval using a jugular or femoral approach [106]. The Option IVC filter is laser cut from one single piece of nitinol. Its conical shape has six struts radiating from the apex and includes a caudal hook for retrieval. Although it only requires a 5 Fr delivery system, the Option filter can be used in a maximal caval diameter of 32 mm. In a multicenter, single-arm clinical trial, 8 % of patients had recurrent PE, 2 % of patients had filter migration, and 3 % had caval thrombosis [106].

Filter Choice

After deciding to place an IVC filter, the clinical scenario should dictate whether a permanent or retrievable filter is used. Beyond this choice, each filter has unique characteristics which may factor into the selection process. Table 13.6 lists specific parameters associated with each commercially available filter. Evaluating filters based on PE prevention rates remains difficult as no clinical trial has directly compared filters and not all individual studies used PE after IVC filter insertion as a reportable outcome. A recent meta-analysis offered some insight into filter performance by reporting PE rates of 0.7 % with ALN, 1.1 % with Celect, 3.4 % with G-2, 1.6 % with OptEase, 4 % with Option, 1 % with Recovery, and 0.9 % with Tulip [28]. For permanent filters, rates of recurrent PE were 2.6 % with stainless steel Greenfield, 3.1 % with titanium Greenfield, 2.9 % with Bird's Nest, 3.8 % with Simon nitinol, 3.8 % with Vena Tech, and 0 % with TrapEase [107]. The same systematic literature review reported on the rate of DVT after IVC filter placement; however, it used variable criteria for the diagnosis of DVT. Several filters were associated with a high incidence of DVT after placement including ALN filters (15.2 %), Option filters (18 %), and titanium Greenfield filters (22 %) [107–109]. The Tulip filter had the lowest rate of DVT [110, 111]. Although the risk of DVT appeared to increase with the duration of use, it remains unclear whether this risk reflects the underlying prothrombotic condition which prompted IVC filter insertion or IVC filter-induced changes in vena cava blood flow [26, 27]. Most filters had a less than 1 % incidence of migration risk with the exception of the G-2 filter which had a 4.5 % rate of migration [28]. Celect filters had the lowest rate of caval thrombosis (0.6 %), while Option filters (8 %) and Vena Tech filters (11.2 %) had the highest rates [28, 107] (Table 13.7).

Randomized clinical trials directly comparing different types of filters will never be conducted as they would require a prohibitively large number of patients to detect any true differences in their low complication rates. Filter selection therefore should be individualized to each patient and clinical setting. The clinician placing the filter can determine which combination of filter device attributes is most important to the patients' successful clinical outcome. Filter efficacy and complication rates also reflect the skill of the interventionist which emphasizes the value of proficiently placing these devices with an appropriately trained team.

Table 13.7 Filter complications by filter type

Complication	High rates (%)	Low rates (%)
Recurrent PE with retrievable IVC filters	G-2 (3.4 %) Option (4 %)	ALN (0.7 %) Tulip (0.9 %) Recovery (1 %) Celect (1.1 %) OptEase (1.6 %)
Recurrent PE with permanent IVC filters	Stainless steel Greenfield (2.6 %) Bird's Nest (2.9 %) Titanium Greenfield (3.1 %) Simon nitinol (3.8 %) Vena Tech (3.4 %)	TrapEase (0 %)
Recurrent DVT	ALN (15.2 %) Option (18 %) Titanium Greenfield (22 %)	Tulip (0 %)
Migration	G-2 (4.5 %)	Most other filters (<1 %)
Caval thrombosis	Option (8 %) Vena Tech (11.2 %)	Celect (0.6 %)

Post-procedural Management and Complications

Rate of DVT and Benefits of Concurrent Anticoagulation

The subject of concomitant anticoagulation therapy following IVC filter placement still generates debate. Although IVC filters protect patients from PE, they do not alleviate the underlying prothrombotic condition and therefore do not alter the risk of DVT formation or propagation. Potential thrombotic complications after placing an IVC filter include venous access site thrombosis and dislodgement or extension of emboli trapped by the filter [26]. To mitigate these thrombotic risks, the AACP recommends starting anticoagulation after placing an IVC filter as soon as a patient's risk of bleeding becomes acceptable (grade 2B evidence). Despite the intuitive appeal of this guideline, evidence supporting the benefit of concomitant anticoagulation is scarce. Yale et al. reported no difference in the rate of recurrent VTE events in patients treated with an IVC filter and concomitant anticoagulation compared to patients managed with an IVC filter alone [112]. Sakuma et al. demonstrated a reduction in 30-day mortality in patients treated with an IVC filter irrespective of concomitant anticoagulation use [113]. The decision to use concomitant anticoagulation after IVC filter placement should be made on a case-by-case basis depending on the underlying prothrombotic state, the extent of the DVT/PE, and the presence or absence of insertion site thrombosis.

Indications for Filter Retrieval

Although IVC filters can prevent PE, they do not prevent or treat DVT, and they may actually pose a thrombotic risk. The previously cited PREPIC study found an increased incidence of DVT in patients with IVC filters during mid- and long-term follow-up. Anticoagulation remains the first-line therapy for DVT treatment and prevention and should be used when clinically feasible. Many patients have only a temporary contraindication to anticoagulation and therefore require the protection of an IVC filter for a finite period of time. For these patients, a permanent IVC filter is a potential liability as it

Table 13.8 Retrieval considerations

IVC filter	Suggested retrieval period	Comments
Gunther Tulip	4 weeks	Success rate: 99 %
	12 weeks	Success rate: 94 % [115]
OptEase	14 days	
Recovery G-2	140 days	Maximum reported retrieval period: 300 days
Celect	12 weeks	Can be retrieved as long as 52 weeks
ALN	No recommendation	Success rate: 100 % at 3 months; attempts at 25 months successful [105, 116]
Option	175 days	[106]

could increase their thrombotic risk, perforate the cava, or migrate over time. Retrieving IVC filters offers a way to realize the short-term benefit of IVC filters while minimizing their long-term risks.

Criteria for IVC filter retrieval vary slightly depending on the indication for placing the filter. Patients with an IVC filter can be categorized into two groups: therapeutic use (patients with a documented DVT/PE) or prophylactic use (patients without a documented DVT/PE). In therapeutic patients, the IVC filter can be retrieved when the patient can tolerate sustained anticoagulation. Filter retrieval can be safely performed without cessation of anticoagulation. In prophylactic patients, the IVC filter can be retrieved whenever the thrombotic risk factors have resolved or the patient can safely receive effective thromboprophylaxis. In general, the sooner the filter retrieval is attempted, the higher the success rate [114] (Table 13.8).

Technical Details of IVC Filter Retrieval

The technique for IVC filter retrieval depends in part on the type of filter used. Most retrievable filters have an apical hook that can be snared from a superior approach through the internal jugular vein. Percutaneous internal jugular vein access is obtained with a micropuncture kit, and a wire is advanced into the IVC under fluoroscopic guidance. Once a larger sheath is exchanged over the wire, a catheter is guided over the wire past the IVC filter, with care taken to not dislodge the filter or become entangled with its legs. A venogram is performed to ensure minimal clot burden within the filter. If thrombus fills more than 30 % of the filter, it should be left in place as removal may precipitate a PE. In this case, the patient may undergo lysis of clot or 3 months of anticoagulation followed by another attempt at filter removal. If there is little or no thrombus in the filter, the apical hook is snared and held under tension. The retrieval sheaths are then advanced to collapse the IVC filter within the sheath. The inner sheath and filter are then completely withdrawn. Collapsing the filter pulls the struts inward and gently dislodges them from the cava, in contrast to pulling on the filter which may tear the IVC. A completion venogram is taken through the remaining outer sheath to ensure that the cava is uninjured and free of residual thrombus. For the OptEase filter, femoral access is obtained, and the snare is used on the caudal hook to recapture the IVC filter in a similar fashion.

Troubleshooting: Retrieval

IVC filters can occasionally be difficult to retrieve because the position of the filter prevents successful snaring of the hook. A significant tilt of the filter can embed the hook into the caval wall or angle it into the orifice of a renal vein. An elusive hook can frustrate efforts to retrieve a filter even when the filter appears to be centered, as anterior/posterior tilt is difficult to appreciate in standard, non-angled fluoroscopy. To correct IVC filter tilt, a large caliber balloon can be advanced from the femoral approach, inflated above the filter, and retracted. The balloon can also be positioned between the IVC filter and the caval wall to push the filter away from the caval wall in an attempt to dislodge and expose the hook [117]. Endobronchial forceps can also be used to directly grasp and pull on the IVC filter to expose its hook. A Glidewire (Terumo, Somerset, NJ) can be passed through the apex of the filter, snared from below, and used as a loop for retraction. The term "loop wire" or "flossing" has been coined to describe this technique aimed at correcting difficult IVC filter tilt [118].

All advanced techniques for IVC filter retrieval should be used with caution since they carry the risk of fracture or entanglement of snares and wires within the IVC filter struts. Difficult IVC filter retrievals warrant the administration of heparin as clot usually builds up around wires. It is always more prudent to leave a filter in place and abandon efforts at retrieval instead of creating situation where open surgical IVC foreign body retrieval is necessary.

Retrieval Rates

Despite the commercial success and theoretic advantages of retrievable IVC filters, the rate of filter retrieval remains low. A single-center study reviewing IVC filter placements and retrievals between 2001 and 2006 found that only 30.4 % of patients had documented plans for filter retrieval. A history of cancer and lack of anticoagulation predicted lower retrieval rates, but 21.6 % of patients without retrieval attempts did not have any contraindications to retrieval [119]. Although technical issues can preclude the retrieval of some filters, most non-retrieval cases result from losing patients in follow-up due to physician inattention or patient noncompliance. Retrieval rates significantly increase with the establishment of dedicated filter clinics which allow for the clinician who placed the filter to arrange for retrieval. Studies on dedicated filter clinics show that the increase in retrieval rate was not related to a decrease in technical failures but reflected more meticulous patient management [120, 121].

FDA Warning

In August of 2010, the FDA issued a warning regarding nearly 1,000 reports of adverse events involving retrievable IVC filters. The warning included the following statements:

> …IVC filters, intended for short-term placement, are not always removed once a patient's risk for PE subsides. Known long term risks associated with IVC filters include but are not limited to lower limb deep vein thrombosis (DVT), filter fracture, filter migration, filter embolization and IVC perforation… The FDA recommends that implanting physicians and clinicians responsible for the ongoing care of patients with retrievable IVC filters consider removing the filter as soon as protection from PE is no longer needed [www.fda.gov/MedWatch/report.htm].

In light of this mandate, and the reported complications of long-term IVC filters, physicians must exercise discretion in selecting patients for IVC filter placement and remain committed to retrieving them if indicated.

IVC Filter Complications and Management

Insertion-site thrombosis occurs more often with large caliber sheaths and can be avoided by using filters with lower-profile delivery systems (Table 13.9) [70, 126]. Catheter-directed thrombolysis and percutaneous mechanical thrombectomy can be used to treat thrombotic IVC filter complications including DVT progression and filter thrombosis with subsequent renal failure [127]. Fracture of the IVC filter can decrease its ability to trap thromboemboli and predispose the device or its parts to embolize [128]. Pulmonary emboli that originate from trapped thrombus in the IVC filter can be managed with anticoagulation. Patients who cannot receive anticoagulation may require a second IVC filter placed above the original device to prevent further PE in these rare cases [122]. Filter migration that results from a megacava or central venous line exchange can induce a potentially fatal dysrhythmia if the dislodged filter travels into the right atrium [129]. A snare through the internal jugular vein can be used to recover an embolized IVC filter; however, immediate surgical extraction may be necessary if the clinical condition deteriorates or the filter migrates further into the pulmonary artery, making percutaneous retrieval difficult or impractical.

Table 13.9 IVC filter complications

Complication	Incidence (%)	Pivotal studies
Perioperative complications		[122–124]
Improper placement	1.3	
Pneumothorax	0.02	
Hematoma	0.6	
Air embolism	0.2	
Arterial puncture	0.04	
Arteriovenous fistula	0.02	
Insertion-site thrombosis	0.4–1.8	
Late complications		[2, 28, 103, 123, 125]
IVC thrombosis	2–9.5	
IVC penetration	4.4	
Migration	1–18	
Filter embolization	2–5	
Filter fracture	2–10	
Recurrent PE	1.3	
Recurrent DVT	6–36	
Mortality	0.12	[5]

Extraluminal penetration of the IVC by a leg of the filter rarely causes symptoms and is typically detected as an incidental finding during radiographic imaging. While the incidence of asymptomatic IVC penetration can be high (40 % for the Greenfield filter and 37 % for the Bird's Nest filter), symptomatic IVC penetration occurs at a much lower rate [103, 130–132]. Reports describing filter legs piercing the aorta, duodenum, or ureter represent serious but rare clinical manifestations of IVC filter penetration. Although some experts recommend surgical treatment for both asymptomatic and symptomatic caval penetrations to avoid unpredictable complications, observation remains the most common management strategy for patients with asymptomatic caval penetration. Percutaneously removing a filter that has penetrated the IVC is often technically difficult due to its incorporation into the wall of the IVC and adjacent tissues. Open surgical intervention is often necessary to remove the filter and repair of adjacent organ injury; however, endovascular approaches to deal with filter complications in specific contexts have also been described [133–137].

Conclusions

Inferior vena caval interruption to prevent PE has evolved over the last 50 years from a morbid open surgical operation with inconsistent results to a 15-min percutaneous procedure with reliable technical success. The ease of placing an IVC filter and the emergence of retrievable filters triggered an exponential increase in filter use. Although IVC filters provide safe and effective protection against PE, the widespread use of filters should not be misinterpreted as an endorsement of their benign nature. IVC filters carry short- and long-term risks which become especially relevant for young patients treated with prophylactic filters. Safe and cost-effective decisions about whether to place an IVC filter should balance the risk of a filter-related complication with the likelihood of a PE without an IVC filter. Despite a growing list of relative indications, the absolute indications for placing an IVC filter remain unchanged and include: a documented VTE with contraindication to anticoagulation, recurrent VTE despite adequate anticoagulation, and discontinuation of anticoagulation due to complications in the context of a documented VTE. In most cases, therapeutic anticoagulation should be started as soon as possible followed by IVC filter removal if it is feasible. If a patient receives a prophylactic IVC filter, it should be removed as soon as the patient can receive effective thromboprophylaxis or when the patient's thrombotic risk returns to baseline. Increasing filter retrieval rates requires the concerted effort of clinicians and institutions to raise awareness of the risks associated with IVC filters and to establish filter clinics and protocols that improve patient follow-up.

Acknowledgements The authors would like to thank Drs. Efthimios Avgerinos and Andrew Leake for their contribution of fluoroscopic images (Fig. 13.2).

References

1. White RH. The epidemiology of venous thromboembolism. Circulation. 2003;107(23 Suppl 1):I4–8.
2. Athanasoulis CA, et al. Inferior vena caval filters: review of a 26-year single-center clinical experience. Radiology. 2000;216(1): 54–66.
3. Kim HS, et al. A comparison of clinical outcomes with retrievable and permanent inferior vena cava filters. J Vasc Interv Radiol. 2008;19(3):393–9.
4. Stein PD, Kayali F, Olson RE. Twenty-one-year trends in the use of inferior vena cava filters. Arch Intern Med. 2004;164(14):1541–5.
5. Becker DM, Philbrick JT, Selby JB. Inferior vena cava filters. Indications, safety, effectiveness. Arch Intern Med. 1992;152(10): 1985–94.
6. Nabseth DC, Moran JM. Reassessment of the role of inferior-vena-cava ligation in venous thromboembolism. N Engl J Med. 1965;273(23):1250–3.
7. Amador E, Li TK, Crane C. Ligation of inferior vena cava for thromboembolism. Clinical and autopsy correlations in 119 cases. JAMA. 1968;206(8):1758–60.
8. Askew AR, Gardner AM. Long-term follow-up of partial caval occlusion by clip. Am J Surg. 1980;140(3):441–3.
9. Burget Jr DE, et al. Inferior vena cava plication for prevention of pulmonary embolism: results in 24 cases. Ann Surg. 1967;165(3): 437–41.
10. Couch NP, Baldwin SS, Crane C. Mortality and morbidity rates after inferior vena caval clipping. Surgery. 1975;77(1):106–12.
11. Harlal A, Ojha M, Johnston KW. Vena cava filter performance based on hemodynamic and reported thrombosis and pulmonary embolism patterns. J Vasc Interv Radiol. 2007;18(1):103–15.
12. Wolf G, Altmann E. [Long-term follow-up of Mobin-Uddin umbrella filter implantation for prevention of pulmonary embolism]. Vasa. 1993;22(1):68–74.
13. Mobin-Uddin K, et al. Transvenous caval interruption with umbrella filter. N Engl J Med. 1972;286(2):55–8.
14. Greenfield LJ, et al. A new intracaval filter permitting continued flow and resolution of emboli. Surgery. 1973;73(4):599–606.
15. Greenfield LJ, Proctor MC. Twenty-year clinical experience with the Greenfield filter. Cardiovasc Surg. 1995;3(2):199–205.
16. Tadavarthy SM, et al. Kimray-Greenfield vena cava filter: percutaneous introduction. Radiology. 1984;151(2):525–6.
17. Guyatt GH, et al. Introduction to the ninth edition: antithrombotic therapy and prevention of thrombosis, 9th ed: American College of Chest Physicians Evidence-Based Clinical Practice Guidelines. Chest. 2012;141(2 Suppl):48S–52.
18. Kearon C, et al. Antithrombotic therapy for VTE disease: antithrombotic therapy and prevention of thrombosis, 9th ed: American College of Chest Physicians Evidence-Based Clinical Practice Guidelines. Chest. 2012;141(2 Suppl):e419S–94.
19. Baadh AS, et al. Indications for inferior vena cava filter placement: do physicians comply with guidelines? J Vasc Interv Radiol. 2012;23(8):989–95.
20. Hirsh J, et al. Executive summary: American College of Chest Physicians Evidence-Based Clinical Practice Guidelines (8th edition). Chest. 2008;133(6 Suppl):71S–109.
21. Kaufman JA, et al. Guidelines for the use of retrievable and convertible vena cava filters: report from the Society of Interventional Radiology multidisciplinary consensus conference. J Vasc Interv Radiol. 2006;17(3):449–59.
22. Ingber S, Geerts WH. Vena caval filters: current knowledge, uncertainties and practical approaches. Curr Opin Hematol. 2009;16(5):402–6.
23. Usoh F, et al. Long-term follow-up for superior vena cava filter placement. Ann Vasc Surg. 2009;23(3):350–4.
24. Watanabe S, et al. Superior vena caval placement of a temporary filter: a case report. Vasc Surg. 2001;35(1):59–62.
25. Ascher E, et al. Lessons learned from a 6-year clinical experience with superior vena cava Greenfield filters. J Vasc Surg. 2000; 32(5):881–7.
26. Decousus H, et al. A clinical trial of vena caval filters in the prevention of pulmonary embolism in patients with proximal deep-vein thrombosis. Prevention du Risque d'Embolie Pulmonaire par Interruption Cave Study Group. N Engl J Med. 1998;338(7): 409–15.
27. PREPIC Study Group. Eight-year follow-up of patients with permanent vena cava filters in the prevention of pulmonary embolism: the PREPIC (Prevention du Risque d'Embolie Pulmonaire par Interruption Cave) randomized study. Circulation. 2005; 112(3):416–22.
28. Angel LF, et al. Systematic review of the use of retrievable inferior vena cava filters. J Vasc Interv Radiol. 2011;22(11):1522–1530.e3.
29. Anaya DA, Nathens AB. Thrombosis and coagulation: deep vein thrombosis and pulmonary embolism prophylaxis. Surg Clin North Am. 2005;85(6):1163–77, ix–x.
30. Geerts WH, et al. A prospective study of venous thromboembolism after major trauma. N Engl J Med. 1994;331(24):1601–6.
31. Meyer CS, et al. Surveillance venous scans for deep venous thrombosis in multiple trauma patients. Ann Vasc Surg. 1995; 9(1):109–14.
32. Winchell RJ, et al. Risk factors associated with pulmonary embolism despite routine prophylaxis: implications for improved protection. J Trauma. 1994;37(4):600–6.
33. Shackford SR, et al. Venous thromboembolism in patients with major trauma. Am J Surg. 1990;159(4):365–9.
34. Geerts WH, et al. Prevention of venous thromboembolism: American College of Chest Physicians Evidence-Based Clinical Practice Guidelines (8th edition). Chest. 2008;133(6 Suppl):381S–453.
35. Kirilcuk NN, et al. Are temporary inferior vena cava filters really temporary? Am J Surg. 2005;190(6):858–63.

36. Antevil JL, et al. Retrievable vena cava filters for preventing pulmonary embolism in trauma patients: a cautionary tale. J Trauma. 2006;60(1):35–40.
37. Quirke TE, Ritota PC, Swan KG. Inferior vena caval filter use in U.S. trauma centers: a practitioner survey. J Trauma. 1997;43(2): 333–7.
38. Cherry RA, et al. Prophylactic inferior vena cava filters: do they make a difference in trauma patients? J Trauma. 2008;65(3): 544–8.
39. Velmahos GC, et al. Prevention of venous thromboembolism after injury: an evidence-based report–part II: analysis of risk factors and evaluation of the role of vena caval filters. J Trauma. 2000; 49(1):140–4.
40. Velmahos GC, et al. Prevention of venous thromboembolism after injury: an evidence-based report–part I: analysis of risk factors and evaluation of the role of vena caval filters. J Trauma. 2000; 49(1):132–8; discussion 139.
41. McMurtry AL, et al. Increased use of prophylactic vena cava filters in trauma patients failed to decrease overall incidence of pulmonary embolism. J Am Coll Surg. 1999;189(3):314–20.
42. Sing RF, et al. Bedside insertion of inferior vena cava filters in the intensive care unit. J Trauma. 1999;47(6):1104–7.
43. Khansarinia S, et al. Prophylactic Greenfield filter placement in selected high-risk trauma patients. J Vasc Surg. 1995;22(3):231–5; discussion 235–6.
44. Carlin AM, et al. Prophylactic and therapeutic inferior vena cava filters to prevent pulmonary emboli in trauma patients. Arch Surg. 2002;137(5):521–5; discussion 525–7.
45. Rodriguez JL, et al. Early placement of prophylactic vena caval filters in injured patients at high risk for pulmonary embolism. J Trauma. 1996;40(5):797–802; discussion 802–4.
46. Spangler EL, Dillavou ED, Smith KJ. Cost-effectiveness of guidelines for insertion of inferior vena cava filters in high-risk trauma patients. J Vasc Surg. 2010;52(6):1537–45.e1–2.
47. Rogers FB, et al. Practice management guidelines for the prevention of venous thromboembolism in trauma patients: the EAST practice management guidelines work group. J Trauma. 2002; 53(1):142–64.
48. Geerts WH. Prevention of venous thromboembolism in high-risk patients. Hematology Am Soc Hematol Educ Program. 2006: 462–6.
49. Austin MS, et al. The inferior vena cava filter is effective in preventing fatal pulmonary embolus after hip and knee arthroplasties. J Arthroplasty. 2007;22(3):343–8.
50. Strauss EJ, et al. The use of retrievable inferior vena cava filters in orthopaedic patients. J Bone Joint Surg Br. 2008;90(5):662–7.
51. Prandoni P, et al. Recurrent venous thromboembolism and bleeding complications during anticoagulant treatment in patients with cancer and venous thrombosis. Blood. 2002;100(10):3484–8.
52. Elting LS, et al. Outcomes and cost of deep venous thrombosis among patients with cancer. Arch Intern Med. 2004;164(15): 1653–61.
53. Schunn C, et al. Inferior vena cava filter placement in late-stage cancer. Vasc Endovascular Surg. 2006;40(4):287–94.
54. Cohen JR, Grella L, Citron M. Greenfield filter instead of heparin as primary treatment for deep venous thrombosis or pulmonary embolism in patients with cancer. Cancer. 1992;70(7):1993–6.
55. Lee AY, et al. Low-molecular-weight heparin versus a coumarin for the prevention of recurrent venous thromboembolism in patients with cancer. N Engl J Med. 2003;349(2):146–53.
56. Eifler AC, et al. Optional or permanent: clinical factors that optimize inferior vena cava filter utilization. J Vasc Interv Radiol. 2013;24(1):35–40.
57. Agnelli G. Prevention of venous thromboembolism in surgical patients. Circulation. 2004;110(24 Suppl 1):IV4–12.
58. Krivak TC, Zorn KK. Venous thromboembolism in obstetrics and gynecology. Obstet Gynecol. 2007;109(3):761–77.
59. Aburahma AF, Mullins DA. Endovascular caval interruption in pregnant patients with deep vein thrombosis of the lower extremity. J Vasc Surg. 2001;33(2):375–8.
60. Matchett WJ, et al. Suprarenal vena caval filter placement: follow-up of four filter types in 22 patients. J Vasc Interv Radiol. 1998; 9(4):588–93.
61. Hamad GG, Bergqvist D. Venous thromboembolism in bariatric surgery patients: an update of risk and prevention. Surg Obes Relat Dis. 2007;3(1):97–102.
62. Goldhaber SZ, et al. A prospective study of risk factors for pulmonary embolism in women. JAMA. 1997;277(8):642–5.
63. Prystowsky JB, et al. Prospective analysis of the incidence of deep venous thrombosis in bariatric surgery patients. Surgery. 2005;138(4):759–63. discussion 763–5.
64. Scholten DJ, Hoedema RM, Scholten SE. A comparison of two different prophylactic dose regimens of low molecular weight heparin in bariatric surgery. Obes Surg. 2002;12(1):19–24.
65. Kalfarentzos F, et al. Prophylaxis of venous thromboembolism using two different doses of low-molecular-weight heparin (nadroparin) in bariatric surgery: a prospective randomized trial. Obes Surg. 2001;11(6):670–6.
66. Birkmeyer NJ, et al. Preoperative placement of inferior vena cava filters and outcomes after gastric bypass surgery. Ann Surg. 2010; 252(2):313–8.
67. Obeid FN, et al. Efficacy of prophylactic inferior vena cava filter placement in bariatric surgery. Surg Obes Relat Dis. 2007;3(6): 606–8; discussion 609–10.
68. Gargiulo 3rd NJ, et al. Experience with inferior vena cava filter placement in patients undergoing open gastric bypass procedures. J Vasc Surg. 2006;44(6):1301–5.
69. Trigilio-Black CM, et al. Inferior vena cava filter placement for pulmonary embolism risk reduction in super morbidly obese undergoing bariatric surgery. Surg Obes Relat Dis. 2007;3(4): 461–4.
70. Gorman PH, Qadri SF, Rao-Patel A. Prophylactic inferior vena cava (IVC) filter placement may increase the relative risk of deep venous thrombosis after acute spinal cord injury. J Trauma. 2009; 66(3):707–12.
71. Richard 3rd H, Widlus DM, Scalea TM. Inferior vena cava filters in trauma: balancing pulmonary embolism prevention with the risk of deep venous thrombosis. J Trauma. 2010;69(4):1003; author reply 1003–4.
72. Savin MA, et al. Placement of vena cava filters: factors affecting technical success and immediate complications. AJR Am J Roentgenol. 2002;179(3):597–602.
73. Danetz JS, et al. Selective venography versus nonselective venography before vena cava filter placement: evidence for more, not less. J Vasc Surg. 2003;38(5):928–34.
74. Isaacson S, Gray RR, Pugash RA. Manipulation by catheter of unopened LGM filter. Can Assoc Radiol J. 1993;44(3): 217–20.
75. Baron HC, et al. Bilateral iliac vein filter deployment in a patient with megacava. Ann Vasc Surg. 1999;13(6):634–6.
76. Chiou AC. Intravascular ultrasound-guided bedside placement of inferior vena cava filters. Semin Vasc Surg. 2006;19(3): 150–4.
77. Conners 3rd MS, et al. Duplex scan-directed placement of inferior vena cava filters: a five-year institutional experience. J Vasc Surg. 2002;35(2):286–91.
78. Garrett JV, et al. Expanding options for bedside placement of inferior vena cava filters with intravascular ultrasound when transabdominal duplex ultrasound imaging is inadequate. Ann Vasc Surg. 2004;18(3):329–34.

79. Jacobs DL, Motaganahalli RL, Peterson BG. Bedside vena cava filter placement with intravascular ultrasound: a simple, accurate, single venous access method. J Vasc Surg. 2007;46(6):1284–6.
80. Proctor MC, Greenfield LJ. Form and function of vena cava filters: how do optional filters measure up? Vascular. 2008;16(1):10–6.
81. Kantor A, et al. Percutaneous insertion of the Kimray-Greenfield filter: incidence of femoral vein thrombosis. AJR Am J Roentgenol. 1987;149(5):1065–6.
82. Roehm Jr JO, Thomas JW. The twist technique: a method to minimize wire prolapse during Bird's Nest filter placement. J Vasc Interv Radiol. 1995;6(3):455–9.
83. Thomas JH, et al. Vena caval occlusion after bird's nest filter placement. Am J Surg. 1998;176(6):598–600.
84. Nicholson AA, et al. Long-term follow-up of the Bird's Nest IVC Filter. Clin Radiol. 1999;54(11):759–64.
85. Murphy TP, et al. LGM vena cava filter: objective evaluation of early results. J Vasc Interv Radiol. 1991;2(1):107–15.
86. Crochet DP, et al. Long-term follow-up of Vena Tech-LGM filter: predictors and frequency of caval occlusion. J Vasc Interv Radiol. 1999;10(2 Pt 1):137–42.
87. Simon M, et al. Simon nitinol inferior vena cava filter: initial clinical experience. Work in progress. Radiology. 1989;172(1):99–103.
88. Leask RL, Johnston KW, Ojha M. In vitro hemodynamic evaluation of a Simon nitinol vena cava filter: possible explanation of IVC occlusion. J Vasc Interv Radiol. 2001;12(5):613–8.
89. Poletti PA, et al. Long-term results of the Simon nitinol inferior vena cava filter. Eur Radiol. 1998;8(2):289–94.
90. Oliva VL, et al. The Jonas study: evaluation of the retrievability of the Cordis OptEase inferior vena cava filter. J Vasc Interv Radiol. 2005;16(11):1439–45; quiz 1445.
91. Schutzer R, et al. Preliminary results of the new 6 F TrapEase inferior vena cava filter. Ann Vasc Surg. 2003;17(1):103–6.
92. Corriere MA, et al. Vena cava filters and inferior vena cava thrombosis. J Vasc Surg. 2007;45(4):789–94.
93. Mahrer A, et al. Retrievable vena cava filters in major trauma patients: prevalence of thrombus within the filter. Cardiovasc Intervent Radiol. 2008;31(4):785–9.
94. Grande WJ, et al. Experience with the recovery filter as a retrievable inferior vena cava filter. J Vasc Interv Radiol. 2005;16(9):1189–93.
95. Oliva VL, et al. Recovery G2 inferior vena cava filter: technical success and safety of retrieval. J Vasc Interv Radiol. 2008;19(6):884–9.
96. Rosenthal D, et al. Retrievability of the Gunther Tulip vena cava filter after dwell times longer than 180 days in patients with multiple trauma. J Endovasc Ther. 2007;14(3):406–10.
97. Millward SF. Gunther Tulip retrievable filter: why, when and how? Can Assoc Radiol J. 2001;52(3):188–92.
98. Millward SF, et al. Gunther tulip retrievable vena cava filter: results from the Registry of the Canadian Interventional Radiology Association. J Vasc Interv Radiol. 2001;12(9):1053–8.
99. Van Ha TG, et al. Techniques used for difficult retrievals of the Gunther Tulip inferior vena cava filter: experience in 32 patients. J Vasc Interv Radiol. 2009;20(1):92–9.
100. Van Ha TG, et al. Use of retrievable compared to permanent inferior vena cava filters: a single-institution experience. Cardiovasc Intervent Radiol. 2008;31(2):308–15.
101. Looby S, et al. Gunther Tulip retrievable inferior vena caval filters: indications, efficacy, retrieval, and complications. Cardiovasc Intervent Radiol. 2007;30(1):59–65.
102. Sangwaiya MJ, et al. Safety and effectiveness of the celect inferior vena cava filter: preliminary results. J Vasc Interv Radiol. 2009; 20(9):1188–92.
103. Bogue CO, et al. Symptomatic caval penetration by a Celect inferior vena cava filter. Pediatr Radiol. 2009;39(10):1110–3.
104. Caronno R, et al. Mid-term experience with the ALN retrievable inferior vena cava filter. Eur J Vasc Endovasc Surg. 2006;32(5):596–9.
105. Imberti D, et al. Clinical experience with retrievable vena cava filters: results of a prospective observational multicenter study. J Thromb Haemost. 2005;3(7):1370–5.
106. Murphy EH, et al. Crux vena cava filter. Expert Rev Med Devices. 2009;6(5):477–85.
107. Kinney TB. Update on inferior vena cava filters. J Vasc Interv Radiol. 2003;14(4):425–40.
108. Johnson MS, et al. The safety and effectiveness of the retrievable option inferior vena cava filter: a United States prospective multicenter clinical study. J Vasc Interv Radiol. 2010;21(8):1173–84.
109. Mismetti P, et al. A prospective long-term study of 220 patients with a retrievable vena cava filter for secondary prevention of venous thromboembolism. Chest. 2007;131(1):223–9.
110. De Gregorio MA, et al. Retrieval of Gunther Tulip optional vena cava filters 30 days after implantation: a prospective clinical study. J Vasc Interv Radiol. 2006;17(11 Pt 1):1781–9.
111. Hoppe H, et al. Gunther Tulip filter retrievability multicenter study including CT follow-up: final report. J Vasc Interv Radiol. 2006;17(6):1017–23.
112. Yale SH, et al. Recurrent venous thromboembolism in patients with and without anticoagulation after inferior vena caval filter placement. Int Angiol. 2006;25(1):60–6.
113. Sakuma M, et al. Inferior vena cava filter is a new additional therapeutic option to reduce mortality from acute pulmonary embolism. Circ J. 2004;68(9):816–21.
114. Binkert CA, Bansal A, Gates JD. Inferior vena cava filter removal after 317-day implantation. J Vasc Interv Radiol. 2005;16(3):395–8.
115. Smouse HB, et al. Long-term retrieval success rate profile for the Gunther Tulip vena cava filter. J Vasc Interv Radiol. 2009;20(7):871–7; quiz 878.
116. Pellerin O, et al. Early and late retrieval of the ALN removable vena cava filter: results from a multicenter study. Cardiovasc Intervent Radiol. 2008;31(5):889–96.
117. Lynch FC. Balloon-assisted removal of tilted inferior vena cava filters with embedded tips. J Vasc Interv Radiol. 2009;20(9):1210–4.
118. Rubenstein L, et al. Loop-snare technique for difficult inferior vena cava filter retrievals. J Vasc Interv Radiol. 2007;18(10):1315–8.
119. Mission JF, et al. Rates and predictors of plans for inferior vena cava filter retrieval in hospitalized patients. J Gen Intern Med. 2010;25(4):321–5.
120. Minocha J, et al. Improving inferior vena cava filter retrieval rates: impact of a dedicated inferior vena cava filter clinic. J Vasc Interv Radiol. 2010;21(12):1847–51.
121. Ko SH, et al. Institutional protocol improves retrievable inferior vena cava filter recovery rate. Surgery. 2009;146(4):809–14; discussion 814–6.
122. Nicholson W, et al. Prevalence of fracture and fragment embolization of Bard retrievable vena cava filters and clinical implications including cardiac perforation and tamponade. Arch Intern Med. 2010;170(20):1827–31.
123. Joels CS, Sing RF, Heniford BT. Complications of inferior vena cava filters. Am Surg. 2003;69(8):654–9.
124. Ray Jr CE, Kaufman JA. Complications of inferior vena cava filters. Abdom Imaging. 1996;21(4):368–74.
125. Grassi CJ, et al. Quality improvement guidelines for percutaneous permanent inferior vena cava filter placement for the prevention of pulmonary embolism. J Vasc Interv Radiol. 2003;14(9 Pt 2):S271–5.
126. Blebea J, et al. Deep venous thrombosis after percutaneous insertion of vena caval filters. J Vasc Surg. 1999;30(5):821–8.

127. Yan BP, et al. Combined pharmacomechanical thrombectomy for acute inferior vena cava filter thrombosis. Cardiovasc Revasc Med. 2008;9(1):36–40.
128. Johnson MS. Vena cava filter fracture: unplanned obsolescence. J Vasc Interv Radiol. 2012;23(2):196–8.
129. Haddadian B, et al. Sudden cardiac death caused by migration of a TrapEase inferior vena cava filter: case report and review of the literature. Clin Cardiol. 2008;31(2):84–7.
130. Proctor MC, et al. Assessment of apparent vena caval penetration by the Greenfield filter. J Endovasc Surg. 1998;5(3):251–8.
131. Feezor RJ, et al. Duodenal perforation with an inferior vena cava filter: an unusual cause of abdominal pain. J Vasc Surg. 2002; 35(5):1010–2.
132. Streiff MB. Vena caval filters: a comprehensive review. Blood. 2000;95(12):3669–77.
133. Shang EK, et al. Delayed complications of inferior vena cava filters: case report and literature review. Vasc Endovascular Surg. 2011;45(3):290–4.
134. Siepe M, et al. Aorto-caval fistula from acute rupture of an abdominal aortic aneurysm treated with a hybrid approach. J Vasc Surg. 2009;49(6):1574–6.
135. Sparrow P. Double whammy: inferior vena cava filter-related perforation and thrombosis of the inferior vena cava and aorta. Circulation. 2011;123(7):e245-6.
136. Veroux M, et al. Late complication from a retrievable inferior vena cava filter with associated caval, aortic, and duodenal perforation: a case report. J Vasc Surg. 2008;48(1):223–5.
137. Becher RD, et al. Late erosion of a prophylactic Celect IVC filter into the aorta, right renal artery, and duodenal wall. J Vasc Surg. 2010;52(4):1041–4.

Part V

Vascular Trauma

Vascular Injuries in the Neck

14

Mathew Adam Schechter, Patrick Joshua O'Brien, and Mitchell W. Cox

Although vascular surgeons, neurosurgeons, and interventional radiologists perform most elective interventions on the vasculature of the head and neck, Cervical trauma remains the province of the general surgeon. While long-term management of severe cervical trauma may require the input of a multidisciplinary team, only the general surgeon must decide what to do when confronted with a patient who is rapidly exsanguinating from a transcervical gunshot wound. In the neck, the close juxtaposition of critical structures including the spine, aerodigestive tract, and cerebral vasculature creates some particularly challenging and high-stress clinical situations. Fortunately, even nonspecialists who not routinely perform elective vascular procedures on the head and neck can evaluate, stabilize, expose, and repair traumatic neck injuries by relying on basic knowledge of the relevant anatomy, imaging modalities, and treatment algorithms.

Initial Evaluation and Imaging

Blunt or penetrating trauma to the vasculature of the neck can often result in immediately life-threatening injuries, with significant potential for exsanguination, airway compression, or ischemic stroke. Given these devastating outcomes, prompt surgical exploration with or without angiography has been the mainstay in evaluation and treatment of penetrating neck injuries for decades. In the past few years, however, new diagnostic and therapeutic strategies have been developed, which allow for prompt identification and management of vascular injuries without mandatory surgical exploration. While the care for neck wounds has undoubtedly improved over the years, the treatment algorithm has also become somewhat more complex.

When confronting a patient in the trauma bay, the evaluation and management of blunt and penetrating injuries proceeds along distinctly different lines, and trauma to the vasculature of the head and neck is no different. The mechanism of injury, presenting symptoms, workup, and management of blunt and penetrating neck injuries are vastly different and worth considering as separate entities.

Penetrating Neck Injuries

Incidence

Penetrating neck injuries account for 1 % of all traumas in the United States and have an associated mortality of 3–6 %. Most of the fatalities result from arterial damage, with 80 % of deaths in these cases resulting from ischemic stroke and the remaining 20 % from exsanguination. Firearms cause 45 % of penetrating injuries, stab wounds account for 40 %, and shotgun injuries cause approximately 4 % [1].

Classification

Penetrating neck injuries have traditionally been classified according to their zone of injury using the anatomic landmarks first described by Roon and Christensen in 1979 [2] (Fig. 14.1). Zone I extends from the clavicles to the cricoid cartilage. Zone II is from the cricoid cartilage to the angle of the mandible. Zone III includes the area above the angle of the mandible to the base of the skull. Zone II injuries are the most common (47 %), with Zone I injuries carrying the highest mortality rate [3]. In more complex penetrating neck injuries, such as blast or high-velocity gunshot wounds, use of this classification system may be limited. These types of injuries often involve multiple zones and can injure structures in the posterior neck (e.g., vertebral arteries), which this classification

M.A. Schechter, MD • M.W. Cox, MD (✉)
Department of Surgery, Duke University School of Medicine, Duke University Medical Center, 2301 Erwin Road, Box 2833, Durham, NC, USA
e-mail: mitchell.cox2@duke.edu

P.J. O'Brien, MD
Department of Surgery, International Heart Institute of Montana, St. Patrick Hospital, 500 W. Broadway, Missoula, MT 59802, USA

V. Gahtan and M.J. Costanza (eds.), *Essentials of Vascular Surgery for the General Surgeon*,
DOI 10.1007/978-1-4939-1326-8_14,

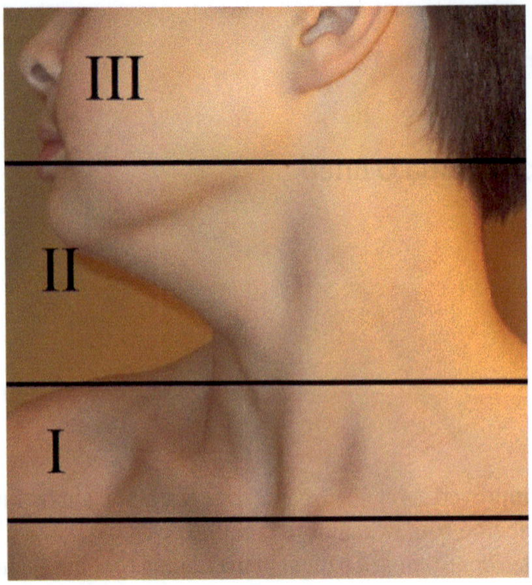

Fig. 14.1 Traditionally defined zones of the neck

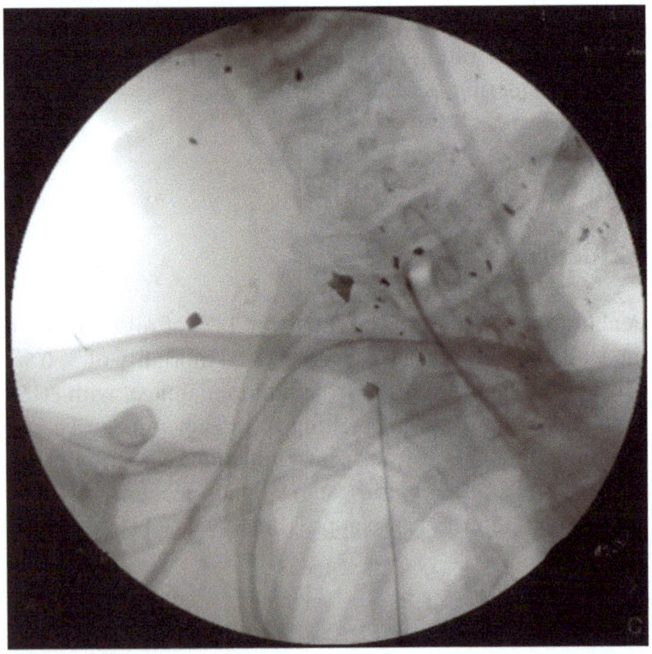

Fig. 14.2 This blast injury with multiple fragments bilaterally in zones I and II defies traditional classification

system largely ignores [4] (Fig. 14.2). The zone classification system has also become less relevant as mandatory exploration for Zone II injuries has fallen out of favor. Zone of injury does help determine the operative approach, and it remains a straightforward way to describe many injuries.

Initial Assessment

As with any significant trauma, initial assessment should proceed according the Advanced Trauma Life Support guidelines (the A, B, Cs) [5]. Patients with neck injuries can decompensate quickly, and the location of the injury puts the airway uniquely at risk. Therefore, securing an airway is essential in these patients, and there should be a very low threshold for intubation. Unfortunately, intubation can be difficult in a patient with a large neck hematoma, and advanced airway management techniques including early cricothyroidotomy or tracheostomy may be required.

Table 14.1 Hard signs of injury

Active bleeding with signs of hemorrhagic shock
Expanding hematoma
Bruit or thrill
Pulse defect
Evolving stroke

These are the classic "hard" signs of injury which are virtually diagnostic of vascular trauma which must be surgically addressed

While active arterial bleeding or an expanding hematoma can be dramatic, assessment for vascular injuries only occurs during the "C" portion of the primary survey. After the airway is secure, an immediate determination must be made as to whether the patient's injuries require urgent surgical attention. If the patient has any hard signs of vascular injury (Table 14.1), prompt surgical intervention will be required, and the remainder of the evaluation can proceed on that basis.

Diagnostic Imaging

The evaluation and management of the stable patient with a penetrating neck injury has evolved over the last couple of decades; however, these cases can still generate some controversy. Historically, the potential for a devastating missed vascular injury was the primary focus, and any Zone II penetrating injury deep to the platysma mandated prompt surgical exploration. Some studies reported injuries in as many as 30 % of patients undergoing surgery, and given the relatively limited morbidity of a neck incision, diagnostic exploration remains a safe course of action [6]. The drawback of mandatory neck exploration is a high rate of nontherapeutic surgery. One study reported a negative neck exploration rate of 98 % in asymptomatic patients [7]. In the mid-1990s, many trauma centers began using a selective approach to Zone II penetrating injuries. Stable patients with minimal symptoms may benefit from additional diagnostic imaging to determine if surgery is necessary. Catheter angiography continues to be the gold standard for detecting arterial pathology, with a sensitivity and specificity for major injuries approaching 100 % [8]. Angiography can accurately evaluate for injuries in all zones of the neck and has the advantage of being therapeutic as well as diagnostic. In the traditional approach to cervical vascular trauma, stable patients with Zone I and III injuries underwent diagnostic angiography, while all patients with

Zone II were surgically explored. Despite its advantages, angiography is an invasive procedure with a 1–2 % risk of complications, including puncture site hematomas, distal embolization of atheromatous plaques or thrombus, and arterial dissection [9]. Catheter angiograms also require technical expertise to perform, and trained personnel may not always be immediately available on-site. Waiting for the requisite support personnel to arrive may delay the diagnosis and treatment of an unstable patient. These limitations coupled with the relatively high negative angiography rates (ranging from 10 to 30 %) have allowed noninvasive imaging modalities to supplant catheter angiography as the preferred initial diagnostic study.

Helical computed tomographic angiography (CTA) has become faster and more available over the last decade allowing it to play a more prominent role in the assessment of penetrating neck trauma. A recent review on imaging for neck trauma which included multiple prospective studies comparing helical CTA to catheter angiography reported that the sensitivity and specificity for helical CTA ranged from 90 to 100 % [10]. A helical CTA of the neck can be done in minutes, with no need for direct physician intervention, thereby reducing the time to diagnose and treat cervical vascular injuries. Widely used standardized protocols have also made this test reproducible, and high-quality studies can be obtained in almost any institution. CTA enables the physician to assess soft-tissue injuries documenting any damage in the head or chest and potentially determine the trajectory of the missile. Tracing the trajectory of injury can facilitate prompt evaluation of injuries to other vital structures in the area including the spinal column and aerodigestive tract [4]. With 64-slice scanners and the most current software, multiplanar reformations and 3-dimensional reconstructions are immediately available, increasing the diagnostic yield of these studies. There have been only occasional reports of major vascular injuries that were missed by CT scan; however, the majority of these have involved venous injuries without significant hemorrhage [11]. Given its speed, immediate availability, and accuracy, CTA has become the de facto first-line study in most institutions for the stable patient with a penetrating neck injury.

Metallic implants or projectile fragments create imaging artifacts which degrade the diagnostic accuracy of CT scans. In these cases, catheter-based arteriography may be required to reach a definitive diagnosis. When multiple studies are required, patients can receive a large contrast load, which may adversely affect renal function. Rarely is there time to assess renal function in a rapidly evolving trauma situation, but if a trauma patient has known renal insufficiency, a directed catheter arteriogram can minimize overall contrast volume.

Although other noninvasive imaging modalities exist, they have a limited role in the evaluation of cervical trauma. Color Doppler ultrasonography has the potential advantage of being a portable, cheap, noninvasive test that does not require the intravenous contrast dye. Its drawbacks include the fact that it is operator-dependent, requires a long examination time, and can rarely evaluate for injuries to Zone I or III. Artifacts within the scanning field and bone or soft-tissue injuries also reduce the ability of ultrasound to evaluate cervical vascular structures. Magnetic resonance angiography (MRA) has occasionally been used to assess vascular injury following penetrating trauma, but it is a time-consuming study that requires MR-compatible equipment and on-site technical expertise for scanning protocols and interpretation. The potential presence of ferromagnetic fragments in the neck after trauma is a contraindication to MRA in many trauma situations.

Blunt Injuries

Incidence and Presentation

Although blunt cerebrovascular injuries occur in less 0.75 % of all trauma patients, they can have devastating consequences. Mortality rates of blunt carotid injuries range from 16 to 59 %, with 24 to 58 % of survivors having severe neurological deficits [12–17]. The extremely variable clinical presentation of blunt cerebrovascular injuries may account for their high morbidity and mortality. Traditional hard signs of vascular trauma are rarely apparent, and concomitant facial and head injuries can limit the physician's ability to pick up subtle alterations in the neurologic exam. There may also be a latent period between time of injury and the appearance of symptoms. Studies suggest that 25–50 % of patients develop symptoms more than 12 h after the traumatic event, and there have even been reports of symptoms presenting several days after the initial injury [13, 16, 17]. In contrast, some patients with minimal trauma due to a minor fender bender or sports injury can sustain a carotid dissection and present with a severe neurologic deficit. Such wide variability in presentation means a blunt cerebrovascular injury may not be readily appreciated or considered in the context of an unstable patient with multisystem blunt injury. While a stab or bullet wound to the neck immediately draws attention to the possibility of a cervical vascular injury, the differential diagnosis for a polytrauma patient with a low Glasgow Coma Score (GCS) is quite long. Evaluation and management should ideally focus on screening the appropriate patient cohort to detect this type of injury early.

Blunt cerebrovascular injury results from one of four mechanisms: hyperextension/rotation, direct force to the vessel, intraoral trauma, or laceration by bony fragments. These forces most commonly cause intimal damage with dissection and thrombus formation. Thrombus can either occlude the vessel completely or embolize to the cerebral circulation, while dissection can lead to pseudoaneurysm formation. In very rare cases, complete transection and exsanguination occurs. Motor vehicle accidents are the most common cause of blunt cerebrovascular injuries (41–70 %), while other mechanisms include pedestrians struck (17–33 %), assault (10–20 %), hanging, and sports injuries [14, 17]. Bilateral injuries occur in 18–41 % of cases [12, 16, 17]. Not surprisingly, blunt cerebrovascular injury is associated with injuries to other important structures, including closed head injuries (48–65 %), facial fractures (22–60 %), thoracic injuries (19–63 %), intra-abdominal injuries (16–30 %), and extremity fractures (25–39 %) [4, 13, 16, 17]. Not only do these associated injuries contribute to the delay in diagnosis, they also complicate subsequent management. A patient's carotid dissection might cause ischemic injury in some cases, but class IV hemorrhagic shock or a tension pneumothorax will cause death in short order, and management of these injuries takes precedence.

Although a majority of patients with blunt cerebrovascular injury have no obvious symptoms upon presentation, there are certain findings that should prompt immediate diagnostic imaging. These symptoms include arterial bleeding from the neck, mouth, ear, or nose; expanding hematoma, a cervical bruit in a patient less than 50 years old; and any lateralizing neurological deficits or Horner syndrome. Other findings on initial evaluation which may not have a high correlation with vascular injury include: high-energy mechanism, near hanging, seat-belt abrasion, cervical vertebral fracture, and diffuse axonal injury. As a general rule, a patient with neurologic deficits not explained by the findings on the initial head CT requires further evaluation. Liberal use of vascular imaging of the neck can avoid missing a cervical vascular injury in the clinical setting of severe blunt trauma and a decreased GCS.

For the asymptomatic blunt force trauma patient, the decision to proceed with neurovascular imaging is more difficult. A number of factors involving mechanism of injury, as well as certain physical findings, have been associated with blunt cerebrovascular injury (Table 14.2). Given the high morbidity and mortality associated with a missed blunt cerebrovascular injury, screening protocols have been developed to help identify asymptomatic patients at risk for these injuries (Table 14.3). The first widely implemented screening protocol was developed at the Denver Health Medical Center [13]. Based on this criteria, 4.8 % of trauma patients were screened, of which 18 % were found to have an injury [14]. Having one of the risk factors predicted a carotid injury in 33–48 % of patients, while all four risk factors predicted 93 % of injuries [14]. The second screening protocol, developed at the University of Tennessee in Memphis, resulted in 3.5 % of all trauma patients getting screened, with 29 % of screened patients found to have an injury [18]. Despite aggressive screening, over 20 % of patients with a blunt cerebrovascular injury will have none of the risk factors identified by these protocols (Table 14.4) [14–17]. A recent meta-analysis of common diagnostic screening criteria (basilar skull fracture, cervical abrasion, GCS <8 with head or neck injury, neurological deficit, and head, cervical spine, thoracic, or abdominal injury) found that only cervical spine and thoracic injury were significantly associated with blunt cerebrovascular injury [19]. This study does not advocate screening only patients with cervical spine or thoracic injuries, as occult blunt cerebrovascular injuries would certainly be missed. Instead, these studies emphasize the importance of considering

Table 14.2 Risk factors for blunt cerebrovascular injury

Arterial bleeding from neck, mouth, ear, or nose[a]
Expanding hematoma[a]
Cervical bruit (if patient less than 50 years old)[a]
Focal neurological deficit (e.g., hemiparesis, vertebrobasilar insufficiency, Horner syndrome)[a]
Unexplained neurologic symptoms[a]
Basilar skull fracture
Facial fractures
Closed head injury
Spinal cord injury (especially cervical spine)
Neck soft-tissue injury
– Stable hematoma
– Hanging or near hanging
– Clothesline-type injury
– The "seat-belt sign"

Classically described clinical findings which may be consistent with blunt cerebrovascular injury are presented
[a]If present, emergent diagnostic imaging required

Table 14.3 Screening protocols for blunt cerebrovascular injury

Denver criteria [13, 14]	Memphis criteria [18]
Signs/symptoms	Cervical spine fracture
Cervical hematoma	Unexplained neurologic deficit
Cervical bruit	Horner syndrome
Focal neurological deficit	Leforte II or III fracture pattern
Unexplained neurological deficit	Basilar skull fracture with involvement of the carotid canal
Risk factors Leforte II or III fracture pattern Basilar skull fracture with involvement of the carotid canal Head injury with GSC <6 Near hanging with anoxic brain injury Any cervical spine fracture[a]	Neck soft-tissue injury (i.e., seat-belt sign, hanging, or hematoma)

Criteria for screening in cases of blunt trauma to the head and neck as suggested by two major trauma centers are listed. The Denver group has documented a 70 % incidence of blunt cerebrovascular injury if any one of the signs and symptoms are evident and a 40 % incidence if any one of the risk factors are present. The Memphis study demonstrated a 29 % incidence of blunt cerebrovascular injury in patients with at least one of the listed criteria for screening. Both groups recommended aggressive screening in patients with evidence of severe head and neck trauma and any one of the listed clinical findings
[a]Risk factor for vertebral artery injury only

Table 14.4 Grading system for blunt cerebrovascular injury [23]

Injury grade	Criteria	Stroke incidence (%)
I	Luminal irregularity with <25 % narrowing	3
II	Intraluminal thrombus, dissection or intramural hematoma with >25 % narrowing	11
III	Pseudoaneurysm	33
IV	Occlusion	44
V	Transection with extravasation	100

the possibility of a cerebrovascular injury in a blunt force trauma patient with unexplained symptoms referable to the head and neck. Figure 14.6 demonstrates a carotid dissection in a patient who presented only with neck pain after sustaining a very minor sports-related trauma.

Diagnostic Imaging

Although arteriography remains the gold standard, CTA has become the screening test of choice for suspected blunt cerebrovascular injury, as evidenced by its integration into the practice guidelines of both the Eastern Association for the Surgery of Trauma [20] and the Western Trauma Association [21]. Most patients who have risk factors for blunt cerebrovascular injury have indications for scanning other regions of the body, and a CTA protocol can easily be incorporated into the imaging plan. The entire noninvasive study can be completed in less than 5 min with a contrast load which is not excessive. While initial studies questioned the sensitivity and specificity of CTA [18], more recent studies with experienced radiologists using 16- or 64-slice CT scanners found that the accuracy of CTA approached that of angiography [15, 22]. Accordingly, CTA has emerged as the test of choice for screening patients with suspected cerebrovascular injuries, with arteriography reserved for equivocal results or high clinical suspicion.

As with penetrating neck trauma, other noninvasive imaging modalities play a limited role in the evaluation of blunt cerebrovascular trauma. Duplex ultrasound by an experienced sonographer will often pick up flow abnormalities due to dissection, but it is an operator-dependent test that can only detect injury in Zone II. Small intimal tears and nonocclusive dissections usually go undetected by duplex ultrasound. MRA provides high resolution images free of bony artifact without the use of IV contrast. Although MRA may detect cerebral infarction earlier, the time required for image acquisition and logistical issues with unstable, ventilated trauma patients make it impractical for general use in the setting of trauma.

Management of Injuries

Initial Approach/Exposure

When confronting a cervical vascular injury, the approach and the incision depend on the clinical situation and the available diagnostic imaging. The first decision point involves determining whether the patient is stable enough for imaging or must proceed directly to the operating room. In the past, this was a more difficult decision, since CT scanning and angiography were prolonged events in remote locations, with a high potential for decompensation and disaster in the radiology department. Now most level-1 trauma centers have 64-slice CT scans located in close proximity to the trauma bay. CT angiograms have a very high diagnostic yield for both arterial and nonvascular injuries, allowing a relatively comprehensive evaluation in a short period of time. As a result, only patients with active exsanguination or rapidly expanding hematoma are taken for immediate neck exploration without any imaging.

Unstable Patients

A surgeon taking an unstable patient directly to the OR will not know the exact nature or location of the injury. This uncertainty highlights the importance of using versatile incisions with the ability to achieve exposure and proximal control rapidly. A standard carotid incision along the anterior border of the sternocleidomastoid muscle or a median sternotomy will be sufficient to address most instances of life-threatening hemorrhage. Fortunately, nearly all general surgeons can perform these exposures.

The traditionally defined zones of the neck provide a useful template for addressing active hemorrhage. A penetrating wound in Zone I or an expanding hematoma just above the clavicle should tip off the trauma surgeon to the need for proximal control in the chest. A median sternotomy provides the safest initial exposure for a Zone I injury. Rapid control of the proximal common carotid or innominate artery can be achieved, and the incision can be extended onto the neck along the sternocleidomastoid as needed for repair. Zone 1 injuries may also unexpectedly involve the subclavian artery, and extension of the incision to an anterior thoracotomy or across the clavicle may be required. Control of the left subclavian artery is difficult but possible through a median sternotomy but is most reliably achieved through an anterior thoracotomy in the third interspace.

With a clear-cut Zone II injury, a longitudinal incision along the anterior border of the sternocleidomastoid muscle, similar to that used for an elective carotid endarterectomy, will be adequate. The incision can be extended down to the sternum or up to the level of the mastoid as needed. The common carotid can either be isolated proximal to the

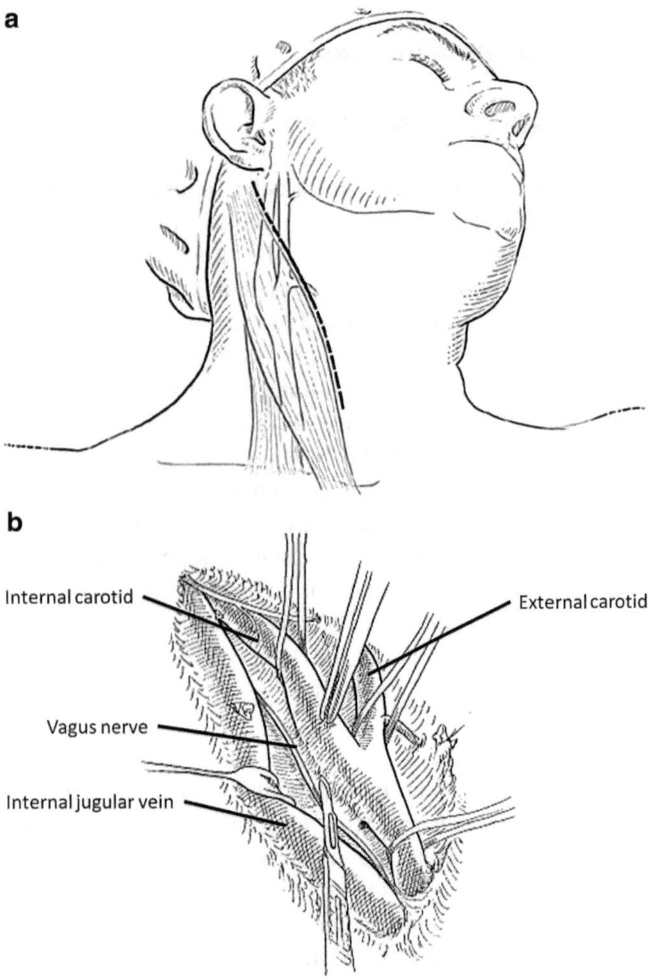

Fig. 14.3 (**a**, **b**) Diagram of a standard carotid/internal jugular exposure by incision along the anterior border of the sternocleidomastoid

injury or controlled with finger pressure as the dissection and identification of the injury proceeds. Most nonvascular injuries can also be addressed through an incision along the anterior border of the sternocleidomastoid muscle. If head and neck surgeons need to repair a laryngotracheal injury, the incision can be extended across the midline at the base of the neck, or a second contralateral incision can be made in the case of bilateral or transcervical injuries (Fig. 14.3).

Exposure of Zone III injuries usually begins with the standard carotid incision followed by a superior extension approximately 1 cm lateral and inferior to the angle of the mandible. True Zone III injuries to the internal carotid can be extremely difficult to control, and there are several well-described adjuncts for distal exposure including subluxation of the mandible or mandibular osteotomy. These maneuvers often require the assistance of maxillofacial surgery or otolaryngology and take time to implement. In practice, aggressive retraction, finger pressure, and Fogarty balloons are usually attempted to gain control in the setting of ongoing hemorrhage. Carotid ligation may, in fact, be the only option if distal exposure and vascular control cannot be achieved.

Stable Patients

Rapidly performed, extensive incisions with a high potential for morbidity can usually be avoided in stable patients. If the patient does not need to go to the operating room immediately, the surgeon has an opportunity to use imaging to define the injury and endovascular adjuncts for control and repair in locations that are difficult to expose. While traditional teaching emphasized surgical exploration for all deep Zone II injuries, preoperative imaging studies may be useful to identify associated nonvascular injuries, plan arterial repair, or even avoid surgery altogether. As mentioned previously, a CTA is usually the initial study of choice to identify and prioritize the various injuries. Repairing arterial injuries may require a combination of open and endovascular techniques, so appropriate imaging support, ideally in an OR with fixed imaging capability, is critical.

Injury to the subclavian artery low in the neck is a classic illustration of how endovascular intervention has almost totally supplanted open surgical approaches and their associated morbidity. Older literature advocated proximal arterial control with a left anterior thoracotomy or median sternotomy, followed by extension of the incision across the clavicle with possible claviculectomy if needed. In contrast, the technique involved in stent grafting a subclavian artery injury is almost trivial. The arterial injury can be excluded with a stent graft delivered percutaneously or via a small cutdown on the brachial or common femoral arteries (Fig. 14.4).

A stable patient with an injury that can be completely controlled through a neck incision along the anterior border of the sternocleidomastoid should have a standard surgical exploration and repair. For injuries to the more proximal carotid or subclavian arteries, or the more distal ICA, an endovascular approach may be indicated. The stability of the patient affords time to consult with vascular, head and neck, or thoracic surgery colleagues to formulate a plan that should only rarely require emergent, highly morbid surgical incisions such as the "open book" thoracotomy.

Arteriovenous Fistula

An arteriovenous fistula represents a rare presentation of penetrating cervical vascular trauma. Although an arteriovenous fistula may present with a bruit or thrill at the time of injury, the diagnosis can often be delayed, and it may only be detected as an incidental finding on CT scan. While a thrill or bruit is one of the hard signs of arterial injury, suspicion of an AVF in the head and neck need not provoke immediate operative exploration if the patient is otherwise stable. The fistula itself is almost never a life-threatening problem, and if neck exploration is not needed immediately to repair aerodigestive injuries, definitive therapy for the arteriovenous fistula can await comprehensive imaging evaluation and formulation of a multidisciplinary surgical plan. Figure 14.5 illustrates a case of carotid-jugular AV fistula after stab wound

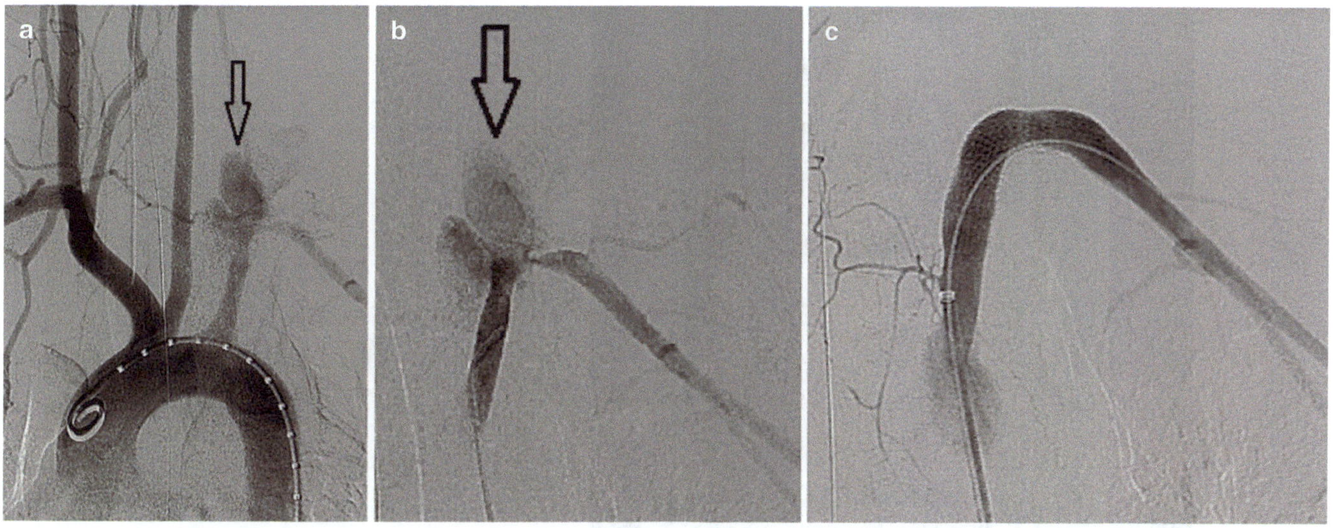

Fig. 14.4 This patient presented with a large hematoma after a stab wound to the neck in Zone I. CTA demonstrated a large pseudoaneurysm of the subclavian artery (arrow), and he was taken for arteriogram (**a**, **b**). The defect was repaired with a stent graft delivered via a femoral artery cutdown (**c**)

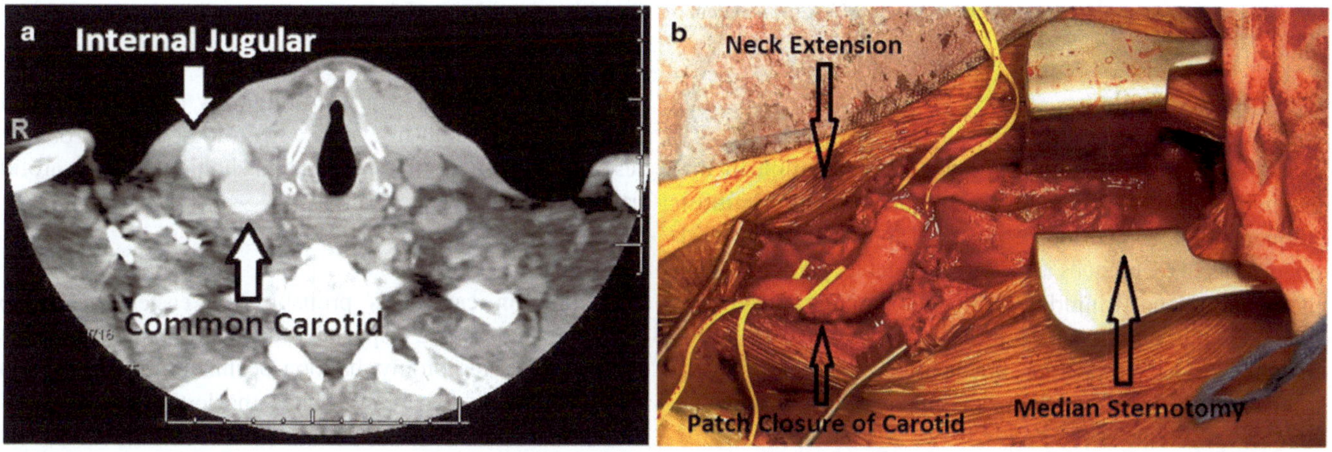

Fig. 14.5 This patient presented several years after a stab wound to the neck with a thrill palpable in Zone I and congestive heart failure. CTA demonstrated a common carotid to internal jugular fistula (**a**), and open repair was performed via a median sternotomy extended up onto the neck along the border of the sternocleidomastoid muscle (**b**). Endovascular repair with a stent graft was not feasible due to the large diameter of the involved vessels

which presented in a delayed fashion as high-output cardiac failure. Vascular injury was suspected based on a palpable thrill in the neck, confirmed by arteriography, and treated with a carotid patch angioplasty. Proximal control was achieved via median sternotomy.

Blunt Trauma

Blunt trauma to the neck causing a vascular injury should be considered in polytrauma patients who have a neurologic deficit in the absence of major intracranial pathology. A CTA of the neck can function as the definitive study, and treatment is almost always anticoagulation. Exceptions to this rule include patients with a fluctuating neurologic deficit or an injury that can be surgically addressed. These patients make up a small minority of cases, as the majority of patients with blunt vascular injury will present with a major fixed neurologic deficit and an occluded artery, or a minimal deficit with carotid dissection noted as an incidental finding on CT scan. A classification system for blunt carotid injury has been proposed by Biffl et al. which correlates the degree of injury with stroke risk [23].

Unfortunately, regardless of injury type or grade, therapeutic options for blunt cervical vascular trauma are limited. The rare patient with a very short intimal flap or a limited segment of severe narrowing may be amenable to stenting to re-expand the true lumen; however, anticoagulation with heparin/warfarin or antiplatelet medication remains the standard of care [24]. Figure 14.6 shows the CTA and arteriogram of a patient who presented with carotid dissection after a minor trauma.

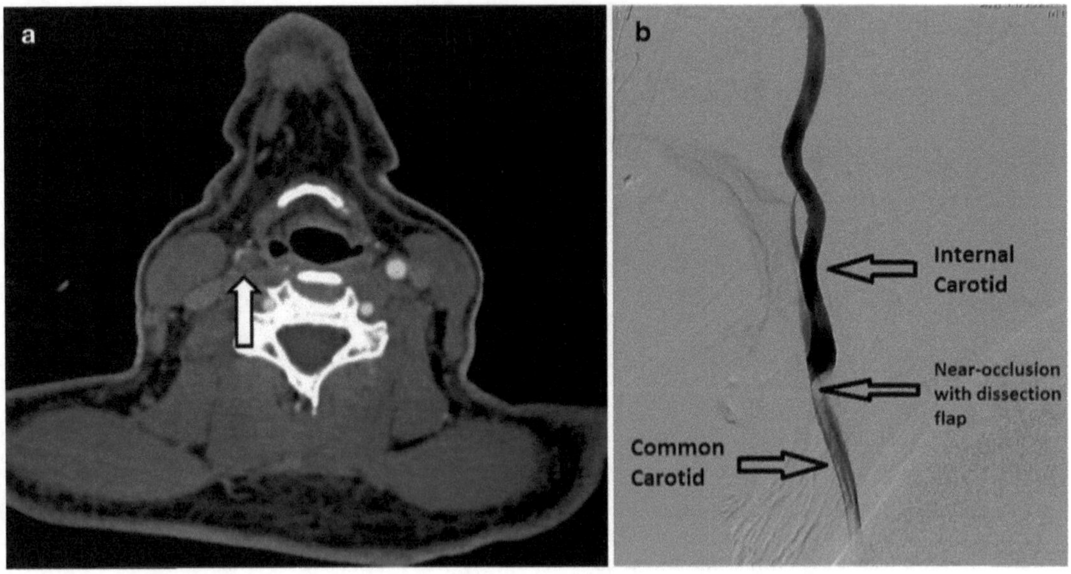

Fig. 14.6 This patient presented with neck pain, but no neurologic deficit after a very minor sports-related neck injury. Near occlusion of the distal common carotid artery (arrow) is seen on CTA (**a**) and demonstrated by arteriogram (**b**). Treatment was with systemic anticoagulation, and the injury healed with eventual restoration of normal arterial diameter and resolution of the neck pain

Operative Repair

Carotid injuries tend to receive the most attention in the evaluation of a polytrauma patient, and they are the most frequently treated with an open surgical approach. Traditional open surgical techniques are often applicable, particularly in the case of Zone II injuries, while endovascular maneuvers may be required to manage injuries in Zones I and III. In the most severe cases, repair may not be indicated at all, although this is a controversial strategy, and making firm recommendations is difficul.

There is no uncertainty regarding the treatment of patients with active bleeding or an expanding hematoma; they always require repair to control the hemorrhage and prevent exsanguination. Decision making and management becomes more challenging for carotid injuries that present with a neurologic defect due to arterial occlusion. Some case series suggest that repair of the carotid artery in the face of a fixed neurologic deficit risks converting a bland ischemic infarction into an intracranial bleed with potentially lethal consequences [25, 26]. In contrast, multiple series report that hemorrhagic conversion is rare and recommend repairing most carotid injuries, even in the setting of a major, fixed neurologic deficit. Overall, patients with a neurologic deficit have a poor outcome; however, the prognosis may be slightly less dismal for the individual patient who undergoes a successful carotid artery repair [27]. Clearly, there is room for discretion in most cases, and a challenging repair is ill advised in a patient presenting several hours post-trauma with a severe fixed neurologic deficit and multiple other injuries. At the other end of the spectrum, a patient presenting shortly after a trauma with a carotid injury, decreased mental status, and a difficult-to-evaluate neurologic exam probably deserves the benefit of the doubt and should undergo carotid artery exploration and repair.

Common Carotid

The common carotid is probably the easiest vessel to approach and repair, especially once proximal control is achieved via sternotomy, balloon occlusion, or an incision low in the neck. Clamping below the level of the carotid bifurcation allows for continued perfusion of the internal carotid via external carotid backflow, and shunting is not typically necessary for a straightforward repair. Primary closure alone may be appropriate for a simple stab wound, but most gunshot wounds and more complex lacerations will require debridement back to normal-appearing vessel and reconstruction. If the arterial defect is very short, mobilization and end-to-end anastomosis may be feasible, but a short interposition graft with PTFE or Dacron is often required and should result in excellent long-term patency. If the surgical field is heavily contaminated, or there is oropharyngeal injury, using an autogenous conduit is probably a safer option. Reversed great saphenous vein taken from the groin is a reasonable choice, even though it may be a size mismatch. Femoral vein offers a closer size match, is almost always available, and rarely causes a harvest-related morbidity.

In a patient with a very limited wound and no associated injuries, systemic heparinization is appropriate during the repair. Regardless of whether systemic heparin is used, it is critical to forward and back flush the proximal and distal vessels after repair to remove any accumulated

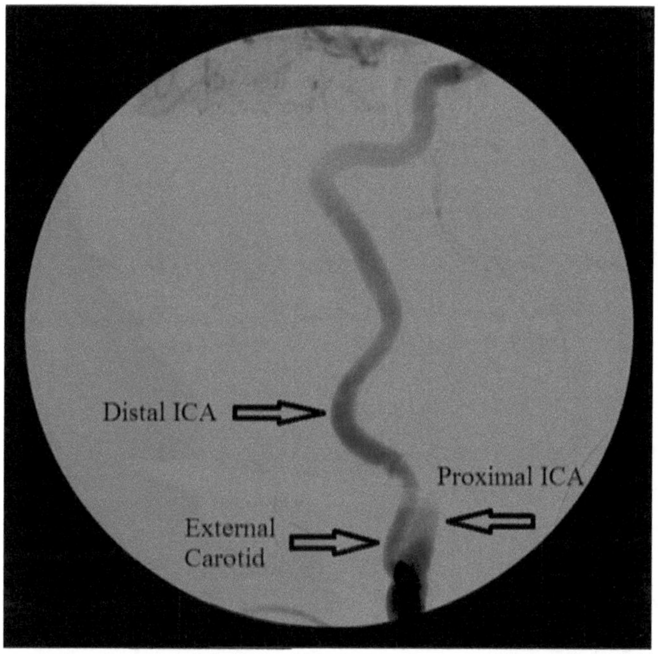

Fig. 14.7 This patient underwent an external-to-internal carotid transposition. The proximal ICA was ligated, with transposition of the external carotid onto the internal carotid. Completion arteriogram is shown

thrombus or air bubbles. If there is any suspicion of thrombus, or poor flow from the proximal or distal vessel, carefully passing a Fogarty balloon is acceptable.

Internal Carotid

Repair of the internal carotid poses more of a technical challenge, even for an experienced vascular surgeon. The internal carotid artery is smaller, shunting may be required, exposure can be difficult, and distal control is often elusive in a bloody surgical field. In addition, there are multiple cranial nerves prone to injury by inadvertent clamping while obtaining control or performing the repair. As is the case with the common carotid, primary repair of a defect may be appropriate for short stab wounds, but most gunshot wounds and complete transections will require interposition grafting. The conduit of choice is a reversed great saphenous vein graft, which is often a good size match and has documented excellent long-term patency. In some cases, a quick and elegant solution for proximal ICA injury is transposition of the external carotid over to the more distal internal carotid (Fig. 14.7).

Shunting is often recommended for patients requiring complex repair of the ICA, and there are a variety of shunts available. Technically, the most straightforward shunt is the Argyle, a straight, 6-in. PVC tube which is passed into the ICA distally and the CCA proximally and held in place at either end with a vessel loop or Rummel tourniquet. If a vein graft repair is required, the shunt can be passed through the vein graft before insertion to facilitate the repair. Shunting can be cumbersome and difficult in an emergency situation, particularly if the surgeon does not perform elective carotid endarterectomy on a regular basis. In practice, the surgeon should do whatever is necessary to complete the repair in the most expeditious fashion, and there is no consensus on the necessity of shunting every patient. If the repair is felt to be complex enough to require a shunt, it may be advisable for the less experienced general surgeon to consult a vascular surgery colleague to assist with the reconstruction.

In any situation, it is essential to confirm that the distal internal carotid is patent with minimal thrombus. If internal carotid artery back bleeding cannot be obtained, the vessel should simply be ligated. Careful passage of a Fogarty balloon to restore flow is acceptable, but the surgeon should be aware that blind passage of the balloon above the level of the skull base can cause intracranial vascular injury or a carotid-cavernous fistula.

External Carotid

The external carotid artery is often ignored in discussions of cervical vascular trauma, because injury rarely produces a significant neurologic deficit. Injury to the external carotid artery can, however, cause a life-threatening hemorrhage which requires surgical or endovascular repair. Although ligation of the external carotid at its origin is technically straightforward, it may not achieve hemostasis in the case of a branch injury given the extensive arterial collateralization that exists around the face. Transcatheter embolization effectively treats external carotid artery branch injuries and eliminates the risk of late hemorrhage. Figure 14.8 shows a pseudoaneurysm of an external carotid branch that was treated with transcatheter embolization.

Vertebral Artery Trauma

Vertebral artery trauma often has a subtle presentation and infrequently requires open surgical repair. Vertebral injury is not common and rarely causes significant morbidity or mortality. The location of the vertebral artery in the posterior neck, within the vertebral foramina, makes it difficult to expose and repair with open surgical techniques. With the exception of the first segment of the vertebral artery which is surgically accessible, most vertebral injuries require an endovascular approach. Given the redundancy of the posterior circulation, transcatheter embolization of an injured vertebral artery is the most common technique. Prior to vertebral artery embolization, it is critical to confirm patency of the contralateral vertebral artery.

Hemorrhage from the first portion of the vertebral artery may require surgical exposure and direct repair. A transverse incision placed above the clavicle and deepened by dividing the clavicular head of the sternocleidomastoid and the anterior scalene muscle will expose the subclavian artery which can be traced back to the vertebral artery origin. Simple ligation

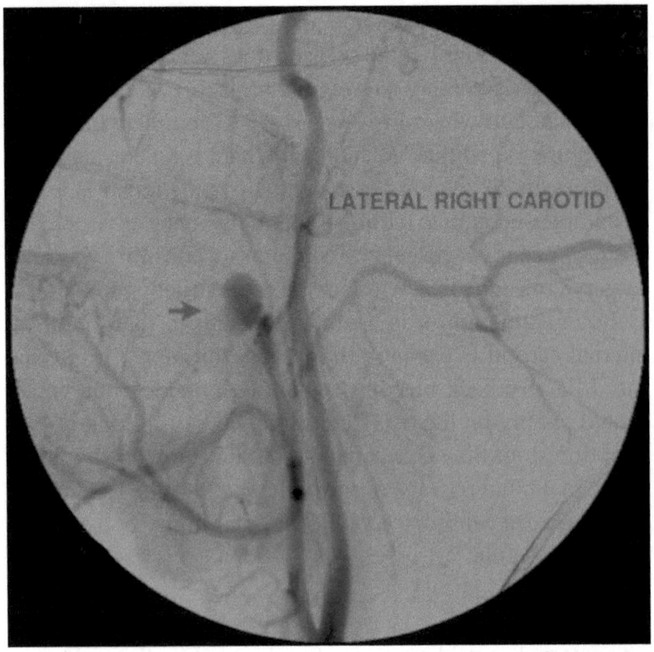

Fig. 14.8 A self-inflicted gunshot wound through the mouth with exit wound in Zone III presented with hemorrhage from the mouth and a pseudoaneurysm of the external carotid (arrow). This was treated with coil embolization

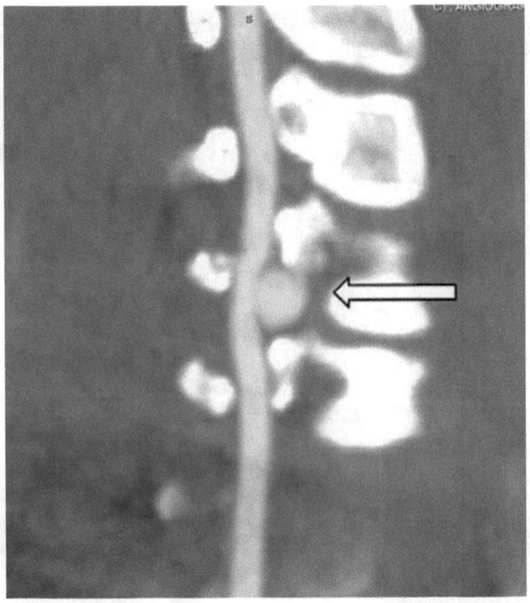

Fig. 14.9 A gunshot wound to the neck produced this pseudoaneurysm of the vertebral artery (arrow). It was treated with a stent graft but also could be addressed with transcatheter embolization

is usually appropriate, but saphenous interposition may be the only option if the contralateral vertebral is occluded, diseased, or hypoplastic. Ligation of the vertebral artery has historically been associated with a 3–5 % stroke rate, which is significant, but in desperate circumstances it may be the only realistic option [27]. A general surgeon should not underestimate the technical difficulty of performing direct repair of vertebral artery, and vascular surgery consultation may be warranted.

Blunt trauma with cervical spine fracture and concomitant vertebral artery occlusion is probably the most common scenario associated with a vertebral artery injury. The injury often represents an incidental imaging finding and requires no treatment, except in cases of active contrast extravasation or pseudoaneurysm formation (Fig. 14.9).

Subclavian Artery

Injury to the subclavian artery in Zone I should be considered when approaching a penetrating neck trauma with active bleeding or contrast extravasation on imaging studies. In the unstable patient, proximal control should be achieved in the chest through either median sternotomy for the right subclavian or a left anterior thoracotomy for the left subclavian. If endovascular expertise is immediately available, rapid control can be achieved with an intraluminal approach to limit the morbidity of the exposure and facilitate repair. In experienced hands and with appropriate imaging support, brachial artery access and placement of a stent graft or occlusion balloon is often just as quick as a thoracotomy or sternotomy.

Open repair of a subclavian artery injury may be necessary when the artery is completely transected. In these cases, the incision used for proximal control must be extended to allow interposition grafting. A supra- and/or infraclavicular incision is usually adequate, but in cases with ongoing severe hemorrhage, resection of the clavicle can give wider exposure to rapidly control venous or arterial bleeding and complete the repair. A segment of the clavicle just lateral to the clavicular head can be excised by extending a median sternotomy incision laterally directly over the proximal clavicle or by making a separate incision just lateral to the clavicular head. After clearing the attached soft tissues with cautery and a periosteal elevator, a 5–10 cm segment of the clavicle can be excised with a saw. Although clavicular resection may result in decreased shoulder stability and strength, limb salvage takes precedence over this minor functional limitation.

A particularly morbid, but classically described, incision for thoracic outlet injuries is the so-called "trapdoor" thoracotomy. This exposure consists of a partial sternotomy extended laterally with both a supraclavicular and a third or fourth interspace anterolateral thoracotomy incision. Opening the "trapdoor" laterally creates a wide exposure of the artery, vein, brachial plexus, and apex of the lung. This type of extensive exposure may be required in the most extensive penetrating trauma such as high-velocity gunshot wounds, shotgun wounds, or blast trauma with shrapnel injury. A damage-control approach is probably most appropriate in this setting, with rapid ligation of venous injuries, control of pulmonary bleeding, and expeditious arterial repair or ligation.

Repairing a subclavian artery with an interposition prosthetic graft is reasonable unless the field is heavily contaminated in which case an interposition saphenous vein graft is preferred. In the most dire circumstances involving an unstable patient and extensive arterial injury, simple ligation offers an effective damage-control strategy. The extensive arterial collateralization in the upper extremity can often maintain its viability in the setting of proximal subclavian artery ligation. Detecting a Doppler signal in the brachial artery distal to the ligation predicts viability in the short term, even without a graft. If a general surgeon does not feel comfortable with a complex arterial reconstruction, or the patient is profoundly unstable, placement of a temporary shunt, with resuscitation and delayed definitive repair, is a reasonable option. A well-placed arterial shunt may remain patent for 24–48 h even without systemic heparin, since these patients are often coagulopathic.

Venous Injury

Major venous injuries account for 40 % of all cervical vascular injuries and are almost exclusively due to penetrating injury [28]. Although an isolated venous injury rarely causes major morbidity, combined arterial and venous injuries are often discovered at the time of neck exploration and can make hemostatic control more difficult. Even an isolated venous injury can pose the threat of exsanguination if there is a large wound and direct pressure is not promptly applied.

Patients with isolated venous injuries rarely have hard signs of vascular injury other than hemorrhage through the wound. Because of the focus on finding an arterial injury, venous injuries are rarely considered during the evaluation of a stable patient with head and neck trauma. A venous injury may manifest only as a neck hematoma on CTA, which raises the suspicion of an arterial injury and may prompt a neck exploration. Encountering an unexpected venous injury during neck exploration can be challenging as they have the potential to be a source of significant blood loss and can be difficult to control.

Much like arterial injuries, treatment of cervical venous injuries depends on the overall status of the patient. The internal jugular, the most frequently injured vein, can be ligated in patients with concomitant arterial injury, shock, or an unsalvageable injury. Ligation of the internal jugular vein does not usually have any clinical sequelae and has not been associated with postoperative edema or venous hypertension [29]. In stable patients, limited venous lacerations involving less than 50 % of the wall can be treated with lateral venorrhaphy which will help establish control of hemorrhage [30]. During neck exploration, a venous injury can bleed as rapidly and profusely as any arterial injury, and the exact source of bleeding can be difficult to localize. Attempts at dissection and exposure near the injury may result in tearing a very thin-walled vein creating more trauma and increased bleeding. Although this can be a frustrating experience, it is important to resist the temptation to blindly place large sutures into the soft tissues of the neck. Pressure applied with fingers or a sponge stick on either side of the injury will almost always staunch the hemorrhage and allow a more careful dissection and an accurate assessment of the extent of the damage. Complex venous reconstructions are unnecessary in penetrating venous injury of the neck, and the only choice to consider is lateral venorrhaphy versus proximal and distal ligation.

References

1. Demetriades D, Theodorou D, Cornwell E, et al. Evaluation of penetrating injuries of the neck: prospective study of 223 patients. World J Surg. 1997;21:41–7; discussion 7–8.
2. Roon AJ, Christensen N. Evaluation and treatment of penetrating cervical injuries. J Trauma. 1979;19:391–7.
3. McConnell DB, Trunkey DD. Management of penetrating trauma to the neck. Adv Surg. 1994;27:97–127.
4. O'Brien PJ, Cox MW. A modern approach to cervical vascular trauma. Perspect Vasc Surg Endovasc Ther. 2011;23:90–7.
5. American College of Surgeons. Committee on Trauma. Advanced trauma life support ATLS: student course manual. 9th ed. Chicago: American College of Surgeons; 2012.
6. Apffelstaedt JP, Muller R. Results of mandatory exploration for penetrating neck trauma. World J Surg. 1994;18:917–9; discussion 20.
7. Insull P, Adams D, Segar A, Ng A, Civil I. Is exploration mandatory in penetrating zone II neck injuries? ANZ J Surg. 2007;77:261–4.
8. Demetriades D, Skalkides J, Sofianos C, Melissas J, Franklin J. Carotid artery injuries: experience with 124 cases. J Trauma. 1989;29:91–4.
9. Willinsky RA, Taylor SM, TerBrugge K, Farb RI, Tomlinson G, Montanera W. Neurologic complications of cerebral angiography: prospective analysis of 2,899 procedures and review of the literature. Radiology. 2003;227:522–8.
10. Patterson BO, Holt PJ, Cleanthis M, et al. Imaging vascular trauma. Br J Surg. 2012;99:494–505.
11. Inaba K, Munera F, McKenney MG, et al. The nonoperative management of penetrating internal jugular vein injury. J Vasc Surg. 2006;43:77–80.
12. Fabian TC, Patton Jr JH, Croce MA, Minard G, Kudsk KA, Pritchard FE. Blunt carotid injury. Importance of early diagnosis and anticoagulant therapy. Ann Surg. 1996;223:513–22; discussion 22–5.
13. Biffl WL, Moore EE, Elliott JP, et al. The devastating potential of blunt vertebral arterial injuries. Ann Surg. 2000;231:672–81.
14. Biffl WL, Moore EE, Offner PJ, et al. Optimizing screening for blunt cerebrovascular injuries. Am J Surg. 1999;178:517–22.
15. Berne JD, Norwood SH. Blunt vertebral artery injuries in the era of computed tomographic angiographic screening: incidence and outcomes from 8,292 patients. J Trauma. 2009;67:1333–8.
16. Desouza RM, Crocker MJ, Haliasos N, Rennie A, Saxena A. Blunt traumatic vertebral artery injury: a clinical review. Eur Spine J. 2011;20:1405–16.
17. Fusco MR, Harrigan MR. Cerebrovascular dissections: a review. Part II: blunt cerebrovascular injury. Neurosurgery. 2011;68:517–30; discussion 30.
18. Miller PR, Fabian TC, Croce MA, et al. Prospective screening for blunt cerebrovascular injuries: analysis of diagnostic modalities and outcomes. Ann Surg. 2002;236:386–93; discussion 93–5.

19. Franz RW, Willette PA, Wood MJ, Wright ML, Hartman JF. A systematic review and meta-analysis of diagnostic screening criteria for blunt cerebrovascular injuries. J Am Coll Surg. 2012;214:313–27.
20. Bromberg WJ, Collier BC, Diebel LN, et al. Blunt cerebrovascular injury practice management guidelines: the Eastern Association for the Surgery of Trauma. J Trauma. 2010;68:471–7.
21. Biffl WL, Cothren CC, Moore EE, et al. Western Trauma Association critical decisions in trauma: screening for and treatment of blunt cerebrovascular injuries. J Trauma. 2009;67:1150–3.
22. Eastman AL, Muraliraj V, Sperry JL, Minei JP. CTA-based screening reduces time to diagnosis and stroke rate in blunt cervical vascular injury. J Trauma. 2009;67:551–6; discussion 5–6.
23. Biffl WL, Moore EE, Offner PJ. Blunt carotid arterial injuries: implications of a new grading scale. J Trauma. 1999;47:845.
24. Cothren CC, Moore EE, Biffl WL, et al. Anticoagulation is the gold standard therapy for blunt carotid injuries to reduce stroke rate. Arch Surg. 2004;139:540–5.
25. Bradley EL. Management of penetrating carotid artery injuries. An alternative approach. J Trauma. 1973;13:248–55.
26. Thal ER, Snyder WH, et al. Management of carotid artery injuries. Surgery. 1974;76:955–62.
27. Thomas GI, Anderson KN, Hain RF. The significance of anomalous vertebral-basilar artery communications in operation on the heart and great vessels. Surgery. 1959;46:747–57.
28. du Toit DF, van Schalkwyk GD, Wadee SA, Warren BL. Neurologic outcome after penetrating extracranial arterial trauma. J Vasc Surg. 2003;38:257–62.
29. Nair R, Robbs JV, Muckart DJ. Management of penetrating cervicomediastinal venous trauma. Eur J Vasc Endovasc Surg. 2000; 19:65–9.
30. Rich NM, Collins Jr GJ, Andersen CA, et al. Venous trauma: successful venous reconstruction remains an interesting challenge. Am J Surg. 1977;134(2):226–30.

15 Vascular Injuries in the Abdomen

Sarah M. Wartman, Vincent L. Rowe, and Shih Yau Grace Huang

Introduction

Abdominal vascular injuries pose a significant challenge to surgeons for a number of reasons. First, the injuries are often lethal: mortality rates for patients sustaining an abdominal vascular injury approach 50 % [1–3]. Second, the majority of patients with abdominal vascular injury present in profound shock secondary to massive blood loss which leads to the potentially fatal triad of acidosis, hypothermia, and coagulopathy. Third, hemorrhage in patients with abdominal vascular injuries cannot be temporarily controlled prior to surgical exploration. In contrast to extremity vascular trauma where digital pressure or tourniquets can slow ongoing hemorrhage, bleeding vessels in the retroperitoneum are not amenable to external compression. Fourth, operative exposure of retroperitoneal injured vessels requires extensive, time-consuming dissection and mobilization of intra-abdominal organs. Rapid execution of the required maneuvers to identify and control the injured vessel in the face of recent or active hemorrhage increases the risk of iatrogenic injuries and continued organ ischemia. Lastly, by virtue of the retroperitoneal location of abdominal vessels and the proximity to adjacent organs, abdominal vascular injuries are associated with numerous injuries to surrounding vascular and nonvascular structures. The time required to repair other critical-associated injuries and the risk of contamination from injuries to hollow viscus organs (e.g., bowel, ureter) escalate not only the complexity of the operation but also the morbidity and mortality for the injured patient [1, 3]. These factors combine to create a complex clinical scenario for surgeons treating patients who have sustained an abdominal vascular injury. Rapid transport to a trauma center, early recognition of the injuries, a thorough knowledge of the anatomy and surgical maneuvers, and practical surgical judgment are crucial elements for improved patient outcomes.

Mechanism of Injury

In civilian series, abdominal vascular injuries comprise approximately 30 % of all vascular trauma treated at urban centers [4, 5]. Penetrating trauma is the most common etiology of abdominal vascular injuries and accounts for 90–95 % of all cases [6]. The mechanism of vascular injury from penetrating objects is due to either direct injury to the vessel or a shock wave cavitation from high-velocity projectiles and blasts.

Blunt trauma leads to abdominal vascular injury much less frequently, comprising only 5–10 % of reported trauma cases. Blunt vascular injury in the abdomen occurs through the following mechanisms:

1. Rapid deceleration, as occurs in a fall from heights or a high-speed motor vehicle accident.
2. Crush injury from direct anterior-posterior forces to the abdomen (i.e., seat belt, direct blow to the abdomen). Vascular injuries caused by crushing occur most commonly at the proximal renal and superior mesenteric arteries.
3. Laceration from a bony fragment. This type of injury is more common in the pelvic area where iliac arteries and veins traverse large bony pelvic structures [7].

S.M. Wartman, MD • S.Y.G. Huang, MD
Division of Vascular Surgery and Endovascular Therapy, University of Southern California, Los Angeles, CA USA

V.L. Rowe, MD, FACS (✉)
Division of Vascular and Endovascular Surgery, Department of Surgery, Keck School of Medicine at University of Southern California, 1520 San Pablo Street, Suite 4300, Los Angeles, CA 90033, USA
e-mail: Vincent.rowe@med.usc.edu

V. Gahtan and M.J. Costanza (eds.), *Essentials of Vascular Surgery for the General Surgeon*, DOI 10.1007/978-1-4939-1326-8_15, © Springer Science+Business Media New York 2015

Incidence

For patients undergoing exploratory laparotomy for trauma, the incidence of a vascular injury is 14.3 % for gunshot injuries, 10 % for stab wounds, and 3 % for blunt trauma [4, 6, 8]. The incidences of arterial and venous injuries in abdominal vascular injuries appear to be evenly divided. In a review of 302 abdominal vascular injuries treated at an urban trauma center, Asensio et al. reported a nearly equal incidence of arterial and venous injuries (49 and 51 %, respectively) [1]. In that series, the most commonly injured abdominal vessel was the inferior vena cava (25 %), followed by the aorta (21 %), iliac arteries (20 %), iliac veins (17 %), and the superior mesenteric artery (10 %).

Clinical Presentation

The clinical presentation of patients who have sustained abdominal vascular injury is mainly determined by whether the bleeding from the injured vessel is contained as a retroperitoneal hematoma or hemorrhages freely into the peritoneal cavity. Patients with contained hematomas appear hemodynamically stable either on initial presentation or shortly after limited resuscitation with intravenous fluids. Conversely, patients with uncontained bleeding into the peritoneal cavity remain severely hypotensive even after aggressive volume repletion. Additional clinical factors affecting the clinical presentation include: specific vessel or vessels injured, extent of the injury, type of injury (i.e., thrombosis, transection), the presence of associated injuries, and time elapsed from the initial traumatic insult. Patients sustaining blunt trauma may present with less overt clinical signs which may be missed on the initial examination. Loss of a femoral pulse in patients with severe pelvic trauma and gross hematuria should alert the surgeon of the possibility of an underlying vascular injury.

Diagnosis and Evaluation

The most crucial factors for the survival of patients with abdominal vascular injuries are rapid transport to the trauma center followed by prompt surgical control of the bleeding. The clinical status and hemodynamic parameters of the patient dictate the amount of time available for diagnostic studies.

Upon arrival to the trauma center, each patient should have a set of laboratory blood tests performed that include an arterial blood gas. Since the majority of patients present to the trauma center in extremis, the results of these laboratory studies may be unavailable during a critical time in the patient's care which limits their value in the early diagnosis of an abdominal vascular injury.

When time allows, plain radiographs of the chest, abdomen, and pelvis provide valuable clinical information. In penetrating trauma, plain films can detail the bullet trajectory and location. For patients sustaining blunt traumatic injuries, plain radiographs detect significant bony fracture fragments and displacements, particularly pelvic fractures, which may injure retroperitoneal vessels.

Computerized tomography (CT) scans have little or no clinical value in the early management of hemodynamically abnormal patients with suspected abdominal vascular trauma due to penetrating injury. In the stable patient, elective contrast-enhanced CT scans can identify arteriovenous fistulas and false aneurysms. In blunt trauma, CT scans are useful to evaluate for retroperitoneal hematomas, vessel occlusions, and false aneurysms and to document renal morphology and function in patients with suspected renal artery injury [7].

Surgical Management

Emergency Department

On arrival in the emergency department, all trauma patients should be evaluated according to the Advanced Trauma Life Support protocols. Securing the airway, placing large-bore venous access, nasogastric tube and Foley catheter insertion, and intravenous fluid administration with balanced saline solutions are the tenets of early resuscitative measures. Of special note, a suspected abdominal vascular injury mandates that venous access be placed in the upper extremities. Hemorrhagic or thrombotic injuries to the iliac veins or inferior vena cava may impair the delivery of fluid given through resuscitation lines placed in the femoral vein. Additionally, should the need for venous cross-clamping arise intraoperatively, intravenous fluid infusion through the ipsilateral femoral line would be interrupted.

Ideally, all patients presenting in extremis should be quickly transported to the operating room for definitive surgical treatment. Some patients have injuries that will be fatal without immediate intervention in the form of an emergency department (ED) thoracotomy. According to the American College of Surgeons Committee on Trauma, ED thoracotomy has little value in blunt trauma and should only be performed if the patient has a witnessed cardiopulmonary arrest. Although ED thoracotomy is recommended for penetrating cardiac and thoracic injuries, it is most successful in patients with penetrating cardiac injuries who have signs of life. If the patient has a known exsanguinating abdominal vascular injury, regardless of mechanism, ED thoracotomy should be performed only if the patient cannot be immediately transferred to the operating room. Cross-clamping the descending thoracic aorta with open cardiac massage may abate intra-abdominal hemorrhage and allow for redistribution of the remaining intravascular volume to coronary and cerebrovascular beds [9–11]. The survival rate for patients with abdominal vascular injuries that undergo an ED thoracotomy is approximately 2 % [3].

Operating Room

In the operating room, all steps to prevent hypothermia should be instituted. Warming blankets, warming mattresses, heated intravenous fluids, and elevated ambient room temperature can help minimize the harmful effects of hypothermia.

Surgical preparation should extend from the mid torso to the knees. Including the proximal thigh in the surgical field ensures availability of an autogenous venous conduit should the need arise (great saphenous or femoral vein). Exploration of the abdomen begins with a generous midline abdominal incision extending from the xiphoid to the symphysis pubis. Initial efforts should focus on immediate control of life-threatening hemorrhage followed by containment of leaking gastrointestinal contents. Should any difficulty arise in obtaining control of the hemorrhage or if a cardiac arrest occurs early in the abdominal exploration, a left anterolateral thoracotomy with aortic cross-clamping must be performed expeditiously.

Control of the exsanguinating hemorrhage allows a systematic evaluation for vascular injury based on the three anatomic zones of the abdominal cavity (Fig. 15.1). Zone 1 begins at the aortic hiatus and ends at the sacral promontory throughout the midline of the abdomen. Zone 1 is subdivided into Zone 1 supramesocolic and Zone 1 inframesocolic. The supramesocolic Zone 1 contains the suprarenal aorta and its major branches, the celiac axis, superior mesenteric artery, renal arteries, the supramesocolic inferior vena cava, and the superior mesenteric vein. The inframesocolic Zone 1 contains the infrarenal aorta and inferior vena cava. The right and left Zone 2 areas each contains the kidneys, paracolic gutters, and renal vessels. Zone 3 begins at the sacral promontory and encompasses the pelvis with the iliac arteries and veins [4, 5, 12, 13]. The portal-retrohepatic region is occasionally referred to as Zone 4 and contains the portal vein, hepatic artery, and retrohepatic vena cava [7].

All surgeons involved in the operative management of trauma patients must be familiar with the anatomic zones and exposure techniques for each area. Any retroperitoneal hematoma caused by a penetrating injury should be explored regardless of the zone. The one possible exception to this rule is a Zone 4 hematoma that is stable and small (Table 15.1). In contrast, most retroperitoneal hematomas caused by blunt trauma do not require exploration. In particular, blunt injury

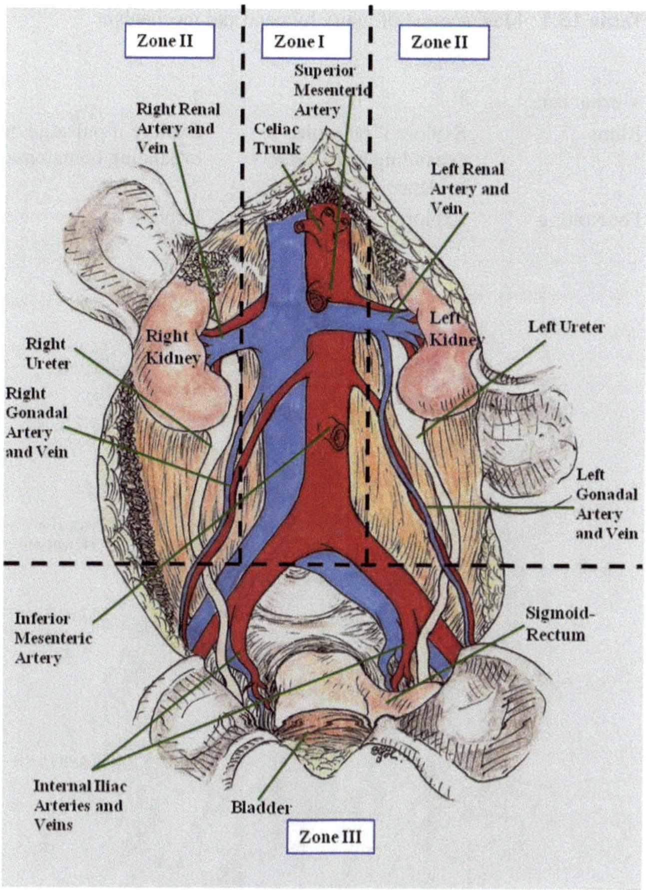

Fig. 15.1 Three anatomic zones of the retroperitoneal space

to Zone 2 and Zone 3 should only be explored if there is a pulsatile or expanding hematoma or an absent femoral pulse. In addition, any evidence of bowel ischemia necessitates exploration of the associated hematoma.

Exposure of the contents in the supramesocolic Zone 1 is best accomplished by left-sided medial visceral rotation (Fig. 15.2). This maneuver first requires incising along the avascular line of Toldt in the left colon and the lienosplenic ligament. The left colon, spleen, tail and body of the pancreas, and stomach are rotated medially, exposing the aortic hiatus, origins of the celiac axis, superior mesenteric artery, and left renal artery [1, 4, 5].

For exposure of the inframesocolic Zone 1 contents, the transverse colon should be retracted cephalad. The small bowel is then eviscerated towards the right upper quadrant and the ligament of Treitz is incised. As the retroperitoneum is opened, the left renal vein must be identified to prevent iatrogenic injury. The remainder of the retroperitoneum is opened inferiorly along the center of the aorta until the aortic bifurcation is reached. The inferior mesenteric artery should be located towards the left side of the aorta approximately 2 cm above the bifurcation. For exposure of the infrarenal IVC, incision of the avascular line of Toldt in the right colon

Table 15.1 Management of injury by zone and mechanism

	Zone			
Mechanism	1	2	3	4
Blunt	Explore if pulsatile, expanding hematoma, evidence of ischemia	Explore if pulsatile or expanding hematoma	Explore if expanding hematoma or absent femoral pulse/evidence of lower extremity ischemia	Explore only if expanding
Penetrating	Explore	Explore	Explore	Explore unless stable, small, and non-expanding

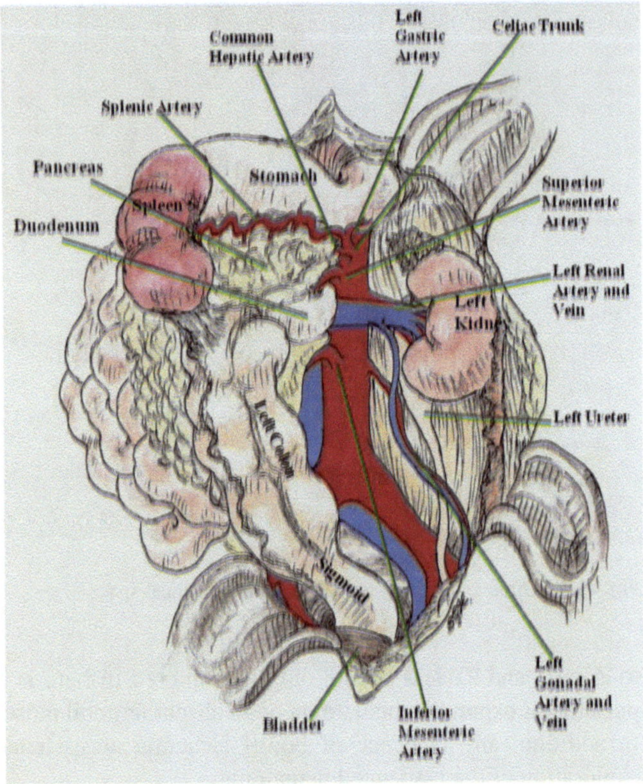

Fig. 15.2 Left medial visceral rotation

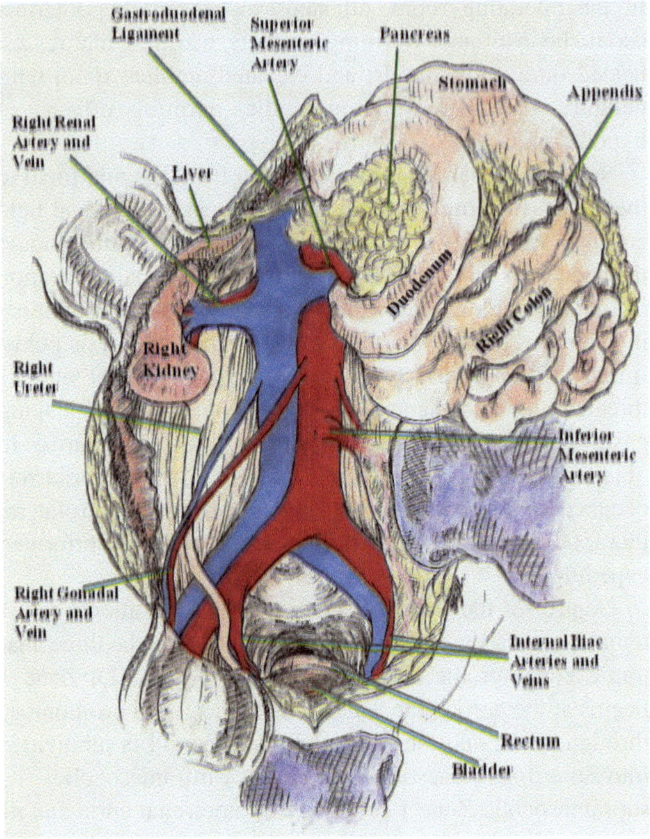

Fig. 15.3 Right medial visceral rotation

is combined with a Kocher maneuver that sweeps the pancreas and duodenum to the left on a superior mesenteric artery pedicle [1, 4, 5].

Zone 2 exposures differ slightly for left-sided and right-sided approaches. On the right, the ascending colon is mobilized from the cecum to the hepatic flexure and combined with a Kocher maneuver (Fig. 15.3). With the infrarenal IVC exposed, the dissection continues cephalad along the right side of the IVC until the right renal vein is identified. Dissection posterior and superior to the right renal vein will expose the right renal artery [1, 4, 5].

On the left side, the descending colon and splenic flexure are mobilized and the small bowel is retracted towards the right upper quadrant. The ligament of Treitz is incised after elevation of the transverse colon, similar to the exposure for the Zone 1 inframesocolic aorta. After transection of the ligament of Treitz, the left renal vein should be identified as it crosses the aorta anteriorly. The left renal artery will typically lay posterior and superior to the left renal vein [1, 4, 5].

Zone 3 vessel exposure should begin by incising the lines of Toldt for the left and right colon and sweeping the colons medially. The common iliac arteries and veins will be directly posterior once the retroperitoneum is incised. Care must be taken to avoid iatrogenic injury to the ureter as it traverses anterior to the distal common iliac artery.

After adequate exposure and hemostatic control, the injury can be classified according to the American Association for the Surgery of Trauma Organ Injury Scale (AAST-OIS) for vascular injuries scoring method (Table 15.2). The AAST-OIS grade of vascular injury correlates with mortality rates: 25 % mortality for Grade II, 32 % for Grade III, 65 % for Grade IV, and 88 % for Grade V injuries [3].

Table 15.2 American Association for the Surgery of Trauma Organ Injury Scale for vascular injuries

OIS grade	Artery injured	Vein injured
I	No named superior mesenteric branches No named inferior mesenteric branches Phrenic Lumbar Gonadal Ovarian Small no named branches requiring ligation	No named superior mesenteric branches No named inferior mesenteric branches Phrenic Lumbar Gonadal Ovarian Small no named branches requiring ligation
II	Hepatic Splenic Gastric Gastroduodenal Inferior mesenteric Primary named vessels of superior mesenteric	Splenic Inferior mesenteric
III	Renal Iliac Hypogastric	Superior mesenteric Renal Iliac Hypogastric Vena cava (infrarenal)
IV	Superior mesenteric (trunk) Celiac axis Aorta (infrarenal)	Vena cava (infrahepatic)
V	Aorta (suprarenal)	Vena cava (suprahepatic) Vena cava (retrohepatic) Portal Hepatic (extrahepatic)

Vascular control also provides the opportunity to thoroughly assess the extent of arterial injury and venous damage before proceeding with definitive repair. The first step involves debriding all macroscopically injured or contused tissue present on the injured vessel to insure the integrity of the vascular repair. In both blunt and penetrating traumatic injuries, the level of intimal damage can extend far beyond the obvious area of injury. Fogarty catheters should be passed gently, both proximal and distal to the arterial injury to remove any intraluminal thrombus. It is extremely important not to overinflate the balloon which could damage the endothelial lining causing arterial spasm or thrombosis. Liberal irrigation with heparinized saline and injury repair with monofilament suture are recommended. If possible, an autogenous vascular reconstruction is preferred especially in the presence of bowel injury and contamination. Repair with a prosthetic graft may be the only practical option for injuries to large-diameter vessels (i.e., aorta, IVC). If the repair requires prolonged clamping of the aorta or iliac vessels, systemic heparin should be considered as long as concomitant injuries do not preclude its use.

Specific Injuries

Abdominal Aorta

Traumatic injuries to the abdominal aorta result from penetrating trauma in the vast majority of cases and blunt trauma in rare cases [14]. In a review of 129 penetrating abdominal aortic injuries, 50 % were infrarenal, 25 % supraceliac, and 25 % visceral aorta [15]. Clinical presentation of the patients depends on the type of injury, the time elapsed from the time of injury, the location and number of associated injuries, and most importantly, whether the bleeding is contained by the retroperitoneum.

Exposure to the supraceliac and visceral aorta involves rotation of the left colon, spleen, pancreas tail, and small bowel to the left, as described for Zone 1 supramesocolic retroperitoneal hematomas. Division of the diaphragmatic crura allows additional exposure of the inferior descending thoracic aorta. For injuries at or above the celiac artery, aortic exposure and cross-clamping via a left anterolateral thoracotomy may be required. Exposure to the infrarenal aorta is the same as Zone 1 inframesocolic retroperitoneal hematoma. Briefly, the transverse colon is elevated cephalad, the small bowel mobilized to the right upper quadrant, the ligament of Treitz incised, and the retroperitoneum opened.

Surgical repair should be performed with monofilament nonabsorbable suture. In cases of side-wall aortic injuries, lateral aortorrhaphy is the primary repair technique. If primary repair causes concentric narrowing, patch angioplasty with bovine pericardium is a suitable alternative, especially in the presence of bowel contamination. In emergent situations, aortic replacement with prosthetic graft is the most practical option. If possible, omental tissue should be placed between the aortic graft and surrounding viscera. In cases of delayed presentation of aortic injury, consideration should be given to aortic replacement with femoral vein harvested from the thigh or cryopreserved aorta [16, 17].

Celiac Artery

As the first major branch of the abdominal aorta, the celiac artery emerges directly anterior from the aorta for 1–2 cm before trifurcating in to the left gastric, common hepatic and splenic arteries. Similar to the aorta, the most common mechanism of injury is penetrating trauma. Exposure of the celiac artery trunk requires a left medial visceral rotation similar to the supraceliac aorta exposure technique. Alternatively, caudad traction on the stomach and entry into the lesser sac allows visualization of the celiac artery and the three proximal branches. Ligation of the main trunk of the celiac artery is well tolerated and the treatment of choice.

Ligation is also the preferred treatment method for each trifurcation branch because rich collateral or alternative source of perfusion (portal vein) is present for each end organ supplied by the celiac branches.

Superior Mesenteric Artery

Penetrating trauma causes most injuries to the superior mesenteric artery (SMA), while blunt trauma accounts for 10–20 % of injuries to the SMA [18, 19]. Clinical presentation of the patient sustaining an injury to the SMA varies from shock secondary to massive intraperitoneal hemorrhage to ischemic bowel secondary to thrombosis of the artery. Superior mesenteric artery injuries are divided into the following four anatomic zones [7]:

- Zone 1: aortic origin to the inferior pancreaticoduodenal branch
- Zone 2: inferior pancreaticoduodenal artery to middle colic artery
- Zone 3: distal to middle colic artery
- Zone 4: segmental intestinal branches

Exposure of the SMA differs slightly for each zone. Left visceral rotation provides clear exposure to Zone 1 of the retropancreatic SMA. Zone 2 SMA exposure requires elevation of the inferior border of the pancreas or careful dissection to the right of the ligament of Treitz combined with a Kocher maneuver. Dissection directly through the mesentery identifies the Zones 3 and 4 SMA segments.

In general, ligation of SMA injuries in Zones 1 and 2 leads to significant ischemia of the entire small bowel and right colon. Ligation of Zones 3 and 4 SMA injuries compromises perfusion to the segment of the small bowel supplied by the arterial arcade ligated. Ligation of any SMA segment should only be considered if bowel ischemia is already present at the time of surgery [7]. Forty percent of injuries to the SMA only require a primary side-wall repair [20]. Injuries requiring complete replacement should be addressed with an autogenous interposition graft (great saphenous vein). Although prosthetic grafts can be effective, an all autogenous reconstruction is preferred in cases with extensive gastrointestinal spillage. Concomitant bowel resection mandates a planned "second-look" laparotomy 24–48 h later.

Renal Artery

Renal artery injuries may occur in both penetrating and blunt trauma. The renal artery is the most commonly injured abdominal vessel in blunt trauma with the left renal artery being injured slightly more often than the right [21, 22]. The hilum of each renal artery is accessible by midline retroperitoneal exposure similar to Zone 2 inframesocolic dissection. For the left renal vasculature, a left visceral rotation allows complete exposure of the renal hilum and parenchyma. On the right side, mobilization of the right colon combined with a Kocher maneuver provides excellent visualization of the renal system.

Management of renovascular trauma varies according to the mechanism of injury and clinical presentation after injury. In penetrating trauma, the diagnosis of renovascular injury is usually made intraoperatively. Zone 2 retroperitoneal hematomas secondary to penetrating trauma warrant exploration with the possible exception of hematomas lateral to the hilum [23]. For renovascular injuries due to blunt trauma, the diagnosis is also made intraoperatively in the unstable patient. In this situation, only expanding Zone 2 retroperitoneal hematomas warrant exploration. In the stable trauma patient, a CT scan allows excellent visualization of renovascular injuries and has the benefit of contralateral kidney assessment. Once the severity of renal injury is determined, the treatment algorithm includes open repair, endovascular intervention, or nonoperative management. Sangthong et al. reviewed patients with blunt renal artery injuries from the National Trauma Data Bank, which is maintained by the Committee on Trauma of the American College of Surgeons. Only 9 % of the 517 patients with a renal artery injury due to blunt trauma underwent revascularization. Of the remaining cases, 73 % had no kidney exploration and 18 % had an immediate nephrectomy. In the group of 87 patients with isolated renal artery injuries, 8 % underwent revascularization, 8 % had early nephrectomy, and 84 % were observed [22]. Nonoperative management should include follow-up for delayed onset of injury-induced renovascular hypertension [21, 24, 25]. Based on the recent success with endovascular management, the authors strongly suggest the endovascular treatment pathway over nonoperative management if feasible [26–28].

General considerations for renal artery repair hinge on the elapsed time from the initial injury and the status of contralateral kidney. Six hours of warm ischemia approaches the limit of tolerance for renal salvage; however, bilateral injuries should extend the time constraints [7]. Interposition grafting with an autogenous conduit is preferred, while direct arteriorrhaphy and patch angioplasty are both reasonable alternatives.

Iliac Artery

The iliac arteries begin their course through the pelvis at the level of the aortic bifurcation, typically at the fourth lumbar vertebra. Penetrating trauma is the most common mechanism of injury for iliac arteries which are not very susceptible to blunt traumatic forces. Blunt trauma can cause a thrombotic injury when severe pelvic fractures disrupt the arterial intima. All hematomas due to penetrating trauma warrant exploration. In blunt trauma, hematomas that are expanding or those associated with an absent femoral pulse require exploration. Exposure of both iliac arteries is as described for Zone 3 retroperitoneal hematomas with additional exposure gained by extending the midline incision towards the groin and dividing the inguinal ligament [29]. Even in the presence of hemorrhage, meticulous dissection is mandatory during operative management of the iliac arteries to avoid iatrogenic injury to the ureter and iliac veins.

Small lacerations can be repaired directly, while interposition prosthetic grafting is preferred for larger disruptions and thrombotic injuries. Debate continues over the use of prosthetic graft for iliac artery repair in the presence of bowel contamination. Although direct bypass with a prosthetic graft offers a straightforward and expeditious repair, the risk of graft infection never completely subsides. The authors still favor minimizing the risk of infection by following the more conservative approach of extra-anatomic bypass in the setting of extensive fecal contamination [30].

Inferior Vena Cava

Originating at the level of the fifth lumbar vertebra, the inferior vena cava (IVC) ascends along the right side of the abdominal aorta, passing anterior to the right renal artery before traveling behind the liver and perforating the diaphragm. The intrathoracic portion is short, extending approximately 2.5 cm above the diaphragm before joining the right atrium. The IVC is one of the most commonly injured vessels in abdominal vascular trauma usually from penetrating trauma [1, 7, 31]. Depending on the location, injuries to this vessel have a mortality rate exceeding 50 %, with some reports as high as 75 % [1, 31].

As with the aorta, all penetrating injuries to the retroperitoneal zones should be explored, with the possible exception of a non-expanding retrohepatic hematoma in a hemodynamically stable patient [7]. Although medializing the right colon alone can expose the infrarenal IVC, full exposure up to and including the suprarenal portion requires a complete right medial-visceral rotation with the Kocher maneuver.

Retrohepatic vena cava injuries represent extremely challenging injuries to control and repair and are nearly universally fatal. These injuries usually require hepatic vascular isolation which involves cross-clamping the supraceliac aorta, followed by isolation and control of the portal triad, infrahepatic IVC, and suprahepatic IVC. Extension of the incision with an additional subcostal incision or a thoracotomy is often necessary. In some cases, an atriocaval shunt can be used for hemostatic control. The technique for an atriocaval shunt includes a sternotomy to expose the right atrium for placement of the tube. The tube (large-bore thoracostomy tube or endotracheal tube) should be passed through a purse-string suture in the right atrial appendage and should be clamped proximally with side holes that line up inside the right atrium. The tube is then advanced inferiorly into the IVC and the suprahepatic and infrahepatic IVC can then be constrained around the tube using umbilical tapes [32].

Venorrhaphy for injuries to the IVC should be performed with nonabsorbable monofilament suture. Anterior lacerations should be repaired in a transverse fashion when possible to minimize vessel narrowing. If a posterior perforation is visualized and accessible through an extended anterior perforation, it can be repaired from inside the IVC. Vascular control of the IVC is best achieved with compression using sponge sticks or manual pressure, if possible, to prevent further damage by attempting to clamp the injured, thin-walled vessel. In hemodynamically unstable patients with extensive injury to the infrarenal IVC, ligation is an option but may result in significant morbidity. Ligation of the suprarenal IVC should be avoided, as it runs the risk of the patient requiring permanent hemodialysis, although limited data exists due to the high mortality in this patient population. It is important to wrap and elevate the extremities in a patient after ligation and observe the patient carefully for lower extremity compartment syndrome. In a recent study of 100 patients who had IVC injuries, 25 % underwent ligation (22 infrarenal, 3 juxtarenal/suprarenal) [31]. Overall mortality was significantly higher in patients who underwent ligation compared to those who underwent repair (59 % vs. 21 %). Patients who required IVC ligation also had a longer length of stay in both the hospital and the intensive care unit and a greater need for lower extremity fasciotomy. Interestingly, none of the patients who survived to discharge had more than trace edema of the lower extremities at an average follow-up of 42 months. Of note, the one patient who survived ligation of the juxtarenal IVC developed acute renal failure requiring temporary dialysis that resolved prior to discharge from the hospital.

Portal Vein

The portal vein is located at the level of the second lumbar vertebra and originates posterior to the neck of the pancreas at the confluence of the splenic vein and the superior mesenteric vein. It then passes through the hepatoduodenal ligament posterior to and between the common bile duct and the hepatic artery.

Injury to the portal vein is often associated with other vascular injuries, and management and survival depend on the location and extent of these injuries. Because portal vein injury rarely occurs in isolation, precise survival data is difficult to apply. In most reports, the mortality of patients sustaining a traumatic injury to the portal vein exceeds 50 % [33, 34].

Exposure of the portal vein requires medial rotation of the right colon and Kocher maneuver, and the Pringle maneuver can help achieve vascular control. If the injury involves the confluence or the retropancreatic portion, division of the pancreas may be required for proper visualization.

Venorrhaphy is preferred when possible. In the event of injury to the hepatic artery, repairing the portal vein should be attempted in order to restore hepatic perfusion. Extensive injury to the portal vein may require an interposition vein graft (great saphenous or internal jugular). Although ligation can be considered as a damage control maneuver if the hepatic artery is not injured, ligating the portal vein can lead to significant bowel edema and possibly bowel ischemia [34]. These cases warrant a second-look operation and aggressive volume resuscitation.

Superior Mesenteric Vein

The superior mesenteric vein (SMV) begins in the right iliac fossa and travels through the mesentery to the right of the SMA. It then passes anterior to the duodenum and posterior to the neck of the pancreas where it joins the splenic vein to become the portal vein.

Injury to the SMV is uncommon and usually accompanied by severe associated injuries due to its proximity to other major abdominal organs and vessels [34, 35]. As with the portal vein, proper exposure may require division of the pancreas.

Although lateral venorrhaphy is the ideal treatment for SMV injuries, in many cases, the only viable option will be ligation. Manual compression of the vein can be performed to maintain hemostasis during surgical repair. As with portal vein ligation, life-saving treatment by ligation of the SMV may lead to venous gangrene of the bowel highlighting the importance of aggressive resuscitation and a second-look operation. In one retrospective study of 51 patients with SMV injury, 59 % underwent ligation and 31 % underwent primary repair, while 10 % died before any definitive repair could be achieved [35]. Survival was 47 % overall and 53 % with isolated SMV injury, with the majority of mortalities occurring in the operating room. Survival was better in the repair group (63 % vs. 40 %), but the ligation group also had a much higher number of associated vascular and nonvascular injuries. None of the surviving patients developed bowel necrosis.

Renal Veins

The renal veins are located anterior to the renal arteries. The left renal vein passes below the origin of the SMA anterior to the aorta to reach the IVC slightly superior to the right renal vein. Exposure of the right renal vein involves medial rotation of the right colon with a Kocher maneuver, while the left renal vein can be visualized with a left-sided medial-visceral rotation. Lateral venorrhaphy is ideal for repairing injuries to the renal veins. Ligation of the left renal vein at the vena cava is tolerated due to collateral circulation via lumbar, adrenal, and gonadal veins. Ligation of the right renal vein requires a concomitant nephrectomy.

Iliac Veins

The internal iliac and the external iliac veins come together to form the common iliac veins at the sacroiliac articulation. The left common iliac vein is longer and travels in a more oblique direction than the right, starting medial to the left common iliac artery and then passing behind the right common iliac artery. The left common iliac vein then joins the right common iliac vein – which is posterior and lateral to the right common iliac artery – to form the inferior vena cava at about the level of the fifth lumbar vertebra.

As with the iliac arteries, the most common mechanism of injury is penetrating trauma. Blunt trauma alone is much less likely to result in an iliac vein injury, but when it does, it is usually associated with a pelvic fracture. Approximately 26 % of patients with iliac vascular injuries have both venous and arterial injuries [7]. Exposure of the veins, particularly at their confluence, is more difficult than that of the arteries due to their posterior location relative to the arteries. Depending on the location of the injury, mobilization of the left and/or right colon medially will provide visualization of the iliac vessels.

In general, ligating the injured iliac vein is safe and should be performed if the patient is hemodynamically unstable or it is not feasible to repair the vein. After iliac vein ligation, patients may develop transient leg edema and they should be monitored closely for signs of compartment syndrome, especially if the iliac artery was also injured. Primary venorrhaphy is a reasonable option if it can be performed without creating a hemodynamically significant stenosis. Venous injury and repair increases the risk of deep vein thrombosis (DVT), and postoperative DVT prophylaxis is advised when it is not contraindicated by other injuries. There is no indication for the use of therapeutic anticoagulation in this setting unless a DVT has been documented. Survival after iliac vein injury approaches 70 % and may be higher when isolated from other vascular injuries [33].

Damage Control

Damage control, or "bail out" as originally described by Stone et al., is the technique of using rapid, temporary measures to maintain life without undertaking definitive repair. Damage control maneuvers include: intraluminal shunting for vascular injuries, abdominal wall closure with prosthetic bridge, ligation of venous injuries, and packing of retroperitoneal bleeding.

These measures attempt to minimize the deleterious effects of hypothermia, coagulopathy, and bowel edema which accompany prolonged life-saving explorations of the abdomen. The usual clinical scenario for damage control consists of coagulopathy, temperature less than 35 °C, base deficit greater than 15 mmol/L, and bowel edema [7]. Current recommendations advise initiating damage control before the aforementioned physiological endpoints are reached, especially in elderly trauma victims and in rural settings with limited resources.

Temporary intraluminal shunting plays an important role when definitive vascular repair must be delayed to address associated life-threatening injuries [36, 37]. Temporary intraluminal shunting restores organ perfusion and decreases the risk of ischemic damage and distal thrombosis. Military literature extensively documents temporary intraluminal shunting in lower extremity trauma; however, the same techniques may apply to abdominal vascular trauma. In a report on the military's experience over 1 year during Operation Iraqi Freedom, the majority of temporary intraluminal shunts were in place for less than 2 h; however, patency was noted in proximal extremity arteries for 18 h without the use of systemic heparin [38]. Any sterile tubing can be used as a temporary shunt, but carotid artery shunts are the most amenable for this application.

Conclusion

The abdomen contains several large-diameter blood vessels in close proximity to each other and other abdominal organs. Blunt or penetrating trauma can injure one or multiple vessels causing potentially fatal hemorrhage. Defying the high mortality rates associated with abdominal vascular trauma requires rapid transport to a trauma center, prompt recognition of the injuries, and expert surgical intervention to control bleeding. Knowledge of abdominal anatomy and vascular exposure techniques can help surgeons control and repair these technically challenging injuries. Practical surgical judgment plays an important role in the management of complicated injuries characterized by persistent hemodynamic instability, extensive vessel damage, or widespread enteric contamination. These clinical scenarios may call for adjunctive maneuvers including damage control laparotomy, temporary intraluminal shunting, and extra-anatomic vascular reconstruction.

References

1. Asensio JA, Chahwan S, Hanpeter D, Demetriades D, Forno W, Gambaro E, et al. Operative management and outcome of 302 abdominal vascular injuries. Am J Surg. 2000;180(6):528–33; discussion 33–4.
2. Asensio JA, Soto SN, Forno W, Roldan G, Petrone P, Gambaro E, et al. Abdominal vascular injuries: the trauma surgeon's challenge. Surg Today. 2001;31(11):949–57.
3. Tyburski JG, Wilson RF, Dente C, Steffes C, Carlin AM. Factors affecting mortality rates in patients with abdominal vascular injuries. J Trauma. 2001;50(6):1020–6.
4. Feliciano D. Abdominal vessels. In: Ivatury R, Cayten C, editors. The textbook of penetrating trauma. Baltimore: Williams and Wilkins; 1996. p. 702–16.
5. Feliciano D, Burch J, Graham J. Abdominal vascular injury. In: Mattox K, Feliciano D, Moore E, editors. Trauma. 4th ed. New York: McGraw Hill; 1999. p. 783–805.
6. Cox EF. Blunt abdominal trauma. A 5-year analysis of 870 patients requiring celiotomy. Ann Surg. 1984;199(4):467–74.
7. Demetriades D, Inaba K. Vascular trauma: abdominal. In: Cronenwett J, Johnston W, editors. Rutherford's vascular surgery. 7th ed. Philadelphia: Saunders; 2010. p. 2343–60.
8. Demetriades D, Velmahos G, Cornwell 3rd E, Berne TV, Cober S, Bhasin PS, et al. Selective nonoperative management of gunshot wounds of the anterior abdomen. Arch Surg. 1997;132(2):178–83.
9. Brotman S, Oster-Granite M, Cox EF. Failure of cross clamping the thoracic aorta to control intra-abdominal bleeding. Ann Emerg Med. 1982;11(3):147–8.
10. Ledgerwood AM, Kazmers M, Lucas CE. The role of thoracic aortic occlusion for massive hemoperitoneum. J Trauma. 1976; 16(08):610–5.
11. Millikan JS, Moore EE. Outcome of resuscitative thoracotomy and descending aortic occlusion performed in the operating room. J Trauma. 1984;24(5):387–92.
12. Asensio J, Hanpeter D, Gomez H, Chahwan S, Orduna S, McDuffie L. Exsanguination. In: Shoemaker W, Greenvik A, Ayres S, Holbrook P, editors. Textbook of critical care. Philadelphia: Saunders; 2000. p. 37–47.
13. Asensio J, Lejarraga M. Abdominal vascular injury. In: Demetriades D, Asensio J, editors. Trauma handbook. Austin: Landes Biosciences; 2000. p. 356–62.
14. Voellinger DC, Saddakni S, Melton SM, Wirthlin DJ, Jordan WD, Whitley D. Endovascular repair of a traumatic infrarenal aortic transection: a case report and review. Vasc Surg. 2001;35(5): 385–9.
15. Lopez-Viego MA, Snyder 3rd WH, Valentine RJ, Clagett GP. Penetrating abdominal aortic trauma: a report of 129 cases. J Vasc Surg. 1992;16(3):332–5; discussion 5–6.
16. Beck AW, Murphy EH, Hocking JA, Timaran CH, Arko FR, Clagett GP. Aortic reconstruction with femoral-popliteal vein: graft stenosis incidence, risk and reintervention. J Vasc Surg. 2008;47(1):36–43; discussion 4.
17. Kieffer E, Gomes D, Chiche L, Fleron MH, Koskas F, Bahnini A. Allograft replacement for infrarenal aortic graft infection: early and late results in 179 patients. J Vasc Surg. 2004;39(5):1009–17.
18. Accola KD, Feliciano DV, Mattox KL, Burch JM, Beall Jr AC, Jordan Jr GL. Management of injuries to the superior mesenteric artery. J Trauma. 1986;26(4):313–9.
19. Asensio JA, Berne JD, Chahwan S, Hanpeter D, Demetriades D, Marengo J, et al. Traumatic injury to the superior mesenteric artery. Am J Surg. 1999;178(3):235–9.
20. Lucas AE, Richardson JD, Flint LM, Polk Jr HC. Traumatic injury of the proximal superior mesenteric artery. Ann Surg. 1981; 193(1):30–4.
21. Haas CA, Spirnak JP. Traumatic renal artery occlusion: a review of the literature. Tech Urol. 1998;4(1):1–11.
22. Sangthong B, Demetriades D, Martin M, Salim A, Brown C, Inaba K, et al. Management and hospital outcomes of blunt renal artery injuries: analysis of 517 patients from the National Trauma Data Bank. J Am Coll Surg. 2006;203(5):612–7.
23. Tillou A, Romero J, Asensio JA, Best CD, Petrone P, Roldan G, et al. Renal vascular injuries. Surg Clin North Am. 2001;81(6): 1417–30.
24. Lock JS, Carraway RP, Hudson Jr HC, Laws HL. Proper management of renal artery injury from blunt trauma. South Med J. 1985;78(4):406–10.

25. Maggio Jr AJ, Brosman S. Renal artery trauma. Urology. 1978; 11(2):125–30.
26. Lee JT, White RA. Endovascular management of blunt traumatic renal artery dissection. J Endovasc Ther. 2002;9(3):354–8.
27. Sprouse 2nd LR, Hamilton Jr IN. The endovascular treatment of a renal arteriovenous fistula: placement of a covered stent. J Vasc Surg. 2002;36(5):1066–8.
28. Villas PA, Cohen G, Putnam 3rd SG, Goldberg A, Ball D. Wallstent placement in a renal artery after blunt abdominal trauma. J Trauma. 1999;46(6):1137–9.
29. Lee JT, Bongard FS. Iliac vessel injuries. Surg Clin North Am. 2002;82(1):21–48, xix.
30. Burch JM, Richardson RJ, Martin RR, Mattox KL. Penetrating iliac vascular injuries: recent experience with 233 consecutive patients. J Trauma. 1990;30(12):1450–9.
31. Sullivan PS, Dente CJ, Patel S, Carmichael M, Srinivasan JK, Wyrzykowski AD, et al. Outcome of ligation of the inferior vena cava in the modern era. Am J Surg. 2010;199(4):500–6.
32. Schrock T, Blaisdell FW, Mathewson Jr C. Management of blunt trauma to the liver and hepatic veins. Arch Surg. 1968;96(5):698–704.
33. Feliciano D, Dente C. Abdominal vascular injury. In: Mattox K, Moore E, Feliciano D, editors. Trauma. 7th ed. New York: McGraw Hill; 2012.
34. Fraga GP, Bansal V, Fortlage D, Coimbra R. A 20-year experience with portal and superior mesenteric venous injuries: has anything changed? Eur J Vasc Endovasc Surg. 2009;37(1):87–91.
35. Asensio JA, Petrone P, Garcia-Nunez L, Healy M, Martin M, Kuncir E. Superior mesenteric venous injuries: to ligate or to repair remains the question. J Trauma. 2007;62(3):668–75; discussion 75.
36. Eger M, Golcman L, Goldstein A, Hirsch M. The use of a temporary shunt in the management of arterial vascular injuries. Surg Gynecol Obstet. 1971;132(1):67–70.
37. Nichols JG, Svoboda JA, Parks SN. Use of temporary intraluminal shunts in selected peripheral arterial injuries. J Trauma. 1986;26(12):1094–6.
38. Rasmussen TE, Clouse WD, Jenkins DH, Peck MA, Eliason JL, Smith DL. The use of temporary vascular shunts as a damage control adjunct in the management of wartime vascular injury. J Trauma. 2006;61(1):8–12; discussion 12–5.

Extremity Vascular Injuries

16

Todd E. Rasmussen and Joseph J. DuBose

Introduction

Trauma to the extremities constitutes one of the most common injury patterns seen in the emergency department and surgical practices. In the evaluation of these injuries, all of the functional components of the affected limb (nerves, bone, soft tissue, and vascular structures) must be considered both individually and as a unit. Complications from these injuries, particularly those of advanced severity, are common. Early recognition and treatment are important in the optimization of outcome.

Epidemiology

The potential etiologies of extremity vascular injuries are diverse. The mechanisms contributing to these injuries include blunt and penetrating trauma and even iatrogenic injury. Severe injuries, or those encountered in the setting of military conflict, are often combined in nature [1, 2]. Regardless of the setting in which they are encountered, penetrating injuries with a significant blunt component are much more likely to be associated with open fracture and nerve, soft tissue, and vascular injury.

The majority of extremity vascular injuries in the civilian setting are due to blunt trauma. Civilian extremity injuries occur most often due to falls (50–60 % of lower extremity injuries and 30 % of upper extremity injuries), industrial or work-related accidents (up to 20 % of upper extremity injuries), and motor vehicle crashes [3]. Among civilians with nonfatal trauma, upper and lower extremity injuries are the most common reason for hospitalization. More than one-third of those hospitalized will have serious or limb-threatening injuries [3, 4].

Extremity injuries are particularly common among casualties of armed or military conflict. Approximately 50 % of wartime injuries recorded in the Department of Defense's Trauma Registry of data from contemporary military casualties involve the extremities [5, 6]. Most extremity wounds experienced during combat have a penetrating component, as they typically result from explosions or gunshot wounds. Only 2 % of extremity injuries during combat are due to isolated blunt trauma [5].

Among civilian patients with extremity fractures, associated vascular injuries occur in less than 1 % of cases [7]. The risk of vascular injury increases with increasing injury severity. In retrospective reviews, the incidence of vascular injury was cited as 5 % for severe extremity fractures [8]. Among patients with arterial injury, bony injuries may be present in over 40 % of patients, according to one recent 5-year review [8]. In the same study, venous injuries were documented in 20 % of patients studied.

Initial Evaluation and Management

Initial evaluation of patients with extremity vascular trauma requires rapid assessment and immediate treatment of life-threatening injuries. Following the protocols developed by

T.E. Rasmussen, MD (✉)
US Army Institute of Surgical Research, Joint Base Fort Sam Houston (San Antonio), San Antonio, TX, USA

US Combat Casualty Care Research Program, 722 Doughten Street, Room 3, Fort Detrick, MD 21702-5012, USA

The Norman M. Rich Department of Surgery, The Uniformed Services University of the Health Sciences, Bethesda, MD, USA
e-mail: todd.e.rasmussen.mil@mail.mil

J.J. DuBose, MD
University of Maryland Health System, R Adams Cowley Shock Trauma Center, United States Air Force Baltimore Center for the Sustainment of Trauma and Readiness Skills (CSTARS), Baltimore, MD, USA

The Norman M. Rich Department of Surgery, The Uniformed Services University of the Health Sciences, Bethesda, MD, USA

Department of Cardiovascular Surgery, University of Texas Houston, Houston, TX, USA

V. Gahtan and M.J. Costanza (eds.), *Essentials of Vascular Surgery for the General Surgeon*, DOI 10.1007/978-1-4939-1326-8_16, © Springer Science+Business Media New York 2015

the Advanced Trauma Life Support (ATLS®) program [9] as part of the American College of Surgeons, Committee on Trauma will optimize patient outcomes following trauma. A significant advance stemming from experience in the wars in Afghanistan and Iraq has been maturation of point of injury care guidelines by the military's Committee on Tactical Combat Casualty Care, or CoTCCC [10]. These strategies outline specific steps for first responders or medics to take to stabilize a complex extremity injury including specific adjuncts such as tourniquets and topical hemostatic agents to control bleeding.

Control of Hemorrhage

External bleeding from an extremity injury represents an emergent threat to life. Initial control is best obtained with the effective utilization of direct pressure. Because prolonged application of direct pressure is problematic in the context of patient transport and the care of multisystem injury, consideration for alternative hemorrhage control adjuncts should be entertained. Approaches that have been utilized include topical agents, external compression clamps, and endovascular occlusion devices. These methods are not, however, widely utilized and are not presently endorsed by the American College of Surgeons in the current version of the ATLS curriculum. Other methods include direct clamping of visible bleeding vessels and tourniquets. Blind clamping of vessels that are not clearly visible should be avoided.

Although it is not novel, tourniquet utilization has increasingly been included in algorithms for control of life-threatening hemorrhage from extremity vascular injuries. Pneumatic tourniquet utilization is a well-established practice of vascular surgery and can effectively be used in the hospital setting to stop extremity bleeding en route to more definitive vascular control. A variety of mechanical tourniquet devices are also available for use. These devices have demonstrated their value very well in the recent military experiences in Iraq and Afghanistan and have low associated risks of ischemia and neurologic complications [11–13]. The Combat Application Tourniquet (CAT), Emergency and Medical Tourniquet (EMT), and the Special Operations Forces Tactical Tourniquet (SOFTT) meet the effectiveness standard of the US military by occluding distal flow in over 80 % of subjects.

Several recent studies provide evidence supporting the use of tourniquets for extremity vascular injury in the prehospital environment. In a review of a combat hospital experience in Iraq, Beekley and colleagues [11] examined 165 patients with extremity hemorrhage. Sixty-seven of these individuals had a tourniquet placed in the prehospital environment. This group of researchers noted that control of hemorrhage significantly improved with the utilization of a tourniquet (83.3 % vs. 60.7 %) with no difference in secondary amputation rate due to ischemia. Another prospective study of 232 combat casualties, conducted by Kragh et al. [12], found a significantly improved survival rate (77 % vs. 0 %) when tourniquet use was undertaken in the early phases after injury. The greatest benefit was noted for those patients who had a tourniquet placed in the prehospital environment. They also noted that tourniquet use resulted in only four nerve palsies, all transient, and no amputations related to tourniquet use. Although these two studies demonstrate the potential for benefits of early tourniquet utilization, civilian trauma systems have only recently adopted their use. The study of civilian tourniquet prehospital use remains a matter of active investigation.

Physical Exam

A brief extremity exam, with control of any hemorrhage, should be performed as part of the primary assessment of a trauma patient. Once other life-threatening injuries have been addressed, the extremity exam should be repeated in greater detail. Evaluation of the injured limb should proceed in an orderly fashion that includes assessment of each functional elements including vasculature, nerves, bones, and soft tissues. Appropriate radiographic tools should be utilized to develop a comprehensive picture of the injury extent and provide a framework for subsequent treatment considerations.

The vascular elements of extremity exam begin with a manual palpation of pulses including the femoral, popliteal, and pedal. During palpation, the provider should not only be cognizant of the presence or absence of the pulse but also its strength compared to the unaffected limb. In some cases, auscultation over the area of injury may reveal a bruit indicative of a partially thrombosed or compressed vessel or an arteriovenous fistula. Finally, because palpation is inherently subjective, the continuous wave Doppler has an important adjunctive role in the setting of extremity injury. In addition to a listening for the presence or absence of an arterial signal over any given extremity artery, the quality of the arterial signal can also be graded as strong and bi- or triphasic or weak and monophasic. Measurement of Doppler occlusion pressures in the injured extremity in relation to a non-injured extremity is also a valuable aspect of the physical exam and will be described in the following section.

In the setting of shock or hypothermia, the extremity vascular exam (palpation and Doppler) should be repeated after resuscitation. Likewise, reduction of joint dislocations or angulated extremity fractures necessitates a repeat assessment of perfusion. In one recent study of combat injuries, these two interventions effectively restored a palpable pulse to a previously ischemic limb in 74 % of patients [14].

During the pulse examination, one should be cognizant of both "hard" and "soft" signs of vascular injury. Hard signs include active hemorrhage, expanding or pulsatile hematoma, bruit or thrill over a given wound, absent distal pulses, and signs of acute extremity ischemia (pain, pallor, paralysis, cold to touch). In the setting of penetrating trauma, the presence of any of these hard signs is highly predictive of a vascular injury requiring surgical repair. These patients should be taken directly to the operating room for operative management. If arteriography is required to clarify the anatomy of injury, it can be performed intraoperatively.

In the setting of blunt trauma, hard signs of vascular injury have a higher false-positive rate compared to penetrating trauma. In the case of a joint dislocation, reduction may change the pulseless limb to one with a palpable distal pulse and a normal arterial Doppler signal. If a pulse deficit persists after reduction and the patient is hemodynamically normal, performance of a Doppler exam including measurement of arterial occlusion pressures should be performed. Quantifying the Doppler occlusion pressure of an injured extremity is also referred to as an injured extremity index, or IEI. If this assessment is performed in the lower extremity, it is often referred to as an ankle brachial index, or ABI. Performance of the IEI and ABI will be described in detail in the following paragraphs. In cases where the pulse deficit or abnormal IEI persists after fracture or dislocation reduction, computed tomography angiography (CTA) or traditional angiography can delineate the location and nature of the vascular injury.

In the absence of hard signs, the sequelae of trauma that raise suspicion for vascular injury constitute "soft signs" which include a stable hematoma or a specific location or type of orthopedic injury. Patients with "soft signs" require a vascular exam and determination of the IEI. Measuring extremity Doppler occlusion pressures is an extension of a thorough physical exam and equivalent to measuring the ABI during evaluation of chronic limb ischemia resulting from vascular disease. This aspect of the exam requires a continuous wave Doppler and a manual blood pressure cuff. The cuff is placed on the extremity proximal to the vessel under Doppler evaluation (e.g., dorsalis pedis, posterior tibial, brachial, radial, or ulnar artery). The cuff is then slowly inflated until the Doppler signal is obliterated and then slowly deflated until the Doppler signal returns. The pressure at which the Doppler arterial signal returns is then recorded. This technique is repeated on the uninjured, contralateral extremity. The IEI is the ratio of the highest occlusion pressure measured in the injured extremity divided by the occlusion pressure measured in an uninjured extremity. As an example, for an injured upper extremity, the higher arterial occlusion pressure between the radial and ulnar artery in the injured extremity would be divided by the occlusion pressure of the contralateral brachial artery.

A normal IEI is 0.9 or greater and has a high negative predictive value for arterial injury. In most instances, patients who have an injured extremity with a normal IEI can be safely managed without additional vascular imaging. An IEI of less than 0.9 is abnormal and indicative of a flow-limiting injury in the limb. It is important to note that measurement of the IEI may be repeated during the early phases of care of the injured patient. This is especially important in patients who are hypothermic or hypotensive during the initial assessment. In such patients, if the initial IEI is abnormal, the exam should be repeated 10–15 min after resuscitation and warming. A persistent value of less than 0.9 is predictive of arterial injury and warrants further vascular imaging or operation.

Vascular Imaging

For patients who have a persistently abnormal IEI, vascular imaging options should be undertaken with consideration for the overall clinical status of the patient and associated injuries. In patients with associated injuries to the head or torso, it may prove useful to combine their required CT imaging of these body regions with CTA of the extremity in question. For patients with isolated extremity injury, an individualized approach may be more practical and useful. Some patients may benefit from immediate surgical exploration and others from digital subtraction arteriography (DSA) instead of a CTA. If the technical expertise is available, duplex ultrasonography is a sensitive and noninvasive method to exclude or characterize extremity vascular injury. In patients who are hemodynamically normal with only soft signs of vascular injury, efforts should be made to avoid reflexively ordering a CTA or angiography as a matter of routine. Frequently, noninvasive tests such as IEI and duplex ultrasound followed by clinical observation are very effective and avoid radiation and contrast exposure.

CTA has replaced DSA in the setting as the initial evaluation of choice for trauma patients with an abnormal IEI. The sensitivity of helical CTA with three-dimensional reconstruction ranges from 90 to 100 %, with specificities of 99 % reported by multiple groups who have studied the subject [15–19]. Newer generation multidetector scanners have sensitivity and specificity approaching 100 % for clinically significant injuries [18, 19]. CTA also has an advantage in patients with multiple injuries, as it is less invasive than conventional angiography and can be performed at the same time as CT imaging of the head, chest, and abdomen. As a single study, CTA is less expensive than most conventional angiographic modalities [19].

Despite the emergence of CTA, conventional digital subtraction arteriography (DSA) still plays an important role in the evaluation of extremity vascular injury. The advent of portable angiographic capabilities and advanced hybrid operating suites has made DSA a useful diagnostic tool and therapeutic adjunct in the care of a polytrauma patient requiring emergent operation [20]. In these cases, DSA can evaluate for a wide range of injuries without having to move the patient which facilitates a more rapid exclusion or characterization of vascular injury. Intraoperative DSA combined with endovascular intervention can be both diagnostic and therapeutic for vascular injuries. In some cases, endovascular techniques function as an adjunct in placing a proximal occlusion balloon to achieve hemostatic control and facilitate a hybrid open repair. In other scenarios, endovascular therapy can provide definitive treatment by stenting or embolizing of specific extremity vascular injuries.

Regardless of the modality used to diagnose extremity vascular injury, specific findings on either CTA or DSA represent indications for treatment. These findings combined with the physical exam and clinical status of the patient dictate the timing or urgency of the required intervention. Specific findings that require surgical or endovascular therapy include extravasation of contrast, pseudoaneurysm, arteriovenous fistula, flow-limiting intimal flap, arterial occlusion, and distal embolism.

Assessment of Nonvascular Structures of the Extremity

In addition to vascular evaluation, other functional elements of the limb must be assessed following trauma. Nerve, bone, and soft tissue disruption due to trauma will, along with the severity of the vascular injury, determine the functional outcome of the limb. These structures should be considered when planning potential operative intervention versus primary amputation.

In the awake and cooperative patient, a neurologic exam facilitates the early identification of associated motor and sensory deficits. In the obtunded patient, gross deficits should be noted including lack of movement in all or part of an extremity or asymmetric movements. Detailed, ongoing evaluation of the extremity can detect specific defects attributable to peripheral nerve injury. Physical exam of the lower extremity should asses the function of the femoral, sciatic, tibial, and peroneal nerves. These nerves are most likely to sustain either direct or ischemic injury in the setting of lower extremity vascular trauma. Historically, plantar sensation was thought to be an indicator of lower extremity viability and long-term function. More recent literature suggests that this finding is not a reliable assessment, as many patients with an insensate foot at initial evaluation subsequently regain elements of function [21].

Familiarity with the neurologic examination of the lower extremity is paramount to the successful evaluation of limb viability. Injury to the sciatic nerve results in decreased sensation of the medial thigh and weakness in hip flexion. Femoral nerve trauma is associated with decreased sensation in lateral thigh and leg, weakness of hip extension, and loss of motor function of the leg and foot. Disruption of peroneal nerve function causes decreased sensation in the first dorsal web space and foot drop. Finally, injury to the tibial nerve is associated with loss of sensation to the heel of the foot, inability to plantar flex the foot, and cavus deformity of the foot. If identified on physical exam, any of the aforementioned injuries should be well documented and considered in decisions regarding limb salvage.

In the upper extremity, the axillary, radial, and median nerves are most prone to injury due to their anatomic location. The game of "rock, paper, scissors" is a rapid and effective way to test the motor function of the median, radial, and ulnar nerves, respectively. The axillary nerve is particularly prone to injury in the context of proximal humerus fracture, an injury pattern which results in loss of arm abduction and an area of paresthesia along the lateral aspect of the upper arm. Radial nerve injury leads to loss of sensation on the dorsum of the hand and weakness of the wrist and finger extensors. Trauma to the median nerve leads to decreased sensation on the palmar aspect of the first three digits and weakness of the thenar musculature.

Injury to soft tissue and bone must also be assessed in order to determine the ability to salvage severely injured limbs. Significant soft tissue defects may be caused by missile injury and exit, tissue avulsion, or skin or muscle flap formation. Significant contamination may lead to considerable risk for infection and soft tissue loss. In penetrating injuries such as high-velocity gunshot or fragmentation wounds, a relatively small external wound may not reflect the severe tissue damage hidden beneath the skin. The muscle compartments of the extremity must also be assessed for the presence of compartment syndrome. Chapter 5 outlines the evaluation and treatment of this entity.

Evaluation for orthopedic injury must also be undertaken. Extremity deformity, point tenderness, ecchymosis, laceration deep to the muscle fascia or near a joint, and joint laxity are all clinical signs of potential fracture. Plain radiography in the early phases of evaluation provides a means for the accurate assessment and characterization of bony injury. When misalignment is identified, splinting and reduction should be undertaken particularly as a precursor to effective vascular evaluation as described previously.

The Mangled Extremity

Although mangled extremities are not common [22], they represent significant management challenges that require careful consideration of complex clinical factors affecting outcome. Limb salvage efforts require extensive resources, prolonged hospitalizations, and comprehensive rehabilitation. Even when successful, multiple reconstruction procedures may be necessary to achieve a functional result. Failed attempts at limb salvage are also associated with increased cost and adverse patient outcomes. For all these reasons, the decision process for the care of a mangled extremity requires a systematic approach that adequately considers all factors.

Many predictors of adverse outcome following mangled extremities have been identified and several groups have proposed the use of predictive scoring systems to determine the need for amputation after these injuries [23–27]. In 1987, Howe et al. [28] performed a retrospective review of 21 injured limbs to determine which variables influenced salvage or loss after trauma. This group found that a Predictive Salvage Index (PSI), consisting of weighted scoring of the level of vascular injury, degree of osseous injury, degree of muscle injury, and warm ischemia time, was 78 % sensitive and 100 % specific in predicting subsequent amputation. In 1990, Johansen and colleagues [29] proposed the utilization of the Mangled Extremity Severity Score (MESS) that was developed through an examination of 25 patients with severe limb injuries. The MESS consists of four primary risk considerations, including skeletal/soft tissue injury, limb ischemia, shock, and age. These investigators then prospectively validated the score in 26 severely injured limbs, concluding that a MESS of greater than or equal to 7 was 100 % predictive of amputation.

A subsequent study conducted by McNamara and colleagues outlined the development and utilization of a nerve injury, ischemia, soft tissue injury, skeletal injury, shock, and age of patient (NISSSA) score which added consideration of the nerve component of injury [25]. The NISSSA score gave the greatest weight to the loss of plantar sensation and also divided tissue injury into soft tissue and skeletal components. In 26 injured limbs, the NISSSA score was found to be both more sensitive (81.8 % vs. 63.6 %) and more specific (92.3 % vs. 69.2 %) than the MESS. Other scoring systems, including the Limb Salvage Index (LSI) proposed by Russell and colleagues in 1991 [30] and the Hannover Fracture Scale [31], have also been utilized to predict the need for amputation after trauma.

Larger prospective studies raised doubts regarding the clinical utility and validity of all the previously described scoring systems. In 2001, Bosse and colleagues conducted a prospective evaluation of available scoring systems in an examination of 556 high-energy lower extremity injuries [21]. They examined the sensitivity, specificity, and area under the receiver operating characteristic curve for MESS, LSI, PSI, NISSSA score, and the Hannover Fracture Scale for both ischemic and nonischemic limbs. Their analysis was conducted in two ways: including and excluding limbs that required immediate amputation. All of the scoring systems demonstrated significant flaws which limit their clinical value. Although all systems had high specificity for prediction of limb salvage when the scores were low, none of the scoring systems proved to be a valid predictor of the need for amputation. Ly and the LEAP study group [32] followed this investigation in 2008 with an analysis of a cohort who participated in a multicenter prospective study of clinical and functional outcomes after high-energy lower extremity trauma. They examined 407 subjects for whom reconstruction was considered successful at 6 months and found that none of the retrospectively validated scoring systems (MESS, LSI, PSI, NISSSA score, or the Hannover Fracture Scale) were predictive of the functional status (as measured by the Sickness Impact Profile) at 6 or 24 months. In addition, none of these scoring systems predicted patient recovery between 6 and 24 months. They concluded that no currently available injury severity score can predict the functional recovery of patients who undergo initial limb reconstruction.

In the absence of a clinically validated scoring system, the management of the patient with a mangled extremity requires a multidisciplinary approach and individualized consideration of complex systemic and limb-related factors. Optimal outcome requires the trauma provider to evaluate these factors systematically, in order to determine the appropriate choice between limb salvage procedures and amputation.

The Unstable Patient: Vascular Management Considerations

Based on ATLS principles, the hemodynamically unstable patient with indications for surgery (positive Focused Assessment with Sonography for Trauma [FAST], hard signs of vascular injury) should be taken to the operating room for identification and control of hemorrhage. Life-threatening injuries to the neck, chest, or abdomen take precedence over extremity injury. A damage control or staged approach to the injured extremity is warranted once external bleeding from the extremity is controlled. In rare cases, the severity of the extremity injury or the delay caused by the need to manage other life-threatening injuries will preclude meaningful attempts at limb salvage. A primary amputation may be the best option in these situations. If the extremity is the primary (or only) injury, a more definitive approach to repair can be pursued from the onset of care.

One valuable damage control adjunct for the treatment of vascular injury, particularly in the polytraumatized patient, is the use of temporary intravascular shunts (Fig. 16.1). These devices have traditionally been used to maintain distal perfusion during carotid endarterectomy and other elective vascular operations. Although the use of temporary vascular shunts for trauma is not new, recent successes in the treatment of military casualties have highlighted their utility [33, 34].

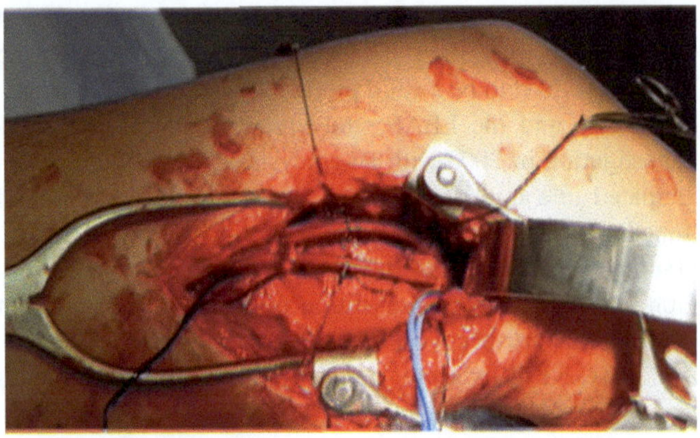

Fig. 16.1 Shunting of left femoral artery and vein in a polytraumatized patient to restore distal perfusion in a damage control setting

Temporary shunts have a variety of applications in the management of extremity vascular trauma. In patients with associated fractures or dislocations, the placement of a temporary vascular shunt allows the orthopedic team to manipulate and fixate the injured extremity without concern for disrupting a vascular anastomosis. The shunt also minimizes ischemic time by providing perfusion during the orthopedic part of the procedure and during vein harvest and preparation. After the reduction and/or fixation, definitive vascular repair can be performed on a stable musculoskeletal platform. Likewise, in hemodynamically unstable patients, placement of a temporary vascular shunt permits more rapid restoration of extremity perfusion mitigating some of the ischemic risks associated with a prolonged vascular repair procedure.

Several vascular shunts are available for utilization. Argyle shunts commonly come in a single container with a variety of sizes making useful for a variety of vessels. Other commercially available conduits, including Javid, Sundt, and Pruitt-Inahara shunts, can also be effective depending upon the size of the vessel and the location of the injury. In extreme circumstances, even intravenous tubing or other soft sterile cylindrical structures can be utilized to temporarily restore perfusion.

The technique of temporary vascular shunt placement requires proximal and distal control of the injured vessel. An embolectomy through the disrupted segment of the artery should then be performed to remove proximal and distal clot and allow temporary restoration of perfusion. Flushing of the vessel with ample quantities of heparinized saline can clear any residual thrombus. Local infusion of heparinized saline rarely contributes to systemic coagulopathy, but should be used cautiously in patients at significant risk for coagulopathy or bleeding from brain, abdominal, or other injuries. Systemic heparinization for isolated extremity injuries without bleeding risk may also be considered; however, the effect of this on the patency of the temporary shunt or the subsequent formal vascular reconstruction has not been well established. Clinical experience, combined with data from animal models of hemorrhage and shock, suggests that temporary vascular shunts placed in the larger, more proximal extremity vessels have high rates of prolonged patency without utilization of systemic anticoagulation [35]. Once positioned, the shunt should be secured both proximally and distally to mitigate the risk of dislodgment during orthopedic manipulation or transportation.

The Stable Patient: Vascular Management Considerations

Patients who are hemodynamically normal can usually tolerate a definitive vascular repair at the time of their initial operation. All repairs begin by gaining vascular control proximal and distal to the site of injury. Once this fundamental surgical tenet has been fulfilled, the injury can be more clearly identified and characterized noting the quality of the injured arterial wall edges. Primary repair may be possible for discrete arterial lacerations with clean, viable injury margins as observed in some stab wounds. Debriding the vessel edges back to healthy, viable tissue is critically important to ensure the integrity of a suture repair or subsequent anastomosis. Because the external appearance of an injured artery may not reflect the extent of intraluminal injury or dissection, adequate debridement requires visualizing the arterial lumen. After debridement, short segments of vessel loss (1–2 cm) may be amenable to mobilization and tension-free primary repair. Longer segments of vessel loss, or the suggestion of tension after mobilization, mandate a vascular interposition graft to restore perfusion.

The choice of conduit, either native vein or synthetic graft, depends on several factors [36]. The diameter of the injured vessel, the degree of wound contamination, and the availability of autologous vein conduit should all be considered. For the majority of injuries, reversed great saphenous vein is the conduit of choice for repair. Although the topic has not been well studied, the preferential use of saphenous vein graft over polytetrafluoroethylene (PTFE) or other artificial materials [37] decreases the incidence of infectious and thrombotic complications associated with the prosthetic grafts. Synthetic grafts provide a reasonable alternative if the great saphenous vein is too small or not available due to injury burden.

The consistent anatomic location of the proximal great saphenous vein makes it easy to harvest for use as a vascular conduit. The incision to expose the vessel begins medial to the femoral pulse, just inferior to the inguinal crease, and travels distally along the anteromedial thigh. It is useful to first identify the saphenofemoral junction in the proximal thigh and then carry the dissection distally to obtain the length of venous conduit required for repair. Isolating the vein circumferentially with a vessel loop can speed the dissection with inadvertently damaging the vein by directly manipulating it. Most surgeons harvest the great saphenous vein from the uninjured (contralateral) lower extremity. Although its clinical importance has not been well established, this practice guards against using a vein that could harbor an unrecognized injury or intimal disruption. Using the contralateral vein also avoids contributing to venous hypertension in the injured limb by preserving its great saphenous vein. In theory, maintaining maximal venous drainage lowers the risk of developing compartment syndrome in the distal injured extremity. The graft should be placed in a reversed configuration to allow unimpeded flow in the direction of the valves. Using the marking pen to draw a series of lines on one side of the vein can help maintain its orientation and avoid twisting the conduit which cuts off flow and causes early thrombosis.

Once a conduit has been selected and properly oriented for interposition, both proximal and distal ends must be sutured into position using nonabsorbable suture on a tapered needle. The size of suture will be dictated by the vessel size, but for extremity injuries, 5-0 or 6-0 Prolene are common choices. Several specific nuances of suturing have been described, including parachute, triangulation, and a simple running suture [38]. All techniques effectively achieve a high-quality anastomosis if properly performed, and the surgeon should use the technique with which he or she is most familiar and facile. Prior to securing the final suture, retrograde and antegrade flushing should be performed by briefly releasing and reapplying the proximal and distal clamps. The anastomosis is then flooded with heparinized saline in an effort to definitively clear the lumen prior to restoration of flow.

At the completion of the repair, distal arterial flow should be assessed by pulse exam and Doppler assessment. Any deficiencies should raise concern for an issue with the graft or anastamosis, either technical error or thromboembolic occlusion. The pulse evaluation should be tempered by the fact that young patients are prone to vascular spasm and peripheral vasoconstriction in the setting of trauma and vessel manipulation. While vasospasm may be ameliorated intraoperatively using intraluminal vasodilators (e.g., low-dose nitroglycerine or papaverine), warming and resuscitation are often required to alleviate this otherwise normal response. A completion arteriogram can be performed by injecting contrast directly into the bypass conduit via a small gauge angiocatheter. This imaging study can confirm the patency of the bypass, distal anastomosis, and outflow. Frequent clinical reevaluation of the extremity in the form of postoperative vascular checks should be initiated and concerns for bypass failure mandate further imaging or re-exploration.

The proven safety and efficacy of endovascular therapy in elective vascular procedures triggered an interest in expanding these techniques to the treatment of vascular trauma and vessel injury [39, 40]. In many cases, endovascular technologies can be seamlessly integrated into the management of vascular extremity trauma. Digital subtraction angiography remains an important diagnostic tool for vascular injury, and modern sheaths and catheters allow select injuries to be treated through the same access site established for DSA with little delay or need for additional manipulation. In hybrid approaches to repair, occlusive endovascular balloons can be utilized to obtain proximal vascular control and decrease blood loss during subsequent open repair. For select injuries, endovascular stent grafting may even preclude the need for open surgery by providing intraluminal coverage of the injured vessel.

Although the role of endovascular technologies in vascular trauma has not been clearly defined, experience with these approaches continues to grow and early results have been encouraging [41–43]. Determining the patency and natural history of endovascular stent grafts placed in young trauma patients requires long-term studies which have not been conducted yet. Despite a lack of long-term follow-up, endovascular therapy will play an increasingly prominent role in vascular extremity trauma. Establishing a multidisciplinary team for the treatment of vascular injuries, including providers with endovascular skills, will help in making treatment decisions for these patients [43].

Considerations for Exposure of Specific Extremity Vascular Injuries

General Principles

Surgical access for vascular injuries should adhere to the basic surgical principle of proximal and distal control and repair of what is in the middle. Accordingly, the initial incision should be amenable to proximal or distal extension if necessary to improve visibility outside the zone of injury. Particularly when a hematoma is present, dissecting back to normal tissue planes frequently improves orientation and visualization allowing more rapid control above and below the injury.

Axillary Artery

Axillary artery exposure begins with an infraclavicular incision that parallels the clavicle and is capable of distal extension onto the arm. The next step requires division of the pectoralis major and minor muscles in sequence. Separating the muscles of the pectoralis major, with the "grain" of the muscle fibers, reveals the deeper pectoralis minor muscle. This muscle can be divided over a clamp just distal to its origin on the coracoid process to expose the underlying axillary artery.

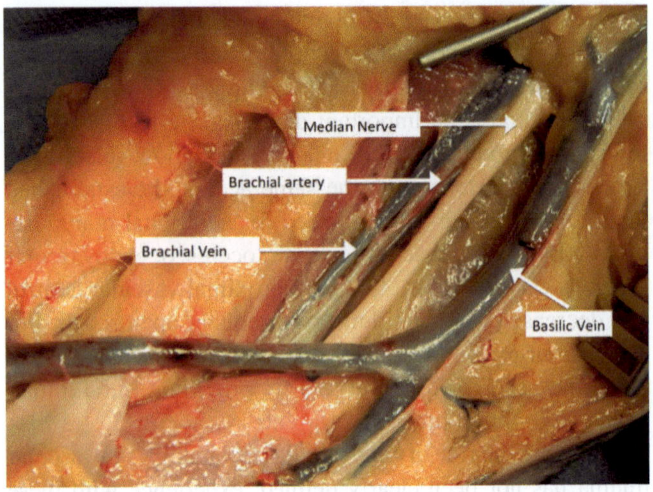

Fig. 16.2 Dissection of the brachial artery in the proximal forearm. The deep brachial fascia has been removed to show vascular structures both superficial and deep to this layer

Brachial Artery

The proximal brachial artery is most readily located via an incision on the medial upper arm in the groove between the biceps and the triceps muscles. In the setting of a large hematoma, care must be taken to avoid injury to the neurovascular bundle, which may be surprisingly superficial. The first structure encountered in the bundle is the median nerve, which should be preserved and protected if it is uninjured.

Distal brachial artery exposure often requires exposure at the antecubital fossa. A sigmoid incision that has its transverse component across the antecubital skin crease is most commonly used. At this location, the artery can be isolated just deep to the biceps tendon. For the sake of access, this tendon can be divided and tagged for later reconstruction. The sigmoid incision can be carried superiorly along the medial aspect of the upper arm to facilitate proximal control or distally for exposure of the brachial artery bifurcation.

Radial and Ulnar Arteries

The bifurcation of the brachial artery can be exposed using a sigmoid incision crossing the antecubital fossa. In the superficial tissues, the median cubital and basilic veins should be identified and preserved if possible. The medial antebrachial cutaneous nerve, which courses along the basilic vein, should also be protected from injury. Opening the deep brachial fascia at this location will reveal the neurovascular bundle, where the median nerve is the first structure encountered. The median nerve can be gently retracted medially, revealing the underlying brachial artery and the more lateral brachial vein (Fig. 16.2).

The bicipital aponeurosis, which overlies the bicipital tendon, is the gateway to the bifurcation of the brachial artery and the proximal radial and ulnar arteries. Division of the bicipital aponeurosis allows exposure of the brachial bifurcation. Distal dissection provides exposure of the ulnar or radial arteries toward the wrist. If either the ulnar or radial artery is injured, an intraoperative Allen's test will be established if single-vessel perfusion of the hand will be adequate for hand viability. In the majority of instances, individual injuries to either of these vessels in isolation can be safely managed with ligation alone.

Femoral Artery

In proximal femoral artery injuries, particularly in unstable patients with complex injury patterns potentially involving the abdomen, the decision to attain proximal vascular control in the abdomen should be considered. If the injury is truly isolated to the groin, however, two options for rapid control are available. The first, and most commonly utilized, is that of a vertical incision over the femoral triangle. This incision can then be extended superiorly with division of the inguinal ligament to establish definitive proximal control. Alternatively, an oblique incision superior and parallel to the inguinal ligament (similar to a renal transplant incision) can expose the external iliac vessels in an extraperitoneal location.

Effective dissection of the groin requires the ability to quickly establish wide exposure and identify and control the common, superficial, and deep femoral arteries and their accompanying veins. The lateral circumflex iliac vein crosses the deep femoral artery very close to its origin and can be injured during looped control of the deep femoral artery. This vein can be isolated, suture ligated, and divided to facilitate adequate exposure.

A medial thigh incision, either as an initial incision if the injury is known or as an extension of a proximal incision, provides the most convenient and facile access to the distal superficial femoral artery, femoral vein, and the proximal popliteal artery. The sartorius muscle, when retracted upward or downward, facilitates identification and opening of Hunter's canal. Controlled dissection can identify and avoid unnecessary injury to the saphenous vein and its accompanying nerve.

Popliteal Artery

Adequate exposure of the popliteal artery can be challenging. Injuries at the popliteal bifurcation are best exposed by a generous incision on the proximal medial calf. Often, adjacent nerves and veins have also sustained injury making the dissection more difficult. More proximal popliteal artery injuries are better accessed by extending the medial thigh incision described above. The great saphenous vein at this location can be superficially located and susceptible to injury. Preserving this vein and protecting it from injury during surgical exposure may promote improved collateral venous outflow should the popliteal vein require ligation due to injury.

The presence of a large hematoma can make it difficult to quickly identify and isolate the injured vessels. Some guidance can be gained from the general principle that major neurovascular bundles of the lower extremities are always located immediately behind the bone. Accordingly, the distal superficial femoral artery and the proximal popliteal artery will be found directly behind the femur, and the popliteal bifurcation and tibioperoneal trunk will be found immediately behind the tibia. At either level, the accompanying vein is often encountered before the artery during dissection.

The Tibioperoneal Trunk

The so-called popliteal trifurcation can be exposed with a medial incision on the proximal calf, just inferior to the edge of the tibia. The dissection is carried down to the medial head of the gastrocnemius muscle which is then divided sharply off the tibia. The attachments of the soleus muscle must also be detached from the tibia to expose the posterior tibial and peroneal vessels adequately.

The medial approach facilitates only proximal control of the origin of the anterior tibial artery. The vessel beyond its origin can be exposed through an anterolateral incision positioned approximately two fingerbreadths lateral to the anterior edge of the tibia. The tibialis anterior and extensor hallucis longus muscles are retracted apart and the anterior tibial artery can be found coursing along the interosseus membrane at the base of the anterior compartment.

Technical Considerations of Extremity Vascular Injury Repair: Key Steps

General Principles

Repair of vascular injuries is a straightforward process that is amenable to an algorithmic approach regardless of injury location. Proximal and distal controls followed by fixing what is "in the middle" remain the basic tenets of safe and effective repair. Utilizing a simple algorithmic approach will yield a successful result in the majority of instances.

Proximal and Distal Control

Using the principles for specific exposures outlined earlier in this chapter will guide the surgeon through exposure and control of injuries at specific locations. The surgeon should always have the ability to extend the initial incision both proximally and distally to establish effective control outside the zone of injury.

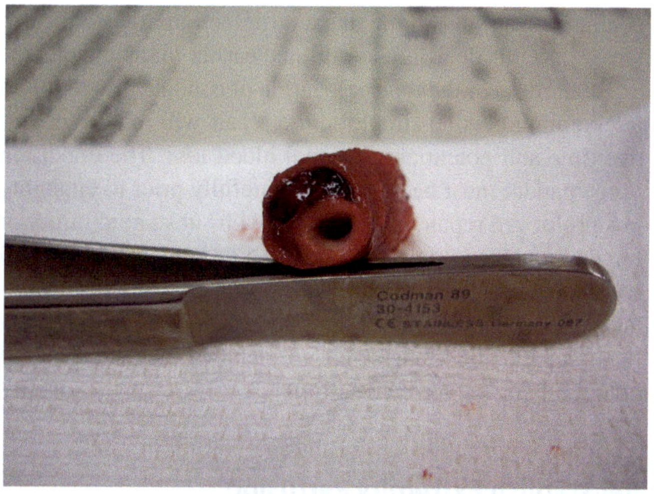

Fig. 16.3 Femoral artery dissection. Note that degree of external alteration may not be reflective of internal injury to the vessel

Characterize Injury Type and Extent

Rapid identification of structures within the zone of injury is often the most challenging step in treating vascular injuries. Hematoma and soft tissue disruption often distort the anatomy extensively. For this reason, it is often advisable to begin the dissection in a more proximal uninjured area and work "from known to unknown" in order to adequately delineate the critical structures.

Characterizing the true extent and severity of injury must include a careful examination of the vessel lumen. The external appearance of the vessel proximal and distal to the obvious injury may not reflect the impact of the injury on the vessel lumen which can be manifested as an associated dissection or intimal disruption (Fig. 16.3). This pitfall often occurs when the vascular injury is discovered at the time of exploration in the absence of preoperative imaging studies.

Feasibility of Definitive Vascular Repair

Once vascular control has been established and the injury has been inspected, nonviable vessel should be debrided back to healthy tissue. The extent of injury will influence the type of repair. Long segments of missing or nonviable vessel will require an interposition bypass to restore distal perfusion. The size of the vessel and the availability of venous conduit will dictate the choice in conduit. The presence of contamination and the anticipated infectious risk will also factor into this decision, as outlined earlier in the chapter.

Regardless of the type or location of conduit, any required intervention beyond simple suture repair will require operative time and potential additional blood loss. The condition of the patient must be considered carefully prior to engaging in a prolonged repair. In the patient with substantial injury or impending physiologic depletion, rapid shunt placement and resuscitation should be undertaken prior to a lengthy vascular repair. If shunting is not an option, ligation (even temporary) should be considered to achieve hemostasis and potentially preserve life over limb.

Reestablish Extremity Perfusion

Prior to restoration of flow by either simple suture repair or interposition conduit, the injured vessel should be cleared of thrombus. Carefully passing Fogarty embolectomy catheters both distally and proximally will facilitate this clearance. Care should be taken to avoid overinflation of the Fogarty balloon so as to minimize the risk of vessel rupture or intimal injury. In addition, the risk of remote perforation and intimal injury increases with each pass of the balloon. The art of Fogarty utilization lies in the feel of pressure and resistance felt at the time of catheter advancement, balloon inflation, and thrombus extraction. Optimal utilization typically requires several clean passes and coordinated control of the balloon, the pressure placed on the inflation syringe, and the tension placed on the vessel during extraction of clot.

Once several passes have failed to retrieve any additional clot, consideration should be given to the use of local heparin infused directly into the vessel (as outlined earlier in this chapter). Although systemic heparinization may help maintain vessel patency, it is frequently contraindicated due to coagulopathy associated with trauma or bleeding risk due to other injuries.

Vascular Reconstruction

Any repair, whether a simple primary repair of a clean laceration or placement of an interposition graft, must be tension-free in nature. The integrity of the repair depends on the presence of healthy tissue from adequate debridement of the injured vessel. Several options for vascular reconstruction exist, as outlined in the previous description of the care of the stable patient. The choice of reconstruction type and conduit must account for the length of the required interposition, vessel size, degree of contamination, and infection risk. For the majority of extremity injuries, reversed great saphenous vein graft is the conduit of choice to provide durable and effective repair. For the sake of expediency, it is useful to take a team approach to the harvest of this conduit, with a partner harvesting and preparing the vein while the primary surgeon is preparing the injured vessel for repair as outlined above.

The saphenous vein should be reversed and gently dilated using an olive-tip catheter on a syringe or a larger diameter soft angiocath. During this maneuver, it is important to look for any leaks in the vessel in the form of side branches that require additional ligation. Unrecognized adherent tissue will also prevent adequate dilation and should be removed until uniform dilation of the vessel is achieved. Marking of one side of the gently stretched vein is advised, as this marking will insure that the vessel is not twisted when secured into position between two suture lines. Such twisting of an interposition graft significantly increases the risk of subsequent conduit thrombosis and should be avoided.

Rarely, only one vessel wall will be injured. Once debrided, these injuries may be repaired with a patch angioplasty. Although the use of patch angioplasty is a common element of elective vascular surgery, the majority of vascular trauma will not prove amenable to this approach.

Immediately prior to tying the final suture throw and closing the vessel, the proximal and distal occlusion should be relieved to flush the vessel. Both forward and retrograde flow should be readily apparent during this maneuver. Any failure to demonstrate reasonable retrograde flow should raise the suspicion of distal thrombosis and warrant an additional distal pass of the Fogarty embolectomy catheter.

Post-Repair Assessment

After the suture line is completed, distal circulation should be assessed. If brisk pulses are restored, the result is reassuring. The gold standard for post-repair evaluation includes the use of intraoperative Doppler ultrasound to document the audible return of a good pulse waveform signal. Particularly in young trauma patients, significant vasospasm may compromise the immediate post-repair assessment. This may be exacerbated by depleted volume status states and hypothermia. As with elective vascular practice, local vessel infusion of nitroglycerine or papaverine in very low doses is utilized by some surgeons prior to suture line closure for this reason. If adequate Doppler signals can be initially documented, however, this vasospasm will almost universally resolve with warming and resuscitation.

Other Considerations

After any extremity vascular reconstruction particularly with known ischemia in excess of 3 h, the need for fasciotomy of distal muscle compartments should be considered.

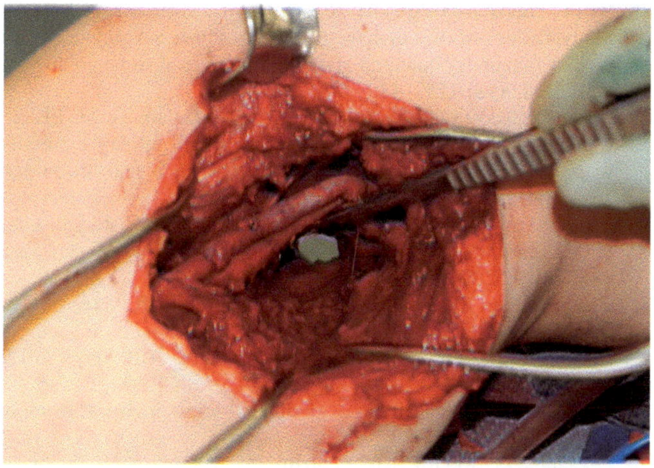

Fig. 16.4 Femoral artery and vein injury following repair with reversed saphenous vein conduits. Mechanism of injury was a high-velocity gunshot wound that resulted in the need for significant debridement of local nonviable tissue. This case illustrates the challenges that can manifest in repair coverage with viable soft tissue

This consideration should be even stronger in the setting of associated vein injury, which may result in venous hypertension exacerbating risk for subsequent compartment syndrome. The specific considerations and techniques of fasciotomy are outlined in Chap. 5 in this text.

Coverage of the vascular repair is also a post-repair priority. Viable soft tissue should be utilized. Failure to achieve closure will increase bleeding and infection risk. Most often, available coverage is found easily within the operative field itself. On occasion, however, specialized flap coverage may be necessary (Fig. 16.4). In these instances, the early involvement of surgical colleagues capable of these maneuvers should be undertaken.

Summary

This chapter is designed to provide reinforcement of the principles and practices required for effective diagnosis and management of vascular injuries to the extremities.

Effective diagnosis requires an algorithmic approach to both examination and the utilization of imaging modalities. Successful treatment is achieved through employment of algorithmic approaches and timely intervention. Optimal outcomes require that the surgeon understand the limitations and benefits of available treatment options.

References

1. Clouse WD, Rasmussen TE, Peck MA, Eliason JL, Cox MW, Bowser AN, Jenkins DH, Smith DL, Rich NM. In theater management of wartime vascular injury: a report from Operation Iraqi Freedom. J Am Coll Surg. 2007;204(4):625–32.
2. White JM, Stannard A, Burkhardt GE, Eastridge BJ, Blackbourne LH, Rasmussen TE. The epidemiology of vascular injury in the wars in Iraq and Afghanistan. Ann Surg. 2011;253(6):1184–9.
3. Mackenzie EJ, Fowler CJ. Epidemiology. In: Feliciano DV, Mattox KL, Moore EE, editors. Trauma. 6th ed. New York: Mcgraw-Hill Medical; 2008. p. 25.
4. Corso P, Finkelstein E, Miller T, Fiebelkorn I, Zaloshnja E. Incidence and lifetime costs of injuries in the United States. Inj Prev. 2006;12(4):212–8.
5. Owens BD, Kragh Jr JF, Wenke JC, Macaitis J, Wade CE, Holcomb JB. Combat wounds in operation Iraqi Freedom and operation Enduring Freedom. J Trauma. 2008;64(2):295–9.
6. Fox CJ, Gillespie DL, O'Donnell SD, Rasmussen TE, Goff JM, Johnson CA, Galgon RE, Sarac TP, Rich NM. Contemporary management of wartime vascular trauma. J Vasc Surg. 2005;41(4):638–44.
7. Schlickewel W, Kuner EH, Mullagi AB, Gotze B. Upper and lower limb fractures with concomitant arterial injury. J Bone Joint Surg Br. 1992;74(2):181–8.
8. Meling T, Harboe K, Soreide K. Incidence of traumatic long-bone fractures requiring in-hospital management: a prospective age- and gender- specific analysis of 4890 fractures. Injury. 2009;40(11):1212–9.
9. Committee on Trauma, American College of Surgeons. ATLS: advanced trauma life support program for doctors. 9th ed. Chicago: American College of Surgeons; 2013.
10. Committee on Trauma, American College of Surgeons and the National Association of Emergency Medical Technicians. PHTLS: pre-hospital life support. 6th ed. Chicago: American College of Surgeons; 2013.
11. Beekley AC, Sebesta JA, Blackbourne LH, Herbert GS, Kauvar DS, Baer DG, Walters TJ, Mullenix PS, Holcomb JB, 31st Combat Support Hospital Research Group. Prehospital tourniquet use in Operation Iraqi Freedom: effect on hemorrhage control and outcomes. J Trauma. 2008;64(2 Suppl):S28–37; discussion S37.
12. Kragh Jr JF, Walters TJ, Baer DG, Fox CJ, Wade CE, Salinas J, Holcomb JB. Survival with emergency tourniquet use to stop bleeding in major limb trauma. Ann Surg. 2009;249(1):1–7.
13. Kragh Jr JF, O'Neil ML, Walters TJ, Jones JA, Baer DG, Gershman LK, Wade CE, Holcomb JB. Minor morbidity with emergency tourniquet use to stop bleeding in severe limb trauma: research, history and reconciling advocates and abolitionists. Mil Med. 2011;176(7):817–23.
14. Burkhardt GE, Cox CM, Clouse WD, Porras C, Gifford SM, Williams K, Propper BW, Rasmussen TE. Outcomes of selective tibial artery repair following combat-related extremity injury. J Vasc Surg. 2010;52(1):91–6.
15. Inaba K, Potzman J, Munera F, McKenney M, Munoz R, Rivas L, Dunham M, DuBose J. Multi-slice CT angiography for arterial evaluation in the injured lower extremity. J Trauma. 2006;60(3):502–6; discussion 506–7.
16. Soto JA, Munera F, Cardoso N, Guarin O, Medina S. Diagnostic performance of helical CT angiography in trauma to large arteries of the extremities. J Comput Assist Tomogr. 1999;23(2):188–96.
17. Soto JA, Munera F, Morales C, Lopera JE, Holguin D, Guarin O, Castrillon G, Sanabria A, Garcia G. Focal arterial injuries of the proximal extremities: helical CT arteriography as the initial method of diagnosis. Radiology. 2001;218(1):188–94.
18. Melvin JS, Dombroski DG, Torbert JT, Kovach SJ, Esterhai JL, Mehta S. Open tibial shaft fractures: I. Evaluation and initial wound management. J Am Acad Orthop Surg. 2010;18(1):10–9.
19. Seamon MJ, Smoger D, Torres DM, Pathak AS, Gaughan JP, Santora TA, Cohen G, Goldberg AJ. A prospective validation of a current practice: the detection of extremity vascular injury with CT angiography. J Trauma. 2009;67(2):238–43; discussion 243–4.
20. Propper BW, Alley JB, Gifford SM, Burkhardt GE, Rasmussen TE. Endovascular treatment of a blunt aortic injury in Iraq: extension

of innovative endovascular capabilities to the modern battlefield. Ann Vasc Surg. 2009;23(5):687.e19-22.

21. Bosse MJ, McCarthy ML, Jones AL, Webb LX, Sims SH, Sanders RW, MacKenzie EJ, Lower Extremity Assessment Project (LEAP) Study Group. A prospective evaluation of the clinical utility of the lower-extremity injury-severity scores. J Bone Joint Surg Am. 2006;87(12):2601–8.
22. Barmparas G, Inaba K, Teixeira PG, et al. Epidemiology of post-traumatic limb amputation: a national trauma databank analysis. Am Surg. 2010;76(11):1214–22.
23. Prichayudh S, Verananvattna A, Sriussadaporn S, et al. Management of upper extremity vascular injury: outcome related to the mangled extremity severity score. World J Surg. 2009;33(4):857–63.
24. Helfet DL, Howey T, Sanders R, Johansen K. Limb salvage versus amputation. Preliminary results of the mangled extremity severity score. Clin Orthop Relat Res. 1990;256:80–6.
25. McNamara MG, Heckman JD, Corley FG. Severe open fractures of the lower extremity: a retrospective evaluation of the mangled extremity severity score (MESS). J Orthop Trauma. 1994;8(2): 81–7.
26. Slauterbeck JR, Britton C, Moneim MS, Clevenger FW. Mangled extremity severity score: an accurate guide to treatment of the severely injured upper extremity. J Orthop Trauma. 1994;8(4): 282–5.
27. Gregory RT, Gould RJ, Peclet M, et al. The mangled extremity syndrome (M.E.S.): a severity grading system for multisystem injury of the extremity. J Trauma. 1985;25(12):1147–50.
28. Howe Jr HR, Poole Jr GV, Hansen KJ, et al. Salvage of lower extremities following combined orthopedic and vascular trauma. A predictive salvage index. Am Surg. 1987;53(4):205–8.
29. Johansen K, Daines M, Howey T, Helfet D, Hansen Jr ST. Objective criteria accurately predict amputation following lower extremity trauma. J Trauma. 1990;30(5):568–72; discussion 572–3.
30. Russell WL, Sailors DM, Whittle TB, Fisher Jr DF, Burns RP. Limb salvage versus traumatic amputation. A decision based on a seven-part predictive index. Ann Surg. 1991;213(5):473–80; discussion 480–1.
31. Durham RM, Mistry BM, Mazuski JE, Shapiro M, Jacobs D. Outcome and utility of scoring systems in the management of the mangled extremity. Am J Surg. 1996;172(5):569–73; discussion 573–4.
32. Ly TV, Travison TG, Castillo RC, Bosse MJ, MacKenzie EJ, LEAP Study Group. Ability of lower-extremity injury severity scores to predict functional outcome after limb salvage. J Bone Joint Surg Am. 2008;90(8):1738–43.
33. Borut LT, Acosta CJ, Tadlock LC, Dye JL, Galarneau M, Elshire CD. The use of temporary vascular shunts in military extremity wounds: a preliminary outcome analysis with 2-year follow-up. J Trauma. 2010;69(1):174–8.
34. Hancock H, Rasmussen TE, Walker AJ, Rich NM. History of temporary vascular shunts in the management of vascular injury. J Vasc Surg. 2010;52(5):1405–9.
35. Chao A, Chen K, Trask S, Bastiansen D, Nelson B, Valentine JC, Borut J, Kang J, Ziegler W, Elshire D. Time to failure of arterial shunts in a pig hemorrhagic shock model. Am Surg. 2012; 78(10):1045–8.
36. Feliciano DV. Management of peripheral artery injury. Curr Opin Crit Care. 2010;16(6):602–8.
37. Felciano DV, Mattox KL, Graham JM, Bitondo CG. Five-year experience with PTFE grafts in vascular wounds. J Trauma. 1985; 25(1):71–82.
38. Ball CG, Feliciano DV. A simple and rapid vascular anastomosis for emergency surgery: a technical case report. World J Emerg Surg. 2009;4:30.
39. DuBose J, Recinos G, Teixeira PG, Inaba K, Demetriades D. Endovascular stenting for the treatment of traumatic internal carotid injuries. J Trauma. 2008;65(6):1561–6.
40. DuBose JJ, Rajani R, Gilani R, Arthurs ZA, Morrison JJ, Clouse WD, Rasmussen TE. Endovascular skills for trauma and resuscitative surgery working group. Injury. 2012;43(11):1785–92.
41. Franz RW, Shah KJ, Halaharvi D, Franz ET, Hartman JF, Wright ML. A 5-year review of management of lower extremity arterial injuries at an urban level I trauma center. J Vasc Surg. 2011;53(6): 1604–10.
42. Carrafiello G, Lagana D, Mangini M, Fontana F, Chiara R, Fillippo P, Carlo P, Piffaretti G, Fugazzola C. Percutaneous treatment of traumatic upper-extremity arterial injuries: a single-center experience. J Vasc Interv Radiol. 2011;22(1):34–9.
43. Franz RW, Skytta CK, Shah KJ, Hartman JF, Wright ML. A five-year review of management of upper-extremity arterial injuries at an urban level I trauma center. Ann Vasc Surg. 2012;26(5): 655–64.

Part VI

Vascular Access

17 Central Venous Access

Kwame S. Amankwah

Indications

VA can be broadly divided into two categories: peripheral and central. Peripheral access is for short-term treatment needs usually involving intravenous (IV) fluids, blood sampling, and infusion of IV medications. Some medications cannot be given though peripheral access because of their tendency to cause vein inflammation (phlebitis). Indications for central VA span a wide range of clinical conditions including:

- Poor vascular access
- Need for hemodynamic monitoring
- Use of medications known to be venous sclerosants
- Repeated venous sampling
- Prolonged administration of chemotherapy, TPN, or antibiotics
- Need for short-term dialysis, aphaeresis, or plasmapheresis
- Emergency situations

Contraindications

Most contraindications to central VA are relative and depend on the urgency of the situation and the available alternatives. Agitated and uncooperative patients may be more safely treated using peripheral access as opposed to trying to cannulate the central veins. Central venous cannulation should be avoided in the presence of overlying cellulitis or infection and at sites with indwelling intravascular hardware such as a dialysis catheter or pacemaker. Distorted anatomy as a result of trauma, surgery, obesity, or previous catheterizations also represents a relative contraindication to central VA.

Central venous access procedures performed on patients with coagulopathy can result in prolonged bleeding from the vein, subcutaneous tunnel, or accidental arterial puncture. Hass et al. evaluated the safety of tunneled central venous catheter insertions in patients with an INR of greater than or equal to 1.5 or a platelet count lower than 50,000/dL [6]. They concluded that a platelet count between 25,000 and 50,000/dL and/or an INR between 1.5 and 2 is safe even without coagulation product transfusion. Other authors have reported that thrombocytopenia (platelets less than 50,000/dL) carries a higher risk of catheter-related bleeding than prolonged clotting times [7]. Overall, coagulopathy represents a relative contraindication to central venous access placement that requires careful consideration of the indications and potential risks and benefits. If possible, patients with coagulopathy should be treated by the most experienced proceduralist available to minimize the bleeding risks. Hemophiliacs who need central venous access require replacement coagulation products, and the correction of clotting factors should be maintained for 48 h prior to the procedure [8].

Patients with cardiac conduction disturbances can have unanticipated complications during placement of a central venous catheter. Contact between the guide wire and the side of the ventricular septum can induce right bundle branch block during the VA procedure [5, 9, 10]. Although this complication rarely causes hemodynamic instability, complete heart block can ensue in patients with preexisting left bundle branch block [10]. An external pacemaker should therefore be available when performing central VA procedures in patients with preexisting left bundle branch block.

Types of Venous Access Devices

Central VA catheters come in a variety of sizes, configurations, and materials. Decisions about the location and type of access catheter should be tailored to the clinical scenario of

K.S. Amankwah, MD, MSc, FACS (✉)
Division of Vascular Surgery, Department of Surgery, SUNY Upstate Medical University, University Hospital, 750 East Adams Street, Syracuse, NY 13210, USA

Department of Surgery and Radiology, Veterans Administration Hospital Upstate Healthcare Network, Syracuse, NY, USA
e-mail: amankwak@upstate.edu

V. Gahtan and M.J. Costanza (eds.), *Essentials of Vascular Surgery for the General Surgeon*, DOI 10.1007/978-1-4939-1326-8_17, © Springer Science+Business Media New York 2015

each patient. Factors that influence the choice of central VA include the predicted duration of the access, the indications for use, and the patient's individual anatomy.

VA devices can be broadly categorized as tunneled catheters (TC) and non-tunneled catheters (Table 17.1). The first decision point in choosing a catheter involves the predicted duration of vascular access. Short-term, temporary access usually warrants placement of a non-TC, while patients needing long-term, permanent access require a TC. Patients with short-term access needs should not be exposed to the risks associated with placement of a TC. In contrast, a patient who requires long-term access for medications such as chemotherapy benefits from a TC with an implanted port. The subcutaneous placement of the port enhances patient comfort by allowing for normal activities in between therapeutic infusion sessions. Implanted ports and TCs have lower rates of infection compared to non-TCs. Potential drawbacks of an implanted port include the inconvenience of needing to puncture the skin for access and the small caliber of the catheter which limits the infusion rate.

Table 17.1 Categorizations of catheters

Tunneled catheters	Non-tunneled catheters
Dialysis catheter with a cuff (permanent)	Dialysis catheters non-cuffed (acute not permanent)
Implantable access ports	Central line
Hickman	Swan-Ganz catheters
Broviac	Peripherally inserted central catheter (PICC)

Vascular access devices have single or multi-lumen catheters. Multi-lumen catheters allow for the simultaneous infusion of more than one blood product or medication. This advantage must be balanced against the increased morbidity associated with multiple lumen catheters as documented in several reports [11, 12]. Decisions regarding the diameter of the catheter depend on the patient's access needs and the clinical scenario. Although large-bore catheters facilitate rapid infusion rates during emergency situations, they have an increased risk of catheter-related thrombosis. In general the smallest-diameter catheter that is feasible for the patient's infusion needs should be chosen [13]. Smaller catheters can often be placed less traumatically and may have a lower risk of triggering venous stenosis [14].

Vascular Access Site Selection

Choosing the location of central VA depends on several factors including: operator skill and preference, catheter and device type, patient anatomy, and indications for placement [7, 15, 16]. The most common sites for central VA are the internal jugular, subclavian, and common femoral veins. Practitioners placing central VA should be familiar with the anatomic landmarks and understand the advantages and drawbacks of each location for central VA (Fig. 17.1). Specific techniques regarding placement will be discussed later.

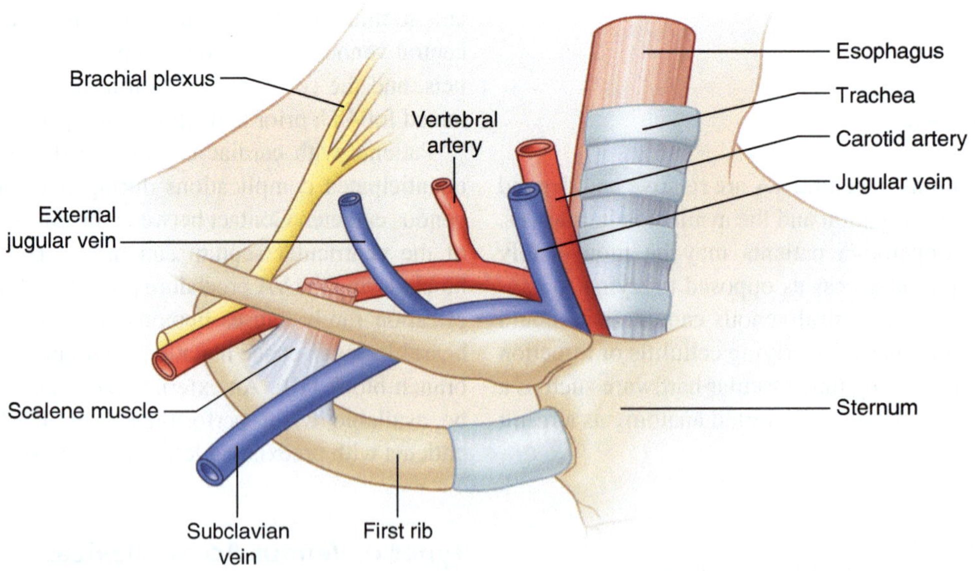

Fig. 17.1 Enlarged view of the anatomy of the subclavian and jugular vein area

Internal Jugular Vein Approach

The internal jugular vein remains the most common site for central VA with a 95–99 % success rate and few complications [17, 18]. Percutaneous access to the internal jugular vein is relatively straightforward compared to the subclavian vein. This technical advantage may explain the lower rate of lung injury (pneumothorax and hemothorax) after internal jugular vein access compared to the subclavian approach [7]. In contrast, a systematic review reported equivalent complication rates for internal jugular and subclavian vein catheters despite a historically higher incidence of complications associated with the subclavian vein approach [4]. The right internal jugular vein follows a straight course into the central venous circulation making the right side the preferred choice over the left side. Internal jugular vein catheterization also poses a lower risk of venous stenosis and thrombosis compared to the subclavian vein [19]. Minimizing the risk of catheter-associated venous stenosis is an important consideration in patients with chronic renal failure in whom central venous stenosis is a leading cause of arteriovenous access failure.

The few drawbacks of internal jugular vein access involve technical challenges associated with placement and patient comfort level. Patients with pain or inadequate sedation during access insertion often tense their sternocleidomastoid (SCM) muscle making it difficult to advance the catheter. Despite being in a compressible location, internal jugular vein puncture can result in a hematoma in a coagulopathic patient potentially compromising the airway. Once in place, non-TCs in the internal jugular vein can cause discomfort during movement of the head and neck.

Ultrasound guidance during VA placement can identify the target vein and provide real-time imaging of the needle entering the vein. Data suggest that using ultrasound to cannulate the internal jugular vein makes the procedure quicker and safer. Lemeris et al. showed that ultrasound guidance reduced failure of catheter placement and complication rates related to insertion by 86 and 57 %, respectively [20]. A large meta-analysis confirmed the enhanced safety profile ultrasound-guided central VA demonstrating significant reductions in the risk of: insertion failure (relative risk [RR] 0.32), complication rates from insertion (RR0.22), and the need for multiple insertion attempts (RR 0.60) [21]. In a prospective study of 900 patients, ultrasound-guided catheter placement in the internal jugular vein not only increased success rates and decreased complication rates but also reduced catheter-associated infections [18]. The well-documented safety track record of ultrasound prompted the UK National Institute for Clinical Excellence (NICE) (www.nice.org.uk) to recommend routine use of ultrasound guidance during internal jugular catheterization.

Subclavian Vein Approach

In the past, surgeons preferentially used the subclavian vein to establish central VA. The subclavian vein is unique in that the vein can be cannulated from an infraclavicular or supraclavicular approach. The supraclavicular technique poses a greater risk of complications, and some authors recommend that only experienced operators attempt this approach [17]. Relative contraindications include bilateral pulmonary disorders, high-pressure ventilation, and altered local anatomy (i.e., after sternotomy). Using ultrasonography to assist with supraclavicular cannulation significantly decreases the risk of placement failure and the need for multiple attempts by up to 86 % [20, 22]. Catheterization of the subclavian vein regardless of the approach has an overall success rate of 90–96 % [23, 24].

Compared to the internal jugular vein, the subclavian vein has a predictable course allowing reliable venipuncture using anatomical landmarks. The subclavian location for central VA has the advantage of easy access to the catheter and a more acceptable cosmetic appearance for the patient. Although observational studies suggest that subclavian vein access decreases infection risk, these results have not been validated in prospective trials [25].

The anatomic location of the subclavian vein has several drawbacks which limit its routine use for VA. The subclavian vein functions as the primary route for venous drainage from the arm. Thrombosis of the subclavian vein from catheter placement can cause acute arm pain and edema requiring treatment with anticoagulation, thrombolytic therapy, or catheter removal [26–28]. Long-term subclavian vein catheter placement increases the risk of venous stenosis which can compromise future arteriovenous access attempts in the same upper extremity [19]. The subclavian vein should therefore be avoided as the site for central VA in patients with renal dysfunction who may eventually require hemodialysis. An exception to this rule would be if the upper extremity were unsuitable for use as a site for dialysis access, for example, a patient with contracture of the arm following a stroke. Other complications associated with subclavian vein cannulation involve injuries that can be sustained during needle puncture. The reported rate of pneumothorax and hemothorax ranges from 0 to 12 % and seems to depend on operator experience [29].

Femoral Vein Approach

The common femoral vein is the easiest site to establish central venous access. With its relatively straight course and large lumen, the common femoral vein allows infusion and removal of large volumes of fluid such as that required in renal replacement therapy or plasmapheresis [7]. In most patients, percutaneous access to the common femoral

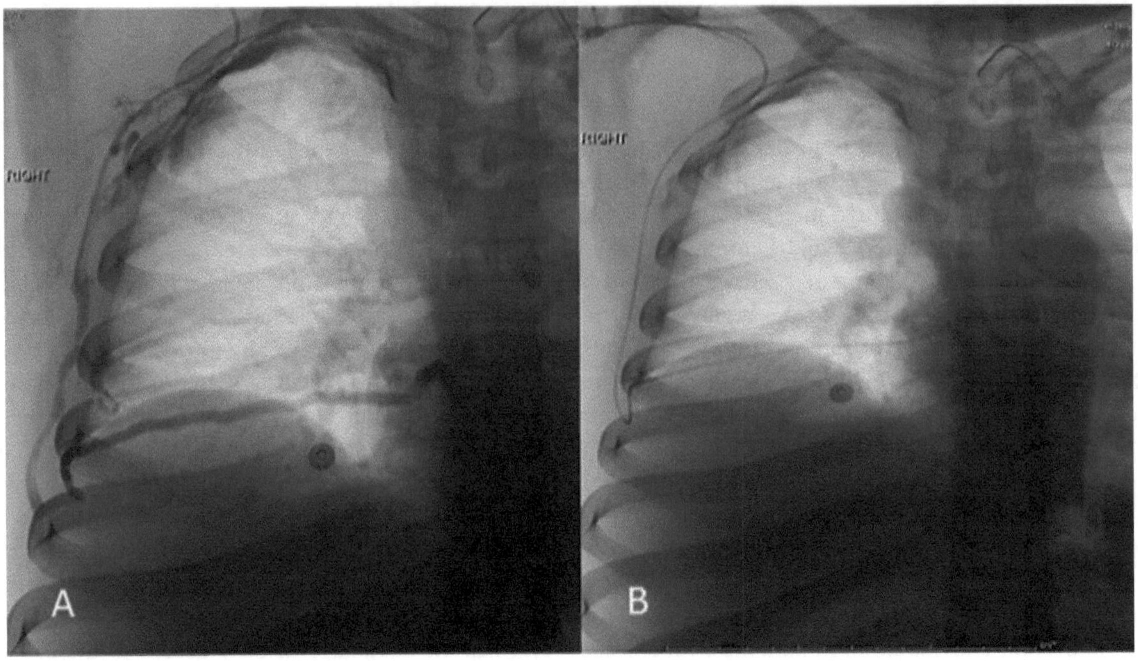

Fig. 17.2 (**a**) Venogram of the right chest intercostal veins with drainage into the vena cava. (**b**) Completion of catheter placement from subclavian, through the intercostal veins with catheter tip in the IVC

vein is straightforward as the vein is close to the skin and relatively isolated from other vital structures. Despite its advantages, the common femoral vein is the least used access site due to the increased incidence of complications, especially infection and thrombosis [30, 31]. Morbid obesity can obscure the anatomic landmarks of the groin making catheterization of the common femoral vein more difficult. Moving the pannus cephalad and to the control lateral side with the aid of an assistant or tape can help determine the appropriate area for percutaneous access to the femoral vein. Similar to other VA sites, ultrasound guidance decreases the risk of failed femoral catheter placement by up to 71 % [20, 22]. Femoral catheters should be removed as soon as possible to minimize the risk of catheter-associated complications.

Alternative Venous Access

Although most surgeons do not place central VA at nonconventional locations, the surgeon must be aware that alternative techniques and access sites do exist. Over time, patients with prolonged central VA often develop stenosis and occlusions of the large veins en route to the central venous system. In these patients, the subclavian and internal jugular veins no longer provide an unobstructed pathway to the central venous system. In the past, overcoming this technical challenge often required open surgical exposure with direct catheter placement in the right atrium, superior vena cava (SVC), or inferior vena cava (IVC) [17]. More recently, central VA routes have been described involving percutaneous access to nonconventional veins including the external jugular, hepatic, intercostal, azygos, and IVC [32–35]. Other techniques involve catheter placement in collateral neck or chest veins or recanalization of chronically occluded veins [36]. Catheters placed at these unconventional sites follow an unusual course when visualized on abdominal or chest radiographs (Fig. 17.2). The distal tip of the catheters terminates in traditional locations such as the right atrium, the lower SVC, or the upper portion of the IVC [37]. Patients receiving long-term hemodialysis or total parental nutrition are more likely to eventually require alternative forms of central VA.

Preparation of the Patient

Consent

Informed consent should be obtained for all elective central VA insertion procedures. A discussion with the patient and/or healthcare proxy should include a description of the procedure as well as its indications, benefits, and acute and long-term complications (Table 17.2). In emergency situations, the consent is implied.

Monitoring

Central VA procedures performed at the bedside or in the angiography suite require some form of monitoring. Cardiac telemetry and pulse oximetry can detect acute changes in the

Table 17.2 Immediate and delayed complications

Immediate	Delayed
Air embolism	Infection
Great vessel perforation/puncture	Venous stenosis
Catheter malposition	Thrombotic
Pneumothorax	

cardiorespiratory status of the patient, such as a dysrhythmia due to wire or catheter placement.

Positioning

Regardless of the access site, the patient's position should fulfill two criteria: (1) maximize the comfort of the patient; and (2) allow the operator to remain comfortable throughout the procedure. The Trendelenburg position facilitates venous filling for internal jugular and subclavian access and may reduce the risk of air embolism [38–40]. Patients who cannot tolerate Trendelenburg but can follow commands should be asked to perform the Valsalva maneuver which temporarily increases the caliber of the internal jugular, subclavian, and femoral veins [41].

Sterile Technique

Minimizing the risk of infectious complications begins with patient preparation and choice of venue. VA procedures should be performed in an environment conducive to aseptic techniques. Randomized controlled trials suggest that prophylactic intravenous antibiotics reduce catheter-related infections (CRI) and sepsis in high-risk immunosuppressed cancer patients; however, current evidence does not support the routine use of antibiotics for central venous catheter placement [42, 43].

Aseptic preparation of the patient and members of the healthcare team plays an important role in infection control. Most institutions mandate the use of surgical masks and caps, sterile gloves and gowns, and a large full-body drape for all central line procedures. Observational studies support the use of these maximal barrier precautions and hand washing as effective measures to reduce the rate of central VA infections [44–46].

Skin preparation options include chlorhexidine, povidone-iodine, and alcohol-based solutions. A study comparing povidone-iodine without alcohol to 2 % chlorhexidine without alcohol reported equivocal findings regarding catheter colonization and catheter-related bacteremia [47]. Studies comparing chlorhexidine with alcohol to povidone-iodine with alcohol have been inconclusive. Consensus from several studies favors the use of chlorhexidine with alcohol for skin preparation [48, 49].

Use of Ultrasound

First described in 1978, ultrasound guidance for central VA now has a solid foundation of evidence supporting its use [22, 50, 51]. Several randomized trials show that using ultrasound for central VA reduces the time to cannulation and decreases the risk of complications and the number of failed attempts [20–22, 50–52]. By clarifying anatomy and providing real-time imaging, ultrasound guidance narrows the performance gap between experienced and inexperienced operators [53]. In the hands of skilled practitioners, ultrasound often proves to be the key to successful catheter placement in patients who are otherwise difficult to cannulate [54]. Current practice guidelines recommend using ultrasound guidance for central VA via the internal jugular and femoral veins when expertise and equipment are available [22, 52]. In contrast, cannulating the subclavian vein does not appear to benefit from ultrasound guidance. Recent studies on subclavian vein access using an axillary and infraclavicular approach have determined that ultrasound does not improve success rate and may increase the time of the procedure when compared to the traditional technique using anatomic landmarks [55–57].

Technique

Internal Jugular Vein

Central Venous Line

After the patient is positioned, the left and right internal jugular veins should be evaluated for patency using the ultrasound. A patent internal jugular vein appears to be a large, echolucent vessel that completely compresses when gentle pressure is applied through the ultrasound probe. The neck and infraclavicular area should then be prepped with chlorhexidine and draped using sterile technique.

The following describes a micropuncture technique; however, using the larger caliber needle provided in most central line kits is also acceptable. When the vein has been localized with ultrasound, the long axis of the probe is placed against the superior portion of the clavicle (Fig. 17.3a) with the image of the internal jugular vein centered on the monitor. Under ultrasound guidance, the area is infiltrated with lidocaine before puncturing the skin with a 21-gauge needle. The angle of puncture is important when using ultrasound guidance. The needle should be almost parallel to the probe, angled only a few degrees from vertical. This permits the tip of the needle to be visualized along its course from skin entry to venipuncture (Fig. 17.3b). The needle is exchanged over a 0.018-in. guidewire for the coaxial 3-French (F) and 5-F micropuncture sheath. The 0.018-in. wire and 3-F dilator are removed from the 5-F micropuncture sheath, and a 0.035-in. wire is inserted with the tip in the SVC. The 5-F sheath is then removed over

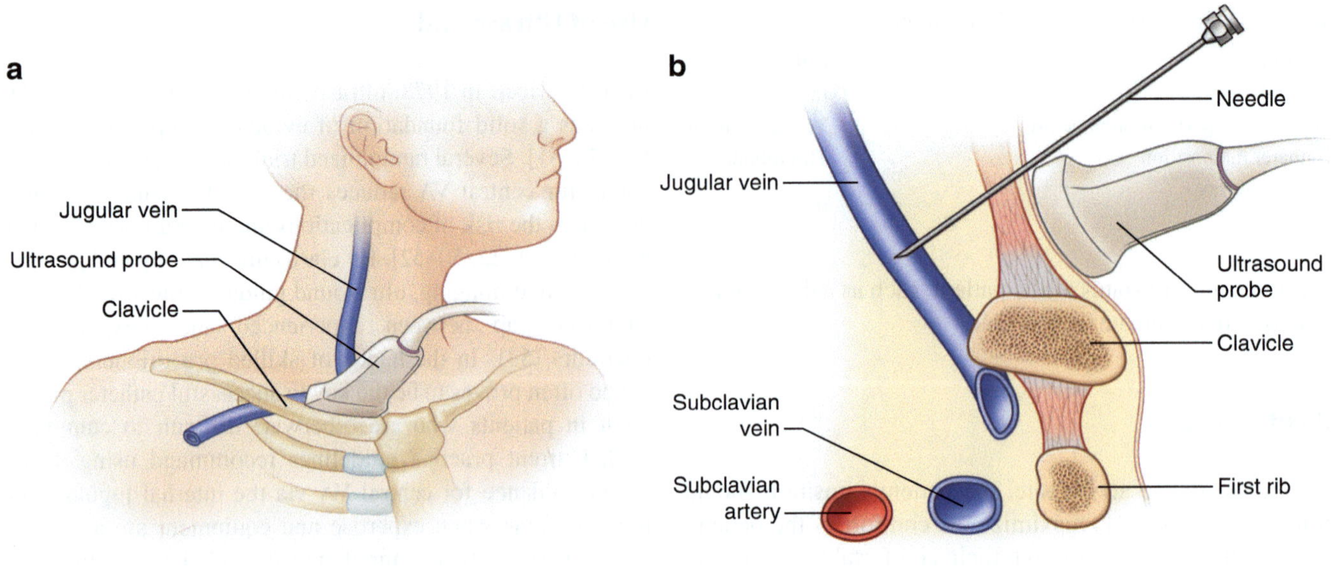

Fig. 17.3 (**a**) Ultrasound use to visualize the jugular vein prior to access placement. (**b**) Sagittal view of the jugular access. The ultrasound is positioned with the inferior portion resting against the clavicle and an acute angle of the needle to the probe to visual the track of the access needle as it enters the jugular vein

the guidewire, and a dilator is inserted to dilate the skin track. The non-tunneled central venous catheter is placed over the guidewire and advanced into the SVC. The guidewire is removed and the catheter secured. All of the catheter lumen should be flushed, and the catheter may be locked with dilute heparinized saline depending on individual hospital protocol. A chest x-ray should be performed to confirm catheter tip location and evaluate for pneumothorax or hemothorax. Procedures performed with ultrasound guidance and under fluoroscopy do not usually require a final chest x-ray.

Chest Port Insertion

Single- or dual-lumen implantable ports are best suited for patients who require intermittent vascular access over a long period of time. Preparation and positioning are the same as described for central venous line placement. The long axis of the ultrasound probe is placed against the superior portion of the clavicle (Fig. 17.3a) with the image of the internal jugular centered on the monitor. Placing the ultrasound probe against the superior portion of the clavicle allows the needle to puncture the internal jugular vein approximately 1 cm above the clavicle. Vein puncture at this level allows the catheter to follow a gentle curve from the vein to its connection with the reservoir on the anterior chest. A higher vein puncture site may cause the catheter to kink, while a lower puncture risks injury to the great vessels and lung. After achieving ultrasound-guided access to the internal jugular vein as previously described, the micropuncture sheath, dilator, and 0.018-in. wire are left in place and temporarily secured to the drape.

The next several steps involve creation of the subcutaneous pocket and tunnel. An imaginary line at an angle of about 45° is drawn from the puncture site in the neck to the anterior chest below the clavicle (Fig. 17.4). This area will be the site of the subcutaneous pocket for the port. After establishing a field block with lidocaine, the skin is incised, and a 1-cm deep pocket is created on the anterior chest wall with blunt finger dissection. The overall size of the pocket should be limited to a few millimeters larger than the port itself. Keeping the subcutaneous pocket small minimizes the chance of the port moving or rotating. The pocket should extend to the level of the fascia for stable fixation points.

The pocket and the neck incision are then connected subcutaneously using the tunneling tool usually provided in the access kit. Attention is then returned to the neck access site. After removing the 3-F dilator and 0.018-in. wire, an 0.035-in. wire is advanced under fluoroscopic guidance into the SVC. Serial dilators are then passed over the wire before placing the peel-away sheath into the SVC. Most peel-away sheaths now have a protective cap, which prevents the sheath from entraining air when the wire and inner dilator are removed. If a protective cap is not in place, caution must be taken to avoid an air embolism when advancing the catheter into the peel-away sheath. The catheter tip should be positioned just within the right atrium. If the catheter triggers cardiac irritability on the monitor, it should be pulled back a few millimeters. The rationale for placing the catheter within the right atrium has to do with the fact that the patient is in a supine position. When the patient is upright, the heart will assume a lower position, and the tip of the catheter will most likely be located at the atrial-caval junction.

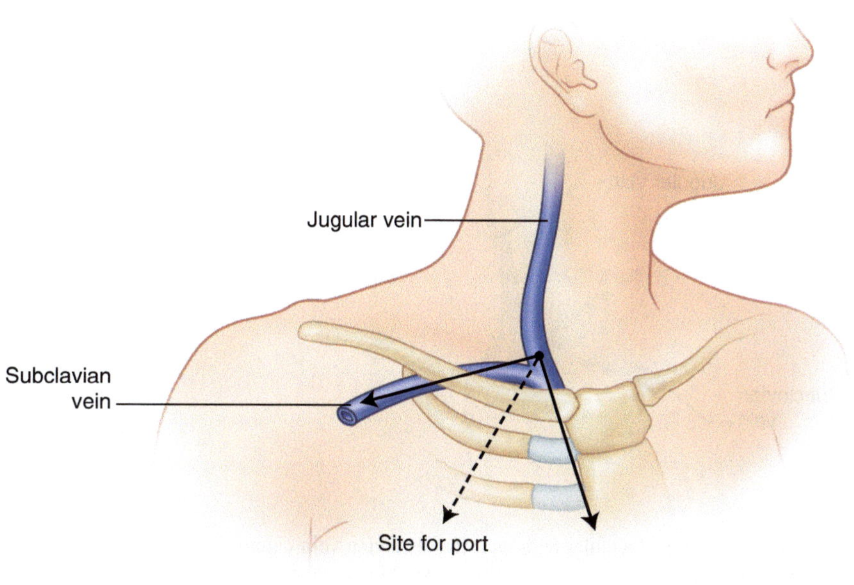

Fig. 17.4 Diagram demonstrates orientation for position of subcutaneous pocket. This can also be utilized for placement of a tunneled catheter

The peel-away sheath can then be partially removed to allow a small straight clamp to be placed on the catheter. The rest of the sheath is then peeled away, and a second clamp is placed on the catheter as it exits the tunnel into the subcutaneous port pocket. Placing these clamps establishes two fixed points on the catheter ensuring that the catheter position cannot be changed and that an appropriate length of catheter remains in the SVC. The catheter can then be attached to the port after trimming its excess length. The port is inserted into the pocket; the small straight clamps are removed; and the port is flushed. The skin incision can be closed with absorbable subcutaneous and subcuticular sutures. If vascular access is needed immediately, a Huber (non-coring) needle can be left in the port. A final fluoroscopic image should document the position of the catheter and port.

Tunneled Catheter Insertion

Most TCs are used for dialysis access, long-term TPN, or chemotherapy. Note that different catheters have been specifically designed for each of these needs. The risk of infection and thrombosis increases with the number of catheter lumens [11, 12]. Therefore, the lowest number of lumens necessary to fulfill the clinical needs should dictate catheter choice.

The technique for inserting a TC parallels the steps described for placing a chest port with a few pertinent details. For internal jugular vein placement, keeping the needle puncture site approximately 1 cm above the clavicle allows the catheter to take a gentle bend as it exits the subcutaneous tunnel and enters the vein. This prevents kinking of the catheter that invariably leads to catheter malfunction. After placing the micropuncture catheter in the vein, fluoroscopy can help choose the appropriate catheter length. The tip of the wire is advanced under fluoroscopy to the desired catheter location; the wire is then marked where it exits the skin, removed, and measured to determine the distance from the atrial-caval junction to the vein puncture site. This distance can be added to the distance from the puncture site to the anterior chest wall to determine the appropriate catheter length. The anterior chest wall is then anesthetized along the route toward the internal jugular puncture site. To minimize bleeding from the tunnel, a purse-string suture can be placed at the chosen chest wall exit site. A small incision is then made in the center of the purse-string suture, and the catheter is tunneled subcutaneously towards the internal jugular puncture site. The catheter is then placed using the peel-away sheath technique previously described. Fluoroscopy during and after catheter placement allows accurate placement of the catheter tip and ensures that the catheter is not kinked [58]. The catheter is then secured in place by tightening and tying the purse-string suture around the hub of the catheter.

Subclavian Vein

Infraclavicular Approach

The anatomic relationship between the subclavian vein and the clavicle changes with shoulder position [59–61]. Magnetic resonance imaging shows that passive retraction of the shoulders by placing a rolled towel between the shoulder blades compresses the subclavian vein between the first rib and clavicle which impedes successful cannulation of the vein [62].

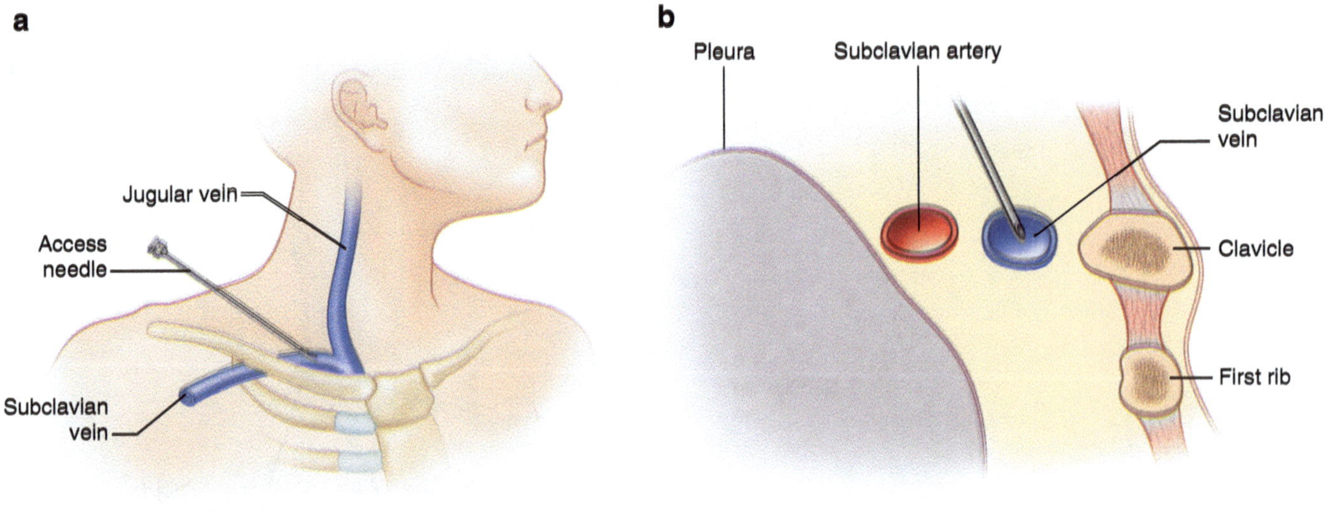

Fig. 17.5 (**a**) Supraclavicular approach to subclavian vein cannulation. (**b**) Cross-sectional view through the medial third of the clavicle. The micropuncture needle is directed anterior to avoid inadvertent injury to the subclavian artery and pleural of the lung

The angle between the subclavian and internal jugular veins increases when the patient's head is rotated to the contralateral side. This change in angle may increase the chance of passing the catheter from the subclavian into the ipsilateral internal jugular vein rather than into the SVC [62]. In other studies, having the patient's head rotated towards the cannulation side failed to improve positioning of the catheter into the SVC [63, 64]. Trendelenburg position does not affect the caliber of the subclavian vein, which is held open in the flat, supine position by the fibrous attachments to the clavicle. Placing the patient in Trendelenburg still provides benefit by increasing venous filling and minimizing the risk of air embolism [65].

In preparation for subclavian vein cannulation, the patient is placed in a supine position in 10–15° of Trendelenburg. Adducting the patient's ipsilateral arm will move the subclavian vein closer to the underside of the clavicle. The shoulders typically assume a more cephalad orientation with the patient in Trendelenburg position which can distort the anatomic landmarks. This tendency should be countered by the use of gentle caudal arm traction.

The goal of subclavian venipuncture is to pass the needle below the clavicle and above the first rib to puncture the subclavian vein as it courses over the first rib. The appropriate course for the needle passes immediately beneath the junction of the medial one-third and lateral two-thirds of the clavicle (Fig. 17.5). This junction or so-called "break" of the clavicle is the point at which the anterior convexity of the medial clavicle transitions into an anterior concavity laterally [65]. The needle should be inserted 1–2 cm inferior and lateral to this transition point, aiming the needle slightly deep to the sternal notch. The needle tip may initially come into contact with the clavicle. The needle should be "walked down" the clavicle to reach its underside. Keeping the needle parallel to the floor (the coronal plane) allows it to slide under the clavicle and enter the vein without injuring the lung or pleura. If the attempt is unsuccessful, these steps should be repeated with the needle pointed more cephalad.

Kilbourne and colleagues examined video recordings of surgery and emergency medicine residents performing subclavian cannulation during trauma resuscitation. They identified six common technical errors, five of which involved anatomic considerations including cutaneous puncture too close to the clavicle, passage of the needle through the clavicular periosteum, too shallow a trajectory beneath the clavicle, failure to identify landmarks properly, and orientation of the needle in a cephalad direction away from the sternal notch. The final error was extravascular displacement of the needle after successful venipuncture but before introducing the guidewire [66]. Being aware of these errors can improve the teaching effectiveness of experienced operators and encourage safe practice among clinicians learning the procedure.

Supraclavicular Approach

Bannon and colleagues published an excellent description of subclavian vein cannulation using a supraclavicular approach (Fig. 17.5a, b) [67, 68]. The essential landmark for the supraclavicular approach is the lateral border of the clavicular head of the SCM muscle as it attaches to the clavicle. Turning the patient's head to the contralateral side accentuates the posterior head of the SCM and provides unobstructed access to the subclavian vein [67]. The point of cutaneous puncture lies 1 cm superior and 1 cm lateral to the SCM attachment site. The junction of the SCM with the clavicle forms the claviculosternomastoid angle. The needle tip should be angled posteriorly 5–15° off a coronal plane and advanced along a line that bisects the claviculosternomastoid angle.

This technique will lead to subclavian venipuncture between the clavicle and the anterior scalene muscle. Other authors suggest cutaneous puncture directly at the claviculosternomastoid angle. The needle is then advanced along the claviculosternomastoid angle bisector parallel and inferior to the clavicle to enter the vein at an insertion depth of 1–2 cm [63]. Anatomic data from three-dimensional computed tomography reconstructions suggest that, with the SCM-clavicular junction as a cutaneous puncture point, the needle should be oriented approximately 11° medially and 35° posteriorly as the needle is advanced approximately 1.4 cm to enter the vein. Unfortunately relatively large variation associated with these mean values limits their clinical utility [69]. In contrast to the infraclavicular approach, supraclavicular subclavian cannulation can be facilitated by ultrasound guidance.

Femoral Vein

The femoral vein is not routinely used for long-term permanent vascular access due to the higher rate of infection and thrombosis compared to the subclavian and internal jugular veins. Despite its drawbacks, femoral vein cannulation can be the only reasonable access site for patients with extensive upper extremity trauma and/or venous thrombosis and in dialysis patients with central venous occlusion (SVC and innominate vein). During cardiopulmonary resuscitation (CPR), the femoral vein has the advantage of allowing cannulation and access placement without interrupting CPR. Other indications for femoral vein access include the emergent need for hemodialysis or plasmapheresis.

To cannulate the femoral vein, the patient is placed in a supine position with the lower extremity extended and slightly abducted at the hip. If available, ultrasound should evaluate the patency of the common femoral vein before preparing the sterile field. A patent femoral vein should completely compress with pressure from the ultrasound probe; if it is not compressible, the contralateral femoral vein should be evaluated and considered for access. If ultrasound is not available, anatomic landmarks should be defined to facilitate femoral vein cannulation. The level of the inguinal ligament can be located by drawing an imaginary line from the anterior superior iliac spine to the top of the pubic tubercle. One or two fingerbreadths below this line mark the inferior border of the inguinal ligament. The maximal pulsation of the femoral artery should be identified, and the access needle should be inserted 1 cm medial to the femoral artery pulse. It is critical to ensure that the femoral vein is punctured below the level of the inguinal ligament. Needle puncture above the inguinal ligament is actually a puncture of the external iliac vein which quickly becomes a deep retroperitoneal structure making it difficult to compress and achieve hemostasis if bleeding occurs [65].

Morbid obesity poses a technical challenge for femoral vein access. A common pitfall is to confuse the inguinal crease formed by the overlying pannus with the inguinal ligament. With the pannus retracted cephalad, the anatomic landmarks marking the inguinal ligament can be identified. Failure to identify the true level of the inguinal ligament often results in an inappropriately low skin puncture which is associated with a higher rate of access failure or inadvertent arterial injury. The previously described micropuncture technique involving a 21-gauge needle, 0.018-in. wire, and coaxial 3- and 5-F catheters can be used for femoral venipuncture as well. Many central line kits also provide an introducer syringe with a wire lumen coming through the plunger of the syringe. The needle and attached syringe should be introduced at a nearly 90° angle. Once the vein has been punctured, the angle should be dropped to 45° to allow the wire to easily advance through the syringe and into the femoral vein. The syringe is then removed, and a small skin incision is made with an 11 blade scalpel. After dilating the skin tract with a series of over-the-wire dilatators, the catheter can be inserted, secured, and flushed. Hemodialysis and plasmapheresis catheters should be long enough to reach the IVC. Short catheters that terminate in the iliac venous system often fail to provide adequate venous flow and are more prone to thrombosis and malfunction.

Ultrasound guidance can increase the safety and speed of femoral venous catheter placement. Using a technique similar to that described for internal jugular vein cannulation, ultrasonography performed during the procedure can identify the femoral vein and provide real-time imaging of the needle puncturing the vein. The femoral vein typically appears as larger caliber, easily compressible structure anteromedial to the pulsatile femoral artery.

Complications

Central VA continues to evolve with improvements in catheter material technology and the widespread acceptance of safer insertion techniques. Despite these advances, central venous catheter placement can still cause acute and delayed complications (Table 17.1). Rare injuries, including brachial plexus and laryngeal palsy, have also been reported during short- and long-term follow-up of patients with central VA [58].

Acute Complications

Air Embolism/Foreign Body Embolism

Air embolism is a rare but potentially lethal complication that can occur during central VA via the internal jugular or subclavian vein. Although it is an entirely preventable problem, air embolism will occur if the practitioner fails to take precautions during central venous catheter placement. In the most common clinical scenario, air enters the vascular system through the needle, dilator, or sheath when the patient suddenly inhales or coughs. Acutely aspirating more than 50–100 mL of air directly into the right atrium and ventricle can cause a fatal obstruction of the right side of the heart. Studies have demonstrated that negative intrathoracic pressure can quickly entrain a large amount of air into the vascular system. A pressure difference of 4 cm H_2O allows 90 mL/s of air to pass through a 4-cm, 18-gauge needle. Intubated patients have a lower risk of air embolism than spontaneously breathing patients due to the absence of negative intrathoracic pressure [7].

To minimize the risk of air embolism, the lumen of the needle, dilator, or sheath should be covered at all times. Asking the patient to hum during catheter insertion decreases the chance of sudden inhalation or coughing [37]. Some catheter manufacturers have developed a sealing valve for the peel-away sheath that prevents air aspiration once the wire and dilator have been removed. Symptomatic air emboli can cause tachyarrhythmias, chest pain, cardiovascular collapse, dyspnea, coughing, and hypoxemia. In the event of an air embolism, the patient should be turned onto their left side and placed into the Trendelenburg position. This maneuver is designed to trap the air in the right ventricular apex; however, its effectiveness has not been rigorously studied. Aspirating through the central venous catheter if it is in place can potentially remove some of the intracardiac air. The patient should also be placed on 100 % oxygen to increase resorption of the air pocket. Supportive measures including fluid resuscitation and adrenergic agents should be used as needed.

Misadventures involving the guidewire or catheter can result in foreign body embolization. During insertion, the guidewire can become knotted or entrapped inside the catheter leading to wire fracture and embolization. The catheter itself can also fracture and embolize due to the shear forces exerted by the wire [70–72]. Embolization of a wire or catheter segment can have severe consequences including perforation or infarction of the heart or occlusion of a great vessel. Retrieving an embolized foreign body can involve endovascular techniques using a loop snare device or open surgery to directly expose the affected vessel [73]. Removal of a small segment of catheter that fractured off and embolized is not always necessary if this foreign body does not pose an obvious danger [7]. Decisions about whether to intervene in these cases requires sound clinical judgment. Guidewires can also become entangled with a previously placed IVC filter causing displacement and structural compromise of the filter. Being aware of the IVC filter and using careful technique can usually prevent this complication [74].

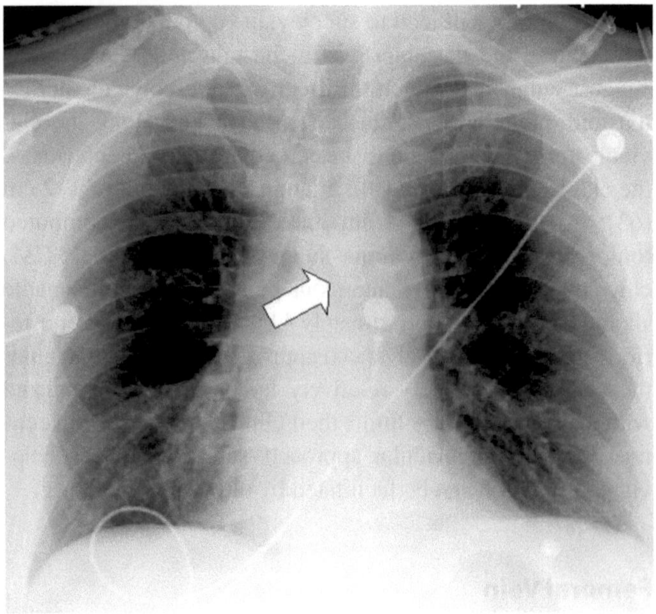

Fig. 17.6 Chest x-ray after placement of jugular line. *Arrow* demonstrates catheter tip crossing midline with respect to the trachea

Great Vessel Perforation/Inadvertent Arterial Catheter Placement

Iatrogenic cardiac perforation and inadvertent injury to the great vessels during central VA placement can result in hemothorax, cardiac tamponade, and mediastinal hematoma. Failure to recognize any of these conditions, alone or in combination, can be fatal. Vessel perforation and arterial misplacement that occur more frequently during internal radiographic signs of these complications include an atypical catheter course and tip position, pleural effusion, or widened mediastinum (Fig. 17.6). Jugular and femoral vein catheter insertion than with subclavian access [4, 30, 75, 76].

Prospective studies report a 6 % incidence of carotid artery puncture during internal jugular vein access [77]. Higher rates of carotid injury (18–25 %) have been reported in the pediatric population [75, 78]. Approximately 40 % of carotid punctures cause a hematoma, and failure to control the bleeding with manual compression can lead to airway obstruction, dissection, arteriovenous fistula, cerebrovascular compromise, and death [77, 79–83]. Puncture of the subclavian artery has a slightly lower incidence, occurring in 0.5–4 % of patients undergoing central VA placement [4, 30]. Hemothorax resulting from inadvertent arterial injury complicates about 1 % of vascular access cases [4]. In an unusual case, a hemothorax following dialysis catheter insertion caused spinal cord infarction and quadriplegia [84].

Perforation or cannulation of the carotid or subclavian artery by large-bore catheters occurs in up to 1 % of central VA procedures [85–87]. This complication can have serious and potentially fatal consequences including hemorrhage and stroke [87–89]. Stroke and other neurological events occur in approximately 27 % of patients who sustain unintentional arterial catheterization with an associated mortality rate of 20–40 % [85, 86].

Minimizing the risk of arterial injury during central venous catheter insertion has two components:

1. Avoiding needle puncture of the artery
2. Recognizing arterial cannulation before dilating or placing a large-bore catheter

Ultrasound guidance offers the most effective safeguard against needle puncture of the artery. Visualizing the tip of the needle when entering the vein lumen with real-time ultrasound imaging significantly decreases the chance of arterial puncture [76, 90, 91]. It is important to understand that inadvertent arterial punctures can still occur even with the use of ultrasound guidance. These events usually involve incorrect identification of the vascular structures or manipulation of the needle after venipuncture. The needle can then penetrate the opposite wall of the vein and puncture the underlying artery. Bright red, pulsatile blood flow from the needle usually alerts the operator that an arterial puncture has occurred. Unfortunately, this warning sign is not always recognized especially in clinical circumstances involving hypotension and hypoxemia. If the location of the needle or micropuncture catheter is unclear, the catheter can be connected to a pressure transducer to confirm low venous pressures and the absence of arterial pulsations before dilating and placing a large-bore catheter [76, 92]. Other methods have been described to identify an arterial puncture; however, none are infallible [80, 93]. Perforation of the aorta during central VA can occur in conjunction with a SVC injury [94]. An injury at the pericardial reflection often leads to cardiac tamponade, which has a mortality rate exceeding 90 % [95, 96]. Aortic injuries can occur as a result of multiple venipuncture attempts or the improper use of large dilators [97, 98]. In a typical clinical scenario, forceful advancement of the dilator causes it to override the wire and perforate the central vein or SVC. The technique of frequently ensuring that the wire moves freely as the dilator is advanced can minimize the risk of this complication.

Recognizing and treating a great vessel injury require a high index of suspicion and prompt diagnostic imaging. A chest x-ray can be misleading while ultrasound provides limited visualization of intrathoracic structures. Diagnosing a central vessel injury can require a contrast-enhanced CT scan or catheter-directed angiography depending on the clinical urgency. Balloon tamponade can provide temporary vascular control while preparing for open surgical repair or endovascular intervention using a stent graft or closure device [99–102].

Pseudoaneurysms and arteriovenous fistulas represent rare complications of inadvertent arterial cannulation or vessel perforation [103, 104]. Arteriovenous fistulas have an incidence of 0.6 and 0.2 % after internal jugular and subclavian vein access, respectively [81, 105]. Clinical signs of an arteriovenous fistula include a palpable thrill or audible bruit in the neck. A pseudoaneurysm is a contained pocket of blood flow associated with an underlying arterial injury. Depending on the size and location, a pseudoaneurysm can present as a pulsatile mass or cause compressive symptoms on adjacent structures. Although fistulas and pseudoaneurysms can cause acute symptoms, they usually have a delayed clinical presentation [106]. Injury to the vertebral artery can also occur during subclavian or internal jugular vein access and may be associated with an adverse neurological event [107].

In the past, open surgical repair was the only treatment option for pseudoaneurysms and arteriovenous fistulas resulting from VA procedures. Endovascular intervention including the use of stent grafts now offers an effective and less invasive alternative in many cases [106, 108]. Ultrasound-guided thrombin injection has been reported in the treatment of a carotid artery pseudoaneurysm; however, this technique should be used with caution because of the potential for cerebral embolization [109].

Catheter Malposition

For upper body central VA, the catheter tip should be positioned at the atrial-caval junction. In the absence of imaging guidance, catheter tip malposition occurs in 25–40 % of cases [76, 110]. The use of ultrasound and fluoroscopic guidance increases the rate of accurate catheter placement to 90–100 % [17]. Advancing the catheter too far so that its tip lies within the heart itself increases the risk of cardiac tamponade and dysrhythmia [91]. At the other extremes, failing to advance the catheter centrally and leaving the tip positioned in the more cephalad SVC can increase the risk of catheter malfunction and thrombosis which can also be life threatening if a pulmonary embolism occurs [169]. The angle of the catheter should also be considered during positioning. The left brachiocephalic vein joins the SVC at nearly a right angle [170]. Catheters inserted from the left side should therefore be advanced further to lie within the proximal right atrium in order to prevent the catheter tip from impinging on the SVC wall.

Catheters placed via the internal jugular veins have fewer prospects for malposition compared to subclavian vein catheters [4]. Misplacement of the catheter from the subclavian vein, retrograde into the ipsilateral internal jugular vein reportedly occurs in up to 15 % of access placement [62, 112]. Maneuvers that can help avoid this complication involve turning the patient's head towards the insertion side and manual compression of the ipsilateral jugular vein during advancement of the wire [113]. Ultrasound guidance can also detect anatomic variation and assist in appropriate placement of the catheter tip in both children and adults [114].

Pneumothorax

Pneumothorax is a common and potentially life-threatening complication of central venous catheterization comprising up to 30 % of all mechanical adverse events [115, 116]. The rate of pneumothorax ranges from 0 to 6 %; however, rates as high as 12 % have been observed with inexperienced operators [117]. The risk of pneumothorax increases with the number of needle passes, emergency access indications, and insertion of large-diameter catheters such as the ones used for hemodialysis [110].

Although symptoms of an iatrogenic pneumothorax can become apparent as early as 6 h post procedure, not all patients have acute symptoms [118]. Delayed pneumothorax reportedly occurs in 0.5–4 % of insertions [116, 119, 120]. Mitigating the risk of a pneumothorax requires heightened awareness and caution especially when catheter insertion proves to be technically challenging. A small pneumothorax often remains asymptomatic and may not require intervention if the visceral pleura is less than 2–3 cm from the parietal pleura [37]. Symptomatic or large pneumothoraces usually resolve after placing a pigtail catheter or small-caliber chest tube with a Heimlich valve. A tension pneumothorax requires urgent decompression with a 14-gauge needle placed in the second intercostal space, midclavicular line followed quickly by chest tube insertion in the standard location. Awareness and observation for re-expansion pulmonary edema should also be part of the pneumothorax treatment algorithm, particularly if the patient is being treated on an outpatient basis [121]. Re-expansion pulmonary edema occurs in 1–14 % of patients with a pneumothorax [122, 123].

Recent literature suggests that clinician performed bedside ultrasound can assist in the immediate diagnosis of a pneumothorax. Ultrasonography has greater sensitivity and accuracy than a supine chest x-ray making it more comparable to a chest CT scan [124–126]. The drawbacks of ultrasound include the dependency on operator skill and the limitations imposed by patient factors and equipment [127].

Delayed Complications

Catheter-Related Infections

Infection, the most common long-term complication of central VA, occurs with an incidence of 5.3 per 1,000 catheter days and has an associated mortality rate as high as 35 % [4, 128, 129]. Multiple factors play a role in the pathogenesis of CRI. Approximately 50 % of CRI involve the patient's skin flora and are caused by coagulase-negative staphylococci. In contrast, gram-negative rods cause most of the infections associated with groin catheter insertions [130]. Although catheter removal is not necessary to eradicate coagulase-negative staphylococcus, CRI caused by *S. aureus*, *Candida*, *Pseudomonas*, or *Stenotrophomonas maltophilia* usually warrant immediate catheter removal [131, 132]. The risk of CRI increases if the insertion site carries a heavy bacterial burden regardless of the aseptic measures taken during catheter placement [134]. During emergency situations with suboptimal sterile preparation, the risk of catheter infection increases, and catheters inserted under these conditions should be replaced or removed as soon as safely possible. Catheter insertion protocols that use maximum sterile barrier precautions reduce the risk of CRI [44–46]. Using chlorhexidine in place of iodine or alcohol appears to be more effective in reducing CRI and is recommended as the preferred method for skin disinfection [47–49].

The risk of CRI increases when thrombus forms around the catheter tip or at the site where the catheter penetrates the vessel wall [135, 136]. Thrombus formation occurs in 30–70 % of patients when the catheter indwelling time exceeds 1 week [135, 137–139]. Although heparin coating may reduce the thrombogenicity of catheters, the potential risk of heparin-induced thrombocytopenia limits their use [140]. The risk of thrombosis also increases with the extent of vessel damage at the time of catheter placement [141].

Catheter indwelling time has a strong association with the risk of infection [130]. The risk of CRI is nearly zero for catheters in place less than 3 days. Infection risk increases to 3–5 % for catheters in place 3–7 days, and the overall cumulative risk is 5–10 % if a catheter is in place more than 7 days [136, 142, 143].

The patient's underlying condition and comorbidities also influence the risk of CRI [144–146]. Patients suffering from neutropenia and those receiving immunosuppressive therapy other than steroids have an increased risk of CRI [145, 147, 148]. Long-term total parenteral nutrition and the presence of malignancy also increase the risk of CRI [149, 150]. Patients with a remote source of infection, such as the lower respiratory tract or urinary tract, are at increased risk for CRI; however, no studies suggest that patients with diabetes have an increased risk of CRI [151].

The physical properties of central venous catheters can affect the risk of infection. Several reports demonstrate that infection rate increases with the number of catheter lumens [11, 12, 136, 154, 155]. This finding may result from the increased manipulation associated with multi-lumen catheters especially in the critically ill patient [4, 153]. Catheters can be made from silicone, polyurethane, Teflon, polypropylene, and polyvinylchloride. Each material has a different thrombotic tendency which may influence the risk of infection [7]. TCs have a Dacron cuff, which allows tissue in growth to immobilize the catheter below the skin surface. In theory, the cuff creates a barrier for bacterial migration which may explain why TCs have a lower risk of infection compared to non-cuffed catheters [128]. TCs offer a low maintenance and relatively durable solution for patients with long-term vascular access needs. Tunneling offers protection when care and maintenance may not be optimal, such as treatment received in the home setting or when the catheter is in proximity to an open wound.

For patients with chronic kidney disease, infection ranks second to cardiovascular disease as a leading cause of death [156]. Non-tunneled dialysis catheters are more susceptible to CRI compared to tunneled dialysis catheters (3.8–6.6 infection episodes/1,000 days vs. 1.6–5.5 infections/1,000 days) [58]. In patients receiving hemodialysis, TCs have a longer functional life span and a decreased incidence of infection [157]. Treatment strategies for catheter-related infections vary with the severity of the infection, the type of catheter involved, and the clinical presentation. Exit site infections may present with erythema, exudate, and crusting of the skin around the catheter. These infections rarely cause systemic illness, and blood cultures remain negative. Non-tunneled dialysis catheters with evidence of an exit site infection should be removed and replaced in 24–48 h under appropriate antibiotic coverage. Tunneled dialysis catheters with limited exit site infection can be treated with local wound care and topical antibiotics. Drainage around the catheter from the tunnel should be cultured and treated with antibiotics. Clinical deterioration of the patients or failure to respond to conservative management mandates immediate removal of the TC.

Bloodstream infections are the most serious manifestation of CRI and represent a potentially lethal complication with an incidence of 1.5–5.5 episodes per 1,000 catheter days [151, 158]. Dialysis patients with catheter-related bacteremia can present with acute onset of fever, chills, or hypoglycemia. Immunosuppressed and elderly patients may present with atypical signs such as confusion, hypothermia, and lethargy. Quantitative cultures from the periphery and the catheter can aid in making the diagnosis. If the cultures from the catheter have five- to tenfold more bacterial colonies than the peripheral blood, the catheter is implicated as the source of infection [159]. All catheter-related bacteremias require antibiotic treatment initially directed at staphylococcus and streptococcus and then adjusted to the final culture results. In selected cases, antibiotic treatment alone may resolve the infection. Marr and associates salvaged 31 % of catheters using antibiotic therapy alone without any evidence of systemic complications [151].

Antibiotics usually fail to eliminate catheter-associated infections because of the presence of biofilm on the catheter surface [160]. The absence of clinical improvement 36 h after initiation of antibiotic therapy warrants removal of the catheter. Several reports support the practice of exchanging the infected catheter over a guidewire as long as the infection does not involve the tunnel track or the exit site. A 2-year prospective observational study of patients with catheter-related bacteremia evaluated three treatment strategies. Patients were treated by guidewire exchange, guidewire exchange with a creation of a new tunnel, and catheter removal and replacement. All three treatment modalities had satisfactory and statistically equivalent cure rates (87.8, 75, and 86.5 %, respectively) [161]. Infections that persist after catheter exchange require removal and a 48–72-h "catheter holiday" before replacement.

Venous Stenosis

Venous stenosis appears to start forming as soon as a catheter is inserted. Damage to the intima during needle puncture (vessel injury), venous stasis (decreased vessel diameter), and hypercoagulability (vessel injury and catheter composition) all contribute to venous stenosis. Subclavian vein catheters may have the highest incidence of stenosis [19]. As discussed earlier in the chapter, subclavian vein stenosis can have a significant negative impact on future attempts to establish ipsilateral upper extremity arteriovenous access. A subclavian vein catheter should therefore be avoided in patients that may require dialysis. Treatment options for venous stenosis have been discussed in Chap. 19.

Thrombotic Complications

Thrombotic complications of central VA vary in severity ranging from a fibrin sheath that forms only around the catheter itself to an occlusive clot that becomes a fatal venous thromboembolism. Several studies report a 33–67 % incidence of thrombus formation for central venous catheters with indwelling times of 1 week or more [137, 138, 162]. Overt symptoms of thrombosis occur in a smaller number of patients since many thrombotic catheter complications remain clinically silent [162]. The rate of catheter-related venous thrombosis appears to be lower in the subclavian vein as opposed to the internal jugular and femoral veins [76]. Trottier et al. reported a 22–29 % rate of thrombosis for femoral vein catheters compared to 2 % for subclavian vein access [163]. Patients with cancer have an even higher rate of catheter-associated vessel thrombosis (41 %) with pulmonary embolism developing in 11 % of patients [164]. Although catheter-related thrombosis in cancer patients often responds to acute treatment, the underlying hypercoagulability makes it difficult to achieve long-term relief [165]. A review of the literature by Vescia and colleagues cautioned against routine prophylactic anticoagulation in cancer patients with venous catheters as a means of preventing catheter-induced thrombosis [166]. They suggested that each institution should assess its rate of catheter-associated thrombosis to facilitate a more individualized approach to thromboprophylaxis in patients with central VA. This clinical strategy can also be applied to patients without cancer.

The pathogenesis of catheter-associated thrombus formation involves injury to the endothelium, disruption of laminar blood flow induced by local trauma, and catheter thrombogenicity [7, 164]. The infusate traveling through the catheter and the patient's underlying disease process may also contribute to thrombus formation [167]. Although a fibrin sheath contributes to catheter malfunction and occlusion, it does not always portend vessel thrombosis [164]. The fibrin sheath is usually present 24 h after catheter insertion originating from the site of catheter insertion and slowly growing with fibrin and platelet deposit until it reaches the end of the catheter. At the catheter tip, the fibrin sheath can cause intermittent obstruction during aspiration while infusion through the catheter remains unimpeded. Postural changes or having the patient perform the Valsalva maneuver can often overcome the fibrin sheath allowing for blood aspiration [7]. If both aspiration and infusion are difficult, slow infusion of tissue plasminogen activator 1 mg/h for a few hours or 5,000–10,000 U of streptokinase may clear the catheter and restore patency [168]. If this fails, exchanging the catheter over a guidewire or stripping the fibrin sheath off of the catheter using an endovascular loop snare offers treatment alternatives.

Conclusion

Although it is often perceived as a minor procedure, placing a central venous catheter can have a significant impact on a patient's well-being. Access to the central venous system allows patients to receive lifesaving and life-sustaining therapy including resuscitation from shock, acute and long-term hemodialysis, total parenteral nutrition, and chemotherapy. Establishing safe and reliable central VA will therefore continue to play an essential role in healthcare delivery. Surgeons charged with placing central venous catheters must be aware of the indications, contraindications, and inherent risks associated with central VA placement. Decisions regarding the type of catheter and the access site location should be individualized based on the patient's specific needs and clinical condition. The most important technical aspects of central VA placement involve appropriate patient positioning, identifying anatomic landmarks, and the use of ultrasound imaging. Ultrasound guidance has a well-documented track record of reducing cannulation time, decreasing failed attempts, and enhancing safety. In many institutions ultrasound imaging for central VA has evolved from an adjunctive technique to the standard of care.

Proper technique and safety precautions can minimize, but not eliminate the risk of catheter-associated complications. Surgeons must recognize and quickly respond to central VA insertion complications to avoid acute cardiovascular collapse. Non-life-threatening complications also require appropriate management to ensure reliable central VA in the long term without compromising future access needs. This chapter clarifies the key concepts and highlights the central role that surgeons play in safely and effectively establishing central VA.

References

1. Aubaniac R. [Subclavian intravenous injection; advantages and technic]. Presse Med. 1952;60(68):1456.
2. Broviac JW, Cole JJ, Scribner BH. A silicone rubber atrial catheter for prolonged parenteral alimentation. Surg Gynecol Obstet. 1973;136(4):602–6.
3. Hickman RO, et al. A modified right atrial catheter for access to the venous system in marrow transplant recipients. Surg Gynecol Obstet. 1979;148(6):871–5.
4. Ruesch S, Walder B, Tramer MR. Complications of central venous catheters: internal jugular versus subclavian access–a systematic review. Crit Care Med. 2002;30(2):454–60.
5. Thomson IR, et al. Right bundle-branch block and complete heart block caused by the Swan-Ganz catheter. Anesthesiology. 1979; 51(4):359–62.
6. Haas B, Chittams JL, Trerotola SO. Large-bore tunneled central venous catheter insertion in patients with coagulopathy. J Vasc Interv Radiol. 2010;21(2):212–7.
7. Polderman KH, Girbes AJ. Central venous catheter use. Part 1: mechanical complications. Intensive Care Med. 2002;28(1):1–17.
8. Bishop L, et al. Guidelines on the insertion and management of central venous access devices in adults. Int J Lab Hematol. 2007; 29(4):261–78.
9. Morris D, Mulvihill D, Lew WY. Risk of developing complete heart block during bedside pulmonary artery catheterization in patients with left bundle-branch block. Arch Intern Med. 1987;147(11):2005–10.
10. Unnikrishnan D, Idris N, Varshneya N. Complete heart block during central venous catheter placement in a patient with pre-existing left bundle branch block. Br J Anaesth. 2003;91(5):747–9.
11. Farkas JC, et al. Single- versus triple-lumen central catheter-related sepsis: a prospective randomized study in a critically ill population. Am J Med. 1992;93(3):277–82.
12. Dezfulian C, et al. Rates of infection for single-lumen versus multilumen central venous catheters: a meta-analysis. Crit Care Med. 2003;31(9):2385–90.
13. Rupp SM, et al. Practice guidelines for central venous access: a report by the American Society of Anesthesiologists Task Force on Central Venous Access. Anesthesiology. 2012;116(3):539–73.
14. Knutstad K, Hager B, Hauser M. Radiologic diagnosis and management of complications related to central venous access. Acta Radiol. 2003;44(5):508–16.
15. Knebel P, et al. Insertion of totally implantable venous access devices: an expertise-based, randomized, controlled trial (NCT00600444). Ann Surg. 2011;253(6):1111–7.
16. Marik PE, Flemmer M, Harrison W. The risk of catheter-related bloodstream infection with femoral venous catheters as compared to subclavian and internal jugular venous catheters: a systematic review of the literature and meta-analysis. Crit Care Med. 2012; 40(8):2479–85.
17. Ganeshan A, Warakaulle DR, Uberoi R. Central venous access. Cardiovasc Intervent Radiol. 2007;30(1):26–33.
18. Karakitsos D, et al. Real-time ultrasound-guided catheterisation of the internal jugular vein: a prospective comparison with the landmark technique in critical care patients. Crit Care. 2006; 10(6):R162.
19. Schillinger F, et al. Post catheterisation vein stenosis in haemodialysis: comparative angiographic study of 50 subclavian and 50 internal jugular accesses. Nephrol Dial Transplant. 1991;6(10): 722–4.
20. Lameris JS, et al. Percutaneous placement of Hickman catheters: comparison of sonographically guided and blind techniques. AJR Am J Roentgenol. 1990;155(5):1097–9.

21. Randolph AG, et al. Ultrasound guidance for placement of central venous catheters: a meta-analysis of the literature. Crit Care Med. 1996;24(12):2053–8.
22. Hind D, et al. Ultrasonic locating devices for central venous cannulation: meta-analysis. BMJ. 2003;327(7411):361.
23. Tripathi M, Tripathi M. Subclavian vein cannulation: an approach with definite landmarks. Ann Thorac Surg. 1996;61(1):238–40.
24. Moran SG, Peoples JB. The deltopectoral triangle as a landmark for percutaneous infraclavicular cannulation of the subclavian vein. Angiology. 1993;44(9):683–6.
25. Lorente L, et al. Central venous catheter-related infection in a prospective and observational study of 2,595 catheters. Crit Care. 2005;9(6):R631–5.
26. Kramer FL, Goodman J, Allen S. Thrombolytic therapy in catheter-related subclavian venous thrombosis. Can Assoc Radiol J. 1987;38(2):106–8.
27. Rooden CJ, et al. Deep vein thrombosis associated with central venous catheters – a review. J Thromb Haemost. 2005;3(11): 2409–19.
28. Macdonald S, et al. Comparison of technical success and outcome of tunneled catheters inserted via the jugular and subclavian approaches. J Vasc Interv Radiol. 2000;11(2 Pt 1):225–31.
29. Lockwood AH. Percutaneous subclavian vein catheterization. Too much of a good thing? Arch Intern Med. 1984;144(7):1407–8.
30. Merrer J, et al. Complications of femoral and subclavian venous catheterization in critically ill patients: a randomized controlled trial. JAMA. 2001;286(6):700–7.
31. Zaleski GX, et al. Experience with tunneled femoral hemodialysis catheters. AJR Am J Roentgenol. 1999;172(2):493–6.
32. Kenney PR, Dorfman GS, Denny Jr DF. Percutaneous inferior vena cava cannulation for long-term parenteral nutrition. Surgery. 1985;97(5):602–5.
33. Kaufman JA, Greenfield AJ, Fitzpatrick GF. Transhepatic cannulation of the inferior vena cava. J Vasc Interv Radiol. 1991; 2(3):331–4.
34. Forauer AR, et al. Placement of hemodialysis catheters through dilated external jugular and collateral veins in patients with internal jugular vein occlusions. AJR Am J Roentgenol. 2000;174(2): 361–2.
35. Meranze SG, et al. Catheter placement in the azygos system: an unusual approach to venous access. AJR Am J Roentgenol. 1985; 144(5):1075–6.
36. Ferral H, et al. Recanalization of occluded veins to provide access for central catheter placement. J Vasc Interv Radiol. 1996;7(5): 681–5.
37. Funaki B. Central venous access: a primer for the diagnostic radiologist. AJR Am J Roentgenol. 2002;179(2):309–18.
38. Parry G. Trendelenburg position, head elevation and a midline position optimize right internal jugular vein diameter. Can J Anaesth. 2004;51(4):379–81.
39. Bellazzini MA, et al. Ultrasound validation of maneuvers to increase internal jugular vein cross-sectional area and decrease compressibility. Am J Emerg Med. 2009;27(4):454–9.
40. Samy Modeliar S, et al. Ultrasound evaluation of central veins in the intensive care unit: effects of dynamic manoeuvres. Intensive Care Med. 2008;34(2):333–8.
41. Beddy P, et al. Valsalva and gravitational variability of the internal jugular vein and common femoral vein: ultrasound assessment. Eur J Radiol. 2006;58(2):307–9.
42. Spafford PS, et al. Prevention of central venous catheter-related coagulase-negative staphylococcal sepsis in neonates. J Pediatr. 1994;125(2):259–63.
43. Vassilomanolakis M, et al. Central venous catheter-related infections after bone marrow transplantation in patients with malignancies: a prospective study with short-course vancomycin prophylaxis. Bone Marrow Transplant. 1995;15(1):77–80.
44. Berenholtz SM, et al. Eliminating catheter-related bloodstream infections in the intensive care unit. Crit Care Med. 2004;32(10): 2014–20.
45. Pronovost P, et al. An intervention to decrease catheter-related bloodstream infections in the ICU. N Engl J Med. 2006;355(26): 2725–32.
46. Warren DK, et al. Preventing catheter-associated bloodstream infections: a survey of policies for insertion and care of central venous catheters from hospitals in the prevention epicenter program. Infect Control Hosp Epidemiol. 2006;27(1):8–13.
47. Maki DG, Ringer M, Alvarado CJ. Prospective randomised trial of povidone-iodine, alcohol, and chlorhexidine for prevention of infection associated with central venous and arterial catheters. Lancet. 1991;338(8763):339–43.
48. Noorani A, et al. Systematic review and meta-analysis of preoperative antisepsis with chlorhexidine versus povidone-iodine in clean-contaminated surgery. Br J Surg. 2010;97(11):1614–20.
49. Darouiche RO, et al. Chlorhexidine-alcohol versus povidone-iodine for surgical-site antisepsis. N Engl J Med. 2010;362(1): 18–26.
50. Troianos CA, et al. Special articles: guidelines for performing ultrasound guided vascular cannulation: recommendations of the American Society of Echocardiography and the Society of Cardiovascular Anesthesiologists. Anesth Analg. 2012;114(1): 46–72.
51. Rabindranath KS, et al. Use of real-time ultrasound guidance for the placement of hemodialysis catheters: a systematic review and meta-analysis of randomized controlled trials. Am J Kidney Dis. 2011;58(6):964–70.
52. Rabindranath KS, et al. Ultrasound use for the placement of haemodialysis catheters. Cochrane Database Syst Rev. 2011;11, CD005279.
53. Geddes CC, et al. Insertion of internal jugular temporary hemodialysis cannulae by direct ultrasound guidance–a prospective comparison of experienced and inexperienced operators. Clin Nephrol. 1998;50(5):320–5.
54. Denys BG, et al. An ultrasound method for safe and rapid central venous access. N Engl J Med. 1991;324(8):566.
55. Abboud PA, Kendall JL. Ultrasound guidance for vascular access. Emerg Med Clin North Am. 2004;22(3):749–73.
56. Fragou M, et al. Real-time ultrasound-guided subclavian vein cannulation versus the landmark method in critical care patients: a prospective randomized study. Crit Care Med. 2011;39(7): 1607–12.
57. O'Leary R, et al. Ultrasound-guided infraclavicular axillary vein cannulation: a useful alternative to the internal jugular vein. Br J Anaesth. 2012;109(5):762–8.
58. Costanza MJ, et al. Angioaccess for hemodialysis. Curr Probl Surg. 2011;48(7):443–517.
59. Fortune JB, Feustel P. Effect of patient position on size and location of the subclavian vein for percutaneous puncture. Arch Surg. 2003;138(9):996–1000; discussion 1001.
60. Tan BK, et al. Anatomic basis of safe percutaneous subclavian venous catheterization. J Trauma. 2000;48(1):82–6.
61. Kitagawa N, et al. Proper shoulder position for subclavian venipuncture: a prospective randomized clinical trial and anatomical perspectives using multislice computed tomography. Anesthesiology. 2004;101(6):1306–12.
62. Unal AE, et al. Malpositioning of Hickman catheters, left versus right sided attempts. Transfus Apher Sci. 2003;28(1):9–12.
63. Jung CW, et al. Head position for facilitating the superior vena caval placement of catheters during right subclavian approach in children. Crit Care Med. 2002;30(2):297–9.
64. Sanchez R, et al. Misplacement of subclavian venous catheters: importance of head position and choice of puncture site. Br J Anaesth. 1990;64(5):632–3.

65. Bannon MP, Heller SF, Rivera M. Anatomic considerations for central venous cannulation. Risk Manag Healthc Policy. 2011;4: 27–39.
66. Kilbourne MJ, et al. Avoiding common technical errors in subclavian central venous catheter placement. J Am Coll Surg. 2009; 208(1):104–9.
67. Nevarre DR, Domingo OH. Supraclavicular approach to subclavian catheterization: review of the literature and results of 178 attempts by the same operator. J Trauma. 1997;42(2):305–9.
68. Cunningham SC, Gallmeier E. Supraclavicular approach for central venous catheterization: "safer, simpler, speedier". J Am Coll Surg. 2007;205(3):514–6; author reply 516–7.
69. Jesseph JM, Conces Jr DJ, Augustyn GT. Patient positioning for subclavian vein catheterization. Arch Surg. 1987;122(10):1207–9.
70. Breznick DA, Ness WC. Acute arterial insufficiency of the upper extremity after central venous cannulation. Anesthesiology. 1993; 78(3):594–6.
71. Casserly IP, et al. Paradoxical embolization of a fractured guidewire: successful retrieval from left atrium using a snare device. Catheter Cardiovasc Interv. 2002;57(1):34–8.
72. Tewari P, Agarwal A. Spring guidewire sticks in the indwelling catheter during internal jugular vein catheterisation. Anaesthesia. 2000;55(8):832.
73. Furui S, et al. Intravascular foreign bodies: loop-snare retrieval system with a three-lumen catheter. Radiology. 1992;182(1):283–4.
74. Streib EW, Wagner JW. Complications of vascular access procedures in patients with vena cava filters. J Trauma. 2000;49(3):553–7; discussion 557–8.
75. Oliver Jr WC, et al. The incidence of artery puncture with central venous cannulation using a modified technique for detection and prevention of arterial cannulation. J Cardiothorac Vasc Anesth. 1997;11(7):851–5.
76. McGee DC, Gould MK. Preventing complications of central venous catheterization. N Engl J Med. 2003;348(12):1123–33.
77. Reuber M, et al. Stroke after internal jugular venous cannulation. Acta Neurol Scand. 2002;105(3):235–9.
78. Verghese ST, et al. Ultrasound-guided internal jugular venous cannulation in infants: a prospective comparison with the traditional palpation method. Anesthesiology. 1999;91(1):71–7.
79. Anagnou J. Cerebrovascular accident during percutaneous cannulation of internal jugular vein. Lancet. 1982;2(8294):377–8.
80. Eckhardt WF, et al. Inadvertent carotid artery cannulation during pulmonary artery catheter insertion. J Cardiothorac Vasc Anesth. 1996;10(2):283–90.
81. Asteri T, et al. Beware Swan-Ganz complications. Perioperative management. J Cardiovasc Surg (Torino). 2002;43(4):467–70.
82. Defalque RJ, Fletcher MV. Neurological complications of central venous cannulation. JPEN J Parenter Enteral Nutr. 1988;12(4): 406–9.
83. Stewart RW, et al. Fatal outcome of jugular vein cannulation. South Med J. 1995;88(11):1159–60.
84. Williams A, et al. Spinal cord infarction following central-line insertion. Ren Fail. 2003;25(2):327–9.
85. Wicky S, et al. Life-threatening vascular complications after central venous catheter placement. Eur Radiol. 2002;12(4):901–7.
86. Robinson JF, et al. Perforation of the great vessels during central venous line placement. Arch Intern Med. 1995;155(11):1225–8.
87. Shah PM, et al. Arterial misplacement of large-caliber cannulas during jugular vein catheterization: case for surgical management. J Am Coll Surg. 2004;198(6):939–44.
88. Kron IL, et al. Arch vessel injury during pulmonary artery catheter placement. Ann Thorac Surg. 1985;39(3):223–4.
89. Jain U, et al. Subclavian artery laceration and acute hemothorax on attempted internal jugular vein cannulation. J Cardiothorac Vasc Anesth. 1991;5(6):608–10.
90. Denys BG, Uretsky BF, Reddy PS. Ultrasound-assisted cannulation of the internal jugular vein. A prospective comparison to the external landmark-guided technique. Circulation. 1993;87(5):1557–62.
91. Gann Jr M, Sardi A. Improved results using ultrasound guidance for central venous access. Am Surg. 2003;69(12):1104–7.
92. Jobes DR, et al. Safer jugular vein cannulation: recognition of arterial puncture and preferential use of the external jugular route. Anesthesiology. 1983;59(4):353–5.
93. Golden LR. Incidence and management of large-bore introducer sheath puncture of the carotid artery. J Cardiothorac Vasc Anesth. 1995;9(4):425–8.
94. Baumgartner FJ, et al. Central venous injuries of the subclavian-jugular and innominate-caval confluences. Tex Heart Inst J. 1999; 26(3):177–81.
95. Greenall MJ, Blewitt RW, McMahon MJ. Cardiac tamponade and central venous catheters. Br Med J. 1975;2(5971):595–7.
96. Collier PE, Goodman GB. Cardiac tamponade caused by central venous catheter perforation of the heart: a preventable complication. J Am Coll Surg. 1995;181(5):459–63.
97. Barton BR, Hermann G, Weil 3rd R. Cardiothoracic emergencies associated with subclavian hemodialysis catheters. JAMA. 1983; 250(19):2660–2.
98. Fangio P, et al. Aortic injury and cardiac tamponade as a complication of subclavian venous catheterization. Anesthesiology. 2002;96(6):1520–2.
99. Walser EM, et al. Percutaneous tamponade of inadvertent transthoracic catheterization of the aorta. Ann Thorac Surg. 1996;62(3): 895–6.
100. Pikwer A, et al. Management of inadvertent arterial catheterisation associated with central venous access procedures. Eur J Vasc Endovasc Surg. 2009;38(6):707–14.
101. Patel SJ, Venn GE, Redwood SR. Percutaneous closure of an iatrogenic puncture of the aortic arch. Cardiovasc Intervent Radiol. 2003;26(4):407–9.
102. Teichgraber UK, et al. Central venous access catheters: radiological management of complications. Cardiovasc Intervent Radiol. 2003;26(4):321–33.
103. Brzowski BK, Mills JL, Beckett WC. Iatrogenic subclavian artery pseudoaneurysms: case reports. J Trauma. 1990;30(5):616–8.
104. Sato O, et al. Arteriovenous fistula following central venous catheterization. Arch Surg. 1986;121(6):729–31.
105. Chloroyiannis Y, Reul GJ. Iatrogenic left subclavian artery-to-left brachiocephalic vein fistula: successful repair without a sternotomy. Tex Heart Inst J. 2004;31(2):172–4.
106. Inamasu J, Guiot BH. Iatrogenic vertebral artery injury. Acta Neurol Scand. 2005;112(6):349–57.
107. Yu NR, et al. Vertebral artery dissection following intravascular catheter placement: a case report and review of the literature. Vasc Med. 2004;9(3):199–203.
108. Bernik TR, et al. Pseudoaneurysm of the subclavian-vertebral artery junction–case report and review of the literature. Vasc Endovascular Surg. 2002;36(6):461–4.
109. Holder R, et al. Percutaneous thrombin injection of carotid artery pseudoaneurysm. J Endovasc Ther. 2002;9(1):25–8.
110. Lefrant JY, et al. Risk factors of failure and immediate complication of subclavian vein catheterization in critically ill patients. Intensive Care Med. 2002;28(8):1036–41.
111. McGee WT, et al. Accurate placement of central venous catheters: a prospective, randomized, multicenter trial. Crit Care Med. 1993;21(8):1118–23.
112. Kidney DD, Nguyen DT, Deutsch LS. Radiologic evaluation and management of malfunctioning long-term central vein catheters. AJR Am J Roentgenol. 1998;171(5):1251–7.
113. Ambesh SP, et al. Manual occlusion of the internal jugular vein during subclavian vein catheterization: a maneuver to prevent

misplacement of catheter into internal jugular vein. Anesthesiology. 2002;97(2):528–9.
114. Lefrant JY, et al. Pulsed Doppler ultrasonography guidance for catheterization of the subclavian vein: a randomized study. Anesthesiology. 1998;88(5):1195–201.
115. Mitchell SE, Clark RA. Complications of central venous catheterization. AJR Am J Roentgenol. 1979;133(3):467–76.
116. Plewa MC, Ledrick D, Sferra JJ. Delayed tension pneumothorax complicating central venous catheterization and positive pressure ventilation. Am J Emerg Med. 1995;13(5):532–5.
117. Sznajder JI, et al. Central vein catheterization. Failure and complication rates by three percutaneous approaches. Arch Intern Med. 1986;146(2):259–61.
118. Tyburski JG, et al. Delayed pneumothorax after central venous access: a potential hazard. Am Surg. 1993;59(9):587–9.
119. Plaus WJ. Delayed pneumothorax after subclavian vein catheterization. JPEN J Parenter Enteral Nutr. 1990;14(4):414–5.
120. Chang TC, Funaki B, Szymski GX. Are routine chest radiographs necessary after image-guided placement of internal jugular central venous access devices? AJR Am J Roentgenol. 1998;170(2):335–7.
121. Gurley MB, Richli WR, Waugh KA. Outpatient management of pneumothorax after fine-needle aspiration: economic advantages for the hospital and patient. Radiology. 1998;209(3):717–22.
122. Rozenman J, et al. Re-expansion pulmonary oedema following spontaneous pneumothorax. Respir Med. 1996;90(4):235–8.
123. Beng ST, Mahadevan M. An uncommon life-threatening complication after chest tube drainage of pneumothorax in the ED. Am J Emerg Med. 2004;22(7):615–9.
124. Maury E, et al. Ultrasonic examination: an alternative to chest radiography after central venous catheter insertion? Am J Respir Crit Care Med. 2001;164(3):403–5.
125. Simon BC, Paolinetti L. Two cases where bedside ultrasound was able to distinguish pulmonary bleb from pneumothorax. J Emerg Med. 2005;29(2):201–5.
126. Zhang M, et al. Rapid detection of pneumothorax by ultrasonography in patients with multiple trauma. Crit Care. 2006;10(4):R112.
127. Sistrom C. US in the detection of pneumothorax. Radiology. 2003;227(1):305–6; author reply 306.
128. O'Grady NP, et al. Guidelines for the prevention of intravascular catheter-related infections. Centers for Disease Control and Prevention. MMWR Recomm Rep. 2002;51(RR-10):1–29.
129. Ryan Jr JA, et al. Catheter complications in total parenteral nutrition. A prospective study of 200 consecutive patients. N Engl J Med. 1974;290(14):757–61.
130. Polderman KH, Girbes AR. Central venous catheter use. Part 2: infectious complications. Intensive Care Med. 2002;28(1):18–28.
131. Mermel LA, et al. Guidelines for the management of intravascular catheter-related infections. Infect Control Hosp Epidemiol. 2001;22(4):222–42.
132. Elting LS, Bodey GP. Septicemia due to Xanthomonas species and non-aeruginosa Pseudomonas species: increasing incidence of catheter-related infections. Medicine (Baltimore). 1990;69(5):296–306.
133. Raad I, et al. Impact of central venous catheter removal on the recurrence of catheter-related coagulase-negative staphylococcal bacteremia. Infect Control Hosp Epidemiol. 1992;13(4):215–21.
134. Snydman DR, et al. Predictive value of surveillance skin cultures in total-parenteral-nutrition-related infection. Lancet. 1982;2(8312):1385–8.
135. Timsit JF, et al. Central vein catheter-related thrombosis in intensive care patients: incidence, risks factors, and relationship with catheter-related sepsis. Chest. 1998;114(1):207–13.
136. Reed CR, et al. Central venous catheter infections: concepts and controversies. Intensive Care Med. 1995;21(2):177–83.
137. Bernard RW, Stahl WM. Subclavian vein catheterizations: a prospective study. I. Non-infectious complications. Ann Surg. 1971;173(2):184–90.
138. Randolph AG, et al. Benefit of heparin in central venous and pulmonary artery catheters: a meta-analysis of randomized controlled trials. Chest. 1998;113(1):165–71.
139. Mickley V. Central vein obstruction in vascular access. Eur J Vasc Endovasc Surg. 2006;32(4):439–44.
140. Laster JL, Nichols WK, Silver D. Thrombocytopenia associated with heparin-coated catheters in patients with heparin-associated antiplatelet antibodies. Arch Intern Med. 1989;149(10):2285–7.
141. Kohler TR, Kirkman TR. Central venous catheter failure is induced by injury and can be prevented by stabilizing the catheter tip. J Vasc Surg. 1998;28(1):59–65; discussion 65–6.
142. Sitzmann JV, et al. Septic and technical complications of central venous catheterization. A prospective study of 200 consecutive patients. Ann Surg. 1985;202(6):766–70.
143. Pittet D, Tarara D, Wenzel RP. Nosocomial bloodstream infection in critically ill patients. Excess length of stay, extra costs, and attributable mortality. JAMA. 1994;271(20):1598–601.
144. McKinley S, et al. Incidence and predictors of central venous catheter related infection in intensive care patients. Anaesth Intensive Care. 1999;27(2):164–9.
145. Howell PB, et al. Risk factors for infection of adult patients with cancer who have tunnelled central venous catheters. Cancer. 1995;75(6):1367–75.
146. Shaul DB, et al. Risk factors for early infection of central venous catheters in pediatric patients. J Am Coll Surg. 1998;186(6):654–8.
147. Donowitz GR, et al. Infections in the neutropenic patient–new views of an old problem. Hematology Am Soc Hematol Educ Program. 2001:113–39.
148. Press OW, et al. Hickman catheter infections in patients with malignancies. Medicine (Baltimore). 1984;63(4):189–200.
149. Mollee P, et al. Catheter-associated bloodstream infection incidence and risk factors in adults with cancer: a prospective cohort study. J Hosp Infect. 2011;78(1):26–30.
150. Armstrong CW, et al. Prospective study of catheter replacement and other risk factors for infection of hyperalimentation catheters. J Infect Dis. 1986;154(5):808–16.
151. Marr KA, et al. Catheter-related bacteremia and outcome of attempted catheter salvage in patients undergoing hemodialysis. Ann Intern Med. 1997;127(4):275–80.
152. Kovacevich DS, et al. Association of parenteral nutrition catheter sepsis with urinary tract infections. JPEN J Parenter Enteral Nutr. 1986;10(6):639–41.
153. Rello J, et al. Evaluation of outcome of intravenous catheter-related infections in critically ill patients. Am J Respir Crit Care Med. 2000;162(3 Pt 1):1027–30.
154. Hilton E, et al. Central catheter infections: single- versus triple-lumen catheters. Influence of guide wires on infection rates when used for replacement of catheters. Am J Med. 1988;84(4):667–72.
155. Lee RB, Buckner M, Sharp KW. Do multi-lumen catheters increase central venous catheter sepsis compared to single-lumen catheters? J Trauma. 1988;28(10):1472–5.
156. Feldman HI, Kobrin S, Wasserstein A. Hemodialysis vascular access morbidity. J Am Soc Nephrol. 1996;7(4):523–35.
157. Schwab SJ, et al. Prospective evaluation of a Dacron cuffed hemodialysis catheter for prolonged use. Am J Kidney Dis. 1988;11(2):166–9.
158. Saad TF. Bacteremia associated with tunneled, cuffed hemodialysis catheters. Am J Kidney Dis. 1999;34(6):1114–24.
159. Fan ST, Teoh-Chan CH, Lau KF. Evaluation of central venous catheter sepsis by differential quantitative blood culture. Eur J Clin Microbiol Infect Dis. 1989;8(2):142–4.

160. Schwab SJ, et al. Vascular access for hemodialysis. Kidney Int. 1999;55(5):2078–90.
161. Beathard GA. Management of bacteremia associated with tunneled-cuffed hemodialysis catheters. J Am Soc Nephrol. 1999; 10(5):1045–9.
162. Mughal MM. Complications of intravenous feeding catheters. Br J Surg. 1989;76(1):15–21.
163. Trottier SJ, et al. Femoral deep vein thrombosis associated with central venous catheterization: results from a prospective, randomized trial. Crit Care Med. 1995;23(1):52–9.
164. Kusminsky RE. Complications of central venous catheterization. J Am Coll Surg. 2007;204(4):681–96.
165. Sprouse 2nd LR, et al. Percutaneous treatment of symptomatic central venous stenosis [corrected]. J Vasc Surg. 2004;39(3):578–82.
166. Vescia S, et al. Management of venous port systems in oncology: a review of current evidence. Ann Oncol. 2008;19(1):9–15.
167. Fontes ML, Barash PG. "AAA" to the rescue? Crit Care Med. 1999;27(12):2827–9.
168. Bagnall HA, Gomperts E, Atkinson JB. Continuous infusion of low-dose urokinase in the treatment of central venous catheter thrombosis in infants and children. Pediatrics. 1989;83(6):963–6.
169. Puel V, Caudry M, Le Metayer P, et al. Superior vena cava thrombosis related to catheter malposition in cancer chemotherapy given through implanted ports. Cancer. 1993;72:2248–52.
170. Gravenstein N, Blackshear RH. In vitro evaluation of relative perforating potential of central venous catheters: comparison of materials, selected models, number of lumens and angles of incidence to simulated membrane. J Clin Monit. 1991;7:1–6.

Arteriovenous Hemodialysis Access

18

Anjuli R. Cherukuri and Vivian Gahtan

Introduction

The goal of placing an arteriovenous fistula or graft is to create a prominent, high flow vascular circuit that can be easily punctured for hemodialysis with minimal complications. To accomplish these goals, the fistula or graft should be at least 6 mm in diameter, have a blood flow rate of 600 ml/min, and be no deeper than 6 mm with discernable margins [1]. To allow multiple needle puncture sites, the usable length of the access should be at least 6 cm, but ideally 10 cm.

Preplacement Evaluation

Timing of Referral

Evaluation for a primary AV fistula should ideally begin at least 6 months in advance of starting dialysis. This time interval allows for evaluation, placement, maturation, and possible revision of an AV fistula. Autogenous fistulas take at least 6 weeks to mature and may require an intervention, such as ligation of competing vein tributaries or angioplasty of a stenotic segment, before being adequate for use. In some patients, a primary fistula never matures and a new fistula must be created. In contrast, an AV graft typically takes only 2 weeks to incorporate into the wound, although it may take slightly longer for the edema to resolve. AV grafts can therefore be placed closer to the time of hemodialysis initiation.

History and Physical Exam

History

A thorough history should be taken prior to dialysis access placement. Particular attention should be paid to conditions which may have damaged the venous integrity including: previous AV access, multiple peripheral intravenous (IV) catheters, peripherally inserted central catheter (PICC) lines, central venous catheters, pacemaker/defibrillator, IV drug abuse, and a history of deep venous thrombosis (DVT) or superficial phlebitis. For example, central venous catheters and pacemakers can lead to central venous stenosis or chronic occlusion. Any known blood pressure asymmetry, prior arterial reconstruction, or history of ischemic steal syndrome must be identified. Choosing the best access site requires knowledge and investigation of anything that could affect the quality of the arteries or veins.

The nondominant arm should be used when possible. If one arm has some disability, such as spastic paralysis or chronic pain, that limb should be avoided for access placement. The patient's pursuits and personal hobbies should be considered as well (e.g., playing guitar, fly fishing, work as an electrician) when selecting the side of the access to avoid interfering with these activities. The patient should be made aware of the potential for functional steal syndrome which may hinder some activities. Any previous surgeries involving the arm, shoulder, or chest should also be noted since they may affect the access location chosen. Table 18.1 lists some pertinent aspects of the history.

Physical

A complete physical examination should be performed giving particular attention to the vascular system. To evaluate the arterial system, bilateral blood pressures and pulses

A.R. Cherukuri, MD
Division of Vascular Surgery and Endovascular Services, Department of Surgery, SUNY Upstate Medical University, Syracuse, NY, USA

V. Gahtan, MD, FACS (✉)
Division of Vascular Surgery and Endovascular Services, SUNY Upstate Medical University, 750 East Adams Street, Suite 8801, Syracuse, NY 13210, USA

Department of Veterans Affairs Healthcare Network Upstate New York at Syracuse, Syracuse, NY, USA
e-mail: gahtanv@upstate.edu

V. Gahtan and M.J. Costanza (eds.), *Essentials of Vascular Surgery for the General Surgeon*,
DOI 10.1007/978-1-4939-1326-8_18, © Springer Science+Business Media New York 2015

Table 18.1 History

History	No	Yes	Comments
Previous AV access			
Previous central catheter, PICC line, pacemaker, or defibrillator			
Previous venous disease (DVT, superficial thrombophlebitis)			
Intravenous drug abuse			
Arm disability, relevant activities			
Previous surgery			
Heart disease or diabetes mellitus			
Anticoagulant therapy or coagulation disorder			
Dominant hand	Right	Left	

AV arteriovenous, *DVT* deep vein thrombosis, *PICC* peripherally inserted central catheter

Table 18.2 Physical exam

Physical exam (vascular)	*Right*	*Left*	*Comments*
Bilateral blood pressures			
Brachial			
Ankle			
Peripheral pulses, +/– Doppler			
Carotid			
Brachial			
Radial			
Ulnar			
Femoral			
Popliteal			
Posterior tibial			
Dorsal pedal			
Allen's test	nl/abnl	nl/abnl	
Tissue loss	yes/no	yes/no	
Edema	yes/no	yes/no	
Discoloration	yes/no	yes/no	
Collateral veins	yes/no	yes/no	
Arm size	nl/abnl	nl/abnl	
Physical exam (other)		*Comments*	
Cardiac	nl/abnl		
Pulmonary	nl/abnl		

nl normal, *abnl* abnormal

should be assessed along with an Allen's test to check for an incomplete palmar arch. A blood pressure difference greater than 15 mmHg between arms is significant and should warrant further testing if the arm with the lower pressure is planned for access placement. In most cases, the arm with the higher blood pressure should be used. Tissue loss in the finger tips or hand should also be noted as this finding could indicate underlying arterial occlusive disease. Since hand perfusion will decrease after access placement, any tissue loss should be resolved before surgery. Venous obstruction can manifest as edema, discoloration, collateral veins on the arms or chest, or a difference in arm size. The cardiopulmonary systems should be evaluated for signs of heart failure. Table 18.2 summarizes the pertinent components of the physical examination.

Imaging

Ultrasound Vein Mapping

As a cost-effective, noninvasive exam that does not require contrast, duplex ultrasound is an ideal imaging modality for evaluating possible autogenous access sites in patients with chronic kidney disease. In addition to measuring the diameter, superficial veins should be assessed for large branches, thrombosis, and thickened walls (evidence of previous phlebitis). The deep venous system should also be evaluated for deep venous thrombosis. A sample vein mapping worksheet is shown (Fig. 18.1) summarizing diameters at multiple points along the upper extremity. In general, a vein diameter of at least 3 mm is preferred for establishing a native arteriovenous fistula.

Venography

Venography should not be routinely performed (especially in patients not on dialysis yet) because it is an invasive exam that requires contrast. Patients who have a pacemaker or a history of central venous catheters (especially subclavian), as well as those with signs of central venous stenosis, should be considered for venography to assess the central veins. Venography to evaluate the veins in the upper extremity should be used selectively.

Order of Site Preference Principles and Guidelines

Fistula First, Catheter Last Principles

The National Kidney Foundation Kidney Disease Outcomes Quality Initiative (NKF-KDOQI) ranks the order in which AV access for dialysis should be attempted, which follows the principles of "fistula first, catheter last". The recommendations generally describe placement of autogenous AV fistulas, followed by grafts in distal to proximal locations in the upper extremities. The first choice is a "snuffbox" radial-cephalic AV fistula followed by more proximal upper extremity AV fistulas, then AV grafts. Once all upper extremity locations have been used, alternative sites, such as axillary and lower extremity fistulas may be considered. Catheters are used for permanent hemodialysis access as a last resort. These guidelines are based on the survival and safety advantages of autogenous AV fistulas over AV grafts and catheters. The order of preferences is summarized in Table 18.3 [1].

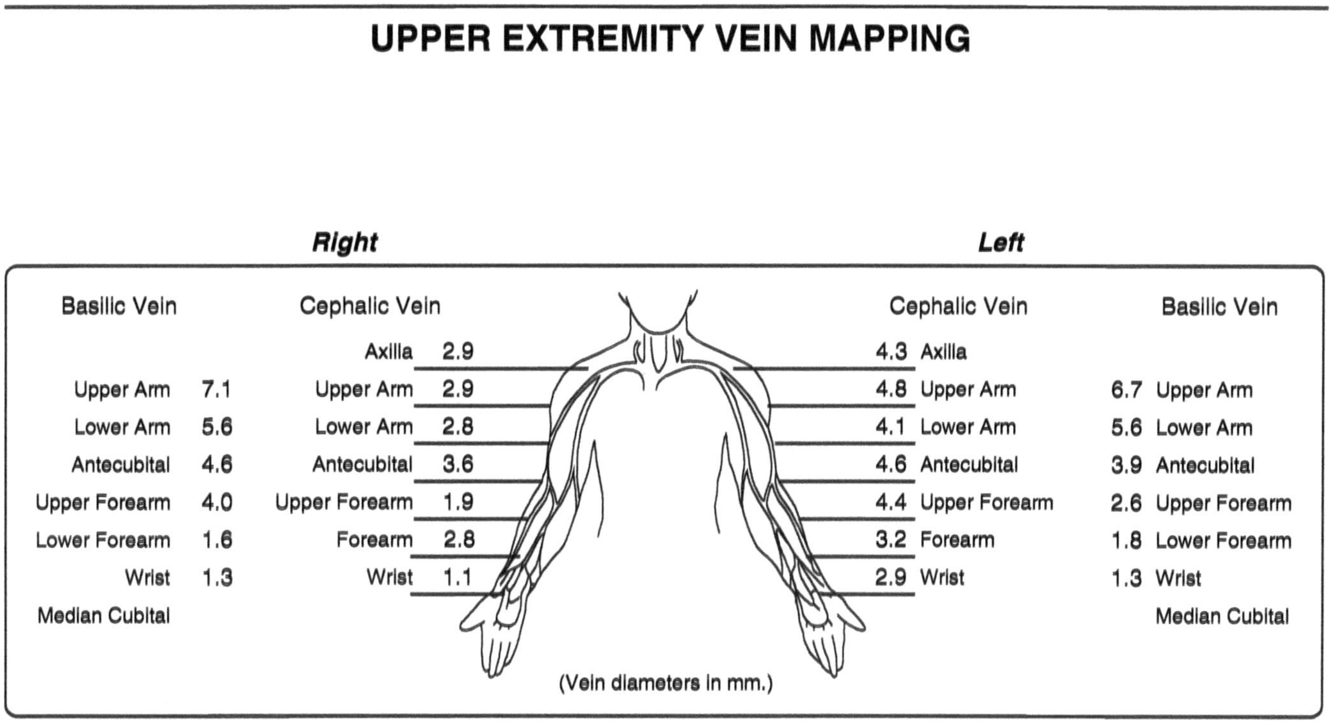

Fig. 18.1 Vein mapping worksheets showing a typical upper extremity mapping of the bilateral basilic and cephalic veins. Note multiple locations for sequential diameters recorded

Table 18.3 Order of preference guidelines for AV access

Fistula/Graft type	Advantages	Drawbacks
Preferred		
Radial-cephalic fistula (snuffbox followed by wrist)	The preferred first location, straightforward procedure, preserves proximal sites	Lower flow, slower maturation, higher risk of hand ischemia
Brachial-cephalic fistula	Higher flow, more reliable maturation	Increased incidence of edema and ischemic steal syndrome may require superficialization
Brachial-basilic (transposition) fistula	Less likely to have been previously accessed due to its deeper and more medial location	Increased pain and edema postop, increased risk of ischemic steal syndrome, kinking if tunneling, requires transposition of length of basilic vein, technically challenging in obese
Acceptable		
Forearm loop AV graft	Shorter lag time, easy cannulation	Infection, thrombosis, postop pain and edema, lower flow than more proximal grafts
Upper arm AV graft (straight or curved followed by loop)	Higher blood flow than distal grafts	Infection, increased risk of ischemic steal syndrome
Femoral AV graft	High blood flow	Infection, ischemia, difficulty positioning for dialysis, difficult if obese
Necklace AV graft		Infection, thrombosis, not for patients who need sternotomy
Avoid if possible		
Tunneled HD catheter	Immediate access	Last resort due to infection and thrombosis

Advantages and Drawbacks of Autogenous AV Fistulas

Patients with autogenous AV fistulas have safer, more effective dialysis and live longer than patients with AV grafts and catheters. AV fistulas are superior to grafts and catheters with regard to infection rate, thrombosis rate, long-term patency, and cost [2]. A drawback of autogenous AV fistulas is their maturation time of at least 6 weeks compared to grafts which require 2 weeks and catheters which are ready for use immediately. Autogenous AV fistulas also have a higher primary failure rate, and some fistulas never mature.

Balloon angioplasty maturation (BAM) has emerged as a promising technique to improve maturation of small caliber autogenous AV fistulas. BAM involves sequential dilation to create a controlled rupture of the vein which then remodels into a large caliber vascular conduit [3].

Technical Details

General Operative Considerations

Anesthesia

AV access placement can be done under general anesthesia, regional block, or local anesthesia with sedation. The author (VG) uses the latter for the vast majority of primary procedures. General anesthesia or regional blocks are generally used for more complex or redo procedures. Selected patients with complicating conditions (e.g., claustrophobia, chronic back pain, psychologic disturbances) may require general anesthesia.

Heparin

Evidence supporting a clear benefit for intraoperative heparin during AV fistula surgery remains elusive. Some studies showed no difference in bleeding complications, and 30-day patency rates with systemic heparin administration [4] and others demonstrated an increased risk of bleeding with heparinization and no benefit in terms of primary patency [5]. The use of systemic heparin in the creation of AV fistulas is therefore based on surgeon preference and experience.

Tunneling

To avoid kinking or twisting of the vein, proper orientation should be maintained by marking the vessel along one surface prior to tunneling. The vein should be tunneled superficially to make it easier to define and puncture for dialysis. It is important to note that the position of the patient's arm during the operation (abduction) is usually different than the more anterior position of the arm during dialysis. Unimpeded access should be possible when the arm is in a natural position for the patient. Access placement issues become more important in patients with redundant tissue or decreased mobility.

Anastomosis

The anastomotic diameter should be limited to minimize the risk of hemodynamic steal syndrome. Although they are not definitive, guidelines for the size of the anastomosis have been proposed. For the brachial artery, the anastomotic diameter should be 4–6 mm [6, 7]. For radial artery fistulas, the anastomotic diameter should be between 5 and 8 mm [8].

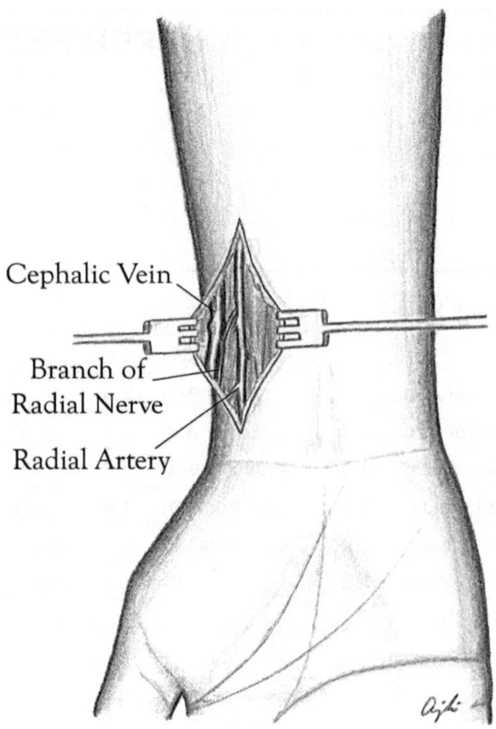

Fig. 18.2 Wrist dissection showing the main structures of the radial artery, cephalic vein, and branch of the radial nerve

Thrill/Pulse

The presence of a thrill over the new AV fistula should be noted both before and after closure of the incisions. A distal pulse should be palpated. If it is not palpable, the pulse should be reevaluated during manual compression of the AVF. If the pulse returns with AVF compression, then the arterial flow is intact. If the pulse does not return, further investigation is warranted for arterial thrombosis or embolus. At a minimum, good distal Doppler signals and capillary refill should be present before leaving the operating room.

Surgical Exposures

This section describes the common exposures for isolating the radial, brachial, axillary, and femoral vessels.

Radial Artery

A longitudinal incision is made along the lateral wrist over or just lateral to the radial pulse (Fig. 18.2). The radial artery is located just lateral to the flexor carpi radialis tendon.

Brachial Artery and Vein

Brachial artery exposure typically involves a transverse incision just distal to the antecubital crease (Fig. 18.3a, b).

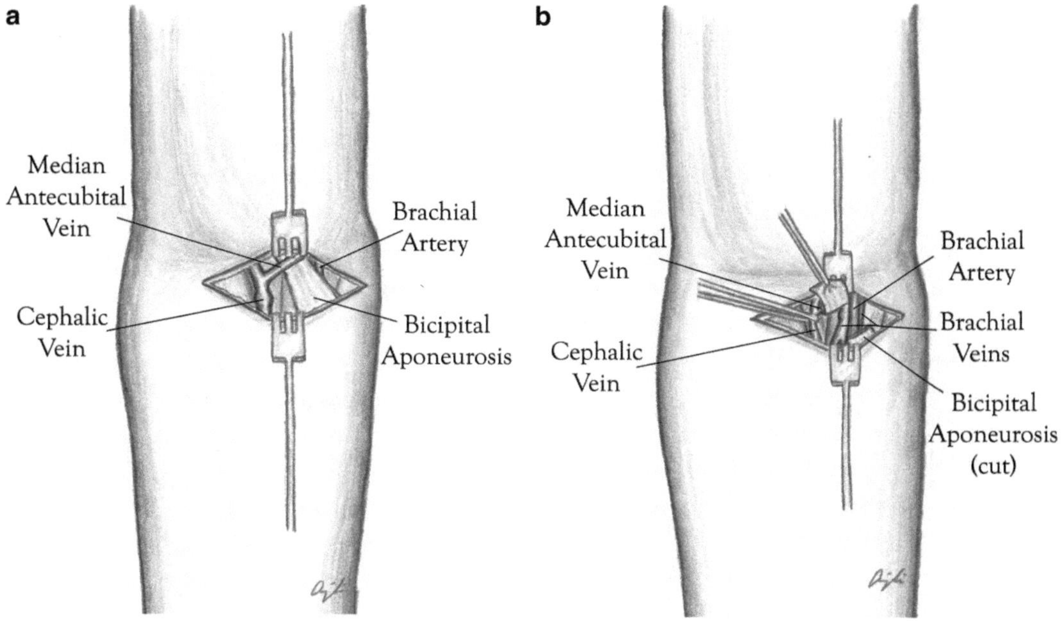

Fig. 18.3 (**a**) Transverse incision just distal to the antecubital crease showing the cephalic vein, median cubital vein, and the bicipital aponeurosis overlying the brachial artery and vein. (**b**) Dissection carried deeper with transaction of the bicipital aponeurosis and exposure of the brachial artery and veins

To expose the brachial artery, the aponeurosis of the biceps tendon is partially divided. The brachial artery should be isolated both proximally and distally with vessel loops. Small arterial branches should also be identified and isolated with vessel loops. The nerve closest to the brachial artery is the median nerve, which is medial to the vessels. This nerve is more prominent during exposure proximal to the antecubital crease.

For dissection proximal to the antecubital crease, the patient's arm is abducted to 90°. A longitudinal incision is made on the medial arm over the groove between the biceps and triceps muscles (Fig. 18.4). The basilic vein can be visualized medial to the brachial sheath. The median and ulnar nerves are usually encountered during the dissection.

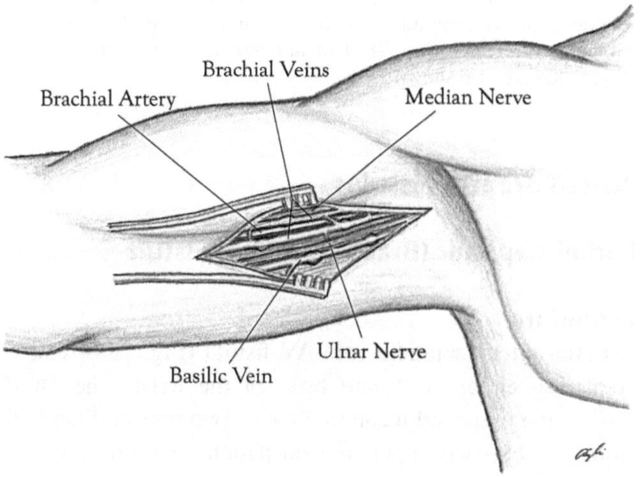

Fig. 18.4 The brachial artery is dissected out proximally. Note the brachial artery and surrounding brachial veins with crossing branches. The median nerve and ulnar nerves can be exposed in this dissection

Femoral Artery and Vein

A longitudinal or oblique incision should be made just distal to the inguinal ligament (Fig. 18.5). The dissection is carried down to the common femoral artery. The femoral bifurcation is identified and isolated. The dissection is then continued medially to expose the femoral veins. The common femoral, deep femoral, proximal femoral, and saphenofemoral junction are isolated and controlled. The femoral nerve is lateral to the artery and should not be visualized during the standard dissection.

Access Types

Common access procedures are described below. Most information regarding access failure and outcome are single-center retrospective reviews. Some representative studies are included to give a general sense of outcome; however, there can be variability between different studies and time periods.

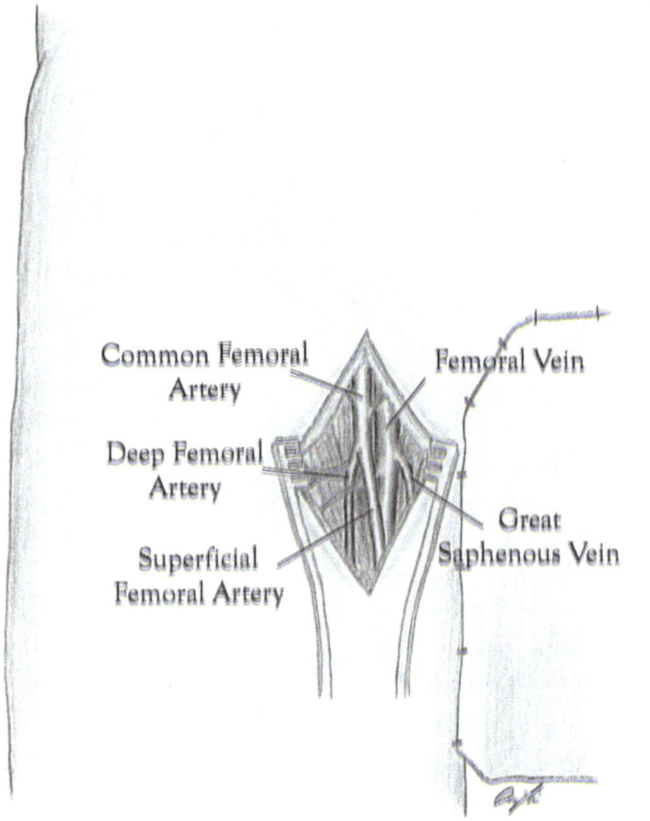

Fig. 18.5 A vertical incision is made over the femoral vessels. The common femoral artery and the bifurcation into the superficial and deep femoral arteries are shown. The medial femoral vein and saphenofemoral junction are also shown

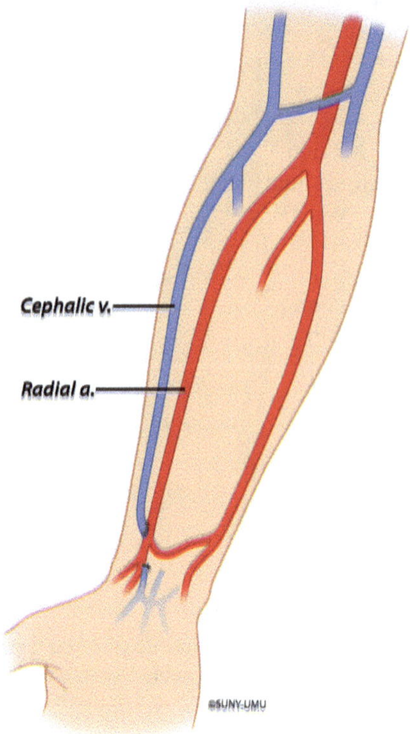

Fig. 18.6 Radial cephalic AV fistula

Wrist/Forearm Fistulas

Radial-Cephalic (Brescia-Cimino) Fistula

Procedure

A radial artery-cephalic vein AV fistula (Fig. 18.6) can be created at either the "snuff box" or the wrist. The "snuff box" is the preferred location. One or two longitudinal incisions can be used depending on patient anatomy and surgeon preference. The cephalic vein is dissected, and side branches ligated and divided so that enough length is obtained to transpose the cephalic vein over to the radial artery. Care should be taken to protect the superficial radial nerve and its branches which lie between the cephalic vein and radial artery. The cephalic vein is then transected, and its distal end suture ligated. When two incisions are used, the natural orientation of the vein must be maintained to avoid twisting and kinking when the vein is tunneled under the skin bridge for the anastomosis with the artery. An end-to-side anastomosis is then created between the end of the cephalic vein and a longitudinal or oblique incision on the radial artery.

Advantages/Drawbacks

A radial-cephalic AV fistula has the advantage of being a straightforward operation with few complications which preserves more proximal vessels for future access.

The drawbacks include a lower blood flow rate and longer maturation time. The overall primary failure rate ranges from 15 to 39 % [9–12] which is higher than brachiocephalic and brachiobasilic AV fistulas [13]. The 1- and 2-year cumulative patency rates for radial-cephalic AVF are 62–69 % and 50–57 %, respectively [9–11]. Because this procedure has an increased risk of hand ischemia, an Allen's test should be performed preoperatively to confirm a patent palmar arch. If a side-to-side anastomosis is performed, venous hypertension in the hand may result. In obese patients, a superficialization procedure may be necessary to make the fistula easier to define and puncture.

Radial-Basilic Fistula

Procedure

A radial artery-basilic vein AV fistula is an uncommon AV access that is used in only a small number of patients compared to the radial artery-cephalic vein AV fistula. A medial incision is made along the length of the forearm to mobilize the basilic vein (Fig. 18.7). The basilic vein is transected near the wrist and transposed anteriorly through

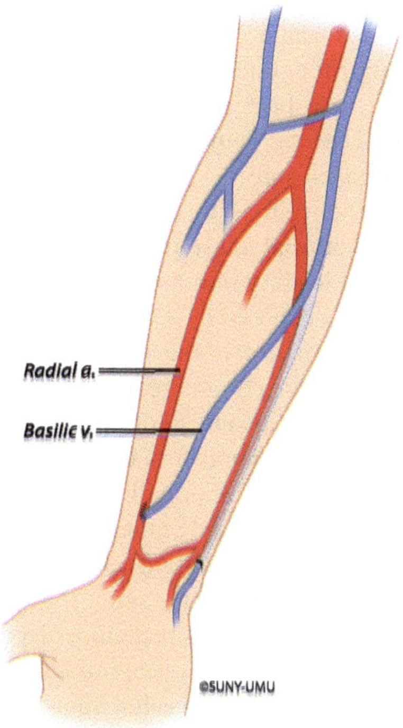

Fig. 18.7 Radial basilic AV fistula

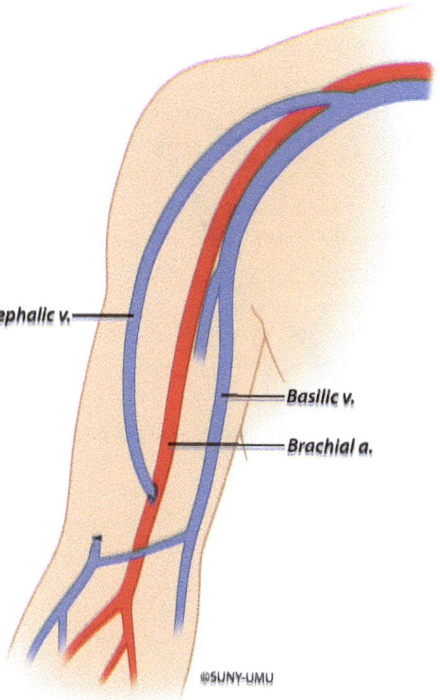

Fig. 18.8 Brachiocephalic AV fistula which is placed proximally to the antecubital crease

a subcutaneous tunnel. The distal end of the basilic vein is then connected to the radial artery by an end-to-side anastomosis. The ulnar artery can also be used for arterial inflow, or the basilic vein can be formed into a loop in the forearm and connected to the brachial artery.

Advantages/Drawbacks

A radial-basilic AV fistula offers another autogenous access option in the forearm before moving on to the upper arm. The maturation rate and patency rates appear relatively comparable to other forearm AV fistulas [14, 15]. The main drawback is the more extensive dissection required to mobilize the basilic vein.

Upper Arm Fistulas

Brachial-Cephalic Fistula

Procedure

A brachial artery-cephalic vein AV fistula can be created through a single transverse incision just proximal or distal to the antecubital fossa or two parallel longitudinal incisions on the upper medial arm (Fig. 18.8). The cephalic vein is dissected and mobilized to gain enough length so that it can reach the brachial artery without tension. The distal end of the cephalic vein is then transected. When using the two-incision technique, the cephalic vein is transposed through a subcutaneous tunnel to create the AV anastomosis. An end-to side anastomosis is then created between the cephalic vein's free end and the side of the brachial artery.

Advantages/Drawbacks

The higher blood flow in brachial-cephalic AV fistulas results in a more reliable maturation rate compared to wrist fistulas. The 1- and 2-year cumulative patency rates were 72–75 % and 75–78 %, respectively [11, 16].

The downside of higher blood flow is a higher incidence of edema and ischemic steal syndrome compared to forearm AV fistulas. The cephalic vein can also be too deep to reliably puncture in obese patients. Since standard dialysis needles are only one inch in length, a superficialization procedure may be necessary if the vein is more than 1 cm deep after arm edema has resolved (usually 4–6 weeks postoperatively). Superficialization is accomplished by either the "fistula elevation procedure", where the vein is dissected free and the subcutaneous tissue is then closed beneath the vein [17], or by lipectomy [18]. These procedures can also be performed on radial-cephalic or brachial-basilic AV fistulas.

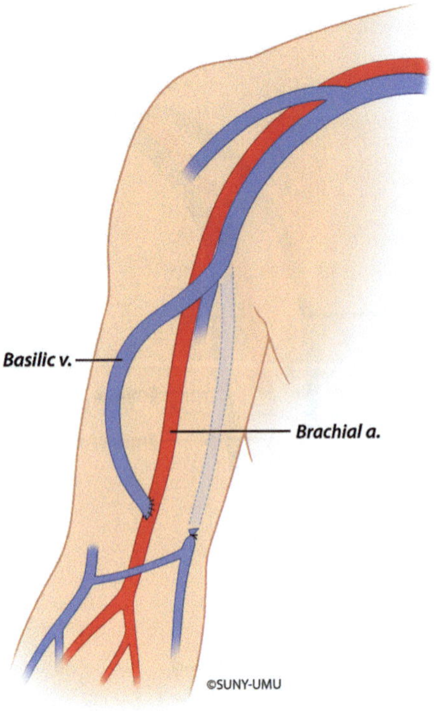

Fig. 18.9 Brachiobasilic AV fistula showing how the basilic vein is mobilized, divided distally and tunneled laterally, and then anastomosed to the brachial artery

Brachial-Basilic (Upper Arm Transposition) AV Fistula

Procedure

A brachial artery-basilic vein AV fistula can be created using a one-stage or two-stage approach. In the one-stage approach, a longitudinal incision on the upper medial arm is used to mobilize the basilic vein from the antecubital crease to its confluence with the brachial vein leading into the axillary vein (Fig. 18.9). Care should be taken to avoid the surrounding nerves. A segment of the brachial artery is then isolated in the distal upper arm. After marking its anterior surface for orientation, the basilic vein is transected distally and tunneled in an anterolateral fashion through the subcutaneous tissue. One or two counter incisions can help facilitate the tunnel. A laterally raised subcutaneous flap can also be used instead of a tunnel. An end-to-side anastomosis is then performed to the brachial artery. Typically a drain is left in the dissection bed.

In the two-stage approach, a single transverse incision is made just distal to the antecubital crease [19, 20]. The basilic vein or the median antecubital vein leading to the basilic vein is transected, and an end-to-side anastomosis is performed to the brachial artery. If, after 4–6 weeks, the basilic vein has reached a diameter of at least 5 mm, a second stage is performed during which the basilic vein is transposed superficially, anteriorly, and slightly laterally. The second stage begins by exposing the upper arm basilic vein with a single longitudinal incision or two incisions with an intervening skin bridge. Although using two incisions adds some time to the vein dissection, this technique can facilitate wound closure by limiting the size of the skin flaps. The basilic vein is then dissected along its entire length from the arterial anastomosis to its confluence with the brachial vein leading into the axillary vein. The basilic vein can then be transposed by securing it in a lateral subcutaneous flap. Alternatively, the basilic vein can be transected, tunneled anteriorly, and reanastomosed to itself. The latter method has the advantage of preserving any crossing structures. If there are a number of crossing nerves, it is usually better to transect the vein, pull the vein out from under the nerves, and reposition and reanastomose the fistula. The authors prefer to perform the transection and reanastamosis within the body of the fistula leaving the original arterial anastomosis undisturbed. This technique decreases the risk of steal since it preserves the original small diameter arterial anastomosis even though the basilic vein may have dilated significantly between the first- and second-stage procedures.

Advantages/Drawbacks

The deep location of the basilic vein makes it less likely to have been accessed or injured prior to fistula creation. In many patients, the upper arm basilic vein is the only healthy superficial vein in the upper extremity.

The drawbacks of a brachial basilic fistula include increased postoperative pain and edema, a longer recovery time, the need for a potentially two-staged procedure, and an increased risk of ischemic steal syndrome [21, 22]. Tunneling can kink or twist the vein, and positioning the vein for unimpeded access can be especially challenging in obese patients.

Transposing the vein has a higher rate of functional success than simply elevating the vein [21]. Additionally, fistulas created using a two-stage procedure may be more successful than fistulas created in one stage [12]. Medium- and long-term patency results for brachial basilic fistulas vary between studies. Segal and colleagues showed an assisted primary patency rate of 64 and 58 % at 1 and 2 years, respectively [23]. In contrast, Humphries and colleagues demonstrated cumulative patency rates of 84 % at 1 year, 73 % at 3 years, 73 % at 5 years, and 52 % at 10 years [24].

Brachial-Median Antecubital Vein Fistula

Procedure

A brachial artery-median antecubital vein AV fistula can be created in a similar fashion to the brachial-cephalic and brachial-basilic fistulas. The median antecubital vein usually lies in close proximity to the distal brachial artery, and both

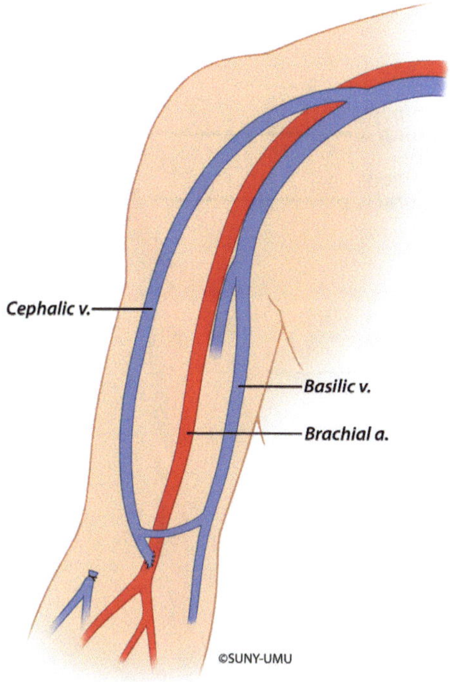

Fig. 18.10 Brachial artery to medial cubital vein AV fistula

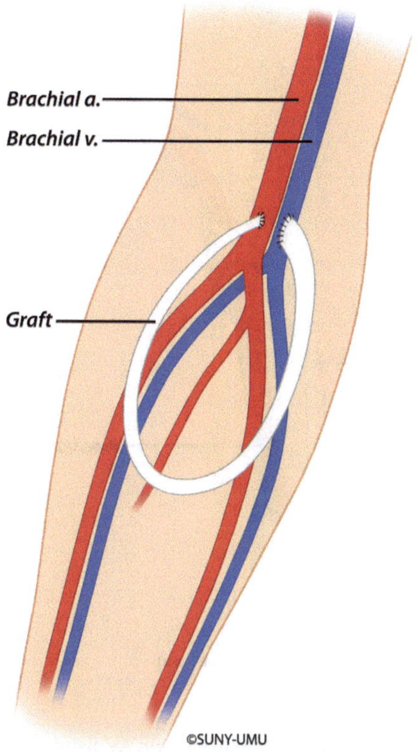

Fig. 18.11 Forearm loop AV graft with the anastomosis to the brachial artery and vein

structures can be isolated through a single transverse incision just distal to the antecubital crease (Fig. 18.10). The median antecubital vein becomes confluent with the upper arm cephalic and basilic veins which are both left intact. After dividing the distal median antecubital vein, it is connected to the brachial artery with an end-to-side anastomosis.

Advantages/Drawbacks

The brachial artery to median antecubital vein fistula has the advantage of preserving flow to both the cephalic and basilic veins. This configuration potentially allows both veins to mature simultaneously for access. Depending on patient anatomy, flow may only occur to one of the two veins using this approach.

Sparks and colleagues showed a patency rate of 80 % at an average follow-up time of 36 months for fistulas created using a perforating median antecubital vein compared to 66 % at 27 months for brachial-cephalic fistulas and 64 % at 7 months for synthetic arm grafts [25].

Prosthetic Grafts

Forearm Loop AV Graft

Procedure

A forearm loop AV graft between the brachial artery and either the cephalic, basilic, median antecubital, or brachial vein can be placed though an incision just distal to the antecubital crease (Fig. 18.11). Once the vessels have been identified and dissected, a small counterincision is made in the mid to distal forearm to aid in tunneling the graft loop through the anterior forearm. Proper orientation of the graft should be maintained while tunneling to avoid kinking, and a semicircular tunneler should be used to maximize the useable length of graft. End-to-side anastomoses are created between one end of the graft and the brachial artery and the other end of the graft and the selected vein. Due to the increased probability of postoperative edema, the authors recommend external sutures for skin closure.

Advantages/Drawbacks

An arteriovenous graft offers an AV access option to patients who lack adequate caliber superficial veins to create a native AV fistula. AV grafts also do not need to mature and can be used as soon as 2 weeks after placement. The larger diameter and superficial location of AV grafts provides an easy and well-defined target for needle puncture.

The drawback of all AV grafts is their higher rate of thrombosis and infection compared to native AV fistulas [1, 2]. Forearm AV grafts also tend to have lower blood flow and increased postoperative edema and pain.

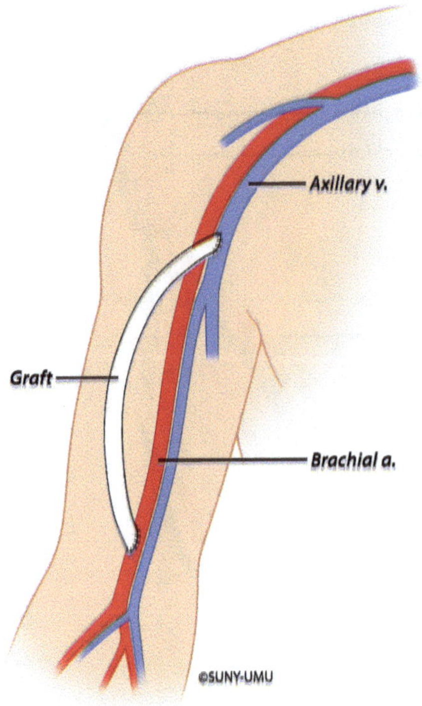

Fig. 18.12 Brachial artery to axillary vein AV fistula

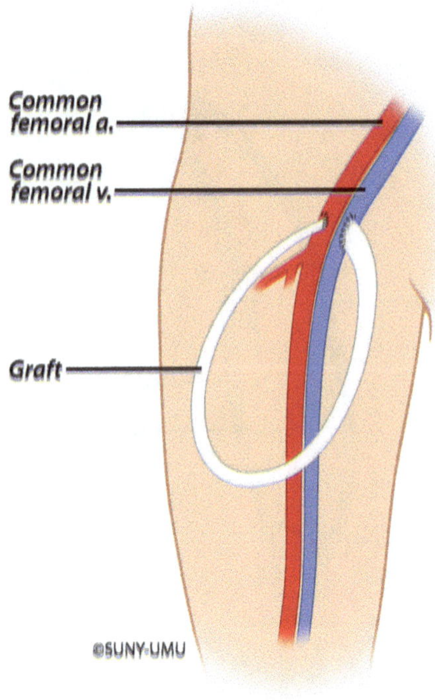

Fig. 18.13 Femoral loop AV graft

Upper Arm AV Graft

Procedure

Upper arm AV grafts can employ a variety of configuration using straight or looped grafts to connect the brachial or axillary artery to the cephalic, basilic, brachial, or axillary vein. A straight graft between the brachial artery and the axillary vein is constructed through two longitudinal incisions: one over the distal arm brachial artery and the other over the axillary vein in the proximal arm (Fig. 18.12). The graft is tunneled through the anterolateral subcutaneous tissue, and end-to-side anastomoses are performed to the artery and vein.

Advantages/Drawbacks

The upper arm AV graft is generally less painful than the forearm loop graft. Because they use larger, more proximal arteries, upper arm AV grafts have a higher rate of hemodynamic steal. In a study examining 193 grafts, Mousa and colleagues did not find a difference in patency rates between forearm and upper arm AV grafts [26]. Whether the graft had a loop or straight configuration also did not affect patency.

Femoral Loop AV Graft

A femoral loop AV graft is usually the next choice of access after exhausting all sites in the upper extremities.

Procedure

A femoral AV graft can be created between the common femoral artery (close to the femoral bifurcation) and the common femoral vein using a transverse or oblique incision in the groin (Fig. 18.13). Typically, the graft used is a 6-mm straight or a 6–8-mm tapered graft, with the smaller end anastomosed to the artery. The graft should be tunneled superficially in a loop configuration on the anterior thigh. Similar to the forearm loop AV graft, a small counterincision helps pass the graft through the tunnel.

Advantages/Drawbacks

In addition to providing access for patients with no upper extremity options, femoral AV grafts have high flow rates. This advantage may account for the reasonable patency rates associated with femoral AV grafts. Tashjian and colleagues reported primary patency rates of 71 and 63 % and secondary patency rates of 83 and 83 % for 1 and 2 years, respectively [27]. Similarly, Geenan et al. found cumulative patency rates to be 75 % at 1 year and 51 % at 5 years [28].

Despite their functionality, femoral AV grafts remain at the bottom of the K-DOQI access preference list because of their high rate of infection and ischemia. Patient selection also plays an important role in femoral AV graft placement. Patients must be able to recline during dialysis, and femoral AV grafts may not be feasible in a patient with a large pannus that overlies the anterior upper thigh.

Alternate Access (Overview)

The more common access procedures have been described above. Other options include the axillary loop AV graft, the "necklace" (axillary artery to contralateral axillary vein AV graft), the mid-thigh loop graft, the femoral vein transposition to distal superficial femoral artery AV fistula, the great saphenous vein AV fistula, and the Hemodialysis Reliable Outflow (HeRO) Device. A brief description of each option follows.

An axillary loop AV graft connects the axillary artery and vein with a graft that loops laterally over the deltoid muscle or medially over the pectoralis major muscle. In a study by Jean-Baptiste and colleagues, axillary loop grafts had a primary patency rate of 51 % at 12 months and a cumulative patency rate of 80 % at 18 months [29].

A necklace AV graft is placed between the axillary artery and the contralateral axillary or internal jugular vein. Since it crosses anteriorly to the sternum, this graft is not appropriate for patients who may need a sternotomy in the future. In a study of 18 patients, the primary patency rate was 83 and 72 % and the cumulative patency rate was 94 and 89 % at 6 months and 1 year from graft placement [30].

A mid-thigh AV graft connects the mid-superficial femoral artery to the femoral vein. This option preserves more proximal femoral vessels for future access or revision and avoids a groin incision. Scott and colleagues found the primary patency rates to be 40 and 18 % and the secondary patency rates to be 68 and 43 % at 1 and 2 years, respectively [31]. Despite the absence of a groin incision, this access configuration still had a high rate of infection resulting in graft removal in 21 % of patients.

The femoral vein transposition (FVT) involves dissecting the femoral vein along its length in the thigh. The vein is then superficially transposed and connected to the distal SFA [32]. Although the patency rates are excellent, FVT has a higher rate of wound complications and ischemia. Wound complications may stem from the deep location of the femoral vein which requires a more extensive dissection. The large size of the vein often leads to a large arterial anastomosis resulting in a higher incidence of hemodynamic steal syndrome. Selectively tapering the femoral vein to reduce its caliber may decrease the incidence of secondary procedures to address ischemia. Hazinedaroglu and colleagues compared the FVT to the femoral loop graft and found a superior 1 year primary patency rate of 87 % for the FVT compared with 38 % for the femoral loop graft. Both types of access had similar infection and ischemia rates [33].

A fistula can be created by forming the great saphenous vein into a loop that connects to the common femoral artery (Fig. 18.14). In a study by Pierre-Paul and colleagues, the mean primary patency was 7 months, the mean primary-assisted patency was 15 months, and the mean secondary patency was 16 months [34]. The GSV did not dilate as much as upper extremity veins, and therefore, the preoperative diameter should be equal or close to the diameter required for successful hemodialysis. Stenoses throughout the body of the AV fistula were common.

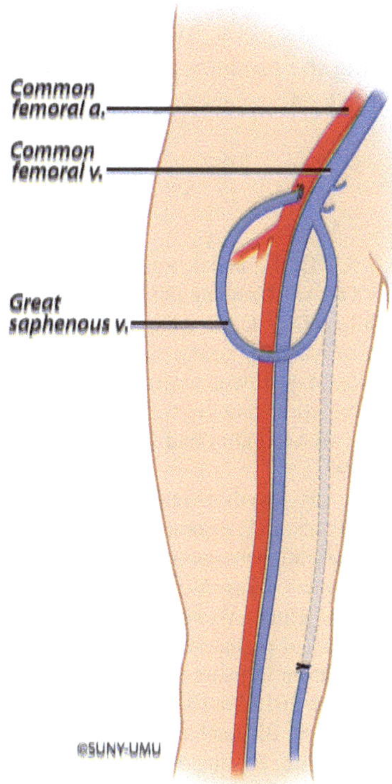

Fig. 18.14 Great saphenous vein to common femoral artery AV fistula

The HeRO is a hybrid device in which a prosthetic graft is anastomosed to the brachial artery, superficially tunneled on the anterior upper arm, and connected to a catheter extending into the internal jugular vein. This access was designed for patients with adequate arterial inflow but no suitable venous outflow proximal to the superior vena cava or right atrium. In a study by Katzman and colleagues, the HeRO device had a primary patency of 39 %, an assisted primary patency of 86 %, and a secondary patency of 72 % at a mean follow-up of 8.6 months [35]. A subsequent study comparing outcomes of the HeRO device to conventional AV grafts showed comparable patency, adequacy of dialysis, and bacteremia rates [36].

Summary

The concept of vascular access for hemodialysis is deceptively simple: arterial inflow connected to venous outflow creates a high blood flow circuit that can be regularly diverted into the dialysis machine. In practice, vascular access can be a challenging problem that often defies a simple solution or a single operation. Planning, persistence, and sound clinical judgment are required to create a functional AV fistula or graft without jeopardizing future access options. This chapter gives surgeons a framework for managing hemodialysis patients by outlining the fundamental procedures and principles for hemodialysis AV access.

References

1. Levin AR. NKF-K/DOQI clinical practice guidelines for vascular access: update 2006. Am J Kidney Dis. 2006;48(suppl):S176–247.
2. Gibson KD, Gillen DL, Caps MT, Kohler TR, Sherrard DJ, Stehman-Breen CO. Vascular access survival and incidence of revisions: a comparison of prosthetic grafts, simple autogenous fistulas, and venous transposition fistulas from the United States Renal Data System Dialysis Morbidity and Mortality Study. J Vasc Surg. 2001;34(4):694–700.
3. De Marco Garcia LP, Davila-Santini LR, Feng Q, Calderin J, Krishnasastry KV, Panetta TF. Primary balloon angioplasty plus balloon angioplasty maturation to upgrade small-caliber veins (<3 mm) for arteriovenous fistulas. J Vasc Surg. 2010;52(1):139–44.
4. Wang BR, Rowe VL, Ham SW, Han S, Patel K, Weaver FA, Woo K. A prospective clinical evaluation of the effects of intraoperative systemic anticoagulation in patients undergoing arteriovenous fistula surgery. Am Surg. 2010;76(10):1112–4.
5. Bhomi KK, Shrestha S, Bhattachan CL. Role of systemic anticoagulation in patients undergoing vascular access surgery. Nepal Med Coll J. 2008;10(4):222–4.
6. Konner K, Nonnast-Daniel B, Ritz E. The arteriovenous fistula. J Am Soc Nephrol. 2003;14:1669–80.
7. Nguyen VD, Griffith CG, Treat L. A multidisciplinary team approach to increasing av fistula creation. Nephrol News Issues. 2003;17:54–7.
8. Jennings WC. Creating arteriovenous fistulas in 132 consecutive patients. Arch Surg. 2006;141:27–32.
9. Rooijens PPGM, Tordoir JHM, Stijnen T, Burgmans JPJ, Smet de AAEA, Yo TI. Radiocephalic wrist arteriovenous fistula for hemodialysis: meta-analysis indicates a high primary failure rate. Eur J Vasc Endovasc Surg. 2004;28(15531191):583–9.
10. Palder SB, Kirkman RL, Whittemore AD, Hakim RM, Lazarus JM, Tilney NL. Vascular access for hemodialysis. Patency rates and results of revision. Ann Surg. 1985;202(2):235–9.
11. Cantelmo NL, LoGerfo FW, Menzoian JO. Brachiobasilic and brachiocephalic fistulas as secondary angioaccess routes. Surg Gynecol Obstet. 1982;155:545–8.
12. Gonzalez E, Kashuk JL, Moore EE, Linas S, Sauaia A. Two-stage brachial-basilic transposition fistula provides superior patency rates for dialysis access in a safety-net population. Surgery. 2010;148(4): 687–93; discussion 693–4.
13. Hakaim AG, Nalbandian M, Scott T. Superior maturation and patency of primary brachiocephalic and transposed basilic vein arteriovenous fistulae in patients with diabetes. J Vasc Surg. 1998;27(1):154–7.
14. Kumano S, Itatani K, Shiota J, Gojo S, Izumi N, Kasahara H, Homma Y, Tagawa H. Strategies for the creation and maintenance of reconstructed arteriovenous fistulas using the forearm basilic vein. Ther Apher Dial. 2013;17:504–9.
15. Weyde W, Letachowicz W, Krajewska MK, Letachowicz K, Watorek E, Kusztal M, Porazko T, Gołebiowski T, Madziarska K, Klinger M. Native forearm fistulas utilizing the basilic vein: an underused type of vascular access. J Nephrol. 2008;21:363–7.
16. Ayez N, van Houten VA, de Smet AA, van Well AM, Akkersdijk GP, van de Ven PJ, Fioole B. The basilic vein and the cephalic vein perform equally in upper arm arteriovenous fistulae. Eur J Vasc Endovasc Surg. 2012;44:227–31.
17. Bronder CM, Cull DL, Kuper SG, et al. Fistula elevation procedure: experience with 295 consecutive cases during a 7-year period. J Am Coll Surg. 2008;206(5):1076–81; discussion 1081–2.
18. Causey MW, Quan R, Hamawy A, Singh N. Superficialization of arteriovenous fistulae employing minimally invasive liposuction. J Vasc Surg. 2010;52(5):1397–400.
19. Francis DM, Lu Y, Robertson AJ, Millar RJ, Amy J. Two-stage brachiobasilic arteriovenous fistula for chronic haemodialysis access. ANZ J Surg. 2007;77(3):150–5.
20. Zielinski CMV, Mittal SK, Anderson P, Cummings J, Fenton S, Reiland-Smith J, Frock JT, Dunlay RW. Delayed superficialization of brachiobasilic fistula: technique and initial experience. Arch Surg. 2001;136:929–32.
21. Hossny A. Brachiobasilic arteriovenous fistula: different surgical techniques and their effects on fistula patency and dialysis-related complications. J Vasc Surg. 2003;37(12663983):821–6.
22. Vascular Access Work Group. Clinical practice guidelines for vascular access. Am J Kidney Dis. 2006;48 suppl 1:S248–73.
23. Segal JH, Kayler LK, Henke P, Merion RM, Leavey S, Campbell DA. Vascular access outcomes using the transposed basilic vein arteriovenous fistula. Am J Kidney Dis. 2003;42(1):151–7.
24. Humphries Jr AL, Colborn GL, Wynn JJ. Elevated basilic vein arteriovenous fistula. Am J Surg. 1999;177:489–91.
25. Sparks SR, VanderLinden JL, Gnanadev DA, Smith JW, Bunt TJ. Superior patency of perforating antecubital vein arteriovenous fistulae for hemodialysis. Ann Vasc Surg. 1997;11(2):165–7.
26. Mousa AY, Patterson W, Abu-Halimah S, Hass SM, Alhalbouni S, Sadek BT, Nanjundappa A, Modak A, Stone PA, Emmett M, AbuRahma AF. Patency in arteriovenous grafts in hemodialysis patients. Vasc Endovascular Surg. 2013;47:438–43.
27. Tashjian DB, Lipkowitz GS, Madden RL, Kaufman JL, Rhee SW, Berman J, Norris M, McCall J. Safety and efficacy of femoral-based hemodialysis access grafts. J Vasc Surg. 2002;35: 691–3.
28. Geenan IL, Nyilas L, Stephen MS, Makeham V, White GH, Verran DJ. Prosthetic lower extremity hemodialysis access grafts have satisfactory patency despite a high incidence of infection. J Vasc Surg. 2010;52:1546–50.
29. Jean-Baptiste E, Hassen-Khodja R, Haudebourg P, Declemy S, Batt M, Bouillanne PJ. Axillary loop grafts for hemodialysis access: midterm results from a single-center study. J Vasc Surg. 2008;47: 138–43.
30. Morsy MA, Khan A, Chemla ES. Prosthetic axillary-axillary arteriovenous straight access (necklace graft) for difficult hemodialysis patients: a prospective single-center experience. J Vasc Surg. 2008;48(5):1251–4, 1254 e1251.
31. Scott JD, Cull DL, Kalbaugh CA, Carsten CG, Blackhurst D, Taylor SM, Snyder BA, York JW, Langan EM. The mid-thigh loop arteriovenous graft: patient selection, technique, and results. Am Surg. 2006;72(9):825–8.
32. Gradman WS, Laub J, Cohen W. Femoral vein transposition for arteriovenous hemodialysis access: improved patient selection and intraoperative measures reduce postoperative ischemia. J Vasc Surg. 2005;41(2):279–84.
33. Hazinedaroglu SM, Tuzuner A, Ayli D, Demirer S, Duman N, Yerdel MA. Femoral vein transposition versus femoral loop grafts for hemodialysis: a prospective evaluation. Transplant Proc. 2004; 36:65–7.
34. Pierre-Paul D, Williams S, Lee T, Gahtan V. Saphenous vein loop to femoral artery arteriovenous fistula: a practical alternative. Ann Vasc Surg. 2004;18(2):223–7.
35. Katzman HE, McLafferty RB, Ross JR, Glickman MH, Peden EK, Lawson JH. Initial experience and outcome of a new hemodialysis access device for catheter-dependent patients. J Vasc Surg. 2009;50(3):600–7, 607 e601.
36. Nassar GM, Glickman MH, McLafferty RB, Kevin CJ, Zarge JI, Katzman HE, Peden EK, Lawson JH, Martinez JM, Thackeray L. A comparison between the HeRO Graft and conventional arteriovenous grafts in hemodialysis patients. Semin Dial. 2014. doi:10.1111/sdi.12173. [Epub ahead of print].

Access Complications

19

Chinenye O. Iwuchukwu and Michael J. Costanza

Introduction

The number of patients who depend on hemodialysis increases every year and already exceeds 400,000 in the USA alone. Creating long-term vascular access for hemodialysis has emerged as one of the most common surgeries with over 500,000 procedures performed annually in the USA. Although an arteriovenous (AV) graft or fistula provides a lifeline for patients with end-stage renal disease, AV access also represents the weakest link in sustaining long-term hemodialysis. Over 25 % of patients who start dialysis die from complications or failure of their vascular access [1]. Vascular access complications cause the most hospitalizations for patients on dialysis and account for over $1.8 billion of Medicare spending each year. The clinical impact of vascular access complications ranges from mild symptoms causing discomfort and inconvenience to catastrophic conditions that endanger life and limb. Recognizing and treating AV access complications can ensure patient safety, improve quality of life, and preserve vascular access function.

C.O. Iwuchukwu, MD, MPH
Department of General Surgery, SUNY Upstate University Hospital, Syracuse, NY, USA

Department of Surgery, SUNY Upstate Medical University, 750 East Adams Street, Syracuse, NY 13210, USA

Department of Veterans Affairs Healthcare Network Upstate New York at Syracuse, Syracuse, NY, USA

M.J. Costanza, MD, FACS (✉)
Division of Vascular Surgery and Endovascular Services, Department of Surgery, SUNY Upstate Medical University, 750 East Adams Street, Syracuse, NY 13210, USA

Department of Veterans Affairs Healthcare Network Upstate New York at Syracuse, Syracuse, NY, USA
e-mail: costanzm@upstate.edu

Bleeding

Bleeding complications usually fall into one of two clinical scenarios: diffuse oozing during vascular access surgery or acute hemorrhage from an existing AV fistula or graft. The inherent coagulopathy of kidney failure prolongs the bleeding time which makes surgical procedures more difficult and time-consuming. Once established, AV grafts and fistulas get punctured three times a week and can potentially bleed from the needle cannulation site, an underlying pseudoaneurysm or an overlying skin ulcer. Efforts to minimize the potentially fatal consequences of vascular access hemorrhage must include preventive measures to decrease the risk of bleeding and appropriate interventions to definitively stop ongoing hemorrhage.

For patients with kidney failure, chronic exposure to toxins associated with uremia causes defective platelet activation, aggregation, and adhesion [2]. Platelet dysfunction impairs primary hemostasis and prolongs the bleeding time, potentially increasing the risk for diffuse intraoperative oozing and postoperative hemorrhage. Dialysis in the perioperative time frame can be a two-edged sword. Although it can improve platelet function by removing some of the uremic toxins, hemodialysis usually requires anticoagulation which can linger if heparin is given close to the time of surgery. Inconsistent results and technical problems have plagued heparin-free dialysis techniques, most of which have failed to gain widespread acceptance [3]. Adequate preoperative hemodialysis should be pursued for elective procedures; however, it cannot be relied on as a stand-alone strategy to prevent all bleeding complications during vascular access surgery.

Anemia represents another chronic condition associated with kidney failure that prolongs bleeding time and undermines normal hemostasis. The loss of red cell mass allows the blood elements to mix homogenously, evenly distributing platelets in the bloodstream. When the hematocrit increases to 27–32 %, hemostasis improves as the increase in red blood

V. Gahtan and M.J. Costanza (eds.), *Essentials of Vascular Surgery for the General Surgeon*,
DOI 10.1007/978-1-4939-1326-8_19, © Springer Science+Business Media New York 2015

cells returns platelets back to the periphery of the bloodstream where they can be in close proximity to interact with the endothelium. Recombinant erythropoietin used to treat anemia may also promote hemostasis by increasing the number of GP-IIb/IIIa receptors on platelets and enhancing the thrombin-induced phosphorylation of platelet proteins [4]. In the setting of elective surgery, preoperative transfusions or erythropoietin to correct chronic anemia can decrease the risk of perioperative bleeding.

Medical therapy has both a therapeutic and prophylactic role in the management of bleeding for patients with kidney disease. Intravenous, subcutaneous, or intranasal administration of desmopressin releases factor VIII and von Willebrand factor (vWF) from the endothelium, shortens the bleeding time, and decreases clinical bleeding. This effect only lasts for 4–8 h, and the efficacy of desmopressin diminishes with repeated doses due to depletion of vWF stores in endothelial cells [5]. Despite its limited durability, desmopressin has proven to be effective in the treatment of active diffuse bleeding and the prevention of anticipated bleeding during surgery or invasive procedures [6]. For intravenous and subcutaneous administration, the dose of desmopressin is 0.3 mcg/kg in 50 ml of saline given over a period of 30 min. The intranasal route requires a tenfold larger dose of 3 mcg/kg.

Conjugated estrogens offer more sustained hemostasis for patients with uremic coagulopathy. To be effective, conjugated estrogen must be given every 24 h for five consecutive days at an oral dose of 25 mg per day or a minimum intravenous dose of 0.6 mg/kg. A significant decrease in bleeding becomes evident 24 h after the first dose, and the effect peaks 5–7 days after treatment. Unlike desmopressin, conjugated estrogens do not increase vWF or restore platelet function. Animal studies suggest that conjugated estrogens promote hemostasis by interfering with the nitric oxide synthetic pathway [7].

Other options for the treatment of uremic coagulopathy include tranexamic acid, recombinant activated factor VII, and factor replacement using cryoprecipitate. These alternative therapies are usually only employed if all other interventions have failed because each has a significant drawback and a spotty track record of success. Tranexamic acid accumulates in renal failure and fails to outperform commonly used therapy [8]. The use of recombinant activated factor VII in "off-label" settings other than hemophilia has had mixed results and may increase the risk of thromboembolic events [9]. Cryoprecipitate generates no response in as many as 50 % of patients and carries the risk of blood-borne disease transmission.

Acute hemorrhage represents a rare but potentially fatal complication of an established AV fistula or graft. The Centers for Medicare and Medicaid Services (CMS) report that vascular access hemorrhage causes 0.4 % of hemodialysis patient deaths; however, this figure significantly underestimates the true mortality rate. A recent review from the Maryland Medical Examiner identified 88 fatal vascular access hemorrhages only one quarter (24 %) of which were included in the CMS data suggesting that bleeding fatalities are underreported to CMS [10]. Fortunately access site bleeding and its consequences can often be prevented or effectively treated by recognizing the signs of impending hemorrhage and intervening appropriately for active bleeding.

Functional AV fistulas and grafts get punctured with two needles three times a week so the high frequency of cannulation site bleeding is not surprising. Initial treatment involves direct, digital pressure at the site of bleeding. The finger provides a safe and effective hemostatic agent as it applies pressure more precisely than a tourniquet or blood pressure cuff without the risk of access thrombosis or skin breakdown. If bleeding persists, a figure of eight monofilament suture (3-0 or 4-0 caliber) placed around the puncture site will stop the bleeding, and the stitch can then be removed the following day or before the next dialysis session. This technique should only be considered if the surrounding skin is intact as sutures will pull through and be rendered ineffective in the setting of a chronic skin ulcer or eschar.

After establishing hemostasis, the focus shifts to determining the cause of bleeding. Venous outflow stenosis leads to prolonged needle site bleeding by increasing the back pressure on the AV graft or fistula. This common condition should be suspected in patients with a history of previous access interventions, high venous pressures at dialysis, and pulsatility instead of a thrill on physical exam. Chronic venous hypertension encourages the formation of pseudoaneurysms at needle puncture sites. A fistulogram can confirm the diagnosis of venous outflow obstruction and provide an opportunity for endovascular intervention. Other, less common causes of prolonged needle site bleeding include coagulopathy and poor technical execution of needle puncture and decannulation.

Patients presenting with an eschar or skin ulcer overlying an AV access have a more complex problem that typically occurs in the setting of a chronic pseudoaneurysm. A pseudoaneurysm forms when repeated needle cannulation at the same site creates a large hole in the fistula or graft. Subcutaneous pressure from the pseudoaneurysm impairs capillary filling of the overlying skin resulting in skin necrosis. The compromised skin provides a thin, tenuous layer covering the hole in the graft or fistula that may eventually give way leading to an acute vascular access hemorrhage (Fig. 19.1).

The presence of a skin ulcer or eschar overlying a vascular access requires prompt surgical intervention. Attempts to suture the friable surrounding tissue will inevitably fail and may precipitate more bleeding by accelerating the rate of skin necrosis. Jaffers and Fasola recently reported uniform

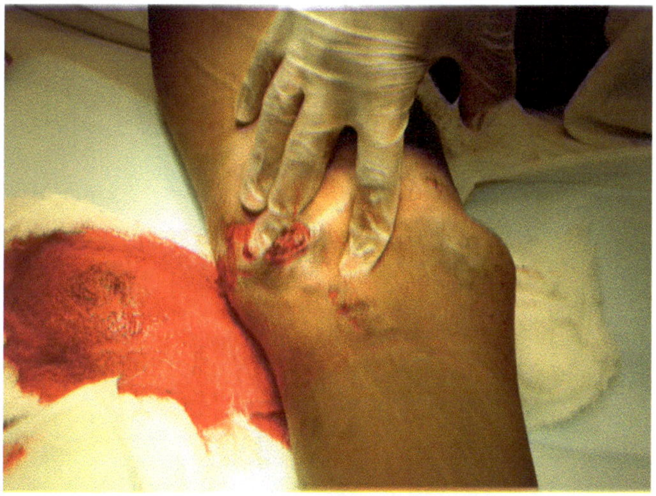

Fig. 19.1 An ulcerated skin ulcer directly overlying an arteriovenous fistula. Hemorrhage from the ulcer is being controlled with manual pressure immediately before surgical repair in the operating room

success in salvaging ulcerated, bleeding autologous fistulas [11]. In most cases, they excised the skin ulcer and primarily repaired the underlying fistula opening. Aneurysmal segments required plication after resection of the anterior fistula wall. All of the fistulas remained functional allowing uninterrupted dialysis. Salvaging an ulcerated AV graft involves excising the overlying skin and tunneling an interposition prosthetic bypass around the area of skin breakdown. Continued dialysis depends on whether the revised AV graft still has a usable segment for cannulation. A temporary dialysis catheter may be required until the interposition bypass has healed allowing more space for needle punctures.

Venous Stenosis

Venous stenosis remains the Achilles heel of vascular access. Triggered by several risk factors, venous stenosis is a common complication that responds poorly to endovascular intervention with a high rate of recurrence. Despite advances in hemodialysis surveillance and endovascular techniques, venous stenosis causes more AV access failures than any other complication. AV grafts typically fail due to stenosis at the venous anastomosis, while fistulas can develop stenosis anywhere including the arterial anastomosis, venous outflow, central veins, and superior vena cava. Depending on the location and severity of the lesion, venous stenosis can have a wide range of consequences including arm edema, superior vena cava syndrome, prolonged bleeding, aneurysm and pseudoaneurysm formation, ineffective dialysis, and vascular access thrombosis. The high prevalence of venous stenosis (16–50 %) coupled with being recalcitrant to definitive intervention creates one of the most vexing problems for vascular access. Management guidelines for venous stenosis therefore consist of prevention, palliative endovascular interventions, and surgical bypass in selected cases.

Central venous catheters remain the most prominent risk factor for the development of central venous stenosis. Catheters injure the venous endothelium inciting an inflammatory and thrombotic response. A vein's response to injury can evolve over time into an organized thrombus associated with smooth muscle proliferation, vessel wall thickening, and formation of a bridge to the catheter. The injury induced by the catheter coupled with the vein's hyperplastic response may create a precursor stenotic lesion which would explain the strong association between central venous catheters and venous stenosis [12]. Other high-risk factors for venous stenosis include multiple catheter placement, long dwell times, and subclavian vein location; however, all catheters, regardless of location or duration, have been linked to venous stenosis. Several studies have documented venous stenosis following internal jugular vein catheters, and even short-term catheters can incite thrombosis, fibrin sheath formation, and stenosis [13]. Therefore, the most effective way to prevent venous stenosis is to avoid the use of central venous catheters altogether [14, 16].

The diagnosis of venous stenosis relies on clinical assessment, hemodialysis monitoring, and imaging studies. Signs and symptoms of venous stenosis include arm edema, loss of a palpable thrill, access pulsatility, and prolonged bleeding after needle decannulation. Dialysis centers track objective measures of access and recirculation over time. Findings which suggest venous stenosis including persistently low flow (less than 600 ml/min), high venous pressure, or ineffective dialysis should prompt imaging studies for confirmation [17, 18]. Duplex ultrasound of the access can often detect venous stenosis; however, it offers limited, indirect evaluation of the central veins. A fistulogram has the highest sensitivity for diagnosing venous stenosis since it can image the entire vascular access from the arterial anastomosis to the right atrium [19].

In addition to being diagnostic, fistulograms also provide an opportunity for endovascular intervention. Balloon angioplasty to dilate stenotic lesions in peripheral and central veins has an immediate technical success rate of 88–94 % [20]. Most peripheral venous lesions require overdilation with angioplasty balloons 10–20 % larger in diameter than the vein being treated. Unlike atherosclerotic arterial disease, stenotic venous lesions consist of endothelial hyperplasia and fibrous tissue [21]. These histologic features may explain why venous stenoses tend to resist balloon angioplasty and recoil after dilation in as many as 64 % of patients as determined by intravascular ultrasound [22]. If the post-angioplasty images show persistent stenosis or immediate recoil, endovascular treatment options include repeat angioplasty using a high-pressure or cutting balloon or stent placement depending on the lesion type and location. Centrally located lesions require a more cautious approach to avoid the risk of potentially fatal central vein perforation [23]. Determining the appropriate balloon size for central venous lesions can be challenging because two-dimensional contrast images often underestimate the true vein diameter. Intravascular ultrasound measures the vessel lumen more accurately and may help in choosing a sufficiently large diameter balloon that will not overdilate the vein. Stent placement can play a role in treating elastic lesions of the central veins that fail to respond to balloon angioplasty or recur within 3 months of treatment [24]. Using self-expanding stents that are slightly larger than the diameter of the vein will assure full-wall apposition and minimize the risk of stent migration. An intravascular ultrasound or pre-procedure CT scan of the thorax provides accurate measurements of the true central vein diameter and ensure appropriate stent sizing.

Limited durability remains the most significant disadvantage of endovascular therapy for venous stenosis. Primary patency following balloon angioplasty for central venous stenosis falls to 25 % and 17 % after 6 months and 12 months, respectively [25]. Balloon angioplasty for peripheral veins results in a similar, slightly less steep, decline in short- and midterm patency. The benefit of stenting appears to be confined to salvaging immediate technical success after an unsatisfactory response to balloon angioplasty [26]. Stents placed in peripheral and central veins fail to prolong primary and secondary patency and may accelerate restenosis in some locations.

The short-lived success of endovascular therapy for venous stenosis mandates regular post-intervention follow-up. Clinical evidence of restenosis including the reappearance of arm edema, prolonged bleeding, high venous pressures, and ineffective dialysis should prompt further investigation with a fistulogram. The treatment of recurrent venous stenosis depends on the time interval to restenosis and the lesion location. Repeated balloon angioplasty may be the most reasonable treatment strategy for patients with peripheral or central venous stenosis who can achieve effective dialysis for at least 3–6 months between endovascular interventions. Although it is not definitive, endovascular therapy can prolong effective patency and allow these patients to avoid or delay the need for surgery and catheter placement.

Surgical revision should be considered if endovascular treatment fails or the stenosis recurs within a short period of time (less than 3 months). Surgical options depend on the extent of the lesion, its location, and the superficial and central venous anatomy. For peripheral venous stenosis, surgery to reestablish venous outflow usually involves patch angioplasty of the venous outflow (Fig. 19.2) or an interposition bypass of the lesion using prosthetic graft (Fig. 19.3). Other surgical options include mobilizing and reimplanting the distal AV fistula on a patent vein or translocating the basilic or cephalic vein. Likewise, a variety of techniques to manage

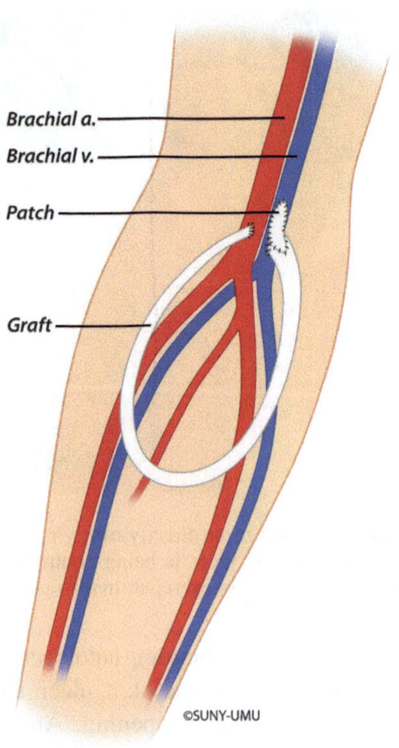

Fig. 19.2 Surgical management of venous outflow stenosis with patch angioplasty of the venous anastomosis

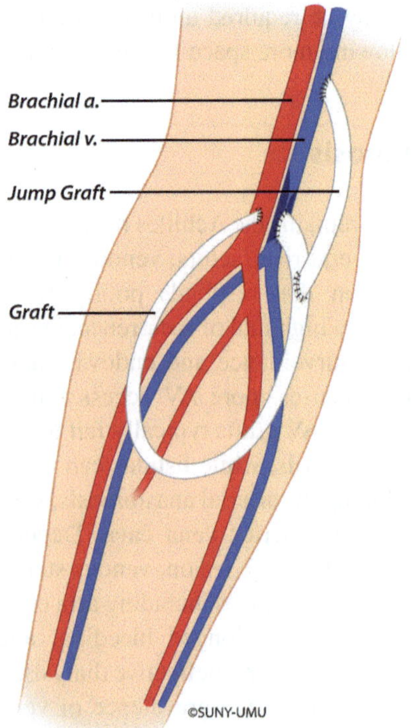

Fig. 19.3 Surgical management of venous outflow stenosis with interposition bypass to a more proximal vein using prosthetic graft

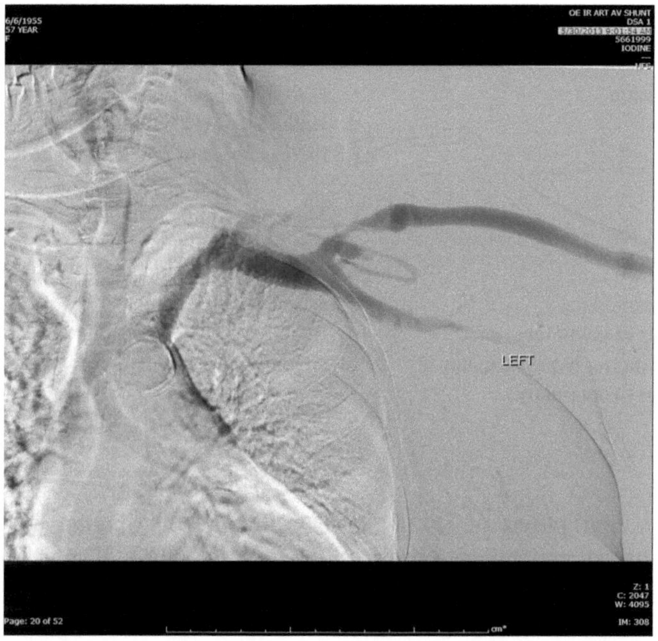

Fig. 19.4 Fistulogram of a left upper arm brachiocephalic AV fistula with stenosis of the cephalic vein in the cephalic arch

recalcitrant subclavian vein lesions have been described including axillary to internal jugular vein bypass, internal jugular to axillary vein transposition, axillary to saphenous vein bypass, and patch angioplasty of the axillosubclavian vein stenosis [27]. A direct bypass to the right atrium offers a solution to central venous occlusion; however, the morbidity and requirement for a thoracotomy makes this procedure appropriate only for highly selected patients with few remaining vascular access options [28, 29].

Venous stenosis at the costoclavicular junction deserves special consideration because of its poor response to balloon angioplasty and stent placement. The musculoskeletal structures surrounding the costoclavicular junction can extrinsically compress the adjacent subclavian vein. Exposure of this anatomically narrowed segment of the vein to turbulent flow from a proximal AV fistula can create a chronic functional injury equivalent to venous thoracic outlet syndrome. According to this theory, endovascular therapy at the costoclavicular junction will fail in the absence of thoracic outlet decompression which usually involves a transaxillary first rib resection. Illig achieved promising early results using a surgical approach for patients with so-called dialysis associated venous thoracic outlet syndrome. He reported an 8-month functional patency of 75 % in a series of 12 selected patients treated with first rib resection [30].

The anatomic area known as the cephalic arch (the final segment of the cephalic vein before its confluence with the axillary vein) is also prone to stenosis and relatively resistant to endovascular intervention (Fig. 19.4). In patients with brachiocephalic AV fistulas, the incidence of cephalic arch stenosis may exceed 77 %, making it a leading cause of vascular access failure [31]. Balloon angioplasty, the widely accepted first-line therapy, has limited durability with a primary 6-month patency of only 42 % [31, 32]. The unique anatomy of the cephalic arch may explain its tendency to form recalcitrant stenotic lesions [33]. After the creation of an AV fistula, all veins react to the hemodynamic changes with intimal hyperplasia and wall thickening. Peripheral veins can usually preserve their lumen diameter because they have the anatomic freedom to dilate and remodel. In contrast, the cephalic arch's pathway over the deltoid muscle creates a constriction limiting fistula dilation and accommodation for intimal hyperplasia. Stenotic lesions develop early in the cephalic arch and usually recoil or quickly recur in response to dilation with balloon angioplasty. Endovascular alternatives for treating cephalic arch stenosis including cutting balloon angioplasty and stent graft placement have shown promising early results in small, selected case series [34, 35, 32]. Surgical revision usually involves rerouting the venous outflow around the cephalic arch by transposing the proximal cephalic vein to the basilic or axillary vein.

Ischemia

Ischemia associated with vascular access goes by several names including hemodialysis access-induced distal ischemia (HAIDI), dialysis-associated steal syndrome, distal hypoperfusion ischemic syndrome, and access-related hand ischemia. All of these terms describe a complication clinically defined as hypoperfusion distal (more peripheral) to an AV fistula or graft [36]. The incidence and severity of HAIDI varies with the type and location of the vascular access. For AV fistulas originating from the brachial artery, the incidence of HAIDI can approach 20 % with over half of the cases classified as severe [37]. Radial artery-based fistulas have a much lower incidence (2 %) and rarely require treatment [38]. The severity of clinical symptoms determines the classification of HAIDI as follows [39]:

- Stage 1: retrograde flow without complaints
- Stage 2: forearm or hand pain with exertion
- Stage 3: forearm or hand pain at rest
- Stage 4: ulceration, necrosis, or gangrene

The pathophysiology of HAIDI provides insight into its prevention, diagnosis, and management. Connecting an artery to a vein for vascular access creates a high-flow, low-resistance circuit. Distal perfusion pressure decreases as an increasing volume of arterial blood flows preferentially through the access into the low-resistance venous outflow. Retrograde flow from the distal artery into the access site occurs during all or part of the cardiac cycle further decreasing pressure in the forearm and hand. Although this "physiologic steal" occurs in virtually all AV fistulas and grafts, only a few

Table 19.1 Techniques for treating hemodialysis access-induced distal ischemia (HAIDI)

Technique	Advantages	Drawbacks
Access ligation	• Maximizes hand perfusion • Technically simple	• Loss of dialysis access • High risk of HAIDI in new access
Banding	• Preserves access • Technically simple	• Increases risk of access thrombosis
Distal revascularization-interval ligation (DRIL)	• Preserves access	• More demanding technically • Brachial artery ligated
Proximalization of arterial inflow (PAI)	• Preserves access • Brachial artery remains in continuity	• Less effective in patients with high access flow or tissue loss • Requires prosthetic conduit
Revision using distal inflow (RUDI)	• Preserves access with shorter bypass conduit • Brachial artery remains in continuity	• Higher failure rate

patients develop significant distal ischemia. The lack of correlation between retrograde flow (steal) and clinical ischemia has fueled speculation that "steal" itself plays only a minor role in the so-called steal syndrome. Scheltinga and Bruijninckx assert that locoregional hypotension, not retrograde flow or steal, is the most critical factor in the onset of HAIDI [40]. The majority of patients overcome "physiologic steal" and other hemodynamic changes by vasodilating inflow arteries, recruiting collaterals, and increasing cardiac output to augment distal perfusion. Ischemia occurs only when these adaptive mechanisms fail to compensate for distal hypoperfusion. The most common clinical scenarios resulting in HAIDI include excessive access flow, arterial occlusive disease, and lack of arterial adaptation or collateral flow.

The first step in preventing HAIDI involves recognizing which patients are at risk. Diabetes emerged as the most predictive factor for developing ischemia in a multivariate analysis of 324 AV fistulas in 309 patients [41]. Other clinical predictors of HAIDI include brachial artery-based access, female gender, age greater than 60, low digital brachial index, and previous operations on the same limb. Unfortunately, none of the preoperative predictors of ischemia has enough predictability to preclude creating an AV access in an "at-risk" patient.

Basing an AV access on the radial artery will decrease the ischemic risk; however, the non-maturation rate increases, and not all patients have an adequate caliber radial artery at the wrist. Whittaker and Bakran reported a low rate of ischemia (2 %) using the proximal radial or ulnar artery as arterial inflow [42]. Through a longitudinal incision in the proximal forearm, they create an end-to-side anastomosis between the median cubital vein and the proximal radial or ulnar artery. This technique offers a reasonable alternative to using inflow from the brachial artery for patients who cannot have a wrist fistula. If the brachial artery must be used, limiting the length of the AV anastomosis to less than 10 mm decreases the risk of developing excessive flow through the access.

Symptoms of HAIDI have a bimodal distribution with half of patients presenting acutely (within 7 days of surgery) and the other half following a more chronic course (presenting after 30 days) [43]. In the acute presentation, the signs and symptoms of HAIDI mirror the classic 6 Ps of acute lower extremity ischemia, namely, pulselessness, pain, pallor, poikilothermia, paresthesias, and paralysis. Chronic symptoms of HAIDI emerge months to years after surgery and include arm fatigue with exertion, hand pain at rest, and tissue loss. Often the tissue loss occurs due to what would otherwise be insignificant skin trauma. The clinical diagnosis of HAIDI relies on both the history and physical examination. Physical exam of a patient with HAIDI usually demonstrates an absent wrist pulse that returns with manual compression of the access; however, this finding cannot be used as the sole diagnostic criteria for HAIDI. In practice, many patients lack a palpable wrist pulse after AV access creation while maintaining adequate perfusion to the arm and hand. At the other extreme, some patients with symptoms of ischemia have a palpable wrist pulse at rest. This apparently contradictory presentation suggests that the upper extremity can develop ischemic symptoms at relatively higher absolute pressures [44].

The timing and type of treatment for HAIDI depend on several factors including symptom severity, type of access, and the patient's clinical condition [45]. Patients with mild symptoms warrant close observation as many will improve over time [46]. Moderate and severe symptoms of HAIDI require prompt intervention to improve perfusion and prevent permanent ischemic injury or tissue loss. The treatment options listed in Table 19.1 should be considered complementary as none of the techniques has universal success nor can any be applied to all clinical scenarios. All interventions should primarily focus on reversing ischemia with a secondary goal of salvaging the vascular access.

Ligation immediately and reliably reverses ischemia at the cost of sacrificing the vascular access. Although symptoms usually improve quickly, paresthesias can persist due to neuropathy related to the initial ischemic injury. Access ligation may serve as a first-line treatment for acute ischemia after a prosthetic AV graft given a graft's predictably short patency. At the other extreme, access ligation can also function as a last resort to reverse ischemia in patients who have failed to improve after a previous remedial procedure. The straightforward nature of access ligation also makes this intervention appropriate for patients with severe comorbidities that preclude more extensive revascularization procedures.

Rarely, treatment for HAIDI involves simply correcting arterial inflow stenosis. Prior to creating the access, a thorough preoperative evaluation should detect and treat inflow lesions. Scali and Huber recommend measuring upper extremity arterial pressure and Doppler waveforms on all potential access patients. Their criteria for a suitable inflow artery include adequate diameter (brachial artery >3 mm; radial artery >2 mm) and absence of hemodynamically significant arterial stenosis based on pressures and waveforms [44]. All patients with symptomatic HAIDI should have complete angiographic imaging of all vessels bringing blood to and from the AV access. The procedure begins by puncturing the AV access in the direction of the arterial anastomosis and advancing a directional catheter over a wire through the arterial anastomosis and into the arterial system as far proximally as the aortic arch. Images and pressure measurements at the aortic arch, subclavian artery origin, axillary artery, and brachial artery (proximal, mid, and pre-anastomotic) are then recorded. Any stenotic lesions encountered can be treated with balloon angioplasty. Redirecting the catheter into the distal arterial runoff can then evaluate for occlusive disease in the forearm and hand.

Most patients do not harbor an arterial inflow lesion of such severity that correcting it alone would alleviate all symptoms of ischemia. Usually HAIDI develops from a combination of excessive access flow and hypotension in the distal arterial system. Reversing ischemia and salvaging the vascular access therefore requires interventions that limit access flow and/or increase distal arterial perfusion. Banding describes a variety of techniques that reduce access flow by increasing resistance in the venous outflow. In its simplest form, banding narrows the venous outflow by suture plication or placement of a restrictive prosthetic cuff. The underlying hemodynamic flaw of banding leads to poor long-term access patency rates. A band that restricts flow enough to reverse ischemia often converts the access into a flow-dependent, high-resistance circuit whose natural tendency is to clot [47]. Miller et al. reported improved results with a modification to traditional banding procedures. The MILLER procedure (minimally invasive limited ligation endoluminal-assisted revision) involves inflating a percutaneously placed 3 or 4 mm diameter angioplasty balloon in the proximal venous outflow. Through a small incision, a suture is passed around the access and tied over the inflated balloon narrowing the access to the diameter of the chosen balloon (Fig. 19.5). The precise band sizing achieved by the MILLER procedure may account for the promising midterm results including a 6-month primary band patency of 75–85 % in a selected series of 183 patients [36].

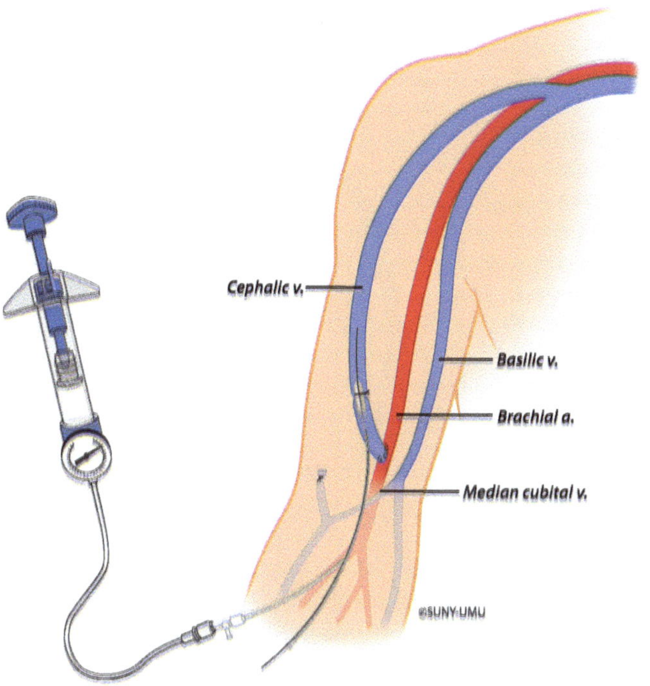

Fig. 19.5 The MILLER procedure for banding an arteriovenous fistula. The percutaneously inserted angioplasty balloon is inflated in the proximal fistula, and a suture is introduced through a small skin incision and tied around the inflated balloon to narrow the vein to the diameter of the chosen balloon

Although banding procedures can decrease access flow, they do not directly increase distal arterial perfusion. The distal revascularization-interval ligation (DRIL) procedure is currently the most accepted method of retaining the AV fistula and improving distal perfusion. DRIL consists of two components in an attempt to address both of these treatment goals. Distal revascularization creates a bypass around the fistula to increase forearm and hand perfusion, while interval ligation of the distal brachial artery cuts off retrograde flow into the access (Fig. 19.6). The great saphenous vein in the thigh and a segment of cephalic or basilic vein from the ipsilateral upper extremity rank first and second in preference as conduits for the brachial bypass. Placing the vein in reverse configuration avoids the need for a valvulotome which can damage thin-walled arm veins. In the absence of an autogenous vein larger than 3 mm in diameter, some access surgeons have reported satisfactory results with a prosthetic graft. In contrast, Scali and Huber avoid using a prosthetic graft opting instead for an alternative revascularization procedure or fistula ligation [44].

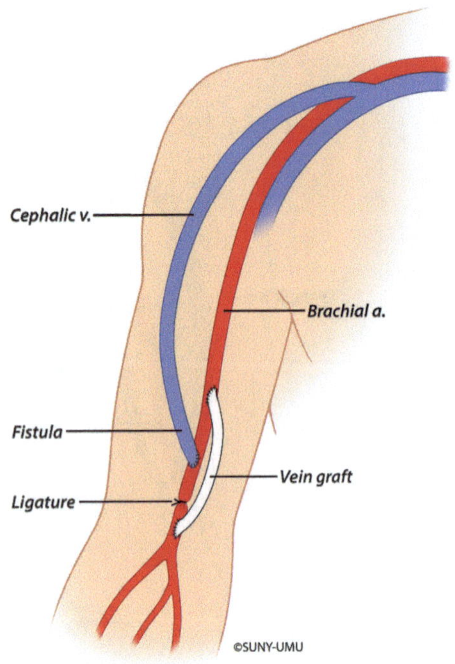

Fig. 19.6 Distal revascularization-interval ligation (DRIL) procedure. A bypass from the proximal brachial artery extends to the brachial artery just distal to the AV fistula anastomosis. The brachial artery is then ligated distal to the AV anastomosis and proximal to the bypass graft

Preparation for a DRIL procedure begins with angiography and brachial artery pressure measurements. In his original description of the DRIL procedure, Schanzer empirically started the brachial bypass 5 cm proximal to the fistula anastomosis [48]. Over the last 25 years, a more clear understanding of the hemodynamics of HAIDI has emerged including the concept of locoregional hypotension. In a series of patients with access-related ischemia, Illig et al. demonstrated a significant pressure drop-off in the brachial artery [49]. They found that this "pressure sink" often extended along the brachial artery more than 5 cm proximal to the fistula anastomosis. To effectively increase distal perfusion, the brachial artery bypass should originate proximal to the "pressure sink." By measuring the distance from the fistula anastomosis to the pressure drop-off, preoperative pressure measurements can identify an appropriate location for the proximal bypass.

The bypass should terminate on the brachial artery just distal to the fistula anastomosis. If the fistula originates from the very distal brachial artery, the fistula anastomosis should be transposed to the more proximal artery to allow space for the distal bypass anastomosis. After ensuring adequate flow through the bypass, the brachial artery is ligated between the anastomoses of the fistula and the distal bypass. Postoperative monitoring in the form of clinical exam and duplex ultrasound seems to be helpful; however, guidelines for the type and frequency of surveillance do not exist. Anaya-Ayala et al. recommend close follow-up in the 30-day postoperative period, especially in patients with suboptimal bypass conduits and microvascular disease [50].

Despite the technical demands, the DRIL procedure appears to be safe and effective. Wound infection is the most common complication, and Scali et al. reported a 30-day mortality rate of 2 % in the largest series of patients [51]. Outcome data after DRIL procedures vary with the definition of clinical success. Relief of presenting symptoms ranges from 78 to 100 % with higher rates reported by authors who overlook residual paresthesias presumably due to the initial ischemic injury [52, 53]. Concerns about the negative impact of ligating the native brachial artery appear to be unfounded. Primary bypass patency ranges from 73 to 100 % at 1 year, while secondary patency exceeds 80 % in most reports [43]. Long-term durability may not be necessary given the limited survival of patients undergoing the DRIL procedure. Anaya-Ayala et al. reported a 1-year mortality of 61 % due to comorbid illnesses unrelated to the DRIL procedure [50], while only 30 % of patients in Scali and Huber's series were still alive 2 years after surgery [44].

Although the DRIL procedure is the most well-known technique, other procedures aimed at reversing ischemia and preserving the access have been described. Proximalization of arterial inflow (PAI) inserts an interposition bypass from the proximal brachial artery near the axilla to the original autogenous access in the antecubital fossa. The bypass consists of a 4–5 mm prosthetic graft which is tunneled in the deep tissue of the upper medial arm (Fig. 19.7). Needle cannulation sites remain on the anterior upper arm along the autogenous venous outflow tract. PAI most likely functions as a flow-limiting procedure as the long, small caliber bypass increases resistance in the access thereby improving distal perfusion [44]. In small case series, PAI resolved ischemic symptoms in 65–84 % of patients [54, 55]. These reports suggest that PAI is less effective in high access flow HAIDI and caution against the use of PAI in patients with severe tissue loss. Other concerns about PAI center around the infectious and thrombotic risk of converting a fistula to a composite prosthetic/autogenous access.

In contrast to PAI, the revision using distal inflow (RUDI) procedure relocates the arterial inflow to a more distal artery. As a first step, the fistula is ligated and transected close to the brachial anastomosis. A short interposition bypass from the radial or ulnar artery to the fistula is then created using a nearby venous collateral or great saphenous vein graft (Fig. 19.8). By switching arterial inflow from the brachial to the radial or ulnar artery, RUDI decreases flow into the fistula and increases distal perfusion. Advantages of RUDI over the PAI and DRIL procedures include the use of a shorter bypass conduit and preservation of uninterrupted flow through the native brachial artery. Fistula failure is the primary drawback of RUDI as the smaller distal artery may fail to supply adequate inflow to the fistula. Although small case

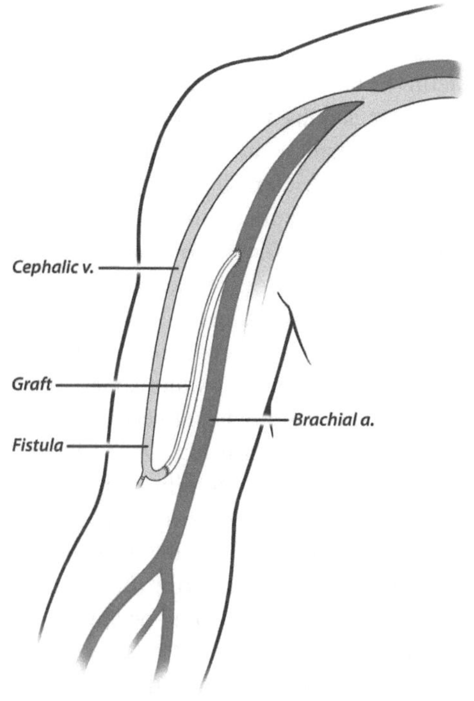

Fig. 19.7 Proximalization of arterial inflow. A long interposition bypass extends from the proximal brachial artery near the axilla to the autogenous access

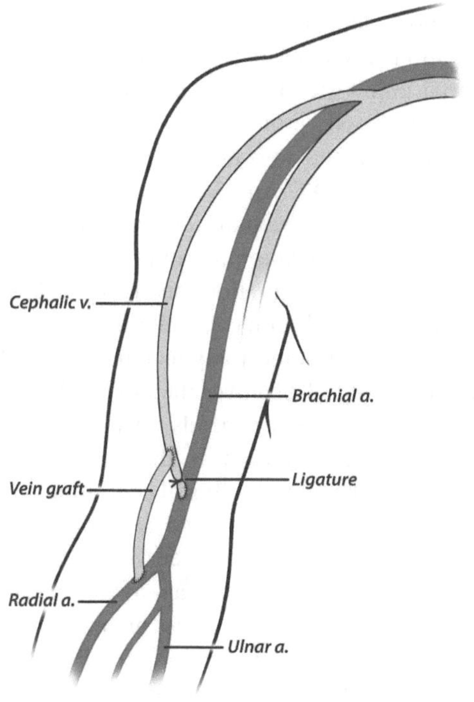

Fig. 19.8 Revision using distal inflow. The fistula is ligated and transected close to the brachial anastomosis. A short interposition bypass is then constructed from the more distal radial (or ulnar) artery

series reported that RUDI resolved ischemic symptoms in nearly all patients, the fistula failure rate ranged from 29 to 43 % [56, 57]. The presence of forearm arterial occlusive disease, especially in the elderly, diabetics, and women, may increase the risk of fistula failure after RUDI.

Ischemic Monomelic Neuropathy

In 1983 Wilbourn coined the term "ischemic monomelic neuropathy" (IMN) to describe an unusual form of ischemia affecting multiple nerves in the same extremity [58]. One of the three patients in his original paper developed IMN after an AV fistula and further experience has demonstrated that IMN is a rare but potentially devastating complication of vascular access with an incidence of 0.5 % [59]. As an unusual form of ischemia, IMN causes nerve damage often resulting in permanent limb dysfunction. The underlying pathology of IMN seems to involve mild, transient ischemia which triggers a disproportionately severe injury to susceptible peripheral nerves [58]. Most reports of IMN describe a diabetic patient who develops intense hand pain and weakness immediately following surgery to create a brachial artery-based AV access. Physical exam typically reveals a well-perfused hand with sensory and motor deficits of all three nerves (radial, ulnar, and median). When the diagnosis is unclear, noninvasive exams can provide valuable supplemental information. Most patients with IMN have digital pressures greater than 50 mmHg, while nerve conduction studies demonstrate reduced or unobtainable sensory and motor nerve action potentials [60]. Although these results support the diagnosis of IMN, noninvasive exams are not necessary in all cases and may serve only to delay treatment when the clinical scenario clearly points to IMN.

Immediate AV access ligation offers the only effective treatment for IMN. Failure to recognize and treat IMN leads to permanent nerve damage and a nonfunctional claw hand in severe cases [61]. Unfortunately, early diagnosis and immediate ligation often fails to completely reverse nerve dysfunction, and most patients require physical and occupational therapy to improve hand function [62]. IMN poses a risk to all patients undergoing AV access surgery making efforts at prevention difficult if not impossible. Although the presence of arterial insufficiency and diabetic neuropathy increases the risk, no preoperative finding or test can predict which patients will develop IMN [63]. Effective management of IMN requires a heightened awareness of its symptoms, early diagnosis in the immediate postoperative period, and prompt access ligation to minimize the long-term effects of the nerve injury.

Thrombosis

Vascular access thrombosis (VAT) is a disruptive and potentially dangerous event in the life of a dialysis patient. VAT interrupts dialysis which can be life-threatening in the setting of hyperkalemia or fluid overload. Salvaging the clotted access involves an invasive procedure with its associated risks, while failure to restore access patency puts the patient in the undesirable position of using a catheter for dialysis. Despite advances in surgery, dialysis surveillance, and endovascular tools, VAT causes more hospital admissions and more vascular access failures than any other complication [64]. Minimizing the negative impact of VAT requires an understanding of the pathophysiology and familiarity with surgical and endovascular thrombectomy techniques.

VAT results from a confluence of thrombotic factors described by Virchow's triad: endothelial cell injury, reduction of blood flow, and hypercoagulability. The first part of the triad, endothelial dysfunction, reflects the underlying intimal hyperplasia which occurs in nearly all forms of vascular access. Intimal hyperplasia involves the proliferation of extracellular matrix, activated cells, and neovascularization which can narrow and ultimately occlude the vessel lumen. Several events commonly encountered in dialysis patients trigger intimal hyperplasia including surgical trauma, hemodynamic shear stress, AV graft bioincompatibility, needle puncture injury, and uremia. The second part of the triad, low blood flow or stasis, usually stems from a problem with access inflow, outflow, or the conduit itself. External compression and systemic hypotension can also compromise flow and predispose to VAT. Hypercoagulability, the third part of the triad, emerges when patients start receiving dialysis. In contrast to the bleeding tendency of uremic patients, patients on dialysis often exhibit hypercoagulability mediated primarily by activated platelets [65]. Exposure to prothrombotic surfaces (extracellular matrix, artificial membrane), coupled with turbulence in the AV access, activates platelets setting off a cascade of events which culminates in platelet deposition and conditions favoring intimal hyperplasia.

Whether inherited hypercoagulable disorders contribute to VAT remains unclear. Several studies reported a higher prevalence of factor V Leiden and the prothrombin 20210 polymorphism in patients with VAT compared to patients without VAT [66, 67]. In contrast, Fekih-Mrissa failed to observe an increased thrombotic risk among dialysis patients with factor V Leiden or prothrombin G20210A mutations [68]. Although a hypercoagulable work-up is probably not necessary in most patients with VAT, an evaluation may be warranted in selected patients especially those with recurrent VAT involving multiple access types.

Comorbid conditions that frequently affect dialysis patients also increase the risk of VAT. Patients with atrial fibrillation have double the risk of VAT which most likely reflects the underlying chronic inflammation associated with atrial fibrillation and hemodialysis [69]. Diabetes increases the probability of AV graft thrombosis to 55 % and 72 % at 6 and 12 months, respectively, compared to 29 % and 49 % in patients without diabetes [70]. Several studies and a recent meta-analysis suggest that the commonly used medication erythropoietin (EPO) triggers intimal hyperplasia and thrombosis [71]. Other acquired thrombotic risk factors include hypertension, malignancy, previous catheter insertion, focal segmental glomerulosclerosis, hyperhomocysteinemia, hypoalbuminemia, and anticardiolipin antibodies. Obesity increases the technical difficulty of cannulation and hemostasis, which may account for the increased risk of VAT [72].

Physical exam demonstrating the loss of a previously palpable thrill and audible bruit provides sufficient evidence to diagnose VAT. Although a duplex ultrasound exam can confirm these findings, this study is not necessary in most cases and should not delay treatment. Once diagnosed, VAT requires prompt treatment to minimize the metabolic and fluid complications related to the interruption of dialysis. Failure to intervene quickly allows the thrombus to grow and increases the contact time between the thrombus and the vessel wall. Thrombectomy procedures become more difficult and less durable as time passes [73]. Reestablishing AV access patency within 48 h can usually return the patient to their routine dialysis schedule without resorting to the use of a temporary catheter.

Interventions for VAT consist of two components: removal of the thrombus and treatment of the underlying cause of access failure. Over 85 % of patients have an underlying venous outflow stenosis which precipitates VAT; however, other conditions can contribute including external compression, arterial inflow stenosis, and pseudoaneurysm [74]. As previously discussed, prothrombotic risk factors such as hypercoagulability and low flow due to hypotension may also play a role in VAT. An AV access thrombectomy can consist of a surgical procedure, an endovascular intervention, or a hybrid combination of both techniques. The wide range of AV access configurations and types makes applying the same strategy to all clinical scenarios difficult. Studies comparing various thrombectomy techniques failed to show universal superiority of one over the others [75]. Therefore, the choice of intervention depends on the practitioner and institution, the type of AV access, the most likely cause of thrombosis, and the patient's clinical condition.

Surgical treatment for a clotted autogenous AV fistula requires exposure of the thrombosed vein in a location that does not encroach on the needle cannulation areas. A transverse venotomy is then made to pass an appropriately sized balloon thrombectomy catheter proximally and distally. After clot removal, an intraoperative fistulogram of the venous outflow and arterial inflow usually suggests the underlying cause of thrombosis. Venous outflow lesions can be treated with balloon angioplasty or surgical revision in the form of a patch angioplasty or interposition jump graft to a patent vein in the upper arm. Severe inflow stenosis usually requires proximal relocation of the arterial anastomosis.

Although initial technical success ranges from 50 to 70 %, surgical thrombectomy for autogenous AV fistulas has a short-term primary patency rate of less than 50 % [76]. This limited durability reflects the underlying endothelial damage which predisposes the access to re-thrombosis. Thrombosis damages the venous endothelium, while a balloon thrombectomy traumatically removes the endothelium, exposing the thrombogenic subendothelial surface. The ideal clinical scenario for a surgical thrombectomy may be a radial-cephalic fistula which clots because of severe juxta-anastomotic stenosis. In this case, venous tributaries usually limit the thrombus to a small segment of cephalic vein which can be easily removed without inflicting widespread endothelial injury. Relocating the arterial anastomosis more proximally can restore adequate inflow and salvage the access.

Endovascular therapy for a thrombosed autogenous fistula has the advantage of nontraumatic thrombus removal. Ultrasound guidance usually helps establish percutaneous access to the clotted vein. Thrombolytic infusion and a variety of percutaneous mechanical thrombectomy devices then remove the thrombus without direct endothelial contact. The procedure can remain completely percutaneous by treating the underlying stenosis with balloon angioplasty and/or stent placement. Minimizing trauma to the endothelium should theoretically translate into improved patency. In practice, this technique still results in a low 6-month primary patency of 19–38 % according to case series reports. Repeat interventions have achieved a reasonable secondary patency of 74 and 69 % at 6 and 12 months, respectively [77]. Convincing evidence to support the use of more costly percutaneous thrombectomy devices instead of thrombolysis and balloon angioplasty does not yet exist.

Surgery for a thrombosed AV graft starts with a balloon thrombectomy after exposure and control of the graft. The suspected cause of the thrombosis and anticipated need for revision determine the location of the incision (Fig. 19.9). After clearing the graft of thrombus, an intraoperative fistulogram should interrogate the access from the arterial anastomosis to the central veins. These contrast images can confirm the cause of the thrombosis and uncover other conditions that could lead to re-thrombosis. In the majority of cases, the culprit lesion lays in the venous anastomosis as a result of intimal hyperplasia. Treatment options include balloon angioplasty or surgical revision with either patch angioplasty or a jump graft to a more proximal vein. Although prosthetic AV grafts thrombose more frequently, they have a better response to thrombectomy compared to AV fistulas. Thrombus is easier to clear from prosthetic conduits because they have no endothelial lining to injure, are uniform in caliber, and can be segmentally replaced if necessary.

The endovascular approach to prosthetic VAT usually begins by placing crossed sheaths into the graft, one toward the arterial anastomosis and the other toward the venous outflow. Percutaneous cannulation of a thrombosed graft can present a challenge since a needle puncture does not usually return blood. In these cases, ultrasound guidance can confirm needle cannulation of the graft, thereby avoiding multiple unsuccessful needle sticks which often bleed after restoring blood flow. In the most well-described technique for endovascular thrombectomy, 2–5 mg of tissue plasminogen activator (tPA) is infused into each sheath and allowed to dwell in the clotted graft for 15–30 min. Balloon angioplasty of the entire graft and venous outflow then debulks the thrombus and dilates areas of stenosis. Complete contrast imaging of the entire access extending to the central veins can then detect any areas of residual stenosis which require further treatment. If thrombus remains in the arterial side of the graft, a balloon thrombectomy catheter should be passed and advanced through the arterial anastomosis. Pulling back on the inflated thrombectomy balloon will restore arterial blood flow by dislodging the arterial plug. Percutaneous mechanical thrombectomy devices such as the Angiojet, the Arrow-Trerotola, and the Hydrolyzer offer an alternative or adjunct to tPA infusion and balloon angioplasty. Although these devices have different methods of fragmenting and aspirating thrombus, some degree of thromboembolization always occurs. Residual thrombotic debris from percutaneous thrombectomy maneuvers ultimately gets released into the pulmonary circulation; however, this event rarely causes any clinical sequelae.

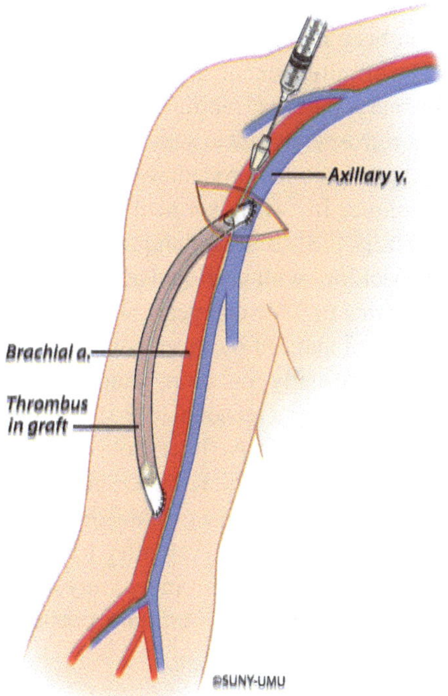

Fig. 19.9 Surgical thrombectomy of an upper arm AV graft. An incision near the venous outflow is used to perform a graft thrombectomy with a Fogarty embolectomy catheter

Prospective studies comparing surgical and endovascular AV graft thrombectomy techniques do not exist. Despite acceptable rates of initial technical success, both approaches have poor primary patency ranging from 30 to 50 % at 6 months. In a retrospective case series, Ito et al. found that endovascular thrombectomy procedures had the same results as hybrid techniques involving surgical thrombectomy with balloon angioplasty [78]. Both techniques proved inferior to surgical thrombectomy with graft revision which achieved a primary patency rate of 23 % at 2 years. The slight advantage of surgery must be balanced by its consumption of "venous capital" which is usually in short supply. Endovascular thrombectomy may offer a reasonable first-line treatment as a repeatable, minimally invasive intervention which does not sacrifice future access sites. The K-DOQI guidelines seemed to support these values when they established a benchmark of 40 % primary patency at 3 months for percutaneous thrombectomy, while surgical thrombectomy was held to a higher standard of 50 and 40 % primary patency at 6 and 12 months, respectively [75].

Pseudoaneurysm

A pseudoaneurysm usually presents as a focal pulsatile mass which forms due to a leaking hole in an artery, vein, or prosthetic graft. The overlying tissues surround and contain a "bubble" of blood flow which enters the pseudoaneurysm cavity and returns to the source vessel with every heart beat. Duplex ultrasound can differentiate a pseudoaneurysm from a true aneurysm or hematoma by demonstrating bidirectional color flow within the mass and a connection to the access vessel or graft, the so-called neck (Fig. 19.10). Although they can develop in autogenous fistulas, pseudoaneurysms occur more frequently in prosthetic grafts with an estimated prevalence of 2–10 % [79]. Pseudoaneurysms that form along the course of the access graft typically represent puncture site injuries, while anastomotic pseudoaneurysms can reflect an underlying infection. A pseudoaneurysm poses a thrombotic, infectious, and hemorrhagic risk, and appropriate treatment depends on its etiology and location as well as the type of access and clinical circumstances.

Prosthetic graft degeneration from repeated needle punctures combined with venous back pressure due to outflow stenosis can lead to a cannulation site pseudoaneurysm. Expansion of the pseudoaneurysm causes necrosis of the overlying subcutaneous tissue and skin which generates multiple problems including difficulty achieving hemostasis upon needle withdrawal, spontaneous bleeding from cannulation sites, severe hemorrhage, and acute graft rupture. The extent of the pseudoaneurysm and the condition of the overlying skin influence treatment decisions. Small puncture site pseudoaneurysms with viable overlying skin often resolve with access rest and observation. Enlarging pseudoaneurysms and those with compromised overlying skin warrant surgery to resect the pseudoaneurysm and create an interposition graft around the site. In most cases, dialysis can continue through the uninvolved graft while the new segment incorporates. More extensive pseudoaneurysms may represent complete destruction of the anterior wall of the graft. Surgical replacement in these cases will not allow continued dialysis through the graft unless it is performed in stages.

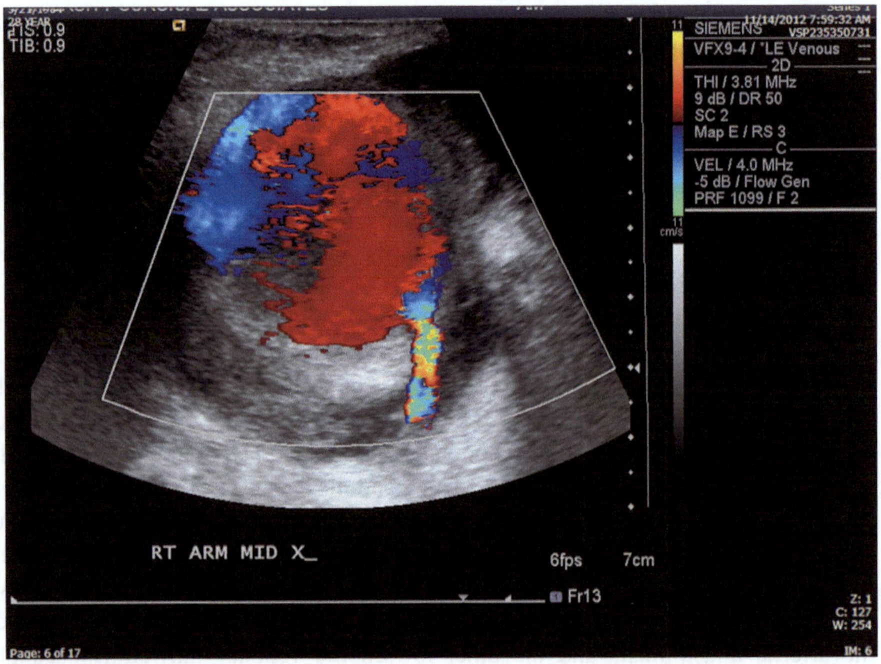

Fig. 19.10 Duplex ultrasound of an AV graft with a large pseudoaneurysm demonstrating characteristic bidirectional flow (*red* and *blue* color)

Since its initial description in 1998, stent graft placement for AV graft pseudoaneurysms has offered an alternative to open surgery [80]. An endovascular approach has the appeal of being able to percutaneously exclude the pseudoaneurysm and address potential venous outflow stenosis without interrupting dialysis or placing a temporary catheter. Several small series reported 100 % procedural success for stent graft placement and excellent 30-day patency which declined to 20–28 % patency at 6 months [81, 82]. Unresolved questions regarding the durability of stent grafts have tempered some of the early enthusiasm for this off-label technique. Stent grafts were not designed to be punctured by dialysis needles, and several reports document stent damage and strut fracture from repeated cannulation [15]. In most cases, safety and durability concerns about stent grafts outweigh their advantages, and endovascular therapy for AV graft pseudoaneurysms remains an inferior alternative to surgical revision.

In autogenous fistulas, distinguishing a pseudoaneurysm from a true venous aneurysm may require a duplex ultrasound exam. Pseudoaneurysms typically occur along cannulation areas due to repeated needle sticks in the same location, so-called one-site-itis. Abandoning the area and adhering to a rotating site or "rope ladder" cannulation strategy usually resolves the problem. The presence of a scab or extremely thin skin overlying the pseudoaneurysm warrants prompt intervention. Hemostasis may be tenuous in this scenario, and the patient is at risk for potentially fatal hemorrhage until the pseudoaneurysm is resected and the fistula can be surgically revised.

Diffuse enlargement of a long-standing autogenous fistula usually reflects a true aneurysm involving all layers of the access wall. If the overlying skin is intact and the aneurysm is free of layered thrombus, it will support continued dialysis and does not require intervention. Surgical intervention may be necessary if the aneurysm compromises the overlying skin or causes obstructive problems from kinking. In many cases resecting the tortuous, aneurismal area and creating a more proximal anastomosis can salvage the fistula. Diameter reduction procedures using a variety of techniques have also achieved technical success with good long-term durability [83, 84].

Infection

Vascular access infection emerged as an important complication with the rise of prosthetic AV grafts in the 1970s. Infection currently ranks second only to thrombosis as the leading cause of access loss, and some studies report that the AV graft infection rate exceeds 30 % [85]. In a survey of dialysis centers, access-related infection occurred in 3.2 % of patients per month which contributes to the 31 % annual incidence of infection related hospitalization among dialysis patients [86]. Although mortality directly attributed to access infection defies accurate reporting, infection in general represents the second most common cause of death in patients with chronic kidney disease [87]. Potentially fatal consequences of vascular access infection include hemorrhage, sepsis, and endocarditis. Prompt diagnosis and aggressive treatment minimizes the clinical impact of infection while preserving the vascular access in selected cases.

Several factors conspire to make dialysis patients more susceptible to infection and more likely to present with an advanced stage of access infection. Uremia causes immunologic dysfunction which interferes with lymphocyte-mediated cellular immunity, slows neutrophil chemotaxis, and impairs phagocytosis and bacterial killing [88]. Common comorbidities among dialysis patients including malnutrition, iron overload, increased intracellular calcium, and diabetes also suppress immune function and increase the risk of infection. Every dialysis session adds to the threat of infection by introducing skin bacteria through the needle puncture sites which explains why most infections begin at the cutaneous access sites of AV grafts. The microbiology of vascular access infections reflects the inherent risk of frequent skin punctures with *Staphylococcus aureus* causing 50–70 % of access infections followed by coagulase negative *Staphylococcus*, *Streptococcus*, and polymicrobial infections with multiple gram-negative bacteria [89].

The signs and symptoms of access infection vary with the severity of infection and the patient's clinical status. Explicit evidence of infection such as a purulent drainage, a sinus tract, and exposed conduit reliably identifies an infected access and rarely cause diagnostic uncertainty. Localized tenderness, erythema, and induration can represent subtle signs of infection; however, these findings also occur in the setting of recent surgery or a cannulation site hematoma. Immunocompromised and elderly patients also present a diagnostic challenge since they cannot mount a localized inflammatory response and may present instead with systemic symptoms related to hypotension, lethargy, and hypoglycemia. If the diagnosis is uncertain, serial exams and duplex ultrasonography can help differentiate an infected access from a hematoma or postsurgical fluid collection. Progressive erythema and induration on serial exams combined with increasing perigraft fluid visualized with ultrasound suggest a vascular access infection. ^{111}Indium-tagged imaging offers a sensitive but nonspecific test whose accuracy is limited by false-positive results due to inflammation from the needle puncture or hematoma.

Treatment for a vascular access infection can range from complete access removal to simple observation. Access type, patency, extent of infection, microbiology, and presenting symptoms guide clinical decision-making and determine the most appropriate intervention. Native AV fistulas rarely become infected, and therefore there is a limited amount of accumulated evidence comparing various treatment options.

Infection confined to the cannulation site of an AV fistula often resolves by stopping needle punctures at the site and resting the arm. More extensive infections require segmental ligation and resection. In some cases, the fistula can be salvaged by relocating the arterial anastomosis to a more proximal site or by replacing the infected segment with an interposition autogenous bypass tunneled through clean tissue planes. Infections associated with bleeding or encroaching on the arterial anastomosis mandate ligation of the AV fistula. Regardless of the planned intervention, all AV fistula infections require broad-spectrum antibiotic coverage (such as vancomycin and an aminoglycoside) for at least 6 weeks [90]. The results of blood and tissue cultures can often narrow the antibiotic coverage.

The rate of prosthetic AV graft infection exceeds that of native fistulas by more than tenfold with an annual incidence ranging from 3 to 19 % [79, 91]. Complete graft removal provides the safest and most effective treatment for an AV graft infection and should be performed for the following indications: systemic sepsis, graft occlusion, *Pseudomonas* or other aggressive bacterial infection, fluid or purulence surrounding the entire graft, recurrent septic pulmonary emboli, and an unincorporated or recently placed graft (less than 30 days old). Surgery to remove an AV graft usually begins by controlling the native vein and artery followed by complete removal of the prosthetic graft and aggressive debridement of the surrounding tissue. While the venous outflow can be occluded and oversewn, preserving arterial perfusion requires an interposition autogenous bypass to replace the infected artery. Failure to adequately debride the infected tissue and vessels leads to recurrent bleeding in 20 % of patients with positive blood cultures [92]. If the severity of the infection and tissue sclerosis precludes safe construction of a bypass, proximal ligation of the native artery may be the only way to achieve hemostasis. Collateral flow provides adequate perfusion, and revascularizaton is usually not necessary after ligating the radial artery or the brachial artery distal to the profunda brachial artery [93].

Oversewing a cuff of graft left on the arterial anastomosis is a reasonable surgical decision provided that the segment of graft remains completely incorporated and uninvolved with the infection (Fig. 19.11). This subtotal graft excision (SGE) technique avoids a potentially difficult dissection and reduces the risk of arterial or nerve injury [94]. Reports of successful SGE emphasize selecting patients with limited infections and confirming complete perianastomotic graft incorporation at the time of surgery. A postoperative regimen involving frequent debridements and twice-daily dressing changes may also decrease the chance of recurrent infection. Although Ryan et al. documented successful SGE in 15 of 15 patients, Schild et al. reported a more sobering outlook as infected prosthetic cuffs accounted for 17 % of their series of vascular access infections [95]. Widespread acceptance of the SGE technique awaits the accumulation of more convincing evidence.

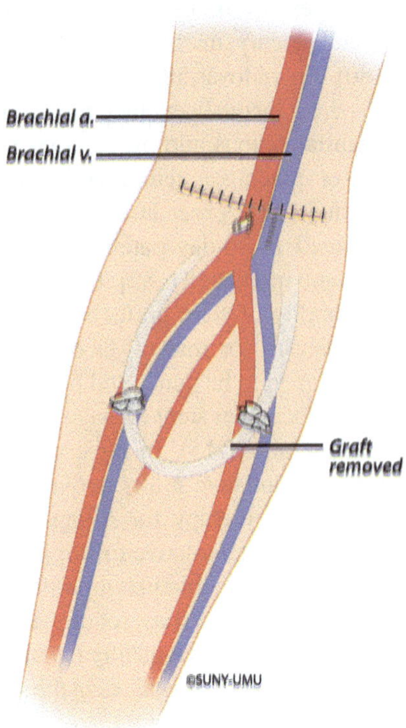

Fig. 19.11 Removal of AV graft with small cuff of graft left in place on arterial anastomosis

Solving the problem of infection with a total or SGE creates a new challenge: lack of hemodialysis access. Immediately following graft removal, patients must endure the limitations and inconvenience of a temporary dialysis catheter. Prospects for a new long-term access are often bleak as patients lack an alternative access site. Avoiding this scenario of access site exhaustion and catheter dependence sparked interest in partial graft excision (PGE) for patients with localized infections. This technique preserves graft patency by replacing the infected segment with an interposition bypass tunneled through clean tissue planes. Surgery for PGE starts by isolating the infected area with adhesive dressings before surgically exposing the incorporated prosthetic graft proximal and distal to the infection. Graft continuity is restored by tunneling an interposition graft well around the infected area and anastomosing it to the proximal and distal uninfected portions of the AV graft (Fig. 19.12). The sterile ends of the infected graft segment can be ligated toward the area of infection to facilitate closure of the tunnel with a purse-string subcutaneous suture. After covering the bypass incisions with occlusive dressings, the infected portion of the graft is then excised through a separate incision. Dialysis can continue through the uninvolved segments of the graft until the interposition bypass heals, and the whole graft can again be accessed.

PGE has the highest chance of success in patients with a localized graft infection who have an ample length of uninvolved graft with no surrounding fluid as confirmed by a preoperative ultrasound. Although the absence of fluid does

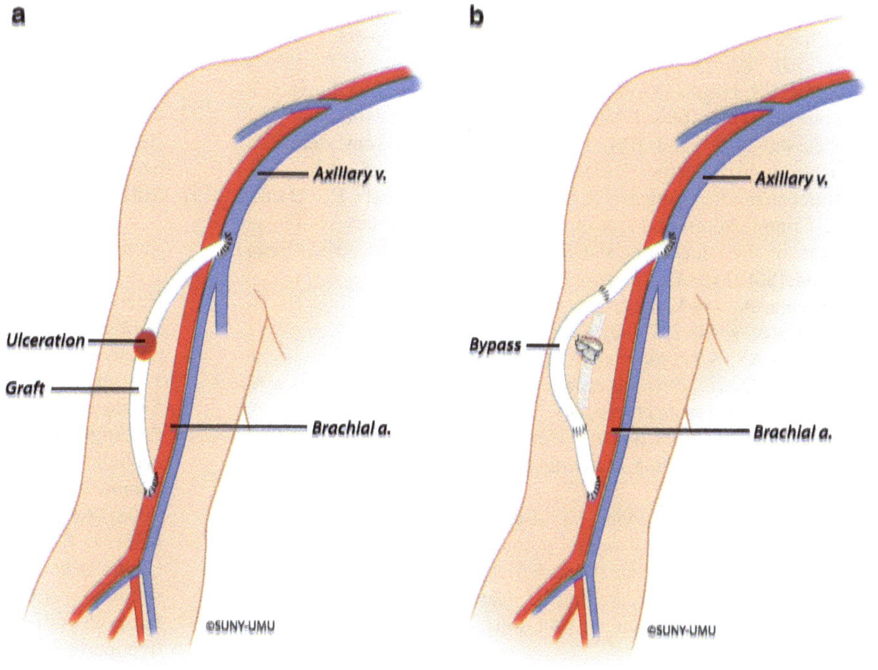

Fig. 19.12 (**a**) Ulcer overlying the upper arm AV graft. (**b**) Partial graft excision. The infected graft segment is removed, and an interposition graft is tunneled around the area and anastomosed to the uninfected portions of the AV graft

not rule out infection, its presence almost always signifies a more extensive infection and should act as a contraindication to PGE. Several authors reported PGE success rates ranging from 74 to 100 % in selected patients [96–98]. Predictors of success and failure for PGE remain unclear because of the relatively small number of patients studied. Although failure of PGE requires total graft excision, it rarely results in a life-threatening complication. In the series reported by Ryan et al., none of the patients who failed PGE presented with hemorrhage or sepsis [95].

Regardless of their patency or function, old prosthetic grafts retain their susceptibility to infection. Abandoned, nonfunctional grafts should be suspected in patients presenting with unexplained systemic infection or resistance to epoetin therapy. An ^{111}Indium-tagged white blood cell or gallium scan usually localizes the abandoned access graft as the site of inflammation. Complete removal of the infected graft provides definitive treatment and should restore the responsiveness to epoetin [75].

Conclusion

The development of reliable vascular access more than 50 years ago transformed end-stage renal disease from a death sentence to a chronic and manageable condition. Nearly half a million patients in the USA now rely on vascular access to receive life-sustaining hemodialysis treatments. For these patients, vascular access complications rival kidney failure itself as a persistent source of morbidity, mortality, and lost quality of life. The clinical impact of vascular access complications ranges from mild symptoms and inconvenience to critical illness, limb loss, and death in severe cases. Insights into the pathophysiology, diagnosis, and treatment of the most common vascular access complications outlined in this chapter will help the vascular access surgeon preserve the quality and extend the length of life for patients receiving hemodialysis.

References

1. U.S. Renal Data System, USRDS 2010 annual data report: atlas of chronic kidney disease and end-stage renal disease in the United States. Bethesda: National Institutes of Health; National Institute of Diabetes and Digestive and Kidney Diseases; 2010.
2. Trainor D, Borthwick E, Ferguson A. Perioperative management of the hemodialysis patient. Semin Dial. 2011;24(3):314–26.
3. Galbusera M, Remuzzi G, Boccardo P. Treatment of bleeding in dialysis patients. Semin Dial. 2009;22(3):279–86.
4. Gawaz MP, Dobos G, Spath M, Schollmeyer P, Gurland HJ, Mujais SK. Impaired function of platelet membrane glycoprotein IIb-IIIa in end-stage renal disease. J Am Soc Nephrol. 1994;5(1):36–46.
5. Canavese C, Salomone M, Pacitti A, Mangiarotti G, Calitri V. Reduced response of uraemic bleeding time to repeated doses of desmopressin. Lancet. 1985;1(8433):867–8.
6. Mannucci PM. Desmopressin (DDAVP) in the treatment of bleeding disorders: the first 20 years. Blood. 1997;90(7):2515–21.
7. Zoja C, Noris M, Corna D, et al. L-arginine, the precursor of nitric oxide, abolishes the effect of estrogens on bleeding time in experimental uremia. Lab Invest. 1991;65(4):479–83.
8. Hedges SJ, Dehoney SB, Hooper JS, Amanzadeh J, Busti AJ. Evidence-based treatment recommendations for uremic bleeding. Nat Clin Pract Nephrol. 2007;3(3):138–53.
9. O'Connell KA, Wood JJ, Wise RP, Lozier JN, Braun MM. Thromboembolic adverse events after use of recombinant human coagulation factor VIIa. JAMA. 2006;295(3):293–8.

10. Ellingson KD, Palekar RS, Lucero CA, et al. Vascular access hemorrhages contribute to deaths among hemodialysis patients. Kidney Int. 2012;82:686–92.
11. Jaffers GJ, Fasola CG. Experience with ulcerated, bleeding autologous dialysis fistulas. J Vasc Access. 2012;13(1):55–60.
12. Agarwal AK, Patel BM, Haddad NJ. Central vein stenosis: a nephrologist's perspective. Semin Dial. 2007;20(1):53–62.
13. Bambauer R, Inniger R, Pirrung KJ, Schiel R, Dahlem R. Complications and side effects associated with large-bore catheters in the subclavian and internal jugular veins. Artif Organs. 1994;18(4):318–21.
14. Vascular Access Work Group. Clinical practice guidelines for vascular access. Am J Kidney Dis. 2006;48 Suppl 1:S248–73.
15. Yevzlin AS, Schoenkerman AB, Gimelli G, Asif A. Arterial interventions in arteriovenous access and chronic kidney disease: a role for interventional nephrologists. Semin Dial. 2009;22(5):545–56.
16. Lacson Jr E, Lazarus JM, Himmelfarb J, Ikizler TA, Hakim RM. Balancing fistula first with catheters last. Am J Kidney Dis. 2007;50(3):379–95.
17. Bosman PJ, Boereboom FT, Eikelboom BC, Koomans HA, Blankestijn PJ. Graft flow as a predictor of thrombosis in hemodialysis grafts. Kidney Int. 1998;54(5):1726–30.
18. Sullivan KL, Besarab A, Bonn J, Shapiro MJ, Gardiner Jr GA, Moritz MJ. Hemodynamics of failing dialysis grafts. Radiology. 1993;186(3):867–72.
19. Lumsden AB, MacDonald MJ, Isiklar H, et al. Central venous stenosis in the hemodialysis patient: incidence and efficacy of endovascular treatment. Cardiovasc Surg. 1997;5(5):504–9.
20. Maskova J, Komarkova J, Kivanek J, Danes J, Slavikova M. Endovascular treatment of central vein stenoses and/or occlusions in hemodialysis patients. Cardiovasc Intervent Radiol. 2003; 26(1):27–30.
21. Gray RJ, Dolmatch BL, Buick MK. Directional atherectomy treatment for hemodialysis access: early results. J Vasc Interv Radiol. 1992;3(3):497–503.
22. Davidson CJ, Newman GE, Sheikh KH, Kisslo K, Stack RS, Schwab SJ. Mechanisms of angioplasty in hemodialysis fistula stenoses evaluated by intravascular ultrasound. Kidney Int. 1991; 40(1):91–5.
23. Siani A, Marcucci G, Accrocca F, et al. Endovascular central venous stenosis treatment ended with superior vena cava perforation, pericardial tamponade, and exitus. Ann Vasc Surg. 2012;26(5): 733 e739–712.
24. Wisselink W, Money SR, Becker MO, et al. Comparison of operative reconstruction and percutaneous balloon dilatation for central venous obstruction. Am J Surg. 1993;166(2):200–4; discussion 204–5.
25. Oderich GS, Treiman GS, Schneider P, Bhirangi K. Stent placement for treatment of central and peripheral venous obstruction: a long-term multi-institutional experience. J Vasc Surg. 2000;32(4): 760–9.
26. Bakken AM, Protack CD, Saad WE, Lee DE, Waldman DL, Davies MG. Long-term outcomes of primary angioplasty and primary stenting of central venous stenosis in hemodialysis patients. J Vasc Surg. 2007;45(4):776–83.
27. Puskas JD, Gertler JP. Internal jugular to axillary vein bypass for subclavian vein thrombosis in the setting of brachial arteriovenous fistula. J Vasc Surg. 1994;19(5):939–42.
28. Doty DB, Baker WH. Bypass of superior vena cava with spiral vein graft. Ann Thorac Surg. 1976;22(5):490–3.
29. El-Sabrout RA, Duncan JM. Right atrial bypass grafting for central venous obstruction associated with dialysis access: another treatment option. J Vasc Surg. 1999;29(3):472–8.
30. Glass C, Dugan M, Gillespie D, Doyle A, Illig K. Costoclavicular venous decompression in patients with threatened arteriovenous hemodialysis access. Ann Vasc Surg. 2011;25(5):640–5.
31. Rajan DK, Clark TW, Patel NK, Stavropoulos SW, Simons ME. Prevalence and treatment of cephalic arch stenosis in dysfunctional autogenous hemodialysis fistulas. J Vasc Interv Radiol. 2003;14(5):567–73.
32. Shawyer A, Fotiadis NI, Namagondlu G, et al. Cephalic arch stenosis in autogenous haemodialysis fistulas: treatment with the viabahn stent-graft. Cardiovasc Intervent Radiol. 2013;36(1):133–9.
33. Miller GA, Friedman A, Khariton A, Preddie DC, Savransky Y. Access flow reduction and recurrent symptomatic cephalic arch stenosis in brachiocephalic hemodialysis arteriovenous fistulas. J Vasc Access. 2010;11(4):281–7.
34. Heerwagen ST, Lonn L, Schroeder TV, Hansen MA. Cephalic arch stenosis in autogenous brachiocephalic hemodialysis fistulas: results of cutting balloon angioplasty. J Vasc Access. 2010; 11(1):41–5.
35. Shemesh D, Goldin I, Zaghal I, Berlowitz D, Raveh D, Olsha O. Angioplasty with stent graft versus bare stent for recurrent cephalic arch stenosis in autogenous arteriovenous access for hemodialysis: a prospective randomized clinical trial. J Vasc Surg. 2008;48(6):1524–31. 1531 e1521–2.
36. Miller GA, Goel N, Friedman A, et al. The MILLER banding procedure is an effective method for treating dialysis-associated steal syndrome. Kidney Int. 2010;77(4):359–66.
37. Leon C, Asif A. Arteriovenous access and hand pain: the distal hypoperfusion ischemic syndrome. Clin J Am Soc Nephrol. 2007;2(1):175–83.
38. Kariya S, Tanigawa N, Kojima H, et al. Transcatheter coil embolization for steal syndrome in patients with hemodialysis access. Acta Radiol. 2009;50(1):28–33.
39. Sidawy AN, Gray R, Besarab A, et al. Recommended standards for reports dealing with arteriovenous hemodialysis accesses. J Vasc Surg. 2002;35(3):603–10.
40. Scheltinga MR, Bruijninckx CM. Haemodialysis access-induced distal ischaemia (HAIDI) is caused by loco-regional hypotension but not by steal. Eur J Vasc Endovasc Surg. 2012;43(2):218–23.
41. Rocha A, Silva F, Queiros J, Malheiro J, Cabrita A. Predictors of steal syndrome in hemodialysis patients. Hemodial Int. 2012;16(4): 539–44.
42. Whittaker L, Bakran A. Prevention better than cure. Avoiding steal syndrome with proximal radial or ulnar arteriovenous fistulae. J Vasc Access. 2011;12(4):318–20.
43. Huber TS, Brown MP, Seeger JM, Lee WA. Midterm outcome after the distal revascularization and interval ligation (DRIL) procedure. J Vasc Surg. 2008;48(4):926–32; discussion 932–3.
44. Scali ST, Huber TS. Treatment strategies for access-related hand ischemia. Semin Vasc Surg. 2011;24(2):128–36.
45. Malik J, Tuka V, Kasalova Z, et al. Understanding the dialysis access steal syndrome. A review of the etiologies, diagnosis, prevention and treatment strategies. J Vasc Access. 2008;9(3):155–66.
46. Papasavas PK, Reifsnyder T, Birdas TJ, Caushaj PF, Leers S. Prediction of arteriovenous access steal syndrome utilizing digital pressure measurements. Vasc Endovascular Surg. 2003;37(3): 179–84.
47. Wixon CL, Hughes JD, Mills JL. Understanding strategies for the treatment of ischemic steal syndrome after hemodialysis access. J Am Coll Surg. 2000;191(3):301–10.
48. Schanzer H, Schwartz M, Harrington E, Haimov M. Treatment of ischemia due to "steal" by arteriovenous fistula with distal artery ligation and revascularization. J Vasc Surg. 1988;7(6):770–3.
49. Illig KA, Surowiec S, Shortell CK, Davies MG, Rhodes JM, Green RM. Hemodynamics of distal revascularization-interval ligation. Ann Vasc Surg. 2005;19(2):199–207.
50. Anaya-Ayala JE, Pettigrew CD, Ismail N, et al. Management of dialysis access-associated "steal" syndrome with DRIL procedure: challenges and clinical outcomes. J Vasc Access. 2012;13(3): 299–304.

51. Scali ST, Chang CK, Raghinaru D, et al. Prediction of graft patency and mortality after distal revascularization and interval ligation for hemodialysis access-related hand ischemia. J Vasc Surg. 2013; 57(2):451–8.
52. Knox RC, Berman SS, Hughes JD, Gentile AT, Mills JL. Distal revascularization-interval ligation: a durable and effective treatment for ischemic steal syndrome after hemodialysis access. J Vasc Surg. 2002;36(2):250–5; discussion 256.
53. Berman SS, Gentile AT, Glickman MH, et al. Distal revascularization-interval ligation for limb salvage and maintenance of dialysis access in ischemic steal syndrome. J Vasc Surg. 1997;26(3):393–402; discussion 402–4.
54. Zanow J, Kruger U, Scholz H. Proximalization of the arterial inflow: a new technique to treat access-related ischemia. J Vasc Surg. 2006;43(6):1216–21; discussion 1221.
55. Thermann F, Wollert U. Proximalization of the arterial inflow: new treatment of choice in patients with advanced dialysis shunt-associated steal syndrome? Ann Vasc Surg. 2009;23(4):485–90.
56. Callaghan CJ, Mallik M, Sivaprakasam R, Iype S, Pettigrew GJ. Treatment of dialysis access-associated steal syndrome with the "revision using distal inflow" technique. J Vasc Access. 2011; 12(1):52–6.
57. Chemla ES, Morsy M, Anderson L, Whitemore A. Inflow reduction by distalization of anastomosis treats efficiently high-inflow high-cardiac output vascular access for hemodialysis. Semin Dial. 2007;20(1):68–72.
58. Wilbourn AJ, Furlan AJ, Hulley W, Ruschhaupt W. Ischemic monomelic neuropathy. Neurology. 1983;33(4):447–51.
59. Ballard JL, Bunt TJ, Malone JM. Management of small artery vascular trauma. Am J Surg. 1992;164(4):316–9.
60. Thermann F, Kornhuber M. Ischemic monomelic neuropathy: a rare but important complication after hemodialysis access placement–a review. J Vasc Access. 2011;12(2):113–9.
61. Miles AM. Vascular steal syndrome and ischaemic monomelic neuropathy: two variants of upper limb ischaemia after haemodialysis vascular access surgery. Nephrol Dial Transplant. 1999;14(2): 297–300.
62. Kirksey L. Ischemic monomelic neuropathy: an underappreciated cause of pain and disability following vascular access surgery. J Vasc Access. 2010;11(2):165–8.
63. Hye RJ, Wolf YG. Ischemic monomelic neuropathy: an under-recognized complication of hemodialysis access. Ann Vasc Surg. 1994;8(6):578–82.
64. Dossabhoy NR, Ram SJ, Nassar R, Work J, Eason JM, Paulson WD. Stenosis surveillance of hemodialysis grafts by duplex ultrasound reduces hospitalizations and cost of care. Semin Dial. 2005; 18(6):550–7.
65. Stolic R. Most important chronic complications of arteriovenous fistulas for hemodialysis. Med Princ Pract. 2013;22:220–8.
66. Knoll GA, Wells PS, Young D, et al. Thrombophilia and the risk for hemodialysis vascular access thrombosis. J Am Soc Nephrol. 2005;16(4):1108–14.
67. Atac B, Yakupoglu U, Ozbek N, Ozdemir FN, Bilgin N. Role of genetic mutations in vascular access thrombosis among hemodialysis patients waiting for renal transplantation. Transplant Proc. 2002;34(6):2030–2.
68. Fekih-Mrissa N, Klai S, Bafoun A, Nciri B, Hmida J, Gritli N. Role of thrombophilia in vascular access thrombosis among chronic hemodialysis patients in Tunisia. Ther Apher Dial. 2011;15(1): 40–3.
69. Chou CY, Chen JY, Liu JH, et al. Atrial fibrillation linked to vascular access thrombosis in chronic hemodialysis patients. J Atheroscler Thromb. 2011;18(6):448–53.
70. Windus DW, Jendrisak MD, Delmez JA. Prosthetic fistula survival and complications in hemodialysis patients: effects of diabetes and age. Am J Kidney Dis. 1992;19(5):448–52.
71. Palmer SC, Navaneethan SD, Craig JC, et al. Meta-analysis: erythropoiesis-stimulating agents in patients with chronic kidney disease. Ann Intern Med. 2010;153(1):23–33.
72. Montagnana M, Meschi T, Borghi L, Lippi G. Thrombosis and occlusion of vascular access in hemodialyzed patients. Semin Thromb Hemost. 2011;37(8):946–54.
73. Reinhold C, Haage P, Hollenbeck M, Mickley V, Ranft J. Multidisciplinary management of vascular access for haemodialysis: from the preparation of the initial access to the treatment of stenosis and thrombosis. Vasa. 2011;40(3):188–98.
74. Kanterman RY, Vesely TM, Pilgram TK, Guy BW, Windus DW, Picus D. Dialysis access grafts: anatomic location of venous stenosis and results of angioplasty. Radiology. 1995;195(7892454):135–9.
75. Levin AR. NKF-K/DOQI clinical practice guidelines for vascular access: update 2006. Am J Kidney Dis. 2006;48(suppl):S176–247.
76. Palmer RM, Cull DL, Kalbaugh C, et al. Is surgical thrombectomy to salvage failed autogenous arteriovenous fistulae worthwhile? Am Surg. 2006;72(12):1231–3.
77. Shatsky JB, Berns JS, Clark TW, et al. Single-center experience with the Arrow-Trerotola Percutaneous Thrombectomy Device in the management of thrombosed native dialysis fistulas. J Vasc Interv Radiol. 2005;16(12):1605–11.
78. Ito Y, Sato T, Okada R, et al. Comparison of clinical effectiveness between surgical and endovascular treatment for thrombotic obstruction in hemodialysis access. J Vasc Access. 2011;12(1):63–6.
79. Zibari GB, Rohr MS, Landreneau MD, et al. Complications from permanent hemodialysis vascular access. Surgery. 1988;104(4):681–6.
80. Hausegger KA, Tiessenhausen K, Klimpfinger M, Raith J, Hauser H, Tauss J. Aneurysms of hemodialysis access grafts: treatment with covered stents: a report of three cases. Cardiovasc Intervent Radiol. 1998;21(4):334–7.
81. Barshes NR, Annambhotla S, Bechara C, et al. Endovascular repair of hemodialysis graft-related pseudoaneurysm: an alternative treatment strategy in salvaging failing dialysis access. Vasc Endovascular Surg. 2008;42(3):228–34.
82. Vesely TM. Use of stent grafts to repair hemodialysis graft-related pseudoaneurysms. J Vasc Interv Radiol. 2005;16(10):1301–7.
83. Pierce GE, Thomas JH, Fenton JR. Novel repair of venous aneurysms secondary to arteriovenous dialysis fistulae. Vasc Endovascular Surg. 2007;41(1):55–60.
84. Woo K, Cook PR, Garg J, Hye RJ, Canty TG. Midterm results of a novel technique to salvage autogenous dialysis access in aneurysmal arteriovenous fistulas. J Vasc Surg. 2010;51(4):921–5. 925 e921.
85. Chavers BM, Solid CA, Gilbertson DT, Collins AJ. Infection-related hospitalization rates in pediatric versus adult patients with end-stage renal disease in the United States. J Am Soc Nephrol. 2007;18(3):952–9.
86. Centers for Disease Control and Prevention. Invasive methicillin-resistant Staphylococcus aureus infections among dialysis patientnited States, 2005. MMWR Morb Mortal Wkly Rep. 2007; 56(9):197–9.
87. Collins AJ, Foley RN, Chavers B, et al. 'United States renal data system 2011 annual data report: atlas of chronic kidney disease & end-stage renal disease in the United States. Am J Kidney Dis. 2012;59(1 Suppl 1):A7. e1–420.
88. Anding K, Gross P, Rost JM, Allgaier D, Jacobs E. The influence of uraemia and haemodialysis on neutrophil phagocytosis and antimicrobial killing. Nephrol Dial Transplant. 2003;18(10):2067–73.
89. Tokars JI, Miller ER, Stein G. New national surveillance system for hemodialysis-associated infections: initial results. Am J Infect Control. 2002;30(5):288–95.
90. Gray RJ, Sands JJ, editors. Dialysis access: a multidisciplinary approach. Philadelphia: Lippincott Williams & Wilkins; 2002. Stevenson KB, editors. Management of hemodialysis vascular access infection

91. Churchill DN, Taylor DW, Cook RJ, et al. Canadian Hemodialysis Morbidity Study. Am J Kidney Dis. 1992;19(3):214–34.
92. Bachleda P, Utikal P, Kalinova L, et al. Infectious complications of arteriovenous ePTFE grafts for hemodialysis. Biomed Pap Med Fac Univ Palacky Olomouc Czech Repub. 2010;154(1):13–9.
93. Schanzer A, Ciaranello AL, Schanzer H. Brachial artery ligation with total graft excision is a safe and effective approach to prosthetic arteriovenous graft infections. J Vasc Surg. 2008;48(3):655–8.
94. Calligaro KD, Veith FJ, Valladares JA, McKay J, Schindler N, Dougherty MJ. Prosthetic patch remnants to treat infected arterial grafts. J Vasc Surg. 2000;31(2):245–52.
95. Ryan SV, Calligaro KD, Scharff J, Dougherty MJ. Management of infected prosthetic dialysis arteriovenous grafts. J Vasc Surg. 2004;39(1):73–8.
96. Palder SB, Kirkman RL, Whittemore AD, Hakim RM, Lazarus JM, Tilney NL. Vascular access for hemodialysis. Patency rates and results of revision. Ann Surg. 1985;202(2):235–9.
97. Taylor B, Sigley RD, May KJ. Fate of infected and eroded hemodialysis grafts and autogenous fistulas. Am J Surg. 1993;165(5):632–6.
98. Raju S. PTFE grafts for hemodialysis access. Techniques for insertion and management of complications. Ann Surg. 1987;206(5):666–73.

Part VII

Complex Vascular Surgery Topics

Arterial Occlusive Disease: Carotid, Mesenteric, and Renal

20

Carlos H. Timaran

Introduction

Atherosclerosis is a systemic disorder that can affect any artery. Atherosclerosis of the carotid, mesenteric, and renal arteries can have debilitating and potentially fatal consequences including stroke, bowel ischemia, hypertension, and renal failure. The prevalence of cardiovascular risk factors ensures that general surgeons will regularly encounter patients with atherosclerotic disease affecting the carotid, mesenteric, and renal arteries. Familiarity with these conditions can help general surgeons to diagnose and manage affected patients and direct them to more specialized care when appropriate. This chapter provides an overview of the clinical presentation, diagnosis, and treatment for carotid, mesenteric, and renal artery disease.

Carotid Artery Stenosis

Despite advances in the medical management of atherosclerosis, stroke continues to be the main cause of disability in most developed countries and the fourth leading cause of death in the United States [1, 2]. Approximately 85 % of all strokes are ischemic, of which 10–30 % may be attributed to extracranial carotid lesions. Carotid artery stenosis is, therefore, one of the main preventable causes of stroke [1]. Several randomized clinical trials have convincingly shown that carotid endarterectomy is a safe and effective procedure for stroke prevention in patients with carotid stenosis [3–6]. Carotid artery stenting (CAS) has also effectively treated patients with carotid stenosis; however, it was initially restricted to high-surgical-risk patients, particularly those with severe comorbidities or a hostile neck from previous surgical procedures or radiation [1]. Recent randomized clinical trials have questioned the restrictions placed on CAS and suggest that CAS may also be feasible in standard risk patients [7, 8].

C.H. Timaran, MD (✉)
Division of Vascular and Endovascular Surgery, Department of Surgery, University of Texas Southwestern Medical Center, 5909 Harry Hines Blvd., Dallas, TX 75390-9157, USA
e-mail: carlos.timaran@utsouthwestern.edu

Clinical Presentation and Symptomatic Status

The presence or absence of symptoms in patients with carotid stenosis is the most important determinant of stroke risk and factors into all treatment decisions. Patients should be considered symptomatic when a clear history of stroke, amaurosis fugax, or transient ischemic attacks (TIA) has occurred within 180 days of the evaluation [9]. Although the 180-day cutoff is controversial, it is based on the timeline defining symptomatic status used in most recent clinical trials dealing with carotid artery disease [7, 10–12]. A TIA represents a focal neurologic deficit that completely resolves or returns to baseline within 24 h [1]. The 24 h limit is an arbitrary definition as most TIAs last only a few minutes. TIAs occur in the hemisphere ipsilateral to the carotid stenosis and therefore manifest as a contralateral motor or sensory deficit. Since TIAs completely resolve, there should be no evidence of cerebral infarction on cerebral imaging studies. Amaurosis fugax occurs secondary to embolism to the ophthalmic artery and manifests as temporary monocular blindness that is ipsilateral to the carotid stenosis. Stroke is defined as any neurologic event lasting greater than 24 h associated with cerebral infarction in the hemisphere supplied by the target vessel [9]. Strokes can be further classified as minor or major. A minor stroke is a new neurological event that persists for more than 24 h but completely resolves or returns to baseline within 30 days, whereas a major stroke is a new neurological event that persists after 30 days. Stroke has also been defined as any neurologic event associated with clear evidence of cerebral infarction on brain imaging with computed tomography (CT) scan or magnetic resonance imaging (MRI). Patients with carotid stenosis that do not meet the definition for symptomatic carotid stenosis are considered asymptomatic.

V. Gahtan and M.J. Costanza (eds.), *Essentials of Vascular Surgery for the General Surgeon*, DOI 10.1007/978-1-4939-1326-8_20, © Springer Science+Business Media New York 2015

This includes those patients with no neurologic symptoms and those with a remote history of neurologic events which have not recurred within the last 180 days. Patients with prior symptoms referable only to the hemisphere contralateral to the target vessel or symptoms in either hemisphere more than 180 days prior to the evaluation should also be considered asymptomatic. Moreover, patients that manifest atypical or non-focal neurologic symptoms (i.e., dizziness, confusion, etc.) or vertebrobasilar symptoms should be considered asymptomatic with respect to carotid artery disease.

Diagnosis

Duplex ultrasound (US) is the preferred imaging modality for the diagnosis of carotid stenosis [1, 13]. The technical details and limitations of the carotid duplex ultrasound exam are discussed in Chap. 2. It is worth reiterating that a duplex ultrasound exam uses blood flow velocity as an indirect measure of carotid artery stenosis. Velocity criteria and categories of stenosis must be established by each vascular laboratory and periodically verified with confirmatory imaging studies. Duplex ultrasound has the advantage of being a noninvasive, convenient, and inexpensive test that does not require exposure to radiation or potentially nephrotoxic contrast agents. These advantages must be balanced against the fact that the quality of a carotid duplex exam depends on the skill of the operator and visualization may be limited in severely diseased or calcified vessels. Moreover, carotid stents often artificially elevate blood flow velocities requiring adjusted velocity thresholds as determined by each individual vascular laboratory [14].

Digital subtraction angiography (DSA) has traditionally been the gold standard to precisely determine the degree of carotid stenosis [1]. The basic concepts of DSA are discussed in Chap. 2. Carotid DSA usually begins with an aortic arch arteriogram followed by catheterization of the aortic arch branches and common carotid arteries. Selective contrast injection into the common carotid artery using two or more imaging projections gives the most complete evaluation of the cervical carotid arteries (common, internal, and external) and the cerebral vasculature. Various techniques have been described for quantifying the degree of internal carotid artery stenosis. In the widely used NASCET method, the parallel tract of the internal carotid artery is used for the reference vessel diameter ("A" in Fig. 20.1), and the minimal lumen diameter ("B" in Fig. 20.1) within the carotid artery is identified for the calculation of the percentage of diameter stenosis [% diameter stenosis = $(1-[B/A])\times 100$] [12, 13]. If near occlusion or a "string sign" is present, the NASCET method should be avoided as the degree of stenosis may be underestimated because of distal underfilling and near collapse of the internal carotid artery.

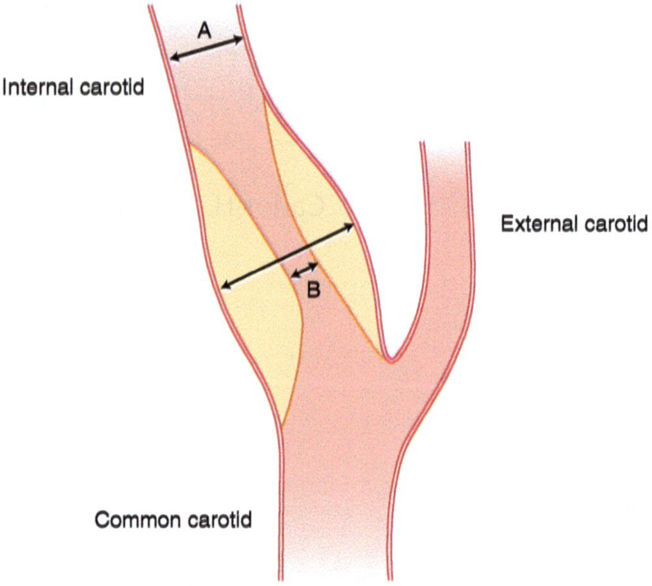

Fig. 20.1 The NASCET method of measuring internal carotid stenosis. The internal carotid artery distal to the stenosis is used as the reference vessel diameter (*A*). The minimal lumen diameter is measured in the proximal internal carotid artery (*B*). The percent stenosis is calculated as % diameter stenosis = $(1-[B/A])\times 100$

As an invasive exam, carotid DSA carries the risk of complications. Catheterization of the aortic arch, aortic branches, and common carotid arteries can dislodge atherosclerotic plaque or generate thromboemboli resulting in a stroke. Other risks common to all forms of angiography include bleeding, pseudoaneurysm, dissection, and contrast reaction. Although the potential risks of carotid DSA have discouraged its use as a purely diagnostic exam, it still plays a role in the management of patients with carotid stenosis. Treatment decisions for carotid disease are now usually based on the results of duplex ultrasonography, CT angiography (CTA), or magnetic resonance angiography. Ensuring the accuracy and reliability of these noninvasive exams requires regular audits to validate and correlate their findings with DSA images. Beyond quality assurance, carotid DSA is also essential for planning and performing carotid artery stenting. Angiographic findings, including aortic arch morphology, vessel tortuosity, plaque ulceration, and angulation, kinking, or coils within the inflow, bifurcation, or outflow vessels of the carotid system have implications for both endovascular and surgical intervention. Cerebral angiography which is usually performed in conjunction with carotid DSA provides information regarding the status of the intracranial circulation.

CTA and MRA provide detailed imaging of the carotid and cerebral circulations and have been increasingly used prior to carotid interventions. The NASCET methodology for determining carotid stenosis (percentage by diameter) should be applied for both CTA and MRA. As previously discussed, validating these imaging modalities requires correlation with the gold standard, i.e., diagnostic angiography including intra- and interobserver variability [15, 16]. Anatomic assessment of the aortic arch, carotid tortuosity and morphology, status of the intracranial circulation, and morphologic characterization of the carotid lesions using CTA and MRA is useful for planning carotid interventions, particularly carotid stenting [15, 16].

Treatment

All patients with carotid stenosis, irrespective of degree of stenosis, symptomatic status, or surgical risk should receive best medical therapy for atherosclerotic disease including risk factor reduction, antiplatelet therapy, and lifestyle modification [1]. The goals of medical treatment should be optimization of both primary risk factors, namely, high systolic blood pressure and elevated low-density lipoprotein (LDL) cholesterol, and secondary risk factors, including diabetes, high non-high-density lipoprotein (non-HDL) cholesterol, smoking, excess weight, and insufficient exercise. Systolic blood pressure should be ideally maintained below 140 mmHg (<130 mmHg in the case of patients with diabetes) and LDL cholesterol levels below 70 mg/dL.

Intervening for carotid stenosis now involves choosing between surgical repair in the form of a carotid endarterectomy (CEA) or endovascular therapy involving carotid angioplasty/stent (CAS). In the past, CEA was considered the treatment of choice for appropriately selected patients with low to moderate surgical risk while CAS was reserved for patients at high surgical risk due to either medical comorbidites or hostile anatomy. Recent evidence suggests that CAS is a feasible form of treatment for patients with carotid stenosis regardless of risk status. Although CEA remains one of the most well studied and widely performed vascular procedures, practice patterns may begin to shift toward endovascular therapy with more patients eligible to receive CAS.

Treatment indications for performing a carotid endarterectomy (CEA) or carotid angioplasty/stent (CAS) vary according to the severity of stenosis and surgical risk. For moderate- and low-risk patients, CAS has the same indications as CEA for both symptomatic and asymptomatic patients. These indications are based on the CREST trial [7] and include:

- Symptomatic carotid stenosis ≥50 % by angiography, ≥70 % by duplex ultrasound, or ≥70 % by computed tomographic angiography (CTA) or magnetic resonance angiography (MRA) if the stenosis on ultrasonography was 50–69 %.
- Asymptomatic carotid stenosis ≥60 % by angiography, ≥70 % by ultrasound, or ≥80 % by CTA or MRA if the stenosis on ultrasonography was 50–69 %.

In practice, the decision to intervene for asymptomatic carotid stenosis is not always as straightforward as these guidelines imply. Medical therapy may be the most appropriate treatment in patients older than 75 or 80 who have stable, asymptomatic carotid stenosis. At the other end of the spectrum, younger patients with more rapidly progressive internal carotid stenosis or an ulcerated plaque usually benefit from an intervention.

High-risk, symptomatic patients have the same treatment indications as conventional risk patients (previously cited), whereas asymptomatic, high-risk patients require greater than 80 % stenosis based on angiography to be considered for treatment with CAS. The higher degree of stenosis required for asymptomatic high-risk patients is solely based on the arbitrary inclusion criteria of the clinical trials and observational studies that the FDA used for the approval of CAS devices in the United States [1, 9, 17]. Most of these studies assumed that CAS was only justified in high-risk patients with severe stenosis even though this has never been assessed or proven by any solid evidence or device trials. The criteria of greater than 80 % stenosis for asymptomatic patients to be considered for CAS will continue because it has been incorporated into the regulatory policies that still dictate reimbursement for CAS.

For patients with carotid stenosis who pose a high risk for surgery, CAS offers an interventional alternative that avoids the morbidity and mortality associated with CEA. High-surgical-risk status can be classified as relating to anatomic factors or medical comorbidities [9]. Anatomic high-risk criteria include restenosis after previous CEA or in-stent restenosis; high or low lesions defined as those superior to the second cervical vertebra or inferior to the clavicle; previous cranial nerve injury (ipsilateral or contralateral); "hostile neck" because of previous radical neck dissection, radiation, presence of a permanent tracheostomy, or a frozen neck; and other associated carotid lesions such as tandem lesions within the same carotid artery or stenosis or occlusion of the contralateral internal carotid artery (ICA). Medical high-risk criteria include class III or IV angina or congestive heart failure, coronary artery disease necessitating revascularization within 4 weeks, and severe chronic obstructive pulmonary disease defined as a forced expiratory volume ≤30 % of predicted or <1 L or the need for home oxygen.

Based on the results of the Carotid Revascularization Endarterectomy versus Stenting Trial (CREST), the FDA recently approved carotid stenting devices for conventional surgical risk patients with carotid stenosis [7, 18]. Although any patient with severe carotid stenosis can now be treated with CAS, reimbursement constraints limit the wide application of CAS. The debate continues as to whether CAS should be considered as a treatment alternative on equal footing with CEA for all patients with carotid stenosis. Recent improvement and refinement in best medical therapies for atherosclerotic diseases have also questioned the benefit of carotid interventions, particularly among asymptomatic high-risk patients. Future clinical trials will help define which patient populations benefit the most from each form of carotid intervention and/or medical therapy. Clinicians will make the most appropriate treatment decisions if they can classify patients with carotid stenosis into one of three categories: patients at high risk for CEA who would benefit from CAS, patients at high risk for CAS that should be treated with CEA, or patients for whom best medical therapy alone may be sufficient.

Mesenteric Ischemia

Mesenteric ischemia results from atherosclerotic stenosis or embolic occlusion of the celiac, superior mesenteric, or inferior mesenteric arteries. Acute mesenteric ischemia (AMI) can result from abrupt embolic occlusion of the superior mesenteric artery (SMA), while chronic mesenteric ischemia usually requires stenosis or occlusion of two of the three arteries supplying the gastrointestinal tract. Mesenteric venous thrombosis and nonocclusive vasospasm can also cause acute mesenteric ischemia.

Multilevel atherosclerotic disease, cardiac arrhythmias, female sex, advanced age, and recent vascular interventions are the most common risk factors for AMI. Despite advances in endovascular therapy and critical care, AMI still has an in-hospital mortality rate as high as 80 % [19]. Several characteristics and conditions conspire to make AMI such a deadly condition including: an ambiguous clinical presentation, delayed diagnosis, long-duration ischemia, reperfusion injury, and medical comorbidities. Chronic mesenteric ischemia (CMI) typically occurs in elderly, frail patients with extensive atherosclerotic disease who present with significant weight loss and malnutrition because of "food fear." Successful management for both acute and chronic mesenteric ischemia requires tailoring the treatment plan to match the severity of ischemia and the patient's coexisting medical problems.

The two mechanisms of AMI are embolism and thrombosis [20]. The most common sources of emboli are cardiac lesions, including left atrial or ventricular mural thrombus, and lesions of the aortic or mitral valves that occur in the setting of atrial fibrillation or myocardial infarction. The embolus usually lodges a few centimeters distal to the ostium of the SMA near the origin of the middle colic artery. In contrast, SMA thrombosis occurs when clot forms within an existing atherosclerotic plaque usually located in the proximal segment of the vessel. Making the clinical distinction between an embolus to the SMA and an SMA thrombosis can be challenging.

Diagnosis

Prompt diagnosis and treatment play an important role in improving the clinical outcome of patients with AMI. Unfortunately, the vague and nonspecific initial clinical presentation of AMI often prevents clinicians from recognizing and treating AMI early in its course. Patients with AMI often present with complaints of abdominal pain that appears to be out of proportion to findings on physical exam. As ischemia progresses, the pain becomes more intense and other gastrointestinal symptoms appear including nausea, vomiting, diarrhea, and abdominal distension. Although it is initially benign, the abdominal examination evolves into an acute abdomen with diffuse tenderness, guarding, rebound, and eventually peritonitis. A detailed history and physical exam should point to the diagnosis of AMI and allow the distinction from CMI. Most patients with AMI have associated dehydration and electrolyte imbalances that require intravenous fluid resuscitation. Other abnormal lab values such as leukocytosis, metabolic acidosis, and amylasemia usually occur in late presentations of AMI and reflect more advanced ischemia.

Patients with CMI typically give a history of postprandial abdominal pain, weight loss, and intermittent diarrhea. They complain of crampy abdominal pain that characteristically occurs 15–45 min after food ingestion. "Food fear" is the term used to describe the behavior of patients with CMI who do not eat in an attempt to avoid postprandial pain. Although "food fear" is pathognomonic for CMI, it is not a required symptom for the diagnosis. Some patients with proven CMI completely deny postprandial abdominal pain and "food fear." Only with specific questioning does it become obvious that these patients restrict their diet to small amounts of specific food (e.g., toast and crackers) that allows them to avoid pain after eating. While CMI itself does not cause intestinal malabsorption, food avoidance and diet restrictions over the protracted course of CMI usually causes malnutrition and frailty in this elderly population. On physical exam, up to two-thirds of patients with CMI have an abdominal bruit on abdominal auscultation [21].

Plain abdominal X-rays for the evaluation of intestinal ischemia are usually nondiagnostic. Nonspecific plain film findings include air in the wall of the intestine or portal venous system in advanced cases of AMI and calcification of the aorta and the visceral arteries in patients with CMI. Duplex ultrasound has limited utility for diagnosing AMI because patients often have an ileus and the dilated, air-filled bowel loops prevent adequate sonographic visualization of the visceral arteries. In contrast, duplex ultrasound has greater than 80 % accuracy for the diagnosis of CMI [21]. Although its accuracy depends on the skill of the operator and requires external validation, the duplex ultrasound has emerged as a useful, noninvasive screening test for patients suspected of having CMI. Moreover, weight loss and the thin body habitus, prevalent among many patients with CMI, allows for technically straightforward ultrasound visualization and interrogation of the visceral vessels. Widely accepted velocity criteria for the diagnosis of stenosis include a peak systolic velocity greater than 275 cm/s for the SMA and greater than 200 cm/s for the celiac artery in a fasting state [21].

CT angiography has replaced catheter-directed DSA as the imaging modality of choice for diagnosing mesenteric ischemia. CTA can be used to confirm the diagnosis in patients suspected of having either acute or chronic mesenteric ischemia. Multidetector CT systems and 3-dimentional-reconstruction software also generate an indispensable guiding road map for planning a mesenteric revascularization [22, 23]. Patients with abnormal renal function may not be candidates for a standard CTA because of the risk of contrast nephropathy. Diagnostic imaging exams that lower the risk of nephrotoxicity include MR angiography (with gadolinium), highly selective diagnostic angiography, or CTA using intra-arterial (as opposed to intravenous) contrast administration.

Treatment

Acute mesenteric ischemia requires early diagnosis and prompt treatment to avoid ongoing bowel ischemia which will ultimately lead to necrosis, perforation, and peritonitis. After confirming the diagnosis treatment begins with systemic anticoagulation with intravenous heparin unless an absolute contraindication exists. The main goal of anticoagulation is to prevent thrombus propagation within the mesenteric vessels. Because AMI can occasionally present as a complication in patients suffering an acute myocardial infarction, an electrocardiogram and cardiac enzymes should be obtained prior to any intervention. Patients with an acute abdomen on physical exam require immediate transfer to the operating room for abdominal exploration.

Over the past several years, endovascular intervention has proven to be a viable treatment option for selected patients with AMI. Ideal patients for endovascular therapy include those who present early in the course of AMI (less than 8 h from the onset of symptoms) without an acute abdomen or evidence of bowel ischemia based on physical examination and laboratory evaluation. Patients with high surgical risk and severe comorbidities may also be considered for endovascular therapy [24]. A combination of catheter-directed mechanical thrombectomy and thrombolysis with or without ultrasound acceleration and balloon angioplasty and/or stenting may be required to restore SMA patency and treat the culprit lesions. Incorporating diagnostic laparoscopy into this minimally invasive approach allows for an evaluation of bowel viability.

Patients with AMI and advanced ischemia or peritonitis require an exploratory laparotomy for bowel resection and surgical revascularization. If a mesenteric embolism is suspected, the SMA is exposed and controlled at the root of the mesentery. Balloon embolectomy catheters are advanced proximally to remove the embolus. Distal arterial branches usually require manual milking of the mesentery to extrude the thrombus. Bowel resection and ostomies are then performed as required. A second-look exploration to assess bowel viability should be performed 24–48 h later regardless of the patient's clinical improvement.

If mesenteric thrombosis or chronic ischemia is suspected or confirmed, the proximal SMA is exposed by mobilizing the fourth portion of the duodenum and incising the ligament of Treitz. A bypass procedure to the SMA is frequently required using antegrade or retrograde inflow. The supraceliac aorta, the infrarenal aorta, or common iliac arteries are the most frequent inflow vessels. Autologous vein graft is preferable in cases of acute thrombosis because of the risk of contamination if bowel viability is compromised. Bypass to both the SMA and the celiac or hepatic artery are frequently performed for chronic mesenteric ischemia using bifurcated prosthetic grafts [23, 24]. The supraceliac aorta is the preferred inflow vessel in these chronic cases as it is rarely affected by advanced atherosclerotic disease. Nonocclusive mesenteric ischemia, which is usually secondary to hypoperfusion in the setting of hypovolemia, vasopressors, or underresuscitation, requires treatment of the underlying condition and occasionally catheter-directed, intra-arterial papaverine infusion. Surgical exploration is indicated if bowel ischemia is suspected.

Endovascular therapy has gained acceptance as a first-line treatment option for CMI because of the reduced periprocedural morbidity and mortality compared to open surgical revascularization [24, 25]. Balloon angioplasty and stenting of one or more visceral vessels can usually be performed with a high technical success rate in excess of 95 %. Although outcomes of endovascular therapy may not be as durable as open revascularization, recent series suggest improved patency rates with covered stents [26]. Moreover, future surgical revascularization remains a treatment option for endovascular failures and for patients in whom endovascular therapy was used as a bridge to promote weight gain and fitness for open surgery.

Renal Artery Stenosis

Renal artery stenosis (RAS) usually results from atherosclerosis (90 % of cases) and may occur in isolation or in combination with hypertension (renovascular hypertension) or chronic kidney disease (ischemic nephropathy) [27]. Although RAS occurs in only 0.1 % of the general population, its prevalence increases to 30 % among patients with coronary artery disease or symptomatic peripheral arterial disease and to 50 % in elderly subjects with atherosclerotic vascular disease [27, 28]. In the United States, 12–14 % of new patients entering dialysis have RAS [29], and ischemic nephropathy due to RAS may be responsible for 5–22 % of end-stage renal disease in patients older than 50 years [15, 16, 29–31]. Among patients with hypertension, up to 4 % will develop RAS [32].

RAS shortens patient survival and increases the risk of stroke and cardiovascular events [30]. In patients undergoing coronary angiography, the 4-year survival rate was 57 % among patients with severe RAS and 47 % in those with bilateral RAS compared to 89 % in patients with normal renal arteries [29]. Efforts to counteract the bleak prognosis associated with RAS have most recently involved renal revascularization in the form of renal artery angioplasty and stenting. The late 1990s witnessed a threefold increase in the number of endovascular renal artery procedures performed on Medicare beneficiaries [28, 33]. Although stenting dramatically improves the angiographic appearance of a stenotic renal artery, the clinical benefit of endovascular therapy for RAS has been more difficult to prove. Critical analysis of patient outcomes after renal artery angioplasty and/or stenting has tempered the initial enthusiasm and popularity of endovascular therapy for RAS [28]. A comparative effectiveness report sponsored by the Agency of Healthcare Research and Quality (AHRQ) reviewed the existing evidence on interventional and medical therapy for RAS. Citing no difference in mortality or cardiovascular event rates, the report concluded that current evidence does not support endovascular or open renal revascularization over medical therapy for the general population of people with RAS [28, 33, 34]. Debate continues as this report included studies with few patients and limited follow-up undermining its ability to make broad generalizations or treatment recommendations.

Clinical Presentation

In most patients RAS causes no symptoms and the renal lesion represents an incidental imaging finding. In this group of patients, hypertension is common but well controlled with one or two medications, and renal function is normal for age, sex, and race. Although disease progression with renal atrophy and loss of function has been documented, asymptomatic RAS has a benign course in 80 % of patients [28]. The risk of renal function loss in patients with asymptomatic RAS is similar to matched controls with normal renal arteries. Similarly, less than 10 % of patients with asymptomatic RAS ultimately require either renal revascularization or dialysis, the exception being asymptomatic patients with bilateral RAS or RAS affecting a solitary functional kidney [33]. Based on current evidence, incidental asymptomatic RAS only requires medical therapy and does not warrant open or endovascular revascularization.

Symptomatic RAS implies an association between the renal lesion and poorly controlled hypertension (despite two or more medications), recurrent flash pulmonary edema, or deteriorating renal function (ischemic nephropathy) [27]. The pathophysiology of symptomatic RAS remains poorly understood as most patients with severe RAS have no symptoms. It is important to recognize that classifying a patient with RAS as symptomatic does not necessarily constitute an indication for renal revascularization. While all patients with symptomatic RAS require medication to reduce cardiovascular risk and prevent disease progression, the indications for renal artery intervention continue to evolve and require careful consideration of the risks and benefits of intervention versus the outcome of best medical therapy [35].

Diagnosis

Duplex ultrasound has replaced renal function scanning as the initial noninvasive imaging of choice to screen for RAS. Although its accuracy exceeds 80 %, ultrasound quality requires a skilled sonographer and frequent external validation [36]. Body habitus and overlying bowel gas can prevent adequate ultrasound visualization of the renal vessels and render the exam nondiagnostic. Widely used sonographic criteria for RAS include a peak systolic velocity greater than 180 cm/s in the main renal artery and the presence of poststenotic turbulence [36].

As with most arterial occlusive lesions, catheter-directed DSA has traditionally been the diagnostic gold standard. Modern management strategies for RAS now rely on CT angiography as the only direct imaging modality before renal revascularization. Most patients who need revascularization for RAS are treated with renal artery angioplasty/stenting and therefore undergo angiography as part of the therapeutic intervention. Diagnostic angiography should be performed in patients being considered for surgical revascularization to confirm RAS and plan the procedure. Both CTA and DSA carry a risk of nephrotoxicity as they both require intravenous (IV) iodinated contrast. Periprocedural hydration and the administration of sodium bicarbonate can mitigate some of the risk associated with contrast, particularly in patients with abnormal or deteriorating renal function. MR angiography offers an accurate and safe imaging alternative for patients with glomerular filtration rate (GFR) greater than 60 mL/min and possibly for patients with moderate renal disease (GFR between 30 and 60 mL/min). The use of gadolinium contrast in MRA can increase the risk of nephrogenic systemic fibrosis in patients with severe renal dysfunction.

Treatment

Patients with RAS should always receive best medical therapy for atherosclerotic disease, including risk factor reduction, antiplatelet therapy, and lifestyle modification [27]. The goal of medical treatment should be to minimize the impact of both primary and secondary risk factors as previously discussed in the section on carotid stenosis. Particular attention should be given to blood pressure control using angiotensin II-converting enzyme inhibitors (ACEIs) and angiotensin-receptor blockers (ARBs) as first-line medications. ACEIs and ARBs interrupt the renin-angiotensin system which forms the underlying pathophysiology in most patients with RAS and hypertension. Blood pressure control usually requires two or more types of medication. Patients with severe bilateral RAS represent a difficult therapeutic dilemma as ACEIs and ARBs may precipitate acute renal failure. In these patients, loop and thiazide diuretics may be a better option to avoid fluid retention due to aldosterone excess. Spironolactone should also be used cautiously in patients with abnormal renal function or when added to ACEIs because of the risk of hyperkalemia.

As previously mentioned, the indications for renal revascularization have evolved with improving medical therapy and a critical analysis of the outcomes after renal intervention. Current evidence suggests that most patients with RAS should not undergo any renal artery intervention. Specific indications for renal revascularization include RAS greater than 60 % associated with:

- Severe, poorly controlled hypertension, usually requiring three or more medications
- Severe hypertension associated with ischemic nephropathy, particularly deteriorating renal function over the last 6 months
- Severe hypertension associated to congestive heart failure, flash pulmonary edema, unstable angina, or neurologic events

Other less widely accepted indications included: unilateral RAS with abnormal renal function, bilateral RAS, and RAS in a solitary functional kidney.

Endovascular therapy for RAS usually involves balloon angioplasty and stent placement in the proximal renal artery [28, 37]. The low profile, rapid exchange balloons and stents currently available have improved the technical success and safety of endovascular intervention compared to the larger caliber, over the wire devices used in the past. Most vascular specialists favor the "no touch" technique which avoids unnecessary manipulation of the renal artery lesion in an attempt to minimize the risk of iatrogenic thromboembolic injury. Guiding catheters that engage just the renal artery ostium are used making it unnecessary to cross the lesion with a large-caliber sheath. This technique also avoids balloon pre-dilation except for near-occlusive lesions in which small-diameter balloon angioplasty can facilitate passage of the stent. Although the use of embolic protection devices has been described, specifically designed filters for renal arteries are not currently available. Dual antiplatelet therapy (aspirin and clopidogrel) is recommended for at least 1 month postprocedure to avoid renal stent thrombosis.

Open surgery for renal artery revascularization is performed less frequently than endovascular interventions. Indications for surgery include severe, complicated RAS or RAS associated with aneurismal or occlusive disease of the aorta which requires operative reconstruction [38]. Although it is durable with a reported 3-year patency rates of 97 %, open revascularization carries a significant risk of morbidity and mortality. The 30-day mortality may be as high as 8 % particularly for revascularizations that involve bilateral RAS or combined aortic reconstruction [28]. Clinical outcomes after open surgery vary and may depend on several factors including the indication for intervention and operative technique. Overall improved blood pressure control can be demonstrated in more than 50 % of patients after surgical revascularization [39]. Nephrectomy has an extremely limited role in the modern management of RAS given the effectiveness of antihypertensive medications and the interventional treatment options. Rare cases warranting a nephrectomy involve uncontrolled hypertension associated with poorly functioning, atrophic kidneys, and unreconstructable arteries.

Conclusion

Atherosclerotic disease affects all arteries and can cause stroke, bowel ischemia, hypertension, and renal failure. Preventing these potentially fatal consequences starts by recognizing the clinical presentation of carotid, mesenteric, and renal disease and confirming the diagnosis with appropriate imaging studies. The rise of endovascular therapy has expanded interventional options and added complexity to the treatment decision-making process. This chapter has reviewed the important concepts of carotid, mesenteric, and renal artery disease to help clarify the management of these important clinical conditions.

References

1. Furie KL, Kasner SE, Adams RJ, et al. Guidelines for the prevention of stroke in patients with stroke or transient ischemic attack: a guideline for healthcare professionals from the American Heart Association/American Stroke Association. Stroke. 2011;42: 227–76.
2. Hoyert DL. 75 years of mortality in the United States, 1935–2010. NCHS Data Brief. 2012;88:1–8.
3. Beneficial effect of carotid endarterectomy in symptomatic patients with high-grade carotid stenosis. North American Symptomatic Carotid Endarterectomy Trial Collaborators. N Engl J Med. 1991; 325:445–53.
4. Endarterectomy for asymptomatic carotid artery stenosis. Executive Committee for the Asymptomatic Carotid Atherosclerosis Study. JAMA. 1995;273:1421–8.
5. Moore WS, Barnett HJ, Beebe HG, et al. Guidelines for carotid endarterectomy. A multidisciplinary consensus statement from the Ad Hoc Committee, American Heart Association. Circulation. 1995;91:566–79.
6. Biller J, Feinberg WM, Castaldo JE, et al. Guidelines for carotid endarterectomy: a statement for healthcare professionals from a Special Writing Group of the Stroke Council, American Heart Association. Circulation. 1998;97:501–9.
7. Brott TG, Hobson 2nd RW, Howard G, et al. Stenting versus endarterectomy for treatment of carotid-artery stenosis. N Engl J Med. 2010;363:11–23.
8. Carotid Stenting Trialists' Collaboration, Bonati LH, Dobson J, Algra A, Branchereau A, Chatellier G, Fraedrich G, Mali WP, Zeumer H, Brown MM, Mas JL, Ringleb PA. Short-term outcome after stenting versus endarterectomy for symptomatic carotid stenosis: a preplanned meta-analysis of individual patient data. Lancet. 2010;376:1062–73.
9. Timaran CH, McKinsey JF, Schneider PA, Littooy F. Reporting standards for carotid interventions from the Society for Vascular Surgery. J Vasc Surg. 2011;53:1679–95.
10. Ederle J, Dobson J, Featherstone RL, et al. Carotid artery stenting compared with endarterectomy in patients with symptomatic carotid stenosis (International Carotid Stenting Study): an interim analysis of a randomised controlled trial. Lancet. 2010;375: 985–97.
11. Ringleb PA, Allenberg J, Bruckmann H, et al. 30 day results from the SPACE trial of stent-protected angioplasty versus carotid endarterectomy in symptomatic patients: a randomised non-inferiority trial. Lancet. 2006;368:1239–47.
12. Mas JL, Chatellier G, Beyssen B, et al. Endarterectomy versus stenting in patients with symptomatic severe carotid stenosis. N Engl J Med. 2006;355:1660–71.
13. Ricotta JJ, Aburahma A, Ascher E, Eskandari M, Faries P, Lal BK. Updated Society for Vascular Surgery guidelines for management of extracranial carotid disease: executive summary. J Vasc Surg. 2011;54:832–6.
14. Cumbie T, Rosero EB, Valentine RJ, Modrall JG, Clagett GP, Timaran CH. Utility and accuracy of duplex ultrasonography in evaluating in-stent restenosis after carotid stenting. Am J Surg. 2008;196:623–8.
15. Edwards MS, Hansen KJ, Craven TE, et al. Associations between renovascular disease and prevalent cardiovascular disease in the elderly: a population-based study. Vasc Endovascular Surg. 2004;38:25–35.
16. Edwards MS, Hansen KJ, Craven TE, et al. Relationships between renovascular disease, blood pressure, and renal function in the elderly: a population-based study. Am J Kidney Dis. 2003;41: 990–6.
17. Yadav JS, Wholey MH, Kuntz RE, et al. Protected carotid-artery stenting versus endarterectomy in high-risk patients. N Engl J Med. 2004;351:1493–501.
18. Mantese VA, Timaran CH, Chiu D, Begg RJ, Brott TG. The Carotid Revascularization Endarterectomy versus Stenting Trial (CREST): stenting versus carotid endarterectomy for carotid disease. Stroke. 2010;41:S31–4.
19. Park WM, Gloviczki P, Cherry KJ, et al. Contemporary management of acute mesenteric ischemia: factors associated with survival. J Vasc Surg. 2002;35:445–52.
20. Ryer EJ, Kalra M, Oderich GS, et al. Revascularization for acute mesenteric ischemia. J Vasc Surg. 2012;55:1682–9.
21. White CJ. Chronic mesenteric ischemia: diagnosis and management. Prog Cardiovasc Dis. 2011;54:36–40.
22. Lee SS, Park SH. Computed tomography evaluation of gastrointestinal bleeding and acute mesenteric ischemia. Radiol Clin North Am. 2013;51:29–43.
23. Oderich GS, Gloviczki P, Bower TC. Open surgical treatment for chronic mesenteric ischemia in the endovascular era: when it is necessary and what is the preferred technique? Semin Vasc Surg. 2010;23:36–46.
24. Sullivan TM, Oderich GS, Malgor RD, Ricotta JJ. Open and endovascular revascularization for chronic mesenteric ischemia: tabular review of the literature. Ann Vasc Surg. 2009;23:700–12.
25. Oderich GS, Bower TC, Sullivan TM, Bjarnason H, Cha S, Gloviczki P. Open versus endovascular revascularization for chronic mesenteric ischemia: risk-stratified outcomes. J Vasc Surg. 2009;49:1472–9 e3.
26. Tallarita T, Oderich GS, Macedo TA, et al. Reinterventions for stent restenosis in patients treated for atherosclerotic mesenteric artery disease. J Vasc Surg. 2011;54:1422–9 e1.
27. Hirsch AT, Haskal ZJ, Hertzer NR, et al. ACC/AHA 2005 Practice Guidelines for the management of patients with peripheral arterial disease (lower extremity, renal, mesenteric, and abdominal aortic): a collaborative report from the American Association for Vascular Surgery/Society for Vascular Surgery, Society for Cardiovascular Angiography and Interventions, Society for Vascular Medicine and Biology, Society of Interventional Radiology, and the ACC/AHA Task Force on Practice Guidelines (Writing Committee to Develop Guidelines for the Management of Patients With Peripheral Arterial Disease): endorsed by the American Association of Cardiovascular and Pulmonary Rehabilitation; National Heart, Lung, and Blood Institute; Society for Vascular Nursing; TransAtlantic Inter-Society Consensus; and Vascular Disease Foundation. Circulation. 2006; 113:e463–654.
28. Balk E, Raman G, Chung M, et al. Effectiveness of management strategies for renal artery stenosis: a systematic review. Ann Intern Med. 2006;145:901–12.
29. Pearce JD, Craven BL, Craven TE, et al. Progression of atherosclerotic renovascular disease: a prospective population-based study. J Vasc Surg. 2006;44:955–62; discussion 62–3.
30. Edwards MS, Craven TE, Burke GL, Dean RH, Hansen KJ. Renovascular disease and the risk of adverse coronary events in the elderly: a prospective, population-based study. Arch Intern Med. 2005;165:207–13.
31. Hansen KJ, Edwards MS, Craven TE, et al. Prevalence of renovascular disease in the elderly: a population-based study. J Vasc Surg. 2002;36:443–51.
32. Davis RP, Pearce JD, Craven TE, et al. Atherosclerotic renovascular disease among hypertensive adults. J Vasc Surg. 2009;50:564–70. 71 e1–3; discussion 71.
33. Balk E, Raman G. Comparative effectiveness of management strategies for renal artery stenosis: 2007. Rockville: Agency for Healthcare Research and Quality (US); 2007.
34. Balk E, Raman G, Chung M, et al. Comparative effectiveness of management strategies for renal artery stenosis. Rockville: Agency for Healthcare Research and Quality (US); 2006.

35. Eagle KA, Guyton RA, Davidoff R, et al. ACC/AHA guidelines for coronary artery bypass graft surgery: executive summary and recommendations: a report of the American College of Cardiology/American Heart Association Task Force on Practice Guidelines (Committee to revise the 1991 guidelines for coronary artery bypass graft surgery). Circulation. 1999;100:1464–80.
36. AbuRahma AF, Srivastava M, Mousa AY, et al. Critical analysis of renal duplex ultrasound parameters in detecting significant renal artery stenosis. J Vasc Surg. 2012;56:1052–9. 60 e1; discussion 9–60.
37. Corriere MA, Pearce JD, Edwards MS, Stafford JM, Hansen KJ. Endovascular management of atherosclerotic renovascular disease: early results following primary intervention. J Vasc Surg. 2008;48:580–7; discussion 7–8.
38. Cherr GS, Hansen KJ, Craven TE, et al. Surgical management of atherosclerotic renovascular disease. J Vasc Surg. 2002;35:236–45.
39. Fleming SH, Hansen KJ. Randomized clinical trials regarding management of atherosclerotic renovascular disease. Semin Vasc Surg. 2010;23:156–64.

Aortic Pathology: AAA, Dissection, and Traumatic Transection

21

David G. Neschis, Marshall E. Benjamin, Justin K. Nelms, and William R. Flinn

Abdominal Aortic Aneurysms

General Considerations

An aneurysm is defined as any artery that dilates to 1.5–2 times greater than the diameter of the adjacent normal artery. Since the abdominal aorta has a normal diameter of 2 cm, a dilation of 3.0 cm or more is considered an abdominal aortic aneurysm (AAA) [1]. The natural history of aortic aneurysms usually involves progressive, clinically silent growth which ultimately leads to rupture, exsanguination, and death. Abdominal aortic aneurysms remain a significant cause of mortality in our aging population: AAAs are the 15th leading cause of death overall and the 10th leading cause of death in men over age 55 [2]. Despite increased public awareness and screening efforts, more than half of patients who die of a ruptured AAA never knew they had an aneurysm. Ruptured aortic aneurysm mortality probably exceeds 80 % with an unknown number of patients dying before they reach the hospital [3]. Of those patients who arrive in the hospital alive with a ruptured AAA, fewer than 50 % survive and return to their original functional state. Preventing AAA-related deaths requires detecting aneurysms prior to rupture when they can be electively repaired with significantly lower mortality and morbidity. Early AAA detection efforts relying on symptoms or physical exam have proven to be ineffective. Few aneurysms generate symptoms prior to rupture, and the physical exam is a notoriously unreliable and insensitive method for diagnosing AAA [4].

Several international studies demonstrated that ultrasound screening populations at risk for aneurysms significantly reduced AAA-related mortality [5, 6]. Aneurysm screening in the United States started in 2006 with the SAAAVE Act which provides a single ultrasound screening for AAA to new male Medicare enrollees who have ever smoked or have a family history of AAA. This Medicare-based screening program does not provide screenings for women or for men beyond their 1-year "Introduction to Medicare" exam window. The exclusions involved in the SAAAVE have limited its ability to address the total US population at risk for AAA [7]. Nevertheless, ultrasound imaging of the aorta is almost universally available to all practitioners in the United States and provides an accurate method for detecting AAAs. As a minimally invasive and inexpensive test, aortic ultrasound has emerged as the preferred exam for AAA detection in patients at risk. Despite efforts to expand AAA screening in this country, most patients with AAAs are still detected as an incidental finding on imaging studies (CT, MRI, US) obtained to evaluate other pathology [8].

The maximal transverse diameter of the aneurysm remains the standard measure of AAA size for the purpose of treatment decision making and for comparison over time. Modalities including ultrasound, CT scan, and MRI all provide accurate measurements of aneurysm diameter [9]. Aortography alone is a poor screening tool as it is an invasive and insensitive exam. In most aneurysms laminated thrombus fills much of the aneurysm sac while blood passes through the flow lumen. The two-dimensional contrast images of aortography only show the blood flow lumen and do not demonstrate the full extent or true diameter of the aneurysm sac (Fig. 21.1). If an arteriogram demonstrates an irregular pathway for aortic flow, additional imaging to evaluate for an aneurysm should be considered.

D.G. Neschis, MD (✉)
Department of Surgery, Baltimore Washington Medical Center, 301 Hospital Drive, Glen Burnie, MD 21061, USA
e-mail: dneschis@bwmc.umms.org

M.E. Benjamin, MD
Department of Vascular Surgery, University of Maryland Baltimore Washington Medical Center, Maryland Vascular Center, University of Maryland, Glen Burnie, MD, USA

J.K. Nelms, MD • W.R. Flinn, MD
Department of Vascular Surgery, University of Maryland Baltimore Washington Medical Center, Maryland Vascular Center, University of Maryland School of Medicine, Glen Burnie, MD, USA

V. Gahtan and M.J. Costanza (eds.), *Essentials of Vascular Surgery for the General Surgeon*, DOI 10.1007/978-1-4939-1326-8_21, © Springer Science+Business Media New York 2015

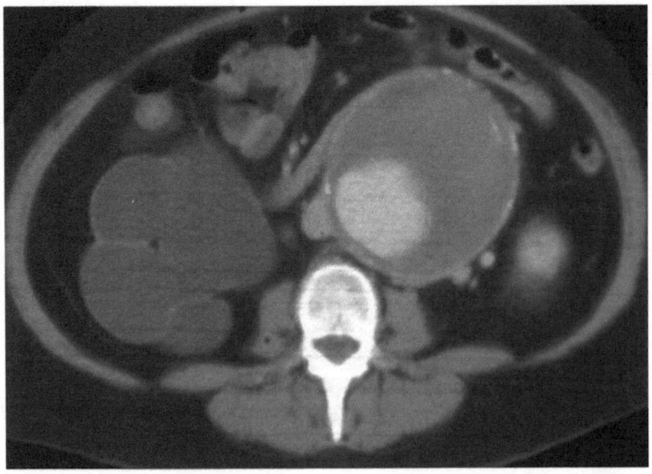

Fig. 21.1 Large abdominal aortic aneurysm. Notice how the majority of this aneurysm is filled with laminated thrombus. The flow lumen is only mildly dilated, and this aneurysm could be missed on angiography alone

Pathophysiology

Although the precise cause of aneurysmal degeneration of the aortic wall remains uncertain, atherosclerosis, cellular inflammation, and metalloproteinases have all been implicated [10]. Men are clearly at a higher risk for AAA, with a ratio of approximately 4:1 compared to women [11]. Other risk factors include age over 60, history of smoking, hypertension, emphysema, history of hernias, and family history. Family history is a particularly strong marker for patients who have a female first-degree relative with an AAA [12].

Developing an appropriate treatment plan for aneurysms requires a clear understanding of the difference between a true aneurysm and a pseudoaneurysm. Technically speaking, the number of vessel wall layers differentiates a true aneurysm from a pseudoaneurysm. Although this definition is precise and useful for pathologists, it cannot be applied clinically nor does it help in treatment planning. A more practical approach defines a true aneurysm as an abnormal expansion of the vessel due to defective structural proteins within the arterial wall. In contrast, a pseudoaneurysm occurs when a focal, transmural defect in the vessel wall allows extravasation of blood out of the artery and into the surrounding soft tissue where it is variably contained. Blood circulates into this "pulsatile hematoma" and back into the arterial lumen creating a characteristic "to-and-fro" flow pattern that is recognizable on color-flow ultrasound exam. Since pseudoaneurysms more accurately represent a contained rupture of the artery, they usually warrant swift intervention. The rate of expansion of pseudoaneurysms may be more rapid and less predictable than true aneurysms making treatment justified at almost any size [13]. In the periphery pseudoaneurysms tend to result from a traumatic injury or iatrogenic puncture. In the abdominal aorta, pseudoaneurysms often resemble a mushroom and stalk in appearance and are sometimes described as "saccular" aneurysms. Aortic pseudoaneurysms are believed to result from a focal rupture of a penetrating atherosclerotic plaque.

Most AAAs develop in the infrarenal aorta leaving a short segment of normal aorta below the renal arteries. This normal aortic segment or "aortic neck" allows for either open or endovascular aneurysm repair without compromising flow to the renal arteries. Juxtarenal aneurysms abut the renal arteries and lack a suitable infrarenal neck. Although surgery to repair juxtarenal aneurysms does not usually involve renal artery bypass or reconstruction, suprarenal clamping is required which increases the risk of postoperative renal dysfunction. Suprarenal aortic aneurysms require both suprarenal clamping and renal revascularization to achieve aneurysm repair and maintain renal blood flow. Repairing thoracoabdominal aortic aneurysms requires exposure in both the chest and abdomen and carries the highest risk of perioperative morbidity and mortality.

Perioperative Evaluation and Indications for Treatment

The risk of AAA rupture increases with the size of the aneurysm. Aneurysms greater than 6 cm in diameter have a rupture risk of approximately 10 % per year and generally warrant repair unless a patient has prohibitive comorbidities or a short life expectancy due to other clinical conditions [14, 15]. The optimal management of smaller aneurysms 4–5.5 cm in diameter has not been completely settled. Historically, patients with AAA greater than 5 cm were recommended for repair; however, several large prospective randomized trials suggest that patients with AAA less than 5.5 cm have a low risk of rupture and can be safely followed with surveillance imaging [16, 17]. Sound clinical judgment must be employed in each case as even small diameter aneurysms can rupture. For patients with a 5 cm AAA who have minimal cardiovascular risks and no evidence of malignancy, the aneurysm represents the single greatest threat to their life and continued well-being. Women and patients with COPD have a higher risk of rupture on a diameter-for-diameter basis and may warrant repair at a smaller AAA size. Likewise, patients with an AAA and symptoms of abdominal or back pain with no other obvious source are thought to have an increased risk of rupture and may require early repair. The morphology of a saccular aneurysm may predispose it to rupture and therefore warrant preemptive repair at a smaller diameter [18].

Aneurysms grow at an average rate of approximately 10 % per year. Aneurysms with a significantly more rapid growth rate should be considered for repair even when they are still small in diameter [19]. Patients who are being followed with surveillance imaging should stop smoking and aggressively control their blood pressure since smoking and hypertension are the only modifiable risk factors associated with aneurysm expansion and rupture [20].

Patients with AAA should be evaluated for aneurysms in other anatomic locations. Popliteal artery aneurysms occur in more than 5 % of patients with AAA, particularly in elderly men [21]. If the popliteal pulse is generous on physical exam, an ultrasound can easily measure the popliteal artery diameter to determine if there is an aneurysm. Recent studies suggest that as many as 25 % of patients with AAA may have a concurrent thoracic aortic aneurysm [22]. Patients with a known AAA being evaluated with CT scan should have a comprehensive scan including the thoracic aorta, particularly women and elderly patients with AAA.

A high-quality CT angiogram should be performed in all patients with AAA who are being considered for treatment, unless they have a major contraindication. In patients with renal dysfunction, a non-contrast CT of the abdomen and pelvis with thin axial cuts (less than 1 mm) can provide valuable anatomic information. CT scanning is essential to determine whether an endovascular repair will be technically feasible, but CT scans also help plan open surgical repair. CT scan demonstrates the proximal extent of the aneurysm to insure that there is no extension above the renal arteries or a coexisting aneurysm involving the distal thoracic aorta or the visceral segment of the abdominal aorta. The celiac trunk and superior mesenteric artery (SMA) should be evaluated to exclude significant mesenteric disease, since the inferior mesenteric artery (IMA) is typically sacrificed as part of the open surgical repair. The presence of severe stenosis or occlusion of the SMA with an enlarged IMA ("meandering mesenteric") might necessitate reimplantation of the IMA into the body of the aortic graft at the time of open repair.

The CT scan can also detect other important abdominal pathology, like an undiagnosed malignancy. The major venous structures should be examined to identify anatomic variants such as a duplicated or left-sided inferior vena cava (IVC), retroaortic renal vein, or a renal venous "ring." These venous anomalies can be the source of troublesome intraoperative bleeding during dissection and proximal aortic control if they are undetected preoperatively.

A CT scan which shows thick, contrast-enhancing soft tissue encompassing the anterior 270° of the aorta may indicate an inflammatory aneurysm which will be discussed in more detail below. Tissue resembling renal parenchyma on the anterior surface of the aorta may represent a horseshoe kidney. Additionally, the aorta should be evaluated for the presence of calcification, particularly at the aortic bifurcation and in the iliac vessels. The iliac vessels themselves should be inspected for the presence of atherosclerotic occlusive disease which could impede passage of an endovascular stent graft or prohibit aortic reconstruction with a prosthetic tube graft. Approximately 10–20 % of patients with an infrarenal AAA have aneurysms involving the common or internal iliac arteries.

Measuring the ankle-brachial index (ABI) provides objective, preoperative documentation of lower extremity arterial perfusion. If the ABI is significantly abnormal, preoperative angiography should be considered to clarify the precise anatomic location and severity of the occlusive lesions. The presence of severe aortoiliac occlusive disease often modifies the plan for surgical repair. Routine noninvasive evaluation of the carotid arteries should also be considered in patients with associated cardiovascular risk factors [23]. Patients with undiagnosed severe internal carotid artery stenosis pose a higher perioperative stroke risk for major open abdominal surgery [24].

In addition to the standard cardiac and non-cardiac risks inherent in any major intracavitary procedure, patients with AAA should be aware of the complications specific to aneurysm repair surgery. Potential complications of AAA surgery include distal embolization or thrombosis in the lower extremities, bowel ischemia, and acute kidney injury. In men, sexual dysfunction in the form of either erectile dysfunction or retrograde ejaculation can occur and appears to be related to the amount of dissection around the autonomic nerves which travel near the infrarenal aorta and left common iliac artery.

Open Surgical Repair

Open AAA repair may be performed through a longitudinal midline or mid-abdominal transverse incision. Retroperitoneal exposure using a left flank incision has also been used and may be favored in cases of hostile abdomen (previous complex abdominal surgery, stoma, etc.) and inflammatory aneurysm (discussed below) and selected patients with severe COPD that are not candidates for an endovascular approach. Advantages of transabdominal exposure are direct evaluation of all intra-abdominal viscera both before and after repair and more predictable access to the right iliac arteries if required. Table 21.1 compares the major advantages and drawbacks of transabdominal and retroperitoneal exposure of the abdominal aorta.

To achieve transperitoneal exposure of the infrarenal aorta, the transverse colon is reflected cephalad and the small bowel is retracted to the patient's right. The retroperitoneal tissue is incised over the aneurysm, and the duodenum is mobilized off the aorta and to the patient's right. The inferior mesenteric vein (IMV) runs parallel to the aorta on the left. Dissection continues superiorly on the anterior surface of the aorta to the level of the left renal vein; if the IMV compromises exposure at that level, it can be divided. In most cases proximal control of normal caliber aorta is possible at the level of the left renal vein. If more proximal aortic exposure is necessary, the left renal vein can be divided toward its

Table 21.1 Advantages and drawbacks of transperitoneal vs. retroperitoneal exposure for open repair of abdominal aortic aneurysm

	Transabdominal	Retroperitoneal
Advantages	Rapid exposure	Avoid hostile abdomen
	Widest access	Better juxtarenal control
	Intra-abdominal evaluation	Shorter ICU stay
Drawbacks	Longer ileus	Poor access to right side
	Greater fluid loss	Flank bulge and incisional pain
	More pulmonary dysfunction	Longer open/close time
	Higher cost	No intra-abdominal evaluation

confluence with the inferior vena cava, taking care to preserve the adrenal and gonadal venous tributaries.

Distal vascular control is then achieved by isolating the common iliac arteries. If the iliac arteries are not involved with aneurysmal or occlusive disease, a tube graft repair of the AAA can be performed. Common iliac artery aneurysms require repair with an aortobi-iliac bypass which is usually anastomosed to the distal common iliac artery or iliac bifurcation. The presence of significant iliac artery occlusive disease usually mandates an aortobifemoral bypass to avoid postoperative lower limb ischemia. This type of vascular reconstruction requires bilateral groin incision for exposure of the femoral arteries.

After suitable proximal and distal control of the vessels has been obtained, systemic heparin is administered prior to clamping. The aneurysm sac is then opened longitudinally and all thrombotic debris removed. Back bleeding from patent lumbar arteries and the IMA can be controlled by oversewing the vessel orifices from inside the aneurysm sac. If the IMA is large (particularly if there is known disease of the SMA) or has sluggish back bleeding, reimplantation of the IMA onto the body of the aortic graft using a Carrell patch should be considered to avoid postoperative colon ischemia.

The prosthetic graft used most often for AAA repair is a woven polyester textile (Dacron) graft, but polytetrafluoroethylene (PTFE) grafts are also available. Grafts are sewn in place with 3-0 or 4-0 nonabsorbable monofilament sutures (usually polypropylene). When graft repair has been completed, the wall of the aneurysm is closed over the graft, and the remainder of the retroperitoneal tissue reapproximated over the aneurysm sac. Prior to wound closure, the viability of the abdominal viscera, particularly the left colon, should be inspected.

Inflammatory Abdominal Aortic Aneurysms

The etiology of inflammatory aneurysms remains uncertain. Patients tend to be younger and more frequently present with abdominal symptoms [25]. The liberal use of CT scanning in modern practice increases the chances of detecting an inflammatory AAA preoperatively. A CT showing a contrast-enhancing, thickened rind of inflammatory tissue around the aneurysm suggests the possibility of an inflammatory AAA. Inflammatory AAA may be associated with retroperitoneal fibrosis with involvement of the ureters and hydronephrosis [26]. Suspicion of an inflammatory AAA based on preoperative imaging studies warrants an endovascular repair if it is anatomically feasible. If open AAA repair is required, a retroperitoneal approach should be considered to avoid dissection in the inflammatory tissue surrounding the anterior aorta.

The typical appearance of an inflammatory aneurysm encountered during transperitoneal exploration is a pearly, milky-white, glistening surface along the entire anterior wall of the aneurysm. This is almost always associated with firm adherence of the duodenum to the aneurysm wall, and no attempt should be made to free the duodenum from this surface. The inflammatory process rarely extends above the body of the aneurysm, and it is often possible to gain proximal infrarenal aortic control. Alternatively, temporary suprarenal or supraceliac aortic control can be used. The inflammatory process frequently involves the common iliac arteries, so direct distal control of those vessels may not be possible. In this situation, control of the iliac arteries is achieved with intraluminal occlusion balloons placed after opening the aneurysm sac with a proximal clamp in place. Graft repair then continues from within the AAA lumen. Following open or endovascular repair of an inflammatory AAA, the retroperitoneal fibrosis may spontaneously resolve [27]. Most aspects of inflammatory AAA including its cause and resolution remain poorly understood.

A mycotic aneurysm of the abdominal aorta is not a true aneurysm but an infected pseudoaneurysm caused by suppurative autolysis of the aortic wall. These rare aneurysms represent a "contained" rupture and should be treated aggressively at any size. Mycotic aneurysms can often be recognized by their atypical morphology on CT scan, appearing as a focal, saccular outpouching along the course of an otherwise disease-free aorta [28]. Suspicion for a mycotic aneurysm should increase in young patients without other risk factors for aneurysm. Patients with mycotic aneurysms may report a prodrome of systemic symptoms (e.g., fever, malaise, gastrointestinal symptoms) prior to presentation. The most common bacteria causing mycotic aortic aneurysms are *Salmonella* species and *Staphylococcus aureus*. If gross purulence is encountered at the time of surgery, it is probably safest to oversew the aorta proximally and distally and debride as much involved aortic wall as possible. Limb revascularization is then provided by constructing an extra-anatomic axillobifemoral bypass [29]. When gross purulence is not present, in situ aortic reconstruction may be considered. This can be performed with an antibiotic-soaked graft (most often rifampin), a cryopreserved aortic homograft, or an autologous reconstruction using deep femoral veins harvested from the legs [30, 31]. In all cases of mycotic aortic aneurysm, long-term antibiotic treatment should continue postoperatively [28].

Primary Aortocaval Fistula

Rarely, brisk venous bleeding from the aortic wall is encountered after opening the aneurysm sac. This clinical scenario represents an aortocaval fistula caused by chronic erosion of the AAA into the adjacent IVC [32]. No attempt should be made to dissect the aortic wall from the IVC as this will likely cause more bleeding. Instead, direct pressure proximal and distal to the fistula can provide temporary hemostasis allowing the defect to be sutured closed from within the aneurysm sac. An aortocaval fistula is almost always associated with a hyperdynamic cardiopulmonary status, so the anesthesiologist should be warned that preload will significantly decrease when the fistula is closed.

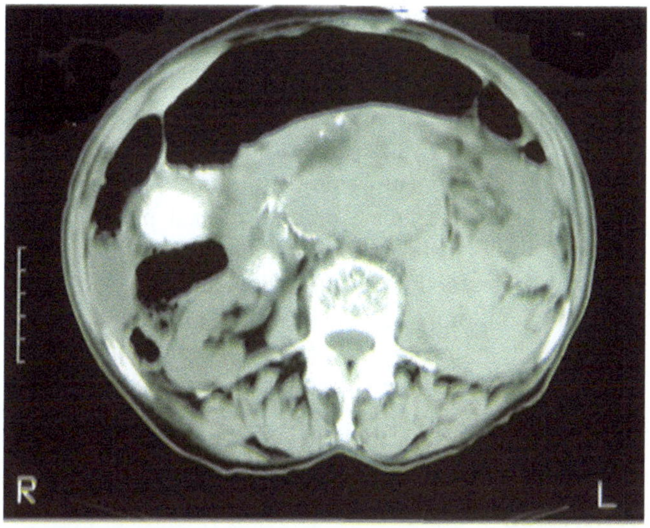

Fig. 21.2 Classic image of a ruptured abdominal aortic aneurysm, which in this case can be seen even without the use of intravascular contrast. Note the lack of symmetry and obliteration of tissue planes in the retroperitoneum on the left. Although contrast is not necessary to diagnose an AAA rupture, it is helpful in determining the candidacy for and planning of endovascular repair

Ruptured Abdominal Aortic Aneurysms

Left untreated, a ruptured AAA is universally fatal. Emergent surgical or endovascular repair offers the only hope of survival. Most modern emergency facilities in the United States have rapid CT scanners capable of imaging the abdominal aorta within minutes. Even without intravenous contrast, a CT scan can diagnose a ruptured AAA and determine the options for repair (Fig. 21.2). In centers with appropriate personnel and equipment, endovascular repair of ruptured AAA has reduced mortality and morbidity [33]. Preparations for an open surgical repair should address several key logistical and technical issues. Blood and blood products (fresh-frozen plasma, platelets) should be readily available. Since patients with ruptured AAAs usually present with hypotension, resuscitation efforts will have already begun in the emergency department. These efforts should be closely monitored with the goal having a responsive patient with a systolic pressure of 70–90 mmHg. Maintaining "permissive hypotension" until bleeding can be definitively controlled is more desirable than aggressive resuscitation which can lead hypertension, increased bleeding, and rapid deterioration of the patient [34].

In the operating room, sterile skin preparation and draping should extend from the upper chest to the knees in cases where exposure and control of the thoracic aorta are required. Ideally, the patient should be prepped and draped prior to induction as muscle relaxation can release the retroperitoneal tamponade causing sudden hypotension or cardiovascular collapse. Proximal control of the aorta is always the initial objective of surgery. In most cases the large retroperitoneal hematoma makes it impossible to directly control the infrarenal aorta without causing a significant venous injury, usually to the left renal vein. Initial proximal control should be achieved at the supraceliac aorta which can be exposed by incising the triangular ligament to retract the left lobe of the liver, dividing the gastrohepatic ligament, and dividing or separating the fibers of the diaphragmatic crus directly overlying the aorta. It is helpful to have a nasogastric or orogastric tube placed for easy identification of the esophagus while dividing the fibers of the crus of the diaphragm.

With a supraceliac aortic clamp in place, a more controlled dissection can be carried down through the hematoma to identify and isolate the normal aortic segment proximal to the aneurysm. The aortic clamp can then be moved to this "aortic neck" to maintain hemostatic control while restoring perfusion to the viscera and kidneys. When infrarenal control has been established, full resuscitation can ensue. The aneurysm sac should be widely opened, and distal control of the iliac arteries can be initially achieved using intraluminal balloon occlusion catheters. If the retroperitoneal hematoma does not extend into the pelvis, direct dissection and control of the iliacs may be possible. Aortic reconstruction with a prosthetic tube graft is usually preferred if it is anatomically possible to decrease the duration of surgery.

Postoperatively patients require close monitoring in the intensive care unit, as the risks of abdominal compartment syndrome and colon ischemia are considerably higher than for elective AAA repair. If there is any concern at the completion of the procedure in terms of tightness of closure or elevation of peak airway pressures, consideration should be given to leaving the abdomen open. These cases are managed in a similar fashion to "damage control" surgery with temporary vacuum-assisted abdominal closure devices and delayed fascial closure when edema resolves [35]. If the abdomen is initially closed but the patient manifests symptoms of abdominal compartment syndrome postoperatively, bladder pressures can approximate intra-abdominal pressure [36]. Persistently high bladder pressures in a patient with elevated airway pressures, abdominal distention, difficulty with ventilation, oliguria, or unexplained hypotension should warrant an immediate return to the operating room. Reopening the abdominal cavity to relieve the abdominal compartment syndrome can be lifesaving.

Conclusion

Abdominal aortic aneurysms remain a serious clinical problem in our aging population. Ultrasound screening of appropriately selected people at risk can significantly reduce AAA-related mortality by detecting aneurysms early in their course. Endovascular therapy (discussed elsewhere) has emerged as a minimally invasive method of AAA repair which significantly reduces morbidity and mortality compared to open repair. Although endovascular surgery now accounts for 60–70 % of all AAA repairs, many patients will still require open surgery because of unsuitable anatomy or clinical circumstances. Surgeons managing these cases must have a working knowledge of the anatomy, techniques for aortic control, and vascular reconstructive alternatives to successfully repair an abdominal aortic aneurysm.

Aortic Dissection

Introduction

Acute aortic dissection is a relatively common condition affecting the thoracic or abdominal aorta that carries a high mortality rate if left untreated. A dissection involves an abnormal blood flow which separates the layers of the vessel wall. A focal intimal tear or injury usually triggers a dissection by allowing blood flow to gain entry and track between the muscular layers of the aortic wall. The extent and clinical severity of a dissection depend on multiple factors including location and size of the intimal injury, systemic blood pressure, and preexisting vascular disease.

The term "dissecting aneurysm" is often the source of considerable confusion and is thus worth addressing. Although a dissection and an aneurysm can occasionally occur in the same patient, it is important to note that they are two completely different clinical entities. The use of this misnomer is probably related to the association between chronic dissection and an increased incidence of aneurysm formation over time. This section will review the classification, epidemiology, physiology, clinical presentation, diagnosis, and treatment of acute aortic dissection, with a focus on care of these patients from the general surgeon's perspective.

Classification

The anatomic location of an acute aortic dissection usually determines its treatment pathway. The Stanford model has emerged as the simplest and most widely used classification system for aortic dissections (Fig. 21.1). A Stanford type A dissection is any dissection involving the ascending aorta, whereas Stanford type B encompasses all dissections which do not involve the ascending aorta. The distinction between Stanford type A and B dissections is of critical importance as the prognosis and management algorithms differ. The DeBakey model offers a slightly more detailed classification system (Fig. 21.3).

Epidemiology

The incidence of acute aortic dissection in the United States ranges from 2.9 to 3.5 per 100,000 person years. Risk factors for developing an aortic dissection include advanced age, hypertension, and smoking. Men are more frequently affected, with a male-to-female ratio of 4:1. Type A dissections occur nearly twice as often as type B dissections (62.5 % versus 37.5 %). Other risk factors for dissection include aortic wall structural abnormalities, the presence of a bicuspid aortic valve, and cocaine abuse. Congenital conditions such as coarctation of the aorta, annuloaortic ectasia, aortic arch hypoplasia, and hereditary collagen vascular conditions (Marfan syndrome and Ehlers-Danlos syndrome) have also been implicated. Marfan syndrome accounts for 50 % of cases of acute aortic dissection in patients younger than 40 years. Pregnancy is also a well-known risk factor for aortic dissection and may be related to the severe hypertension that occurs in women with preeclampsia.

Pathophysiology

A dissection can occur in any artery and is almost always related to an intimal injury or tear which acts as an entry point to the space between the layers of the arterial wall. Systemic arterial pressure drives blood flow between the arterial muscle layers causing the dissection to propagate. The extent and severity of the dissection depend on the size of the intimal tear, systemic arterial pressure, proximity to

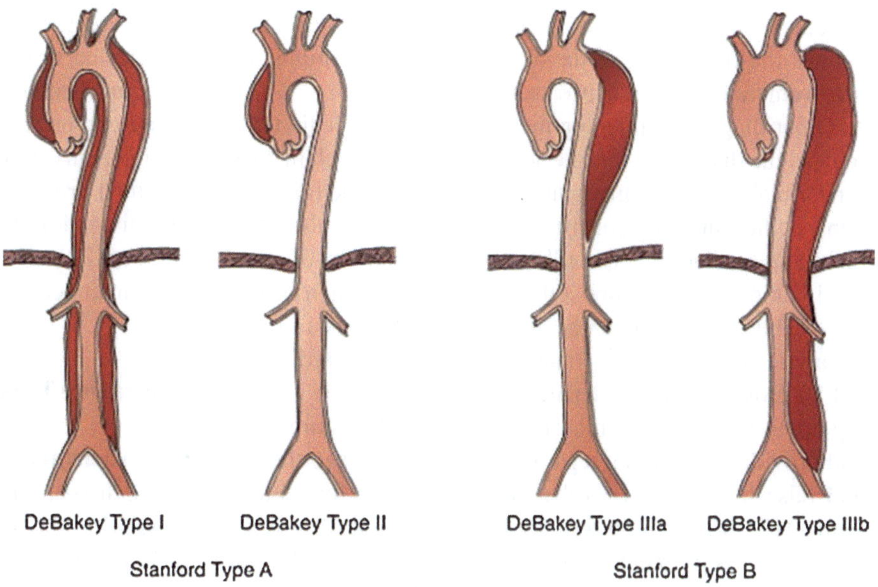

Fig. 21.3 Classification system for thoracic aortic dissection

branch points, and the development of reentry pathways. The dissection plane is referred to as the "false lumen" to differentiate it from the normal pathway for blood flow or "true lumen." In type B dissections, the intimal tear most commonly occurs at the level of the left subclavian artery because it is exposed to the greatest pressure fluctuations and shear stress. The dissection plane usually extends distally along the left posterolateral aspect of the aorta with the celiac, superior mesenteric, and right renal arteries being perfused by the true lumen, while the left renal artery arises from the false lumen. Although this is the most common flow pattern, any combination of visceral artery involvement is possible.

In type A dissection, the dissection flap starts in the ascending aorta and may propagate retrograde. Mortality in type A dissection typically involves one of four possible mechanisms: (1) The dissection flap may propagate into the coronary arteries, causing flow compromise and acute myocardial infarction. (2) The dissection flap may result in expansion of the pericardial sac causing cardiac tamponade. (3) The dissection may disrupt the valve apparatus causing severe aortic insufficiency. (4) The dissection may extend into the carotid arteries resulting in acute stroke.

Aortic branch compromise causing malperfusion represents a severe and potentially fatal complication of all types of acute aortic dissection. Any branch of the aorta may be affected, and the overall incidence of aortic branch compromise is 31 %. Propagation of the dissection into or adjacent to the ostium of a branch causes flow-limiting stenosis or complete branch occlusion depending on the local hemodynamics. The severity of malperfusion depends on the degree of branch compromise as well as the anatomic location and presence or absence of collateral blood flow.

Clinical Presentation

Approximately 93 % of patients with acute aortic dissection present with back, abdomen, or chest pain. Most patients describe the abrupt onset of a ripping or tearing sensation so severe that it prompts them to seek urgent treatment. About 5–10 % of patients present with syncope. Other acute clinical symptoms may represent manifestations of malperfusion related to branch vessel compromise. Abdominal pain out of proportion to the exam suggests possible mesenteric ischemia, while unilateral flank pain can indicate renal compromise. Upper extremity symptoms, such as pain, weakness, or paresthesias, can result from subclavian artery involvement, while lower extremity symptoms indicate compromise of the common iliac, external iliac, or common femoral arteries. Neurologic symptoms can result from cerebrovascular involvement or spinal cord ischemia which occurs in 2–10 % of patients.

Severe hypertension is the most consistent physical finding in patients presenting with acute aortic dissection. It is important to measure blood pressure in both upper extremities as dissection involving a subclavian artery can falsely depress the pressure in that arm. A comprehensive pulse and neurologic exam of the extremities helps evaluate for frequently encountered peripheral vascular complications triggered by the dissection.

Diagnostic Evaluation

CT angiography has emerged as the gold standard diagnostic imaging exam for acute aortic dissection with a sensitivity of 83–95 % and a specificity of 87–100 %. In addition to being extremely accurate, a CT of the thorax, abdomen, and pelvis defines the full extent of the dissection and determines the involvement of any branch vessels.

Other diagnostic imaging modalities can play adjunctive roles in the diagnosis of acute aortic dissection. A plain chest x-ray obtained in the emergency department can demonstrate nonspecific findings consistent with an aortic dissection including cardiac or aortic silhouette, displacement of aortic calcifications, and pleural effusions. Although a transthoracic echocardiogram can be useful in the diagnosis of type A aortic dissection, a transesophageal echocardiogram (TEE) provides a more detailed examination of the ascending aorta. A TEE can demonstrate the site of the intimal tear and provide information regarding flow dynamics in the true and false lumens. TEE is the standard of care for patients with a type A dissection who are being prepared for surgical repair. MRI is probably equivalent to CTA in terms of imaging quality; however, its limitations include lack of immediate availability and long examination times.

Treatment

Acute aortic dissection is a life-threatening condition that demands swift diagnosis and prompt treatment. Patients presenting to the emergency department with suspected acute aortic dissection should have a CT angiogram to establish the definitive diagnosis. Classifying the dissection as Stanford type A or B is the first branch point in the treatment algorithm. Patients with type A dissections require urgent surgical repair which will be briefly discussed in the next section. Patients with type B dissections should be evaluated for the presence of malperfusion with a thorough physical exam and review of imaging and lab results. Evidence of ischemia affecting the viscera, kidneys, or extremities warrants immediate surgical or endovascular intervention to treat the dissection or bypass the occluded branch vessel. Fortunately, most patients with acute type B dissections do not have any signs of malperfusion and require aggressive medical therapy to quickly control their hypertension.

Medical management of hypertension begins by establishing two large-bore IVs to begin intravenous infusion of antihypertensive agents. Heart rate control is also important because a reduced heart rate generates less shear stress and may minimize the propagation of the dissection. An intensive care unit (ICU) is usually the most appropriate setting for patients being treated for aortic dissection. Beta-blockers in combination with vasodilators as needed are the first-line agents used to achieve a goal of less than 120 mmHg for systolic blood pressure with a heart rate of less than 65 beats per minute. Sodium nitroprusside is a quick and effective antihypertensive and should be employed if beta-blockers fail to achieve adequate heart rate and blood pressure control. ICU care should include serial neurovascular exams and monitoring urine output. Once patients with type B dissections are hemodynamically stable with no evidence of end organ compromise, they should be followed regularly with imaging surveillance. The first follow-up CT scan should be obtained prior to discharge from the hospital to ensure that the dissection has not propagated. Following discharge, another CT scan at 3 months and then at 6-month intervals is recommended.

Operative Treatment of Aortic Dissection

Open Surgical Treatment

Acute dissection of the ascending thoracic aortic is an immediately life-threatening condition that requires emergent surgical repair. Left untreated, a type A dissection has a high early mortality rate that increases 2–3 % per hour. Cardiac surgeons usually repair type A dissections by resecting the aortic tear and replacing the ascending aorta with a prosthetic graft. The procedure usually requires hypothermic circulatory and may also require aortic valve replacement and reimplantation of the coronary arteries.

Surgical management of an acute type B aortic dissection differs from a type A dissection in terms of indications for surgery and urgency of repair. As discussed earlier, the first-line therapy for an acute type B dissection involves medical therapy to lower the blood pressure and reduce the heart rate. Indications for surgery include aortic rupture, end organ ischemia, or persistent pain despite adequate blood pressure control. In the modern era, open surgery for type B dissection is rarely performed and usually reserved for cases in which endovascular therapy fails or is not available. Surgical intervention involves a thoracotomy, proximal and distal control of the aorta, and replacement of the descending aorta with a prosthetic graft.

Endovascular Treatment

Endovascular therapy revolutionized the surgical management of acute descending thoracic aortic dissections. Intraluminal coverage of the intimal tear with an aortic endograft allows depressurization of the dissection plane and eventual thrombosis of the false lumen. The aortic endograft can be inserted remotely through the common femoral artery which is surgically exposed or percutaneously accessed. As a minimally invasive technique that does not require a thoracotomy or aortic clamping, endovascular therapy significantly reduces perioperative morbidity and mortality compared to open surgery. Commercially available aortic endografts have been approved for the treatment of patients with type B dissections who have an indication for surgery.

Some vascular specialists advocate endovascular repair for all patients with acute type B dissections regardless of symptoms or response to medical therapy. Preemptive placement of an endograft could theoretically prevent future complications and degeneration of the dissection into an aneurysm. Although this aggressive, interventional approach has intuitive appeal, clinical studies have not shown a benefit for endovascular repair over medical management for patients with uncomplicated type B aortic dissections. Current guidelines recommend endovascular therapy only for patients with type B dissections who have an indication for surgery as detailed in the previous section.

Although endovascular therapy for aortic dissections is safer than open surgery, complications can still occur. Spinal cord ischemia resulting in weakness or permanent paralysis is an uncommon but devastating complication that can occur despite a technically successful endovascular repair. Blood flow to the spinal cord involves the vertebral, intercostal, lumbar, and internal iliac arteries, and any interruption of this segmental blood supply can lead to spinal cord ischemia. Covering a long length of thoracic aorta with a stent graft increases the risk of spinal cord ischemia by occluding intercostals arteries. Likewise, patients who have had a previous aortic aneurysm repair may have lost perfusion to several lumbar arteries and one or both internal iliac arteries making them more prone to spinal cord ischemia. In some cases the stent graft intentionally covers the origin of the left subclavian artery in order to seal the proximal intimal tear. Loss of antegrade flow through the left subclavian and left vertebral arteries detracts from segmental spinal cord perfusion and could increase the risk for spinal cord ischemia. Depending on the clinical scenario, a carotid-subclavian bypass may be appropriate to maintain perfusion to the left subclavian and left vertebral arteries in patients who require proximal placement of the stent graft. Other measures to reduce the risk of spinal cord ischemia include placing a lumbar drain and maintaining an adequate blood pressure. Spinal cord perfusion can be calculated by subtracting the cerebrospinal pressure from the mean arterial pressure. By allowing controlled drainage of cerebrospinal fluid, a lumbar drain can maintain a low cerebrospinal pressure and augment spinal cord perfusion. Efforts to maintain adequate mean arterial pressure with intravascular volume and vasopressors as necessary will also help maintain spinal cord perfusion.

Malperfusion syndrome associated with acute aortic dissection usually requires adjunctive procedures to restore perfusion to the compromised branch. Surgical bypasses route blood flow around the occluded branch orifice and can restore perfusion to the carotid, subclavian, common femoral, mesenteric, or renal arteries. In some cases, endovascular interventions can also restore flow to critical aortic branches. These advanced endovascular techniques involve manipulating wires, balloons, and stents to create and maintain a fenestration through the dissection flap and into the affected branch vessel.

Outcomes

The high mortality after open surgery for type B aortic dissection (ranging from 6 to 67 %) reflects the magnitude of surgery and the fact that most procedures are performed under emergency circumstances [37]. After aortic stent grafts became widely available, multiple case series reported lower mortality rates after endovascular repair of aortic dissection. The EuroSTAR (European Collaborators on Stent/Graft Techniques for Aortic Aneurysm Repair) registry accumulated a large data set on 131 patients with aortic dissection who were treated with stent grafts. Primary technical success was achieved in 89 % with a 30-day mortality of 8.4 %, a postoperative paraplegia rate of 0.8 %, and a 1-year survival rate of 90 % [38]. Although these results are promising, an accurate evaluation of the durability and overall value of endovascular therapy for aortic dissection requires larger studies with longer follow-up.

Natural History and Follow-up

The most common late complication of aortic dissection is aneurysmal degeneration. An estimated 25–40 % of patients who survive an acute aortic dissection develop aneurysmal dilation of the affected segment despite adequate medical management. Long-term follow-up should include a CT scan every 3–6 months for the first 2 years after the initial diagnosis. If the involved segment of aorta is relatively stable after 2 years, surveillance imaging can be performed less frequently.

Conclusion

Acute dissection represents a common but treatable condition that can affect any segment of the aorta. Successful management of acute aortic dissection begins with clinical acumen to suspect the diagnosis and confirmatory imaging to classify the dissection as involving the ascending or descending thoracic aorta. Ascending aortic dissections always require immediate surgical repair performed by cardiac surgery. In contrast, the treatment of dissections involving the descending thoracic aorta varies according to the symptoms and arterial flow patterns. Uncomplicated dissections which maintain perfusion to the aortic branches call for medical therapy to control blood pressure followed by surveillance imaging. Malperfusion caused by compromised blood flow to the bowel, kidneys, or extremities warrants emergent surgical or endovascular intervention to restore perfusion. Chronic dissections that become aneurysmal may require elective intervention to halt the growth of the aneurysm and prevent rupture. Endovascular therapy appears to be an effective and safer alternative to open surgical repair for thoracic aortic dissections.

Traumatic Aortic Injuries: Endovascular Repair

Introduction

Since its first description in 1997, endovascular repair has emerged as the treatment of choice for traumatic aortic injury (TAI) [39]. In 2007 approximately 65 % of trauma centers performed endovascular repair for patients with TAI compared with none just 10 years earlier [40]. The minimally invasive nature and ability of endovascular therapy to improve clinical outcomes has been the driving force behind its rapid rise in popularity. Prospective multicenter reviews and meta-analyses reported significantly reduced mortality rates for patients with TAI undergoing an endovascular repair compared to traditional open surgery [41–43]. Although overall mortality for all TAI repairs (excluding patients presenting in extremis) decreased from 22 to 13 %, mortality in the endovascular treatment group dropped even lower to 7.2 %. Endovascular repair had a more profound impact on the complication of spinal cord ischemia decreasing the rate of paraplegia by a factor of 10 from 8.7 to 0.8 % [40].

Early in its development, endovascular repair for TAI involved the use of stent grafts which were designed for treating thoracic aneurysms and dissections in large atherosclerotic aortas. Applying these devices to the normal, small-caliber aortas typically encountered in young trauma patients created technical problems related to excessive oversizing and inflexibility of the graft. Despite reducing mortality and paraplegia rates, endovascular therapy had a disconcertingly high rate of graft-related failure during the early experience [42]. While endoleaks caused most endovascular treatment failures (approximately 15 % of cases), stent graft collapse, often requiring explantation, was also regularly reported [42, 44]. Endovascular technology continues to evolve as demonstrated by the current generation of stent grafts which come in a wide range of diameters and are designed to conform to the acute angulation at the aortic arch in young patients.

Initial Evaluation and Imaging

Approximately 85 % of patients who sustain a TAI die at the scene of injury. If TAI is not immediately fatal, bleeding from the aorta is contained by the vessel wall and mediastinum allowing some patients to survive to reach the hospital. Although these patients have temporary hemostasis with regard to their aortic injury, the majority will die within 24–48 h in the absence of treatment [45]. Motor vehicle crashes cause most cases of TAI; however, any trauma involving sudden deceleration of the chest, such as a pedestrian struck or a fall from height, can result in a similar injury [46]. The magnitude of energy necessary to inflict a TAI often results in concomitant, potentially fatal injuries of the head, abdomen, and musculoskeletal system. Contrary to popular belief, hypotension in patients with TAI who survive to reach the hospital is almost always caused by these associated injuries, not the aortic injury. One of the principles for managing multiply injured patients with TAI is to promptly treat whichever injury poses the most immediate threat to life. Following this guideline may involve giving priority to surgery for head, abdominal, or orthopedic injuries while delaying intervention for the relatively stable TAI. Often TAI occurs in association with a pulmonary contusion which limits the ability to ventilate a patient on one lung, further complicating potential open repair of the aortic injury.

Modern rapid CT scanners now available in most emergency departments have allowed CT angiography (CTA) to replace catheter-directed angiography as the screening exam of choice for TAI. In contrast to catheter-directed angiography, CTA is a noninvasive, readily available exam that does not require calling in a specialized clinical team. CTA proves to be more sensitive than catheter-based angiography and has the advantage of evaluating for other coexisting injuries [47]. Other imaging modalities include MRI, intravascular ultrasonography, and transesophageal echocardiography. The latter two modalities can be particularly useful in cases where the mechanism of injury or the chest radiograph raises the suspicion of a TAI, but the patient requires immediate transfer to the operating room for surgery to address other life-threatening injuries before a chest CTA can be completed.

Timing of Treatment

Consensus opinion on the time course for treating TAI has changed over the past 40 years. Clinical observations provide strong support for the notion that patients who present with a stable, contained TAI can be managed medically in the short term to allow treatment of other life-threatening injuries [46, 48, 49]. Medical treatment involves both inotropic and blood pressure control to reduce aortic wall stress until the TAI can be definitively repaired. This treatment strategy can create a dilemma in patients with traumatic brain injury in whom elevation of the systemic blood pressure is required to improve cerebral perfusion. These patients are ideal candidates for prompt endovascular repair of the TAI. Once the endovascular stent graft is placed, arterial blood pressure control can be liberalized to allow treatment of other injuries including optimizing cerebral perfusion. Endovascular therapy also offers an expeditious, minimally invasive treatment for patients with numerous coexisting injuries and for frail and elderly patients who present a prohibitively high risk for open surgical repair.

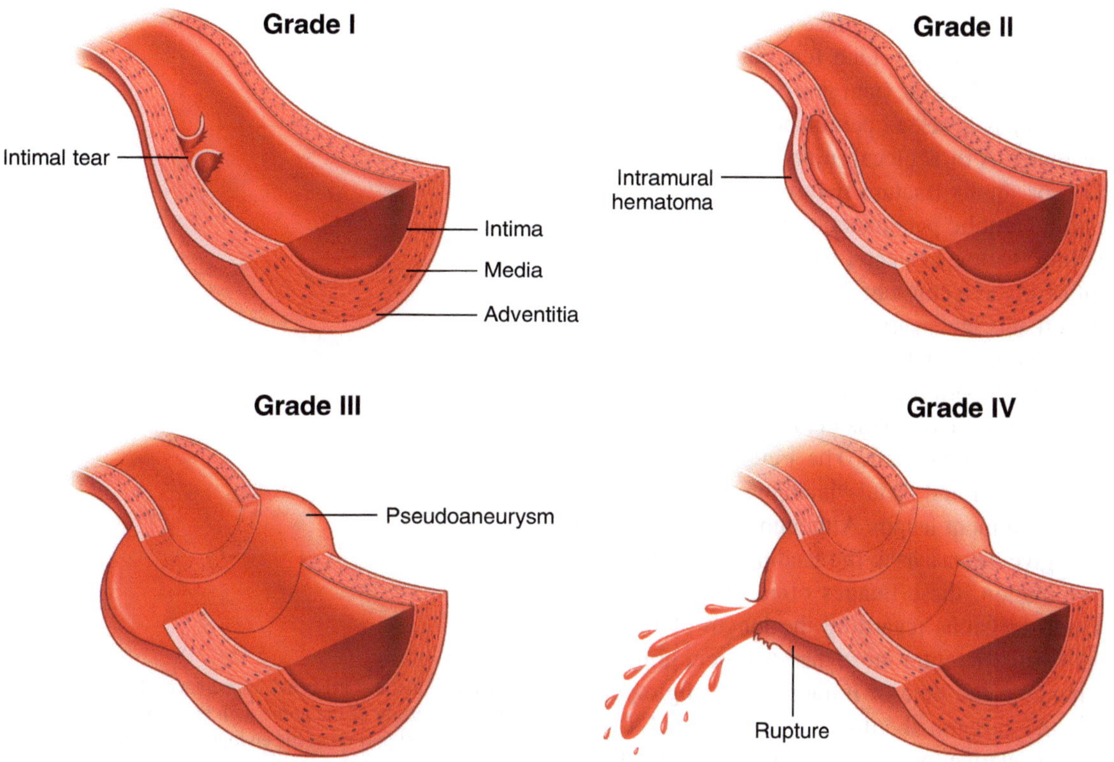

Fig. 21.4 Classification system for traumatic aortic injury (Adapted from Azizzadeh et al. [55])

Minimal Aortic Injury

A patient with TAI and a CT scan showing a large aortic wall defect, pseudoaneurysm, and/or mediastinal blood clearly requires definitive repair usually in the form of an endovascular stent graft. Improved image resolution now allows CTA to identify more subtle lesion and irregularities of the thoracic aorta. The definition and optimal treatment for these so-called minimal aortic injuries remains unclear. One classification scheme defines a type I injury as an intimal defect, type II as a hematoma, type III as an aortic pseudoaneurysm, and type IV as rupture of the aorta (Fig. 21.4). Most vascular specialists would follow type I lesions with surveillance imaging and repair type II through IV lesions. Patients with small pseudoaneurysms (1 or 2 mm diameter), and no associated hematoma may have a minimal aortic injury that does not require repair. Although reports suggest that up to 50 % of minimal aortic injuries develop into pseudoaneurysms within 8 weeks of injury, it remains unclear whether endovascular repair is indicated given the potential long-term complications of the stent graft, particularly among young trauma victims [50].

The location of small aortic pseudoaneurysms (1–2 mm in diameter) and the associated aortic anatomy may help guide treatment decisions. Favorable anatomy for placing a stent graft usually predicts a successful and durable outcome after endovascular repair. In contrast, attempting to place a stent for lesions in proximity to an angulated aortic arch with a short proximal landing zone often results in device failure [44]. If the anatomy appears unfavorable for endovascular repair, these small lesions may be followed with serial imaging and considered for open repair only if they enlarge over time.

Preoperative Planning

Preoperative planning for endovascular TAI repair starts by assessing the nature and severity of coexisting injuries. It is particularly important to identify intracranial or intra-abdominal bleeding which could be exacerbated by the use of anticoagulation during endovascular repair. Elevated intracranial pressure in patients with brain injuries may render them intolerant of the supine position. Although it is feasible to elevate the patient's upper body and still successfully perform an endovascular repair, it requires foresight to secure a flexible table that allows fluoroscopic imaging. Thoracic endovascular procedures performed with a patient's upper body elevated can be complicated by strokes due to air emboli. In this situation, meticulous measures must be followed to avoid introduction of air during angiographic imaging and stent graft deployment.

Vascular access for endograft placement usually involves the common femoral arteries. One femoral artery is surgically exposed to introduce the stent graft, while the contralateral femoral artery is accessed percutaneously to advance a diagnostic catheter. A direct local injury or groin hematoma from a pelvic or femur fracture may compromise femoral artery access and require percutaneous access to the left brachial artery. Introducing a catheter from this location has the advantage of acting as a constant fluoroscopic marker for the origin of the left subclavian artery.

Choosing an appropriately sized endograft requires careful review of the preoperative CTA. The diameter of the normal aorta just proximal and just distal to the injury determines the diameter of the stent graft. The longitudinal distance between the proximal and distal "landing zones" estimates the total aortic treatment length. Although composite reconstructions can give a sense as to the landing zone length and degree of angulation, these images often oversimplify the anatomy. Final decisions regarding the length of the stent graft and the requirement for more than one stent graft often have to be made at the time of intraoperative angiography. Additionally, the surgeon should be aware that a CT scan obtained during relative hypotension can underestimate the true diameter of thoracic aorta and access vessels [51].

Stent graft placement should also take the vertebral artery anatomy into consideration. Achieving an adequate proximal seal may require covering the origin of the left subclavian artery with the stent graft to lengthen the proximal landing zone. Patients with a dominant left vertebral artery are at risk for cerebrovascular ischemia if an aortic stent graft suddenly interrupts antegrade flow through the left subclavian artery. A left carotid-subclavian artery bypass performed before placing the endograft can decrease the risk of this complication.

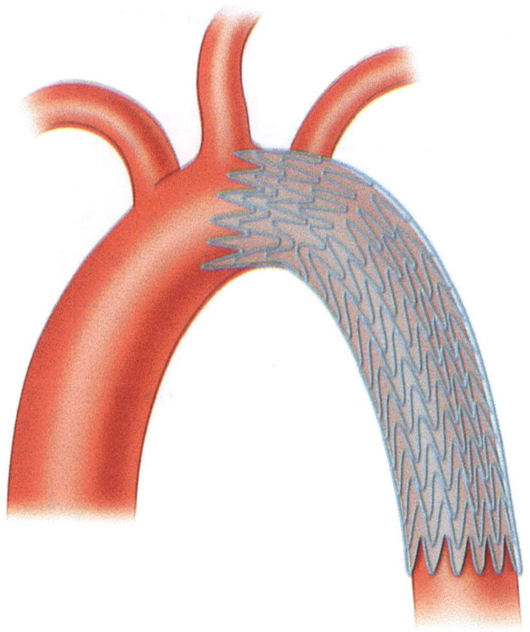

Fig. 21.5 Classic "bird-beak" appearance when endograft extends into the horizontal portion of the aortic arch resulting from incomplete apposition of the proximal portion of the endograft to the lesser curvature of the aorta. When severe, this lack of apposition can lead to device collapse

Operative Approach

General anesthesia for endovascular TAI repair optimizes the quality of intraoperative imaging by minimizing patient movement and providing the ability to suspend respirations at critical times during graft placement. A lumbar drain to decrease the risk of spinal cord ischemia is not routinely used. Most TAI pose a low risk for postoperative paralysis because they are relatively focal injuries that require a limited length of endograft coverage and rarely affect the distal thoracic aorta.

After obtaining vascular access, a diagnostic catheter with radiopaque markers is advanced into the proximal aortic arch to perform an arch aortogram. The initial aortogram maps the location of the injury and its proximity to the left subclavian artery so that a proximal landing site can be chosen. Before committing to an endovascular repair, the aortogram should be carefully reviewed to evaluate the angulation of the aorta particularly where the proximal most portion of the endograft will lie. In some cases it may be necessary to accept a shorter landing zone instead of extending the endograft into the horizontal portion of the aortic arch. Placing a stent graft with its leading edge extending beyond the curve of the aorta results in a "bird-beak" effect (Fig. 21.5). The hemodynamic forces imposed on the "bird-beak" portion of the endograft can lead to catastrophic complications including fatal stent graft collapse [52]. Patients with a combination of a severely angled aortic arch and a short proximal landing zone should be strongly considered for primary open repair if they have a reasonably low risk for surgery.

Regardless of the aortic pathology, an endovascular stent graft placed in a short landing zone has a higher risk of device-associated failure. A shorter landing zone may be acceptable in TAI because the rest of the aorta is normal and the stent graft only needs to cover the focal injury to allow it to heal. Thoracic aortic aneurysms present a greater technical challenge since they require the endograft to establish a permanent seal to the aorta which is often diffusely enlarged. Although aortography with a marker catheter is accurate for length measurements, it is an unreliable way of determining aortic diameter. The diameter of the stent graft should be based on diameter measurements from the CT scan. Intravascular ultrasound performed at the time of surgery can also be used to measure or confirm the aortic diameter.

As noted above, the access vessel of choice is usually the common femoral artery. Although young trauma patients often have small-caliber femoral arteries, they are usually free of disease and elastic allowing insertion of the large stent graft delivery sheath. Fortunately, advances in endovascular technology have reduced the size of thoracic endograft introduction systems. Some devices (e.g., the Gore TAG stent graft) can be advanced into position without a sheath provided the patient has relatively straight, disease-free vessels.

During the initial phases of vascular access, the wire can unintentionally enter the area of injury or coil in the aortic pseudoaneurysm instead of advancing into the proximal aortic arch. To avoid this obstacle, the pigtail catheter should be formed in the distal thoracic aorta and advanced in coiled configuration across the area of injury. Extra stiff wires that are typically used for endovascular aneurysms may be too stiff to negotiate the tight aortic arch angulation of a young patient. We have found the Amplatz wire is a reasonable compromise between stiffness and flexibility [53].

Thoracic aortic endografting usually warrants intraoperative systemic anticoagulation with heparin. In patients with serious head injuries or solid organ bleeding, it may be reasonable to forego anticoagulation. Ideally these patients would have straightforward aortic anatomy which allows for a short procedure time. If systemic anticoagulation is not used, the sheaths and the access vessels should be liberally flushed with heparinized saline solution to reduce the risk of local thrombosis.

Potential complications of left subclavian artery coverage during endograft treatment include left upper extremity ischemia and stroke, particularly if the left vertebral artery is dominant. In practice, most patients with TAI do not require complete coverage of the left subclavian artery to achieve a successful endovascular repair. In our experience, only 21 % of patients undergoing endovascular TAI repair required partial or complete left subclavian artery coverage, and there were no complications associated with coverage [44].

In young patients the aorta often has hyperdynamic arterial pulsations which can alter the position of the stent graft as it is deployed. When endograft placement requires precision measured in millimeters, there are times when temporary cessation of cardiac pulsations is desirable. Temporary cardiac arrest to facilitate stent graft placement was felt to be necessary in approximately half the cases using older devices. Rapid ventricular pacing or adenosine can be used to create temporary asystole. Administering an 18 mg dose of adenosine usually achieves a temporary arrest lasting several seconds.

After positioning and deploying the stent graft, a completion aortogram should be performed to confirm the patency of the arch vessels and verify the exclusion of the aortic injury or pseudoaneurysm. Balloon dilatation is generally not performed unless an endoleak is present which could be resolved by device dilation.

Following successful endovascular TAI repair, follow-up CT angiography is generally performed within a week of surgery and before the patient's hospital discharge. Patients return for a follow-up visit within 2 weeks after discharge for evaluation of the groin incision and to establish a point of contact for future visits. Follow-up CT angiography and frontal and lateral chest radiographs are obtained at 6 months and then yearly thereafter. Because of concerns about radiation exposure from CT scans in young patients, intervals between visits are extended to more than 1 year in cases where the stent graft appears to be stable [54].

Available Thoracic Endovascular Stent Grafts

The only thoracic devices approved for treatment of TAI are the Conformable TAG (CTAG) device manufactured by Gore and the Medtronic Valiant Thoracic Stent Graft with the Captivia delivery system. The Zenith TX2 device has been approved for treatment of thoracic aortic aneurysms but does not have clearance for treatment of TAI. The stent grafts are now available in a wide range of diameters and lengths, including tapered configurations. In contrast to the early stent grafts, these devices have been designed to conform to angulated aortic arches and resist device collapse.

Conclusion

Endovascular therapy has revolutionized the treatment of traumatic aortic injury. Both retrospective and prospective studies clearly demonstrate that endovascular therapy for TAI reduces the mortality and paraplegia rate compared to open surgical repair. Although the success of stent grafts must be tempered by reports of technical complications and graft collapse, endovascular therapy shows no sign of receding. Redesigned stent grafts now available promise to expand the treatment indications and dramatically reduce the rate of device failure. The most significant unresolved issue regarding endovascular repair involves the long-term durability and natural history of stent grafts placed in young patients. Regular follow-up is recommended; however, this can be difficult in the population of trauma patients who are more mobile and do not typically seek extended medical care after recovering from their injuries. Over the next several decades, follow-up studies are necessary to detect long-term complications of stent grafts and quantify the radiation exposure incurred by imaging surveillance.

References

1. Johnston KW, Rutherford RB, Tilson MD, Shah DM, Hollier L, Stanley JC. Suggested standards for reporting on arterial aneurysms. Subcommittee on Reporting Standards for Arterial Aneurysms, Ad Hoc Committee on Reporting Standards, Society for Vascular Surgery and North American Chapter, International Society for Cardiovascular Surgery. J Vasc Surg. 1991;13(3):452–8.
2. Silverberg E, Boring CC, Squires TS. Cancer statistics, 1990. CA Cancer J Clin. 1990;40(1):9–26.
3. Adam DJ, Mohan IV, Stuart WP, Bain M, Bradbury AW. Community and hospital outcome from ruptured abdominal aortic aneurysm within the catchment area of a regional vascular surgical service. J Vasc Surg. 1999;30(5):922–8.
4. Craig SR, Wilson RG, Walker AJ, Murie JA. Abdominal aortic aneurysm: still missing the message. Br J Surg. 1993;80(4):450–2.
5. Fleming C, Whitlock EP, Beil TL, Lederle FA. Screening for abdominal aortic aneurysm: a best-evidence systematic review for the U.S. Preventive Services Task Force. Ann Intern Med. 2005;142(3):203–11.
6. Darwood R, Earnshaw JJ, Turton G, et al. Twenty-year review of abdominal aortic aneurysm screening in men in the county of Gloucestershire, United Kingdom. J Vasc Surg. 2012;56(1):8–13.
7. Lee ES, Pickett E, Hedayati N, Dawson DL, Pevec WC. Implementation of an aortic screening program in clinical practice: implications for the Screen For Abdominal Aortic Aneurysms Very Efficiently (SAAAVE) Act. J Vasc Surg. 2009; 49(5):1107–11.
8. Chervu A, Clagett GP, Valentine RJ, Myers SI, Rossi PJ. Role of physical examination in detection of abdominal aortic aneurysms. Surgery. 1995;117(4):454–7.
9. Pavone P, Di Cesare E, Di Renzi P, et al. Abdominal aortic aneurysm evaluation: comparison of US, CT, MRI, and angiography. Magn Reson Imaging. 1990;8(3):199–204.
10. Ailawadi G, Eliason JL, Upchurch Jr GR. Current concepts in the pathogenesis of abdominal aortic aneurysm. J Vasc Surg. 2003; 38(3):584–8.
11. Melton 3rd LJ, Bickerstaff LK, Hollier LH, et al. Changing incidence of abdominal aortic aneurysms: a population-based study. Am J Epidemiol. 1984;120(3):379–86.
12. Webster MW, Ferrell RE, St Jean PL, Majumder PP, Fogel SR, Steed DL. Ultrasound screening of first-degree relatives of patients with an abdominal aortic aneurysm. J Vasc Surg. 1991;13(1):9–13; discussion 13–4.
13. Vorp DA, Raghavan ML, Webster MW. Mechanical wall stress in abdominal aortic aneurysm: influence of diameter and asymmetry. J Vasc Surg. 1998;27(4):632–9.
14. Nevitt MP, Ballard DJ, Hallett Jr JW. Prognosis of abdominal aortic aneurysms. A population-based study. N Engl J Med. 1989; 321(15):1009–14.
15. Sterpetti AV, Cavallaro A, Cavallari N, et al. Factors influencing the rupture of abdominal aortic aneurysms. Surg Gynecol Obstet. 1991;173(3):175–8.
16. Lederle FA, Wilson SE, Johnson GR, et al. Immediate repair compared with surveillance of small abdominal aortic aneurysms. N Engl J Med. 2002;346(19):1437–44.
17. United Kingdom Small Aneurysm Trial Participants. Long-term outcomes of immediate repair compared with surveillance of small abdominal aortic aneurysms. N Engl J Med. 2002;346(19):1445–52.
18. Faggioli GL, Stella A, Gargiulo M, Tarantini S, D'Addato M, Ricotta JJ. Morphology of small aneurysms: definition and impact on risk of rupture. Am J Surg. 1994;168(2):131–5.
19. Limet R, Sakalihassan N, Albert A. Determination of the expansion rate and incidence of rupture of abdominal aortic aneurysms. J Vasc Surg. 1991;14(4):540–8.
20. Lederle FA, Johnson GR, Wilson SE, et al. The aneurysm detection and management study screening program: validation cohort and final results. Aneurysm Detection and Management Veterans Affairs Cooperative Study Investigators. Arch Intern Med. 2000; 160(10):1425–30.
21. Dent TL, Lindenauer SM, Ernst CB, Fry WJ. Multiple arteriosclerotic arterial aneurysms. Arch Surg. 1972;105(2):338–44.
22. Hultgren R, Larsson E, Wahlgren CM, Swedenborg J. Female and elderly abdominal aortic aneurysm patients more commonly have concurrent thoracic aortic aneurysm. Ann Vasc Surg. 2012;26(7): 918–23.
23. Waterhouse DF, Cahill RA, Sheehan F, Sheehan SJ. Concomitant detection of systemic atherosclerotic disease while screening for abdominal aortic aneurysm. World J Surg. 2006;30(7):1350–9.
24. Qureshi AI, Alexandrov AV, Tegeler CH, Hobson 2nd RW, Dennis Baker J, Hopkins LN. Guidelines for screening of extracranial carotid artery disease: a statement for healthcare professionals from the multidisciplinary practice guidelines committee of the American Society of Neuroimaging; cosponsored by the Society of Vascular and Interventional Neurology. J Neuroimaging. 2007;17(1):19–47.
25. Nitecki SS, Hallett Jr JW, Stanson AW, et al. Inflammatory abdominal aortic aneurysms: a case-control study. J Vasc Surg. 1996; 23(5):860–8; discussion 8–9.
26. Tennant WG, Hartnell GG, Baird RN, Horrocks M. Radiologic investigation of abdominal aortic aneurysm disease: comparison of three modalities in staging and the detection of inflammatory change. J Vasc Surg. 1993;17(4):703–9.
27. Baskerville PA, Blakeney CG, Young AE, Browse NL. The diagnosis and treatment of peri-aortic fibrosis ('inflammatory' aneurysms). Br J Surg. 1983;70(6):381–5.
28. Gomes MN, Choyke PL, Wallace RB. Infected aortic aneurysms. A changing entity. Ann Surg. 1992;215(5):435–42.
29. Reddy DJ, Shepard AD, Evans JR, Wright DJ, Smith RF, Ernst CB. Management of infected aortoiliac aneurysms. Arch Surg. 1991;126(7):873–8; discussion 8–9.
30. Oderich GS, Panneton JM, Bower TC, et al. Infected aortic aneurysms: aggressive presentation, complicated early outcome, but durable results. J Vasc Surg. 2001;34(5):900–8.
31. Clagett GP, Bowers BL, Lopez-Viego MA, et al. Creation of a neo-aortoiliac system from lower extremity deep and superficial veins. Ann Surg. 1993;218(3):239–48; discussion 48–9.
32. Brewster DC, Cambria RP, Moncure AC, et al. Aortocaval and iliac arteriovenous fistulas: recognition and treatment. J Vasc Surg. 1991;13(2):253–64; discussion 64–5.
33. Egorova N, Giacovelli J, Greco G, Gelijns A, Kent CK, McKinsey JF. National outcomes for the treatment of ruptured abdominal aortic aneurysm: comparison of open versus endovascular repairs. J Vasc Surg. 2008;48(5):1092–100, 100 e1–2.
34. Alric P, Ryckwaert F, Picot MC, et al. Ruptured aneurysm of the infrarenal abdominal aorta: impact of age and postoperative complications on mortality. Ann Vasc Surg. 2003;17(3):277–83.
35. Akers Jr DL, Fowl RJ, Kempczinski RF, Davis K, Hurst JM, Uhl S. Temporary closure of the abdominal wall by use of silicone rubber sheets after operative repair of ruptured abdominal aortic aneurysms. J Vasc Surg. 1991;14(1):48–52.
36. Loftus IM, Thompson MM. The abdominal compartment syndrome following aortic surgery. Eur J Vasc Endovasc Surg. 2003;25(2): 97–109.
37. Bortone AS, Schena S, D'Agostino D, Dialetto G, Paradiso V, Mannatrizio G, et al. Immediate versus delayed endovascular treatment of post-traumatic aortic pseudoaneurysms and type B dissections: retrospective analysis and premises to the upcoming European trial. Circulation. 2002;96 suppl 1:234–40.
38. Harris PL, Vallabhaneni SR, Desgranges P, Becquemin JP, van Marrewijk C, Laheij RJ. Incidence and risk factors of late rupture, conversion, and death after endovascular repair of infrarenal aortic

aneurysms: The EUROSTAR experience. J Vasc Surg. 2000; 32:739–49.
39. Semba CP, Kato N, Kee ST, et al. Acute rupture of the descending thoracic aorta: repair with use of endovascular stent-grafts. J Vasc Interv Radiol. 1997;8(3):337–42.
40. Demetriades D, Velmahos GC, Scalea TM, et al. Operative repair or endovascular stent graft in blunt traumatic thoracic aortic injuries: results of an American Association for the Surgery of Trauma Multicenter Study. J Trauma. 2008;64(3):561–70; discussion 70–1.
41. Tang GL, Tehrani HY, Usman A, et al. Reduced mortality, paraplegia, and stroke with stent graft repair of blunt aortic transections: a modern meta-analysis. J Vasc Surg. 2008;47(3):671–5.
42. Demetriades D, Velmahos GC, Scalea TM, et al. Diagnosis and treatment of blunt thoracic aortic injuries: changing perspectives. J Trauma. 2008;64(6):1415–8; discussion 8–9.
43. Xenos ES, Abedi NN, Davenport DL, et al. Meta-analysis of endovascular vs open repair for traumatic descending thoracic aortic rupture. J Vasc Surg. 2008;48(5):1343–51.
44. Neschis DG, Moainie S, Flinn WR, Scalea TM, Bartlett ST, Griffith BP. Endograft repair of traumatic aortic injury-a technique in evolution: a single institution's experience. Ann Surg. 2009;250(3): 377–82.
45. Parmley LF, Mattingly TW, Manion WC, Jahnke Jr EJ. Nonpenetrating traumatic injury of the aorta. Circulation. 1958;17(6):1086–101.
46. Fabian TC, Richardson JD, Croce MA, et al. Prospective study of blunt aortic injury: Multicenter Trial of the American Association for the Surgery of Trauma. J Trauma. 1997;42(3):374–80; discussion 80–3.
47. Fabian TC, Davis KA, Gavant ML, et al. Prospective study of blunt aortic injury: helical CT is diagnostic and antihypertensive therapy reduces rupture. Ann Surg. 1998;227(5):666–76; discussion 76–7.
48. Kipfer B, Leupi F, Schuepbach P, Friedli D, Althaus U. Acute traumatic rupture of the thoracic aorta: immediate or delayed surgical repair? Eur J Cardiothorac Surg. 1994;8(1):30–3.
49. Pate JW, Fabian TC, Walker W. Traumatic rupture of the aortic isthmus: an emergency? World J Surg. 1995;19(1):119–25; discussion 25–6.
50. Malhotra AK, Fabian TC, Croce MA, Weiman DS, Gavant ML, Pate JW. Minimal aortic injury: a lesion associated with advancing diagnostic techniques. J Trauma. 2001;51(6):1042–8.
51. van Prehn J, van Herwaarden JA, Muhs BE, Arnofsky A, Moll FL, Verhagen HJ. Difficulties with endograft sizing in a patient with traumatic rupture of the thoracic aorta: the possible influence of hypovolemic shock. J Vasc Surg. 2008;47(6):1333–6.
52. Idu MM, Reekers JA, Balm R, Ponsen KJ, de Mol BA, Legemate DA. Collapse of a stent-graft following treatment of a traumatic thoracic aortic rupture. J Endovasc Ther. 2005;12(4):503–7.
53. Neschis DG, Moaine S, Gutta R, et al. Twenty consecutive cases of endograft repair of traumatic aortic disruption: lessons learned. J Vasc Surg. 2007;45(3):487–92.
54. Brenner DJ, Hall EJ. Computed tomography–an increasing source of radiation exposure. N Engl J Med. 2007;357(22):2277–84.
55. Azizzadeh A, et al. Blunt traumatic aortic injury: initial experience with endovascular repair. J Vasc Surg. 2009;49:1403–8.

Non-atherosclerotic Vascular Disease: Vasculitis, Popliteal Entrapment, Hypercoagulable

22

Linda M. Harris and James Lukan

Hypercoagulable Disorders

Introduction

Hemostatic disorders increase the risk of perioperative and intraoperative complications. For patients with hypercoagulable states, the risk of venous thromboembolic (VTE) complications depends on the specific abnormality as well as the presence of additional stressors such as surgical intervention and immobilization. Table 22.1 shows the risk of the first VTE episode associated with various hypercoagulable states [1]. Approximately 60–80 % of patients with decreased anticoagulant activity have a VTE episode by 45 years of age [2]. Abnormalities that affect the arterial system are also relevant to surgeons who treat patients with arterial disease, including, for example, patients who require arteriovenous access for hemodialysis (Table 22.2) [3–5]. Although patients with bleeding disorders should also be assessed preoperatively, these conditions are not covered in this chapter.

Normal hemostasis involves a series of events culminating in platelet plug formation and thrombin generation. Abnormalities at any stage of this cascade can increase the risk of abnormal bleeding or thrombosis. Hypercoagulable disorders result from either an increase in procoagulant activity or a decrease in anticoagulant activity. Although abnormalities associated with decreased anticoagulant are rare, occurring in less than 1 % of the population, they place patients at higher risk for thrombosis than the more commonly encountered disorders associated with increased procoagulant activity [6].

L.M. Harris, MD (✉)
Division of Vascular Surgery, Department of Surgery, Kaleida Health Buffalo General Medical Center, 100 High Street B-7, Buffalo, NY 14203, USA
e-mail: Lharris@KaleidaHealth.org

J. Lukan, MD
Department of Surgery, Erie County Medical Center, University of Buffalo, Buffalo, NY, USA

Despite being recognized for centuries, the first hereditary hypercoagulable state, antithrombin deficiency, was not characterized until 1965 [7]. Over the last 50 years, additional hypercoagulable disorders have been identified including: protein C deficiency, protein S deficiency, factor V Leiden (or activated protein C resistance), prothrombin gene mutation (or G20210A), dysfibrinogenemia, and hyperhomocysteinemia. It is clear that other coagulation disorders exist but remain unspecified and undetectable by the currently available diagnostic tests. Therefore, patients with prior clotting episodes or a strong family history of thrombosis despite "negative" workups should be considered at higher risk for thrombosis when they are placed in prothrombotic situations such as surgery.

Hypercoagulable testing should be considered for patients with unexplained, recurrent, or atypically located VTE and for patients with a strong family history of VTE. Testing should generally be delayed until the thrombotic episode has resolved and the patient can safely stop anticoagulation. Most hypercoagulable disorders cannot be detected during the acute phase of thrombosis or during active anticoagulation therapy (Table 22.3). Patients with a VTE that was provoked by temporary or ongoing prothrombotic conditions usually do not benefit from hypercoagulable testing. Aside from hypercoagulable disorders, unexplained arterial or venous thromboembolism also raises the possibility of an occult cancer. Likewise, patients with a prior history of malignancy who develop a first-time or recurrent VTE episode should be assessed for cancer recurrence.

Reduced Level of Anticoagulants

Antithrombin (AT) Deficiency

The clinical manifestation of AT deficiency is usually deep vein thrombosis (DVT), but it can also cause arterial thromboses on rare occasions. AT deficiency increases the risk of a first-time VTE event by 20-fold [8]. Since AT acts as a cofactor for heparin, patients with AT deficiency often require exces-

V. Gahtan and M.J. Costanza (eds.), *Essentials of Vascular Surgery for the General Surgeon*, DOI 10.1007/978-1-4939-1326-8_22, © Springer Science+Business Media New York 2015

Table 22.1 Relative risk of first VTE based upon hypercoagulable disorder

	Protein C deficiency	Protein S deficiency	Antithrombin III deficiency	Factor V Leiden	Prothrombin gene mutation
Relative risk of first VTE	10	10	25	4	2.5

Table 22.2 Tests for arterial hypercoagulable states

Abnormality
Lupus anticoagulant
Anticardiolipin antibody
B2 glycoprotein-1 antibody
Lipoprotein (a)
Sticky platelet syndrome
Homocysteine

Table 22.3 Timing of testing for VTE hypercoagulable states

Hypercoagulable state	Timing
Factor V Leiden	No restriction
Prothrombin mutation	No restriction
B2 glycoprotein-1 antibody	No restriction
Dysfibrinogenemia	No restriction
Antithrombin III deficiency	After cessation of anticoagulation
Protein C deficiency	After cessation of anticoagulation
Protein S deficiency	After cessation of anticoagulation
Lupus anticoagulant	When no sign of active infection
Cardiolipin antibodies	When no sign of active infection
Elevated Factors VIII, IX, XI	After resolution of inflammation – in concert with ESR/CRP

sively high doses of heparin to achieve therapeutic anticoagulation. Resistance to anticoagulation with heparin raises the possibility of AT deficiency and should prompt further testing. Unfortunately, diagnosing AT deficiency at the time of the acute VTE event is usually impossible because AT levels normally decrease in the postoperative and postpartum periods and during anticoagulation with heparin and sometimes warfarin. Assessment for AT deficiency should therefore be pursued after the acute thrombotic event has resolved and the patient has stopped anticoagulation therapy. Subclassifications of AT deficiency describe the underlying pathophysiology and include reduced AT activity levels, reduced AT antigen and activity levels, and a defective heparin-binding site.

Protein C Deficiency

Patients with Protein C deficiency have a tenfold increased risk of VTE and frequently develop recurrent DVT [9]. As a vitamin K-dependent enzyme produced in the liver, protein C is affected by liver disease, disseminated intravascular coagulation (DIC), and warfarin therapy [10]. Warfarin decreases protein C levels more quickly than it inhibits procoagulant factors (Factors II, VII, IX, and X) making patients with protein C deficiency temporarily hypercoagulable and at risk for warfarin-induced skin necrosis. Preventing this complication is the rationale behind overlapping heparin and warfarin therapy during the initial stages of anticoagulation. Testing for protein C deficiency should occur after the VTE event has resolved and the patient has stopped taking oral anticoagulation. Antigen or activity levels can be used to detect protein C deficiency.

Protein S Deficiency

Protein S deficiency is associated with DVT which can occur in atypical locations [11, 12]. Protein S functions as a cofactor for protein C, and patients with protein S deficiency have a comparable thrombotic risk to those with protein C deficiency [9]. Like protein C, protein S is a vitamin K-dependent enzyme produced by the liver. Patients with protein S deficiency are therefore at risk for warfarin-induced skin necrosis if they are not appropriately transitioned from heparin to warfarin therapy. Although protein S deficiency is a hereditary disorder, functional deficiencies can occur during inflammatory states due to increased C4b-binding protein which lowers free protein S levels. Other conditions that can lower protein S levels include liver disease, DIC, pregnancy, estrogen hormonal therapy, and acute VTE. Tests for protein S deficiency usually measure total protein S activity or free activity levels and should be performed after cessation of anticoagulation therapy.

Increased Levels of Procoagulants

Factor V Leiden

Factor V Leiden or activated protein C resistance is the most commonly identified hereditary disorder associated with VTE. The vast majority of thrombotic complications from this disorder involve DVT and pulmonary emboli (PE) [13]. Homozygotes for Factor V Leiden have a 50-fold increased risk of VTE and account for about 1.5 % of VTE events [14]. Factor V Leiden heterozygotes have a fourfold increased risk of VTE and account for 16 % of first-time VTE events and 7 % of all cases of VTE (initial and recurrent) [15–17]. Factor V Leiden predominantly affects Caucasians, with people of Scandinavian origin having the highest prevalence [18]. Some studies suggest that an acquired form of Factor V Leiden can also develop with estrogen use, pregnancy, and elevated levels of Factor VIII [19–22]. The risk of VTE associated with Factor V Leiden deficiency increases in the presence of other hypercoagulable states, including hyperhomocysteinemia, prothrombin gene mutation, protein C or S deficiency, and AT deficiency [23–27]. Prolonged airplane travel, immobility, and surgical interventions can also provoke thrombotic episodes. The laboratory diagnosis of Factor V Leiden involves a second-generation clotting assay which is 85 % specific and 100 % sensitive and usually requires PCR or genetic testing for confirmation [14, 28]. Diagnostic testing is not affected by the presence of an acute thromboembolic episode and may be performed at any time.

Prothrombin Gene Mutation

Patients with prothrombin gene mutation have a 2.5-fold increased risk for VTE [29]. Simioni and Ridker estimated a twofold increased risk of recurrent VTE similar to Factor V Leiden; however, other reports contradict this finding [30–33]. Patients with prothrombin gene mutation are also at increased risk for arterial complications associated with the coronary or cerebrovascular systems [34]. The disorder is essentially nonexistent in African American and Asian populations, and diagnostic testing is not affected by acute VTE [35].

Elevated Factors VIII, IX, and XI

Elevated levels of Factors VIII, IX, and XI can result in lower extremity DVT or PE [36]. Diagnosing these disorders can be challenging because common conditions such as bleeding and inflammation normally increase the levels of procoagulant factors. Laboratory tests to measure Factor VIII, IX, and XI levels should be performed in conjunction with an ESR or CRP to evaluate for concomitant inflammation [37, 38]. If the ESR or CRP levels are also elevated, the procoagulant factor levels must be considered nondiagnostic because of the potentially confounding presence of inflammation. Confirming that elevated levels of Factors VII, IX, and XI reflect a hypercoagulable state and not a temporary, acquired abnormality requires two tests at different time points demonstrating procoagulant factor elevations above the 90th percentile.

Hyperhomocysteinemia

Hyperhomocysteinemia increases the risk of peripheral arterial disease, as well as arterial and venous thrombosis [39–42]. Several studies reported a 2–8-fold increased risk of stroke and myocardial infarction in patients with hyperhomocysteinemia [43, 44]. Although vitamin and folate replacement can reduce serum levels of homocysteine, normalizing the laboratory value of homocysteine does not affect clinical outcome or reduce cardiovascular risk. The only purpose of diagnosing hyperhomocysteinemia is to identify patients at higher risk for cardiovascular and thrombotic events. Patients with atypical arterial thromboses or premature atherosclerosis warrant an evaluation for hyperhomocysteinemia; however, measuring homocysteine levels in patients with VTE is not usually indicated.

Acquired Hypercoagulable States

Antiphospholipid Antibody Syndrome

Antiphospholipid antibody syndrome usually causes recurrent miscarriages in young women or lower extremity DVT; however, this syndrome also increases the risk of arterial thrombosis [45, 46]. The risk of recurrent VTE increases 4–7.7-fold after the initial episode, with the recurrence frequently localized to the site of the initial event [47–49]. Depending on the subtype of antiphospholipid antibody syndrome, the risk of initial DVT can be as high as 3.6-fold [50]. First-time VTE risk increases up to tenfold in patients who have antiphospholipid antibody syndrome and other concomitant hypercoagulable conditions [50]. Laboratory examination for antiphospholipid antibody syndrome involves two different assays: anticardiolipin antibody for IgG and IgM antibodies and anti-β2 glycoprotein 1 screening. Although ongoing infection and underlying malignancy can create erroneous test results, the presence of acute VTE does not affect test accuracy.

Cancer

In 1865, Trousseau first recognized that cancer increased the risk of VTE. The most common thrombotic manifestations of cancer are DVT and PE, and the risk of VTE ranges from 7- to 20-fold for patients with metastatic disease on chemotherapy [51, 52]. Multiple factors influence the risk of thrombotic complications in patients with cancer including: the type and stage of cancer, surgical vs. chemotherapy, comorbid conditions, immobility, and presence of central venous catheters. Some cancers cause vascular complications by exerting extrinsic compression on adjacent blood vessels. The risk of arterial thrombosis and embolization also increases in cancer patients including cerebral, myocardial, and peripheral thromboembolic episodes.

Low-molecular-weight heparin (LMWH) is more effective than warfarin at preventing thrombotic recurrence or propagation in patients with cancer [53, 54]. Patients with VTE and active cancer should be therefore maintained on long-term LMWH. Although newer anticoagulants may be equally effective in patients with cancer, more supporting data is required before they can be recommended for widespread use. Anticoagulation therapy in patients with cancer must be carefully monitored as bleeding complications occur more frequently in this population [55].

No specific testing for hypercoagulable conditions is recommended for cancer patients.

Pregnancy

Hypercoagulable disorders associated with pregnancy are the leading cause of maternal death in the United States with over half of the VTE episodes occurring postpartum [56–58]. Pregnancy creates a prothrombotic state by increasing fibrinogen and Factor VIII levels while decreasing fibrinolytic activity and the level of protein S. As the gravid uterus enlarges, it compresses the inferior vena cava and the left iliac vein which explains why the majority of DVTs during pregnancy occur in the left lower extremity [59–62]. Patients with any inherited coagulation disorder have a markedly increased risk of DVT during pregnancy and the postpartum period [63]. Hellgren et al. reported that 60 % of pregnant patients with VTE had Factor V Leiden deficiency [19]. Patients who develop VTE during pregnancy should be assessed for underlying hypercoagulable disorders to assess their overall thrombotic risk status and to determine the risk of recurrent VTE during future pregnancies.

Heparin-Induced Thrombocytopenia (HIT)

Patients with HIT develop heparin-induced antibodies directed against platelet factor-4. The antibodies trigger the activation and aggregation of platelets which ultimately releases prothrombotic platelet particles into the circulation. The clinical manifestation of HIT can include either venous or arterial thrombosis despite low levels of platelets [64]. HIT typically occurs 3–5 days after exposure to unfractionated heparin; however, HIT can also occur following treatment with LMWH. In patients with prior heparin exposure, HIT can occur as early as 24 h after receiving heparin.

All patients being treated with any form of heparin should have platelet monitoring for at least 5 days. The diagnosis of HIT should be considered in patients who develop thrombocytopenia or have a significant decrease in the platelet count after exposure to heparin. Any thrombotic event that occurs after heparin initiation should also raise the possibility of HIT. If HIT is suspected on clinical grounds, all forms of heparin should be stopped immediately and anticoagulation should continue using a direct thrombin inhibitor (argatroban, lepirudin) or anti-Xa inhibitor (fondaparinux). If HIT is confirmed, anticoagulation should transition to warfarin only when the platelet count normalizes. Testing for HIT can include a serotonin release assay or enzyme-linked immunosorbent assay (ELISA) which has a diagnostic accuracy approaching 100 % when used in combination [65].

Clinical Management

All surgeons regularly encounter patients suspected of having a hypercoagulable disorder. Effective management of these patients must address the following issues: thromboprophylaxis for patients undergoing procedures, appropriate length of treatment for patients who have a VTE, and indications for and timing of testing to diagnose hypercoagulable states.

Thromboprophylaxis

At least half of VTE events that occur in patients with hypercoagulable disorders are provoked by the clinical circumstances. This finding suggests that thromboprophylaxis could reduce the incidence of VTE for hypercoagulable patients who face clinical settings which are associated with an increased thrombotic risk such as surgery and immobility [9, 14, 66]. Multiple guidelines attempt to stratify the VTE risk of patients to determine the appropriate thromboprophylaxis for surgical procedures [67, 68]. Mechanical thromboprophylaxis includes early ambulation and intermittent compression stockings, while pharmacologic thromboprophylaxis typically involves unfractionated heparin, LMWH, or anti-Xa inhibitors. Current American College of Chest Physicians (ACCP) guidelines provide comprehensive recommendations for thromboprophylaxis based on the type of surgical intervention and risk stratification of the patient [69]. These consensus-based guidelines are updated every few years and should be familiar to all surgeons. Approximately one half of VTE events occurring in young patients are associated with inherited hypercoagulable states [70]. Estrogen replacement and hormonal methods of birth control add to the hypercoagulable state and should be avoided in this high-risk patient population [66].

Duration of Therapy

The optimal duration of anticoagulation for patients with hereditary hypercoagulable disorders varies depending on the clinical scenario. The average risk of recurrent VTE is about 5 %, and recurrence seems to be lower for patients with a provoked vs. spontaneous VTE [70]. Patients with a provoked VTE due to transient thrombotic risk factors such as surgery should be treated with a finite period of anticoagulation of 3–6 months [67]. In contrast, current treatment recommendations for patients with a spontaneous VTE are less specific ranging from 2 years to lifelong anticoagulation [32, 67]. The risk of bleeding complications and the high cost of therapy make lifelong anticoagulation an unappealing treatment option [71, 72]. Warfarin has a 3 % risk of significant bleeding per year and a 0.6 % risk of a fatal hemorrhage [6]. Since patients with hypercoagulable disorders have a less than 3 % risk of primary VTE, the risk-benefit calculation usually comes out against lifelong anticoagulation. Based upon these assumptions, few patients have an absolute indication for lifelong anticoagulation.

Regardless of whether the thrombotic episode was provoked or spontaneous, the majority of patients with hypercoagulable disorders should be treated in a similar fashion to patients without clotting abnormalities. This universal treatment strategy is

Table 22.4 Indications for hereditary hypercoagulable disorder testing

VTE episode at age younger than 45
Unprovoked VTE
VTE in atypical location
Strong family history of VTE
Women with multiple miscarriages

based on the hypothesis that most, if not all patients, who develop thrombotic complications have abnormalities in the clotting cascade and that most, if not all, episodes of VTE are provoked. The only difference in clinical scenarios may be the clinician's ability to diagnose the hypercoagulable disorder or detect the often subtle instigating event [73].

Testing

Diagnosing hereditary hypercoagulable disorders may be more important for the family and progeny of the affected individual. Knowledge of an increased VTE risk can help determine the need for thromboprophylaxis in patients who face high-thrombotic-risk situations such as pregnancy, hormone use, surgery, and prolonged air travel. Testing for hereditary hypercoagulable disorders should be considered in several scenarios listed in Table 22.4. Prophylactic anticoagulation is not recommended for asymptomatic individuals found to have hypercoagulable states.

Popliteal Artery Entrapment

Introduction

Popliteal artery entrapment syndrome (PAES) encompasses a group of anatomic anomalies that cause compression of the popliteal artery and occasionally the popliteal vein. The hemodynamically significant stenosis that occurs in PAES usually manifests as claudication but can cause progressive ischemia and limb loss if not diagnosed and appropriately treated. Stuart first described the anatomy of popliteal artery entrapment in 1879, but the associated clinical manifestations of PAES were not recognized until 1958 [74, 75]. Although the incidence remains unclear, PAES appears to be the most common cause of claudication symptoms in young people. Bouhoutsos et al. reported a 0.165 % prevalence of PAES in young men entering the Greek military while Turnipseed et al. reported that PAES caused atypical claudication in 0.15–4 % of young patients, and Gibson et al. reported a 3.5 % prevalence of PAES in postmortem specimens [76–79].

Pathophysiology

During embryologic growth, the popliteal artery normally develops after the medial head of the gastrocnemius muscle has migrated to the medial femoral condyle. Derangements in the timing and sequence of these events lead to the various types of PAES. Abnormally, early development of the popliteal artery or delayed migration of the medial head of the gastrocnemius causes compression and medial displacement of the artery by the gastrocnemius muscle (Type I). In Type II PAES, early development of the popliteal artery interferes with the normal migration of the medial head of the gastrocnemius muscle causing abnormal muscle insertion into the femur. If mesodermal remnants of the medial head of the gastrocnemius fail to involute, they form abnormal fibrous bands or muscle slips that compress the popliteal artery (Type III). These bands can attach to the femoral condyles or the intercondylar space. The rarest form of PAES, Type IV, involves persistence of the primitive axial artery which is compressed by the popliteus muscle. Compression of the vein and artery by any mechanism is classified as Type V.

Type VI PAES can be a catch all term for other anatomic variants or it can designate functional popliteal artery entrapment. The term functional PAES is usually applied when none of the anatomic abnormalities are present, but arterial compression is documented by radiologic imaging during positions of stress or activity. The etiology, incidence, natural history, and treatment of functional PAES remain controversial. Leading theories regarding the pathophysiology of functional entrapment speculate that compression results from muscular hypertrophy or the soleal sling [80]. Pillai et al. reviewed MRI findings and found that patients with functional PAES had more extensive attachment of the medial head of the gastrocnemius muscle to the midline of the bone and the intercondylar notch as well as greater muscle bulk adjacent to the neurovascular bundle [81]. Other imaging studies have questioned the clinical relevance of functional PAES by showing that some form of compression occurs in up to 80 % of healthy adults during forced plantar flexion of the foot [80, 82, 83].

Regardless of the mechanism or PAES type, external compression of the popliteal artery gradually damages the vessel leading to fibrotic occlusion in advanced stages. As the popliteal artery slowly narrows, some patients form a poststenotic aneurysm with thrombus formation and distal embolization. Tibial nerve involvement has also been reported.

Clinical Presentation

PAES should be considered in patients younger than 50 who present with claudication or exertional calf muscle pain. The majority of patients with PAES present before 30 years of age and the male-to-female ratio is about 2:1 [84]. Roche-Nagle et al. found that young athletes participating in basketball, football, rugby, or martial arts were most commonly affected by PAES and 25 % of patients had bilateral involvement [85, 86].

All forms of PAES cause repetitive trauma to the artery which can potentially lead to aneurysmal degeneration, thrombosis, or distal embolization. The clinical signs and symptoms depend on the stage at which the patient seeks medical attention. A delayed presentation of PAES frequently occurs when young patients dismiss muscle cramps as a sign of being "out of shape" and primary care physicians overlook early signs and symptoms of arterial insufficiency. If weakness, paresthesias, and edema are also present, PAES may involve simultaneous nerve and or vein compression. In some patients, the discomfort caused by walking paradoxically improves with more vigorous exercise. These atypical claudication symptoms can create a confusing clinical picture causing further delays in the diagnosis of PAES.

Claudication symptoms due to PAES may not occur until the patient has walked for miles. The onset of exertional leg pain depends on the extent of arterial compression and the physical conditioning of the patient. Due to their young age, long walking distance, and lack of atherosclerotic risk factors, many patients with PAES are initially referred to orthopedic or sports medicine physicians, and a vascular etiology for their symptoms is not considered until late in the course of disease. The sudden onset of severe claudication usually signifies acute occlusion of the popliteal artery. Although critical limb ischemia (CLI) can result from popliteal artery occlusion or emboli to the tibial vessels, only 20 % of patients with PAES present with symptoms of CLI [87, 88]. In most patients, the entrapped popliteal artery undergoes gradual injury allowing time for collateral formation, similar to that seen in atherosclerotic occlusive disease.

The differential diagnosis of PAES should include compartment syndrome and popliteal adventitial cystic disease. Eliminating adventitial cystic disease from the differential diagnosis is usually straightforward since it does not have a predisposition to athletes and usually occurs in less active young patients. Several studies reported that PAES was the cause of symptomatic claudication in up to 60 % of young athletes [87, 89]. In contrast, Turnipseed et al. found that functional entrapment accounted for only 4 % of cases of claudication in young patients with chronic compartment syndrome causing the majority of symptoms [79]. Different referral patterns may explain the contradictory conclusions reached by these studies. Other non-atherosclerotic vascular complications in young, otherwise, healthy athletes can include exercise-induced fibrosis of the external iliac artery most often described in avid cyclists and arterial thoracic outlet syndrome that can occur in baseball pitchers and other athletes engaged in repetitive overhead arm motion.

Diagnosis and Treatment

Patients with PAES typically have palpable pedal pulses at rest which decrease or disappear with active plantar flexion of the foot. Any patient with suspected PAES should undergo exercise testing in the noninvasive vascular lab. Unless the patient is presenting with an advanced stage of entrapment, the popliteal and tibial arteries should have normal triphasic waveforms when the leg is in the neutral position. Active knee extension and forced plantar flexion of the foot occlude the popliteal artery in most patients with PAES. Likewise, a normal ABI at rest (greater than 1.0) should fall to less than 0.9 with exercise in patients with PAES. Well-conditioned athletes with PAES may need to perform more vigorous exercise than the standard vascular lab protocol to induce changes in ABI. Similarly, patients with functional entrapment frequently are usually athletes who develop symptoms at distances measured in miles, not blocks.

MRA or CTA imaging studies can confirm the diagnosis of PAES, identify specific muscular or tendinous abnormalities, and detect the presence of aneurysmal degeneration which warrants repair of the artery. Assessment of the contralateral limb should also be performed as the prevalence of bilateral PAES ranges from 30 to 67 % [90–93]. Angiography usually helps determine whether an arterial bypass is necessary by assessing the extent of intimal damage and identifying distal runoff vessels. All diagnostic modalities should attempt to reproduce the popliteal artery compression that occurs during exercise. Unless the popliteal artery is already occluded or anatomic abnormalities for PAES identified, images of the leg in neutral position should be compared to images obtained with forced active dorsiflexion of the foot against resistance with the knee fully extended. Failure to perform these maneuvers may lead to a false-negative result. Eliminating compartment syndrome from the differential diagnosis may involve taking pressure measurements in the muscle compartments of the lower leg. Left untreated, PAES can acutely occlude the popliteal artery which causes severe, short-distance claudication. DiMarzo et al. and Levien also found a higher rate of distal embolization in patients who had delayed diagnosis and treatment of PAES [87, 94].

Functional Entrapment

In 1985, Rignault described functional popliteal artery entrapment syndrome (FPAES) in symptomatic young military recruits who had no anatomic abnormality [80]. Lower extremity MRI demonstrated compression of the popliteal artery in positions of stress which appeared to result from hypertrophy of the muscles in the popliteal fossa. Other studies confirmed the two levels of compression described by Rignault: one between plantaris and medial head of the gastrocnemius and the other between the popliteus and plantaris muscles. Turnipseed further defined FPAES by identifying hypertrophy of the gastrocnemius as the primary etiology [83, 90, 95]. Although partial resection of the medial head of gastrocnemius muscle provides symptomatic relief for patients with FPAES, Deshpande found that decreasing activity alone obviated the need for surgical intervention in patients willing to abstain from extreme athletics [96].

Treatment

Treatment for PAES should be performed by experienced surgeons with a detailed understanding and experience operating in this area. Surgery is the only effective treatment for anatomic PAES (Types I through V). Percutaneous, catheter-directed thrombolysis has a limited role in the treatment of PAES which involves restoring patency to an acutely occluded popliteal artery in anticipation of definitive surgical repair. Unlike arteries affected by atherosclerotic disease, the popliteal artery in patients with PAES is fibrotic and usually resists dilation with balloon angioplasty and stent placement. Endoluminal interventions are also destined to fail because they do not relieve the underlying problem of extrinsic compression.

All symptomatic patients with confirmed PAES should have surgery to resect the offending muscle or band. Surgery usually involves resection of the gastrocnemius medial head which can be guided by intraoperative duplex assessment of the vessel to confirm successful decompression. This procedure alone may provide definitive treatment for patients with early-stage PAES in whom the artery has not degenerated. Surgery for early-stage PAES can be performed with a posterior popliteal approach using a lazy "S" incision. An adequate length of artery should be exposed to evaluate for other fibrous compressive bands. If the medial head of the gastrocnemius muscle is causing compression of the popliteal artery or vein, it should be divided from its insertion on the medial femoral condyle. Techniques for excising the plantaris muscle, soleal sling, and popliteus muscle have also been described.

Advanced-stage PAES which causes occlusion or aneurismal dilation of the popliteal artery mandates treatment with an intersegmental arterial bypass, generally using the small saphenous or great saphenous veins as a bypass conduit. Some patients have chronic occlusion of the popliteal artery without symptoms of vein or nerve compression. These patients do not require division of the muscle bands and can be treated from a medial approach with the vein bypass tunneled subcutaneously, not anatomically.

Prophylactic intervention for patients with contralateral PAES should be performed electively if imaging studies confirm early-stage compression of the popliteal artery without vessel injury. Early surgical decompression can avoid the need for vascular repair or bypass. Surgical intervention usually allows young patients with PAES to resume their sports and athletic endeavors.

Outcomes

Follow-up information is somewhat limited to relatively small series. Kim et al. followed 22 bypasses in 18 patients with PAES dividing the patients into those with short-segment occlusions and those with occlusion extending beyond the popliteal artery [97]. Both posterior and medial surgical approaches were used in this series. Overall graft patency was 75 % at 3 and 5 years. Patients who had a bypass originating from the distal superficial femoral artery had a significantly lower patency compared to patients with a bypass originating from the above-knee popliteal artery (30 % vs. 86 % at 5 years).

A recent meta-analysis by Sinha et al. attempted to describe the clinical presentation, natural history, and treatment outcome of patients with PAES. Claudication was the most common symptom of PAES with 38 % of patients having bilateral disease, 23 % exhibiting functional entrapment, and only 11 % of patients presenting with critical limb ischemia [84]. At the time of presentation, 24 % of the popliteal arteries were occluded and 13.5 % had aneurismal degeneration. The median duration of symptoms prior to diagnosis was 12 months; however, there was no association between duration of symptoms and presence of significant arterial damage. Three studies in the meta-analysis reported outcomes on a handful of patients treated nonoperatively for PAES: 1 patient required amputation, 1 patient reoccluded 2 months after thrombolysis requiring bypass, 1 patient had persistent symptoms, and 1 patient with functional entrapment had symptom resolution. Although surgery had an overall success rate of 77 %, surgical complications included amputation, wound infection, hematoma, seroma, and deep vein thrombosis. Fewer reports exist for popliteal vein entrapment, and clinical outcomes may differ from PAES due to the predominantly female patient cohort [93, 98, 99].

Thromboangiitis Obliterans

Thromboangiitis obliterans (TAO) was first recognized in 1879, but not well described until 1908 when Leo Buerger published the pathologic findings of the disease that now bears his name. TAO or Buerger's disease is a vasculitis characterized by segmental thrombotic inflammatory changes [100].

TAO involves medium- and small-sized arteries, which are infrapopliteal or infrabrachial in location. Three pathologic phases have been described [101].

1. Acute phase which involves an occlusive cellular thrombus. Microabscesses and multinucleated giant cells may be seen.
2. Subacute phase involves organization of the thrombus.
3. Chronic phase characterized by organized thrombus and fibrosis. This may be more difficult to differentiate from atherosclerotic disease.

Etiology and Presentation

Despite extensive clinical and pathologic studies, the etiology of TAO remains unclear. Although tobacco use is central to the disease process, immunologic factors, hereditary disposition, and endothelial dysfunction may also play a role in the pathophysiology of TAO. Patients with TAO typically present with ischemic symptoms caused by occlusive small-vessel disease of the lower leg, forearm, or both. The most characteristic clinical scenario for TAO involves a man under the age of 40 who smokes and has digital ischemia. TAO occurs less commonly in women and rarely affects other vascular beds. Superficial thrombophlebitis and rheumatologic symptoms such as arthralgias, arthritis, and carpal tunnel syndrome have also been described as clinical manifestations of TAO [101, 102].

Diagnosis

The diagnosis of TAO begins with a thorough physical exam including palpation of distal pulses, auscultation for bruits, inspection of the digits, and evaluation for superficial venous thrombophlebitis. Ankle brachial indices (ABIs) should be obtained to detect and quantify the severity of arterial occlusive disease. A neurologic exam should be performed, as up to 70 % of patients have sensory findings [103]. Clinical diagnostic criteria for TAO include [103]:

- Age younger than 45
- Recent tobacco use
- Distal extremity ischemia
- Absence of autoimmune disease, thrombophilia, diabetes, or proximal embolic source
- Consistent radiographic findings

Adjunctive diagnostic studies for TAO include arterial duplex, CTA, MRA, or catheter-directed angiography. These imaging studies can exclude a proximal embolic source and confirm that the occlusive lesions only involve arteries distal to the elbow or knee. Although corkscrew collateral vessels have been associated with TAO, this pattern is not specific to TAO and may occur in other types of arterial occlusive disease.

Treatment and Outcomes

Smoking cessation is the primary treatment strategy for patients with TAO. Patients who completely stop smoking have significantly more favorable outcomes than patients who continue to smoke. In a relatively large study, no amputations were performed on patients with TAO who stopped smoking, while 43 % of active smokers required an amputation [104]. Endovascular and surgical interventions have limited success in patients with TAO due to the distal nature of the disease. Small studies have described the use of vasodilators for TAO including iloprost, alpha-blockers, calcium channel blockers, and sildenafil. The use of sympathectomy to relieve the symptoms of TAO has not proven to be successful.

Vasculitis

Introduction

Vasculitis refers to inflammation of the blood vessel wall that can lead to arterial damage in the form of aneurismal degeneration or thrombosis of the involved vessel. This inflammatory process can occur in several different types of arteries affecting patients from a variety of demographic groups. Vasculitis therefore encompasses an uncommon group of disorders with a wide range of pathologic features and clinical presentations that can be challenging to concisely summarize. Despite the rarity and complexity of vasculitis, general surgeons should be familiar with the diagnosis and initial management of this group of vascular diseases. Patients with vasculitis often present with vague symptoms that require immediate recognition and appropriate treatment to avoid potentially devastating complications such as thrombosis, aneurysm rupture, blindness, and hemoptysis. Mistakenly treating vasculitis as a manifestation of atherosclerotic disease can have significant adverse consequences.

The diagnosis and management of some forms of vasculitis remains controversial with considerable disagreement between and within medical disciplines. Debate continues over even the most fundamental issues including whom to biopsy, when to initiate steroids, and how long to continue therapy. Because of this lack of consensus, surgeons often take the lead in determining the indication for a biopsy and the timing of medical treatment. Surgeons must also recognize the appropriate role for revascularization because it is clear that patients with vasculitis do not follow the same clinical course as patients with atherosclerotic disease. The following section will review the different classes of vasculitides with attention to presentation, pathophysiology, diagnosis, and treatment options. Particular attention will be paid to giant cell or temporal arteritis (GCA), as it is one of the more commonly encountered forms of vasculitis and one that stimulates considerable debate regarding diagnosis and treatment.

Classification and Pathophysiology

Vasculitis can be classified by the size of arteries it affects: large, medium, or small. Parameters to subclassify vasculitis include ANCA status (positive or negative) and patient age at presentation. The more common forms of vasculitis can be summarized as follows (some less common vasculitides have been omitted for clarity) [105]:

Large-vessel disease	
Takayasu's arteritis	(Age<30)
Giant cell (temporal) arteritis	(Age>50)
Medium-vessel disease	
Kawasaki's disease	(Age<5)
Behcet's disease	(Age 20–40)
Polyarteritis nodosa	
Small	
Henoch-Schonlein purpura	
Arteritis of connective tissue disease	
Wegener's granulomatosis	(ANCA+)

Large-Vessel Vasculitis

As the name implies, large-vessel vasculitis involves the aorta and its major branches; however, GCA can also affect small vessels such as the temporal, ophthalmic, retinal, and ciliary arteries. While Takayasu's arteritis is more prevalent in the Mediterranean and Asia, GCA is more common among patients in North America [106].

An accurate diagnosis and prompt treatment is paramount to achieving a good clinical outcome in patients with GCA. Delayed treatment puts patients at risk for blindness due to ischemic optic neuropathy. Other consequences of untreated arteritis include an increased incidence of peripheral arterial disease, the development of aortic aneurysms (particularly of the ascending aorta), an increased risk of cardiovascular events, and potentially increased mortality [107]. The complex pathophysiology of GCA involves recruitment and activation of CD-4 T cells by local dendritic cells. Macrophages damage the vessel resulting in luminal narrowing. Histologic findings include granulomatous changes and multinucleated giant cells [108].

Giant Cell Arteritis Diagnosis

GCA affects patients over the age of 50 with a higher prevalence in patients in their seventh and eighth decades. Although the disease process of GCA remains poorly understood, more women are diagnosed than men (female-to-male ratio 3:1), and genetics seems to have an etiologic role. The clinical diagnosis of GCA can be challenging because patients present with a variety of signs and symptoms. Arterial occlusive disease affecting the brachial or femoral arteries in the absence of atherosclerotic disease or risk factors should raise suspicion for GCA. Patients may also have fever of unknown origin and complain of headache, jaw pain, and vision changes. The physical exam in patients with GCA may demonstrate prominent, tender temporal arteries or scalp ischemia. Biochemical markers can provide supporting evidence for diagnosis of GCA in patients with relatively nonspecific findings from the history and physical exam. Estimated sedimentation rate (ESR) greater than 50 and C-reactive protein (CRP) greater than 2.45 g/dL are both predictive of a positive biopsy result for GCA [109]. Elevated platelet counts, although nonspecific, may be predictive as well.

Ultrasonography can function as a valuable diagnostic tool for evaluating patients with suspected GCA. An ultrasound exam of the temporal arteries in patients with GCA often demonstrates a hypoechoic line within the vessel wall. This line or "halo" appears to be related to edema and inflammation and has a sensitivity of 68–73 % and a specificity of 91–100 % for the diagnosis of GCA. Specificity increases when bilateral halos are present, while sensitivity diminishes after the initiation of steroids as the halo fades away and completely disappears after 14 days of therapy [107, 110]. Given the ease, availability, and noninvasive nature, ultrasonography is an excellent starting point for diagnosing patients with GCA. A positive ultrasound exam should prompt treatment and may obviate the need for a temporal artery biopsy. A negative ultrasound result may require further evaluation depending on the clinical scenario. Other imaging studies such as MRI and PET scanning may assist in the diagnosis of GCA; however, their role in general practice remains poorly defined [106, 107].

Temporal artery biopsy was first described in 1932 and is often invoked as the gold standard for diagnosing GCA [108]. Despite the widespread use and recognition of temporal artery biopsy, this technique has several shortcomings and still generates debate regarding its necessity as a diagnostic exam. According to some studies, temporal artery biopsy has a 20–40 % false-negative rate, possibly related to the initiation of steroids before biopsy or inadequate specimen. No consensus has ever been reached regarding the minimal length of the specimen or the need for unilateral versus bilateral temporal artery biopsy. The presence of skip lesions highlights the need to obtain an adequate length of temporal artery to avoid a false-negative biopsy result.

In 1990, the American College of Rheumatologists (ACR) proposed that patients meeting three of the following five clinical criteria could be diagnosed with GCA:

1. Age>50
2. New-onset headache

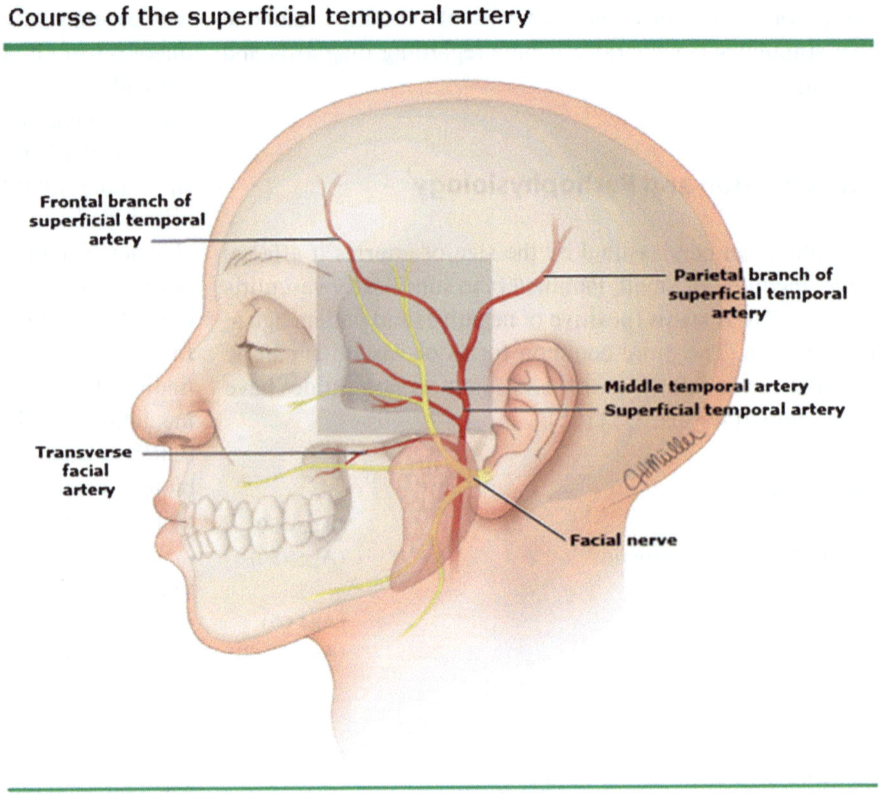

Fig. 22.1 Course of the superficial temporal artery. Danger zone delineated by box showing proximity of frontal branch of facial nerve to the frontal branch of superficial temporal artery (Illustration courtesy of Marie Kim. Iowa Head and Neck Protocols, Iowa City, IA. http://wiki.uiowa.edu/display/protocols/Home)

3. Temporal artery tenderness or decreased temporal artery pulse
4. ESR greater than 50 mm/h
5. Abnormal temporal artery biopsy

Although the ACR guidelines suggest that a temporal artery biopsy is not always necessary, the issue has not been settled. The titles of two recent journal articles demonstrate how polarized this issue remains: "Temporal artery biopsy is not required in all cases of suspected giant cell arteritis" versus "Temporal artery biopsy: skip it at your patient's peril" [110, 111]. A recent abstract questioned the value of a biopsy by reporting that steroids were stopped in only 36.5 % of patients with a negative biopsy result [112]. It seems hard to justify a nontherapeutic intervention that carries a small risk of facial nerve injury if the requesting physician has no intention of altering the treatment plan based on the biopsy results.

Until wider consensus can be achieved, the diagnosis of GCA requires an individualized approach. Patients with clinical findings and elevated biochemical markers consistent with GCA should begin treatment without waiting for confirmation with a temporal artery biopsy. An ultrasound exam demonstrating a halo sign can then confirm the diagnosis and a biopsy can be reserved for patients with a negative or nondiagnostic ultrasound in whom the diagnosis remains unclear. Initiating steroid treatment 2 weeks or more in advance does not appear to affect the diagnostic accuracy of a temporal artery biopsy in patients with clinical indications of active disease [113].

Although a temporal artery biopsy is a minor procedure, potential adverse outcomes include a nondiagnostic result and injury to the facial nerve. These complications can be avoided by adhering to a few sound techniques when performing the biopsy. To increase the diagnostic yield, the biopsy should be performed on the symptomatic side or the side with a diminished or absent temporal artery pulse. Before beginning the procedure, a Doppler probe can locate and mark the path of the temporal artery as it courses superiorly from its origin anterior to the ear [114]. Figure 22.1 shows the course of the temporal artery. Making the incision over the parietal branch of the artery within the patient's hairline decreases the risk of injuring the facial nerve. The incision should be long enough to remove a 2–3 cm segment of the artery to ensure that an adequate sample is obtained for diagnosis [115]. Skin closure using subcuticular absorbable sutures gives the best cosmetic result.

Giant Cell Arteritis Treatment

First described in 1953, glucocorticoid treatment for giant cell arteritis has significantly reduced the number of patients who go blind because of GCA. Steroids should be started as soon as possible because a delay of more than 24 h past symptom recognition reduces the rate of visual symptom resolution from 50 % to only 6 % [107]. The initial recommended dose of prednisone is 0.8–1.0 mg/kg/day. Protocols to taper the steroid dose usually target resolution of symptoms and normalization of biochemical markers over a time period of less than 6 months [107]. Unfortunately, steroids can cause significant side effects including diabetes, hypertension, infection, fractures, and heart failure. In some studies, high-dose steroids for longer than 6 months increased mortality, although confounding variables were present [107]. The fact that steroids are nonspecific mediators of the immune system with an unfavorable side effect profile has sparked interest in more directed medical therapy including the use of methotrexate, TNF-alpha antagonists, azathioprine, hydroxychloroquine, cyclophosphamide, dapsone, and cyclosporine. While these alternative agents can mitigate the systemic effects of GCA and prevent blindness, their ability to reduce the vascular morbidity remains unclear. Low-dose aspirin may also play a role in decreasing the rate of cerebrovascular events in patients with GCA [18].

Takayasu's Arteritis Diagnosis

Takayasu's arteritis involves large arteries such as the aorta and its branches, resulting in stenosis, occlusion, and aneurysm formation. One of the diagnostic criteria for Takayasu's arteritis is age younger than 40 and most cases occur in patients 20–40 years of age [108]. Takayasu's arteritis should be considered in young patients with unexplained bruits or decreased pulses on physical exam and in patients with hypertension related to renal artery stenosis. The initial presentation of Takayasu's arteritis can include stroke, cerebrovascular symptoms, and upper extremity pain with exertion. Stenosis involving the lower extremity and visceral arteries and aneurysm formation are less common clinical manifestations of Takayasu's arteritis.

Takayasu's Arteritis Treatment

Although steroids can effectively treat Takayasu's arteritis, symptoms often relapse during attempts to taper the steroid dose [116]. Alternative pharmaceutical agents may allow for steroid sparing and more targeted therapy; however, supporting evidence for these treatment strategies remains insufficient. Surgical intervention for Takayasu's arteritis requires careful consideration given the increased risk of technical failure and the relatively high rates of restenosis and recurrent aneurysm. Cardiac risk in patients with Takayasu's arteritis may also be higher than age-matched controls [117]. If surgery is necessary, it should be performed in the quiescent stage of the disease, and steroid treatment plays an important role in preoperative preparation. Significant doubt remains as to whether endovascular interventions have any role in the treatment of Takayasu's arteritis.

Medium-Vessel Vasculitides

Several vasculitides are described below – Kawasaki's vasculitis, Behcet's disease, and Polyarteritis nodosa.

Kawasaki's vasculitis is an example of a medium-vessel vasculitis that typically occurs in children younger than five although there have been reports of adult disease. The American Heart Association guidelines for the diagnosis of Kawasaki's vasculitis include:

- Fever of unknown origin
- Bilateral bulbar conjunctival injection
- Oral mucous membrane and tongue changes
- Erythema of the palms and soles
- Rash
- Lymphadenopathy

The treatment for Kawasaki's disease consists of intravenous immunoglobulin and high-dose aspirin early in the course of the disease in an effort to prevent complications such as coronary artery disease, heart failure, and coronary artery aneurysms. Echocardiography and nonspecific serum markers such as CRP can be useful in the diagnosis and monitoring of the disease process.

Behcet's disease affects people between the ages of 20 and 40 and has a higher incidence in the Middle East. Affected arteries including the aorta, renal, pulmonary, and peripheral vessels can thrombose or become aneurismal, while veins can develop deep vein thrombosis or thrombophlebitis [18]. Many patients with Behcet's disease have recurrent skin ulcers as well as oral and genital ulcers [116]. One of the unique diagnostic criteria for Behcet's disease is pathergy, which is defined as development of a pustule after a prick of the skin. Like the other vasculitides, a delay in the diagnosis of Behcet's disease can result in blindness. Immunosuppression forms the mainstay of therapy for Behcet's disease. The benefit of long-term anticoagulation in these patients remains unclear [18].

Polyarteritis nodosa is a necrotizing vasculitis of medium vessels that can lead to thrombosis and aneurysm formation. Symptoms of mesenteric ischemia often occur.

Small-Vessel Vasculitis

Wegener's granulomatosis is a small-vessel vasculitis characterized by necrotizing and granulomatous changes affecting arteries or veins. In addition to the general treatment strategies already discussed, statins may help reduce inflammation; however, clear evidence for this is lacking [18].

Fibromuscular Dysplasia

Introduction and Pathophysiology

Fibromuscular dysplasia (FMD) is a non-atherosclerotic, noninflammatory disease that can result in stenosis, thrombosis, emboli, and aneurysm formation in numerous arterial beds. Although FMD was first described in 1938, this disease remains poorly understood. Pathologically, FMD can be classified into one of four types based on the predominant layer of the arterial wall involved in the disease process: [118]

- Intimal fibroplasia – A less common type that typically occurs in the younger population, intimal fibroplasia is characterized by subendothelial deposits of collagen within the intima. Radiographic findings include long, smooth stenotic segments.
- Medial hyperplasia – The rarest type is characterized by an increase in medial smooth muscle and may appear as concentric stenosis in the mid-renal artery. Some consider this type of FMD a precursor to medial fibroplasia and therefore do not include it as a distinct category.
- Medial fibroplasia – This type accounts for 80–90 % of diagnoses and is what most people think of when referring to "FMD." Medial fibroplasia most commonly occurs in women between the ages of 30 and 50. Pathologically, the lesions consist of media with fibrous tissue, collagen, and ground substance. The alternating thickening and thinning of the media results in the radiographic string of beads appearance and may lead to aneurysm formation.
- Perimedial dysplasia – The second most common type of FMD involves accumulation of elastic tissue between the media and adventitia; however, perimedial dysplasia is not associated with aneurysm formation. Perimedial dysplasia may present as multiple high-grade renal artery stenotic lesions in young patients.

Etiology and Presentation

The etiology of FMD may involve multiple factors including mechanical stress and relative ischemia to the vasa vasorum as well as patient-specific factors such as smoking, hormone levels, and genetics [119]. Although FMD can occur in numerous arterial beds, it most commonly affects the renal and cerebrovascular systems, specifically the mid to distal internal carotid artery. Screening for intracranial aneurysms should be considered, as the reported prevalence ranges from 7 to 50 % [119]. Overall, the prevalence of FMD is 4 %; however, the number of incidentally identified lesions will most likely rise as the volume and quality of radiographic studies increase [120].

Presenting symptoms for FMD vary. Olin et al. suggest that the diagnosis of FMD should be considered in patients with any of the following clinical conditions [120]:

- Onset of hypertension <35 years of age
- Resistent hypertension
- Epigastric bruit and hypertension
- Cervical bruit at <10 years of age
- Pulsatile tinnitus
- Severe and recurrent headaches
- TIA or stroke in those <60 years of age
- Peripheral dissection
- Intracranial or visceral aneurysm
- Aortic aneurysm in those <60 years of age
- Subarachnoid hemorrhage
- Renal infarction

Diagnosis and Treatment

The clinical circumstances usually raise the possibility of FMD. Imaging studies including ultrasound duplex, CTA, MRA, conventional angiography, or IVUS often demonstrate characteristic stenotic lesions further supporting the diagnosis of FMD [121]. Treatment for FMD depends on the symptoms. Asymptomatic patients should be started on aspirin 81 mg daily and educated to recognize signs and symptoms that could indicate cerebrovascular or renal disease. These patients should also be informed that FMD increases the risk of arterial dissection associated with participation in contact sports, physical activities, and chiropractic manipulations. A CT scan of the head to screen for intracranial aneurysms should be considered since patients with FMD appear to have a greater risk for these aneurysms than the general population [118]. Although it does not have strong supporting evidence, systemic anticoagulation remains a widely used treatment strategy for patients with a carotid dissection due to FMD [119]. Symptomatic arterial occlusive lesions caused by FMD respond well to percutaneous balloon angioplasty, and endovascular intervention represents a first-line therapy despite a lack of randomized controlled studies. Endovascular stent grafts have also successfully treated cerebrovascular pseudoaneurysms and aneurysms caused by FMD; however, comparative studies have not been performed. Open surgical repair and revascularization is a reasonable treatment option in patients with complex lesions that are not amenable to endovascular intervention [118].

Conclusion

Vascular disease is not always confined to elderly patients with a history of smoking and systemic atherosclerosis. Patients with non-atherosclerotic vascular disorders come from a wide range of demographic groups and have a different presentation, natural history, and treatment compared to patients with traditional vascular disease. Failure to recognize and treat these non-atherosclerotic vascular diseases can have significant and potentially fatal consequences. General surgeons who are familiar with non-atherosclerotic vascular disease can recognize and appropriately manage patients with these rare conditions.

References

1. Kearon C, Crowther M, Hirsh J. Management of patients with hereditary hypercoagulable disorders. Annu Rev Med. 2000; 51:169–85.
2. Rao AK, Sheth S, Kaplan R. Inherited hypercoagulable states. Vasc Med. 1997;2:313–20.
3. Ray SA, Rowley MR, Loh A, et al. Hypercoagulable states in patients with leg ischemia. Br J Surg. 1994;81:811–4.
4. Eldrup-Jorgensen J, Flanigan DP, Brace L, et al. Hypercoagulable states and lower limb ischemia in young adults. J Vasc Surg. 1989;9:334–41.
5. Donaldson MC, Weinberg DS, Belkin M, et al. Screening for hypercoagulable states in vascular surgical practice: a preliminary study. J Vasc Surg. 1990;11:825–31.
6. Crowther MA, Kelton JG. Congenital thrombophilic states associated with venous thrombosis: a qualitative overview and proposed classification system. Ann Intern Med. 2003;138(2):128–34.
7. Egeberg O. Inherited antithrombin deficiency causing thrombophilia. Thromb Diath Haemorrh. 1965;13:516–30.
8. Mateo J, Oliver A, Borrell M, et al. Laboratory evaluation and clinical characteristics of 2,132 consecutive unselected patients with venous thromboembolism. Results of the Spanish Multicentric Study on Thrombophilia (EMET-study). Thromb Haemost. 1997;77:444.
9. Van Den Belt AGM, Huisman MV, Hirsh J. Familial thrombophilia: a review analysis. Clin Appl Thromb Hemost. 1996; 2(4):227–36.
10. Weiss P, Soff GA, Halkin H, et al. Decline of protein C and S and factors II, VII, IX and X during the initiation of warfarin therapy. Thromb Res. 1987;45(6):783–90.
11. Borgel D, Gandrille S, Aiach M. Protein S deficiency. Thromb Haemost. 1997;78:351.
12. Clark DA, Williams WL, Marlar RA. Mesenteric vein thrombosis associated with famlilal deficiency of free protein S. Arch Pathol Lab Med. 1991;115:617.
13. Baglin T, Gray E, Greaves M, et al. British Committee for Standards in Haematology. Clinical guidelines for testing for heritable thrombophilia. Br J Haematol. 2010;149:209–20.
14. Rodeghiero F, Tosetto A. Activated protein C resistance and factor V Leiden mutation are independent risk factors for venous thromboembolism. Ann Intern Med. 1999;130:643–50.
15. Rees DC, Cox M, Clegg JB. World distribution of factor V Leiden. Lancet. 1995;346:1133–4.
16. Koster T, Rosendaal FR, de Ronde H, et al. Venous thrombosis due to poor anticoagulant response to activated protein C: Leiden thrombophilia study. Lancet. 1993;342:1503–6.
17. Leroyer C, Mercier B, Escoffe M, et al. Factor V Leiden prevalence in venous thromboembolism patients. Chest. 1997;111:1603–6.
18. Springer J, Villa-Forte A. Thrombosis in vasculitis. Curr Opin Rheumatol. 2012;24:1–7.
19. Hellgren M, Svensson PI, Dahlback B. Resistance to activated protein C as a basis for venous thromboembolism associated with pregnancy and oral contraceptives. Am J Obstet Gynecol. 1995;173:210.
20. Olivieri O, Friso S, Manzato F, Guella A, Bernardi F, Lunghi B, Girelli D, Azzini M, Brocco G, Russo C. Resistance to activated protein C in healthy women taking oral contraceptives. Br J Haematol. 1995;91:465–70.
21. Henkens CMA, van der Bom JG, van der Meer FJ. Lowered activated protein C-sensitivity ratio related to increased factor VIII-clotting activity. Thromb Haemost. 1995;74:1198–9.
22. Cumming AM, Tait RC, Fildes S, Young A, Keeney S, Hay CR. Development of resistance to activated protein C during pregnancy. Br J Haematol. 1995;90:725–7.
23. Vandenbroucke JP, Koster T, Briet E, et al. Increased risk of venous thrombosis in oral-contraceptive users who are carriers of factor V Leiden mutation. Lancet. 1994;344:1453–7.
24. McColl MD, Ramsay JE, Tait RC, et al. Risk factors for pregnancy associated venous thromboembolism. Thromb Haemost. 1997;78:1183–8.
25. Ridker PM, Hennekens CH, Selhub J, et al. Interrelation of hyperhomocyst(e)inemia, factor V Leiden, and risk of future venous thromboembolism. Circulation. 1997;95:1777–82.
26. Gandrille S, Greengard JS, Alhenc-Gelas M, et al. Incidence of activated protein C resistance caused by the ARG 506 GLN mutation in factor V in 113 unrelated symptomatic protein C-deficient patients. Blood. 1995;86:219–24.
27. Zoller B, Holm J, Svensson P, Dahlback B. Elevated levels of prothrombin activation fragment 1+2 in plasma from patients with heterozygous Arg506 to Gln mutation in the factor V gene (APC resistance) and/or inherited protein S deficiency. Thromb Haemost. 1996;75:270–4.
28. Lane DA, Mannucci PM, Bauer KA, et al. Inherited thrombophilia: part 2. Thromb Haemost. 1996;76(6):824–34.
29. Ridker PM, Hennekens CH, Miletich JP. G20210A mutation in prothrombin gene and risk of myocardial infarction, stroke and venous thrombosis in a large cohort of US men. Circulation. 1999; 99:999–1004.
30. Ridker PM, Miletich JP, Stampfer MJ, et al. Factor V Leiden and risks of recurrent idiopathic venous thromboembolism. Circulation. 1995;92:2800–2.
31. Simioni P, Prandoni P, Lensing AWA, et al. The risk of recurrent venous thromboembolism in patients with an $Arg^{506}Gln$ mutation in the gene for factor V (factor V Leiden). N Engl J Med. 1997; 336:399–403.
32. Kearon C, Gent M, Hirsh J, et al. A comparison of three months of anticoagulation with extended anticoagulation for a first episode of idiopathic venous thromboembolism. N Engl J Med. 1999; 340:901–7.
33. Eichinger S, Pabinger I, Stumpflen A, et al. The risk of recurrent venous thromboembolism in patients with and without factor V Leiden. Thromb Haemost. 1997;77(4):624–8.
34. Doggen CJ, Cats VM, Bertina RM, Rosendaal FR. Interaction of coagulation defects and cardiovascular risk factors: increased risk of myocardial infarction associated with factor V Leiden or prothrombin 20210A. Circulation. 1998;97(11):1037–41.
35. Rosendaal FR, Doggen CJM, Zivelin A, et al. Geographic distribution of the 20210 G to a prothrombin variant. Thromb Haemost. 1998;79:706–8.
36. Koster T, Blann AD, Briet E, et al. Role of clotting factor VIII in effect of von Willebrand factor on occurrence of deep-vein thrombosis. Lancet. 1995;345:152.
37. O'Donnell JO, Tuddenham EGD, Manning R, et al. High prevalence of elevated factor VIII levels in patients referred for thrombophilia screening: role of increased synthesis and relationship to acute phase reaction. Thromb Haemost. 1997;77:825.
38. Kamphusien PW, Eikenboom JCJ, Bertina RM. Elevated factor VIII levels and the risk of thrombosis. Arterioscler Thromb Vasc Biol. 2001;21:731.
39. Stampfer MJ, Malinow MR, Willett WC, et al. A prospective study of plasma homocyst(e)ine and risk of myocardial infarction in US physicians. JAMA. 1992;268:877–81.
40. Clarke R, Daly L, Robinson K, et al. Hyperhomocysteinemia: an independent risk factor for vascular disease. N Engl J Med. 1991;324(17):1149–55.
41. den Heijer M, Koster T, Bloom HJ, et al. Hyperhomocysteinemia as a risk factor for deep vein thrombosis. N Engl J Med. 1996;334:759–62.
42. Simioni P, Prandoni P, Burlina A, et al. Hyperhomocysteinemia and deep-vein thrombosis: a case controlled study. Thromb Haemost. 1996;76:883.

43. Arnesen E, Refsum H, Bonaa KH, et al. Serum total homocysteine and coronary heart disease. Int J Epidemiol. 1995;24:704–9.
44. Nygard O, Nordrehaug JE, Refusum H, et al. Plasma homocysteine levels and mortality in patients with coronary artery disease. N Engl J Med. 1997;337:230.
45. Lim W, Crowther MA. Antiphospholipid antibodies: a critical review of the literature. Curr Opin Hematol. 2007;14:494.
46. Miyakis S, Lockshin MD, Atsumi T, et al. International consensus statement on an update of the classification criteria for definite antiphospholipid syndrome (APS). J Thromb Haemost. 2006; 4:295.
47. Turiel M, Sarzi-Puttini P, Peretti R, et al. Thrombotic risk factors in primary antiphospholipid syndrome. A 5 year prospective study. Stroke. 2005;36:1490.
48. Rosove MH, Brewer PMC. Antiphospholipid thrombosis: clinical course after the first thrombotic event in 70 patients. Ann Intern Med. 1992;117:303.
49. Khamashta MA, Cuadrado MD, Mukic F, et al. The management of thrombosis in the antiphospholipid antibody syndrome. N Engl J Med. 1995;332:993.
50. de Groot PG, Lutters B, Derksen RH, et al. Lupus anticoagulants and the risk of a first episode of deep venous thrombosis. J Thromb Haemost. 2005;3:1993.
51. Trousseau A. Phlegmasia Alba Dolen. In: Clinique Medicale De L'Hotel-Dieu de Paris. Paris: JB Balliere; 1865. p. 654.
52. Blom JW, Doggen CJ, Osanto S, Roendaal FR. Malignancies, prothrombotic mutations and the risk of venous thrombosis. JAMA. 2005;293:715–22.
53. Lee AY, Levine MN, Baker RI, et al. Low-molecular-weight heparin versus a coumarin for the prevention of recurrent venous thromboembolism in patients with cancer. N Engl J Med. 2003; 349(2):146–53.
54. Hull RD, Pineo GF, Brant RF, et al. LITE Trial Investigators. Long-term low-molecular-weight heparin versus usual care in proximal-vein thrombosis patients with cancer. Am J Med. 2006; 119:1062.
55. Prandoni P, Lensing AW, Piccioli A, et al. Recurrent venous thromboembolism and bleeding complications during anticoagulant treatment in patients with cancer and venous thrombosis. Blood. 2002;100:3484.
56. Heit JA, Kobervig CE, James AH, et al. Trends in the incidence of venous thromboembolism during pregnancy or postpartum: a 30 year population-based study. Ann Intern Med. 2005;143:697.
57. Andres RL, Miles A. Venous thromboembolism and pregnancy. Obstet Gynecol Clin North Am. 2001;28:613.
58. James AH, Tapson VF, Goldhaber SZ. Thrombosis during pregnancy and the postpartum period. Am J Obstet Gynecol. 2005; 193:216.
59. Faught W, Garner P, Jones G, et al. Changes in protein C and protein S levels in normal pregnancy. Am J Obstet Gynecol. 1995;172:147.
60. Comp PC, Thurnau GR, Welsh J, et al. Functional and immunologic protein S levels are decreased during pregnancy. Blood. 1986;68:881.
61. Johnson CM, Mureebe L, Silver D. Hypercoagulable states: a review. Vasc Endovascular Surg. 2005;39(2):123–33.
62. Ginsberg J, Brill-Edwards P, Burrows RF, et al. DVT during pregnancy: leg and trimester presentation. Thromb Haemost. 1992; 67:519.
63. Martinelli I, DeStafano V, Taioli E, et al. Inherited thrombophilias and first venous thromboembolism during pregnancy and puerperium. Thromb Haemost. 2002;87:791–5.
64. Warkentin TE. Clinical presentation of heparin-induced thrombocytopenia. Semin Hematol. 1998;35(4 Suppl 5):9.
65. Warkentin TE, Elavathil LJ, Hayward CP, et al. The pathogenesis of venous limb gangrene associated with heparin-induced thrombocytopenia. Ann Intern Med. 1997;127:804.
66. Simioni P, Sanson BJ, Prandoni P, et al. Incidence of venous thromboembolism in families with inherited thrombophilia. Thromb Haemost. 1999;81:198–202.
67. Antithrombotic therapy and prevention of thrombosis, 9th ed: American College of Chest Physicians evidence-based clinical practice guidelines. Chest. 2012;141(2 suppl):7S–47S.
68. Caprini JA. Risk assessment as a guide for the prevention of the many faces of venous thromboembolism. Am J Surg. 1991; 1S:S3–10.
69. Geerts WH, Bergqvist D, Pineo GF, Heit JA, Samama CM, Lassen MR, Colwell CW, American College of Chest Physicians. Prevention of venous thromboembolism: American College of Chest Physicians Evidence-Based Clinical Practice Guidelines (8th Edition). Chest. 2008;133:381S–453.
70. Anderson JA, Weitz J. Hypercoagulable states. Crit Care Clin. 2011;27:933–52.
71. Landefeld CS, Beyth RJ. Anticoagulant-related bleeding: clinical epidemiology, prediction, and prevention. Am J Med. 1993;95: 315–28.
72. Palareti G, Leali N, Coccheri S, et al. Bleeding complications of oral anticoagulant treatment: an inception-cohort, prospective collaborative study (ISCOAT). Lancet. 1996;348:423–8.
73. Schafer AI, Levine MN, Konkle BA, et al. Thrombotic disorders: diagnosis and treatment. Hematology. 2003;520–39.
74. Stuart TP. Note on a variation in the course of the popliteal artery. J Anat Physiol. 1879;13:162.
75. Hamming JJ. Intermittent claudication at an early age, due to an anomalous course of the popliteal artery. Angiology. 1959;10: 369–70.
76. Bouhoutsos J, Daskalakis E. Muscular abnormalities affecting the popliteal vessels. Br J Surg. 1981;68:501–6.
77. Gibson MHL, Mills JG, Johnson GE, et al. Popliteal entrapment syndrome. Ann Surg. 1977;185:341–8.
78. Turnipseed WD. Popliteal entrapment syndrome. J Vasc Surg. 2002;35:910–5.
79. Turnipseed WD. Clinical review of patients treated for atypical claudication: a 28-year experience. J Vasc Surg. 2004;40:79–85.
80. Rignault DP, Pailler JL, Lunel F. The "functional" popliteal entrapment syndrome. Int Angiol. 1985;4:341–3.
81. Pillai J. A current interpretation of popliteal vascular entrapment. J Vasc Surg. 2008;48:61S–5.
82. Chernoff DM, Walker AT, Khorasani R, et al. Asymptomatic functional popliteal artery entrapment: demonstration at MR imaging. Radiology. 1995;195:176–80.
83. Turnipseed WD, Pozniak M. Popliteal entrapment as a result of neurovascular compression by the soleus and plantaris muscles. J Vasc Surg. 1992;15:285–94.
84. Sinha S, Houghton J, Holt P, et al. Popliteal entrapment syndrome. J Vasc Surg. 2012;55(1):252–62.
85. Roche-Nagle G, Wong KT, Oreopolulos G. Vascular claudication in a young patient: popliteal entrapment syndrome. Hong Kong Med J. 2009;15(5):388–90.
86. Ehsan O, Darwish A, Edmundson C, et al. Non-traumatic lower limb vascular complications in endurance athletes. Review of literature. Eur J Vasc Endovasc Surg. 2004;28:1–8.
87. Levien L. Popliteal artery thrombosis caused by popliteal entrapment syndrome. In: Greenhalgh RM, Powell JT, editors. Inflammatory and thrombotic problems in vascular surgery. London: WB Saunders Co Ltd; 1997. p. 159–68.
88. Gibson MHL, Mills JG, Johnson GE, et al. Popliteal entrapment syndrome. Ann Surg. 1997;185:341–8.

89. Murray A, Halliday M, Croft RJ. Popliteal artery entrapment syndrome. Br J Surg. 1991;78:1414–9.
90. Di Cesare J, Marsili L, Marino G, Masciocchi C, et al. Stress MR imaging for evaluation of popliteal artery entrapment. J Magn Reson Imaging. 1994;4:617–22.
91. Collins PS, McDonald PT, Lim RC. Popliteal artery entrapment: an evolving syndrome. J Vasc Surg. 1989;10:484–90.
92. Zund G, Brunner U. Surgical aspects of popliteal artery entrapment syndrome: 26 years of experience with 26 legs. Vasa. 1995; 24:29–33.
93. DiMarzo L, Cavallaro A, Mingoli A, et al. Popliteal artery entrapment syndrome: the role of early diagnosis and treatment. Surg. 1997;122:26–31.
94. DiMarzo L, Cavallaro A, Sciacca V, et al. Natural history of entrapment of the popliteal artery. J Am Coll Surg. 1994;178: 553–6.
95. Akkersdijk WL, de Ruyter JW, Lapham R, et al. Colour duplex ultrasonographic imaging and provocation of popliteal artery compression. Eur J Vasc Endovasc Surg. 1995;10:342–5.
96. Deshpande A, Denton M. Functional popliteal entrapment syndrome. Aust N Z J Surg. 1998;68:660–3.
97. Kim SY, Min SK, Ahn S, et al. Long-term outcomes after revascularization for advanced popliteal artery entrapment syndrome with segmental arterial occlusion. J Vasc Surg. 2012;55(1): 90–7.
98. Papaioannou S, Tsitouridis K, Giataganas G, et al. Evaluation of popliteal arteries with CT angiography in popliteal artery entrapment syndrome. Hippokratia. 2009;13:32–7.
99. Rich NM, Collins Jr GJ, McDonald PT, et al. Popliteal vascular entrapment. Its increasing interest. Arch Surg. 1979;114: 1377–84.
100. Espinoza LR. Buerger's disease: thromboangitis obliterans 100 years after the initial description. Am J Med Sci. 2009;337(4): 285–6.
101. Piazza G, Creager M. Thromboangitis obliterans. Circulation. 2010;121:1858–61.
102. Puechal X, Fiessinger JN, Kahan A, et al. Rheumatologic manifestations in patients with thromboangitis obliterans. J Rheumatol. 1999;26:1764–8.
103. Olin JW. Thromboangitis obliterans. N Engl J Med. 2000;343: 864–9.
104. Ohta T, Ishioashi H, Hosaka M, et al. Clinical and social consequences of Buerger disease. J Vasc Surg. 2001;39:176–80.
105. Jayne D. Update on the European Vasculitis Study Group trials. Curr Opin Rheumatol. 2001;13:48–55.
106. Luqmani R. Large vessel vasculitides. Update for the cardiologist. Curr Opin Cardiol. 2012;27(6):578–84.
107. Devauchell-Pensec V, Jousee S, Destombe C, et al. Epidemiology, imaging and treatment of GCA. Joint Bone Spine. 2008;75(3): 267–72.
108. Weyand C, Liao JY, Goronzy JJ, et al. The immunopathology of GCA: diagnostic and therapeutic implications. J Neuroophthalmol. 2012;32(3):259–65.
109. Wlavick MD, Walvick MP. GCA: laboratory predictors of a positive temporal artery biopsy. Ophthalmology. 2011;118:1201–4.
110. Danesh-Meyer H. Temporal artery biopsy: skip it at your patient's peril. Am J Ophthalmol. 2012;154(4):617–9.
111. Quinn EM, Kearney DE, Keohane C. Temporal artery biopsy is not required in all cases of suspected GCA. Ann Vasc Surg. 2012;26(5):649–54.
112. Cowey S, Reynolds C, Joglekar S, et al. Does temporal artery biopsy influence management of GCA? Int J Surg. 2010;8:501.
113. Achkar AA, Lie JT, Hunder GG, O'Fallon WM, Gabriel SE. How does previous glucocorticosteroid treatment affect the biopsy findings in giant cell (temporal) arteritis? Ann Intern Med. 1994; 120:987–92.
114. Dastgir G, Gutman J, Shinder R. Facial nerve injury: a complication of superficial temporal artery biopsy. Am J Ophthalmol. 2011;153(1):187.
115. Ypilantis E, Courtney ED, Chopra N, et al. Importance of specimen length during temporal artery biopsy. Br J Surgery. 2011; 98:1556–60.
116. Scafer V, Zwerina J. Biologic treatment of large vessel vasculitides. Curr Opin Rheumatol. 2012;24(1):31–7.
117. Talwar KD, Kumar K, Copra P, et al. Cardiac involvement in nonspecific arteritis. Am Heart J. 1991;122:1666–70.
118. Curry TK, Messina LM. Fibromuscular dysplasia: when is intervention warranted? Semin Vasc Surg. 2003;16(3):190–9.
119. Bornak A, Milner R. Diagnosing and treating atypical arterial pathologies of aortic arch vessels: dissection and fibromuscular dysplasia. Semin Vasc Surg. 2011;24:36–43.
120. Olin JW, Froehlich J, Xiaokui G, et al. The United States registry for fibromuscular dysplasia results in the first 447 patients. Circulation. 2012;125:3182–90.
121. Weinberg I, Jaff MR. Nonatherosclerotic disorders of the lower extremities. Circulation. 2012;126:213–22.

Surgical and Endovascular Complications: Infection and Hemorrhage

23

Mark G. Davies

Diagnosis and Management of Hemorrhage: Retroperitoneal, Cervical, and Groin

In all cases of hemorrhage, the Advanced Trauma Life Support (ATLS) algorithm should be followed, with prompt recognition, rapid resuscitation, and immediate decision making and action [1].

Retroperitoneal Hemorrhage

Etiology

Retroperitoneal hematoma (RPH) describes bleeding into the potential space between the peritoneum and the musculoskeletal elements of the back. Several conditions can cause RPH including ruptured aortic aneurysm, traumatic vascular injury, retroperitoneal neoplasms, and coagulopathy. RPH occurs most frequently as a complication of percutaneous femoral artery puncture for interventional procedures. The reported incidence of RPH after cardiac catheterization is 0.15 % for diagnostic procedures, 0.8 % for balloon angioplasty, and 3 % for coronary stents. Three dichotomous variables were identified as independent predictors of RPH: female gender (odds ratio [OR] 5.4), body surface area (BSA) less than 1.73 m^2 (OR 7.1), and high femoral artery puncture site (OR 5.3) [2]. Twenty-five percent of retroperitoneal bleeds were remote from the femoral artery puncture site, with the majority of these being contralateral to the side of the puncture.

M.G. Davies, MD, PhD, MBA (✉)
Vascular and Endovascular Surgery, Houston Methodist DeBakey Heart & Vascular Center, Houston Methodist Hospital, 6550 Fannin, Smith Tower, Suite 1401, Houston, TX 77030, USA
e-mail: MDavies@tmhs.org

Presentation

The diagnosis of retroperitoneal hematoma requires clinical acumen, and an awareness of the scenarios in which this complication is likely to occur. Patients with significant groin, flank, abdominal, or back pain or hemodynamic instability following an interventional procedure should be evaluated for a retroperitoneal hematoma. The nonspecific symptoms associated with RPH often delay the diagnosis. Approximately 23–54 % of retroperitoneal hematoma patients have documented clinical evidence of femoral neuropathy caused by compression of the femoral nerve [3]. Seventy-five percent of cases presented within the first 3 h after conclusion of the procedure, with a rapid decline in frequency after this time period [4]. Spontaneous hemorrhage usually occurs in patients receiving anticoagulation. Idiopathic retroperitoneal hematoma may present symptomatically in the form of acute abdominal pain, nausea, and anorexia. Upon physical examination, the patient may have a tender abdomen and hypovolemic shock.

Imaging

Contrast-enhanced computed tomography (CT) scan is the imaging modality of choice to identify and categorize a retroperitoneal hemorrhage (Fig. 23.1).

Treatment

Although a widely accepted consensus on the management of patients with RPH does not exist, a reasonable treatment algorithm is shown in Fig. 23.2.

Conservative Therapy

Hemodynamically stable patients with RPH can be managed with fluid resuscitation, correction of coagulopathy, and blood transfusion. Non-interventional therapy mandates close observation for the development of abdominal compartment syndrome (ACS) which can be fatal if it is not promptly recognized and treated. ACS is defined as sustained intra-abdominal pressure greater than 20 mmHg with end-organ dysfunction manifested as respiratory insufficiency, oliguria, and decreased venous return resulting in severe hypotension.

V. Gahtan and M.J. Costanza (eds.), *Essentials of Vascular Surgery for the General Surgeon*,
DOI 10.1007/978-1-4939-1326-8_23, © Springer Science+Business Media New York 2015

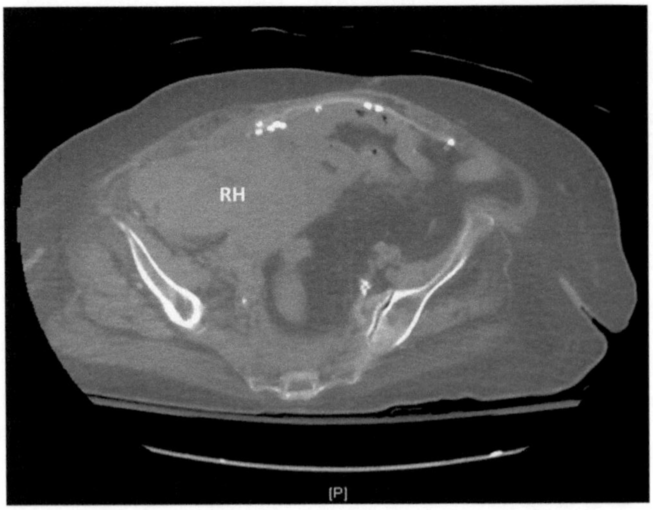

Fig. 23.1 CT scan without contrast showing a retroperitoneal hematoma (*RH*)

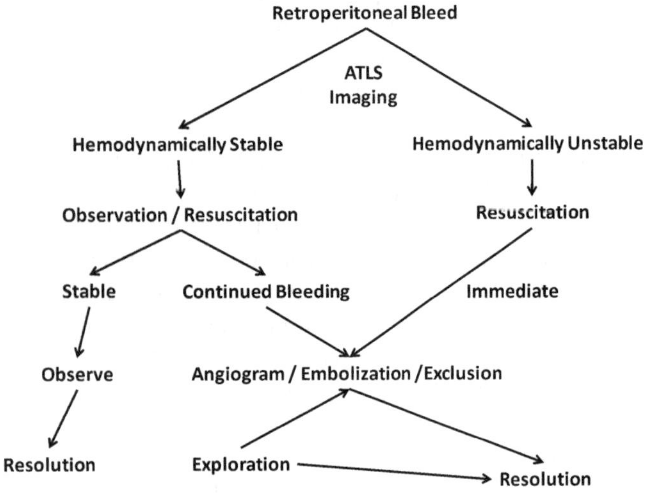

Fig. 23.2 Algorithm for the treatment of a retroperitoneal bleed. *ATLS* Advanced Trauma Life Support

Endovascular Intervention

Hemodynamic compromise that persists or fails to respond to resuscitation indicates the need for more definitive intervention. Endovascular therapy for RPH requires arteriography and selective vessel catheterization. Selective embolization of a bleeding arterial branch or exclusion of an injured vessel segment with a stent graft can provide definitive hemostasis. Balloon occlusion offers temporary control of the bleeding, while surgical exploration is undertaken. If there is no arterial injury, venography should be considered.

Exploration

Open surgical repair of retroperitoneal bleeding should be reserved for cases when conservative management fails or endovascular measures are either not available or do not control the bleeding. The surgical procedure begins with retroperitoneal exploration and packing. Proximal and distal vascular control is then obtained followed by careful exploration and definitive primary repair or replacement of the injured vessel.

Outcomes

RPH is a potentially deadly condition that carries a mortality rate of 18–60 %. Although there is no level I evidence to guide the management of patients with RPH, it is clear that delayed diagnosis and inappropriate treatment increase the risk of death, and this may account for the wide range in reported mortality rates. Angiography and selective embolization have emerged as effective methods for treating RPH. Several case series document that the technical success of embolization for RPH approaches 100 % resulting in immediate and sustained (greater than 24 h) hemodynamic improvement in more than 90 % of patients. Despite these promising initial results, some patients still require additional hemostatic surgery, and all-cause mortality at 1 month ranges from 32 to 75 % [5]. The ability of embolization to stabilize hemodynamic parameters may depend on the rate of administration of packed red blood cells and fresh frozen plasma (FFP), as well as the systolic blood pressure (SBP) immediately before embolization. Predictors of mortality from RPH include the number of injured sites, SBP before embolization, the need for vasopressive drugs before embolization, and hemodynamic recovery after intervention.

Cervical (Neck) Hemorrhage

Etiology

The most common causes of cervical hemorrhage are traumatic injury, postoperative issues related to specific organs, and the sequelae of therapy for cancer. Projectiles and blades cause most traumatic neck injuries, while postsurgical hemorrhage (including post carotid endarterectomy [CEA] hematoma) represents a common nontraumatic cause of cervical hemorrhage. Penetrating neck trauma represents approximately 5–10 % of all trauma cases that present to the emergency department. About 30 % of these cases are accompanied by an injury outside of the neck zones [6]. In contrast, blunt injury to the carotid and vertebral arteries is rare, occurring in only 1 % of patients with blunt trauma to the face and head. The natural history of blunt neck injuries remains unclear, and the optimal treatment continues to evolve. Biffle et al. proposed a grading scheme for the severity of blunt cerebrovascular injury [7]:

- Grade I – intimal irregularity with <25 % narrowing
- Grade II – dissection with >25 % luminal narrowing
- Grade III – pseudoaneurysm
- Grade IV – occlusion
- Grade V – transection with extravasation

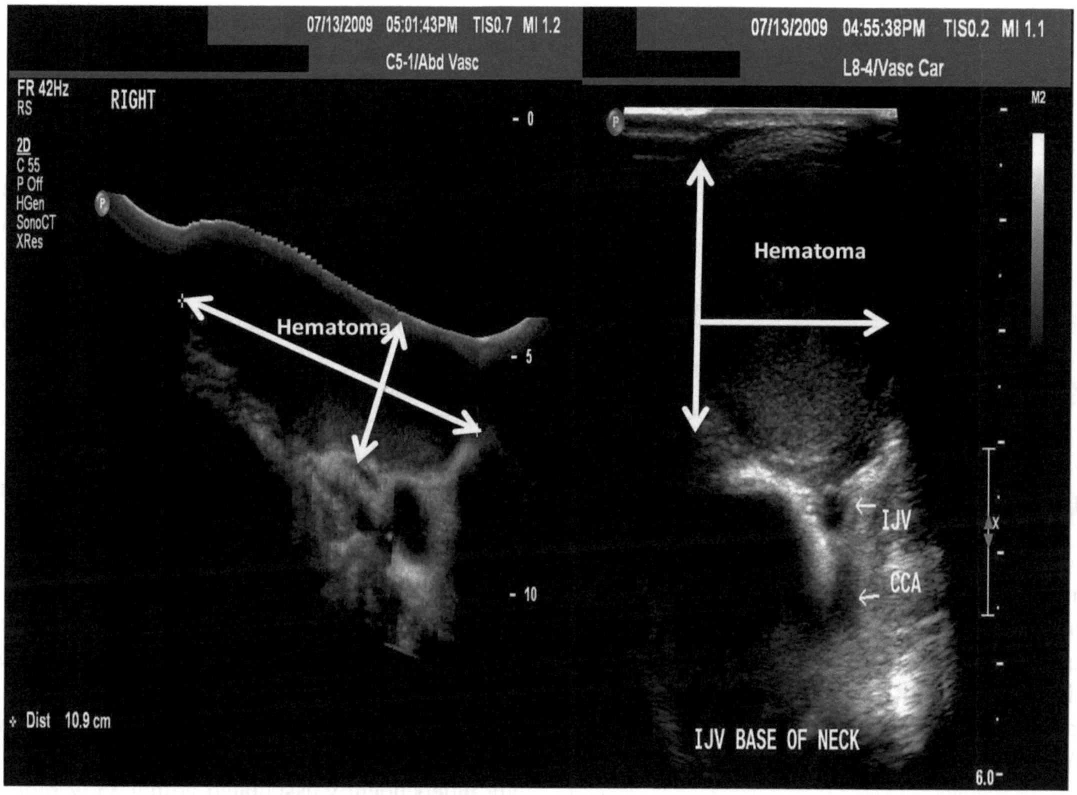

Fig. 23.3 Duplex ultrasound showing a postoperative hematoma in two views (*arrow*) after line placement. *IJV* internal jugular vein, *CCA* common carotid artery

The ability to accurately describe and classify blunt cerebrovascular injuries will advance research efforts aimed at determining the best treatment strategy.

Carotid blowout syndrome (CBS) is a potentially fatal hemorrhagic complication that occurs in 3–4 % of patients with head and neck cancer [8]. The clinical severity for CBS has been classified into three categories: acute, impending, and threatened [9]. Acute CBS involves complete rupture of the vessel with profuse hemorrhage not controlled with surgical packing. The patient's condition rapidly deteriorates if immediate resuscitation and stabilization is not achieved before definitive treatment. Impending CBS manifests as short episodes of sentinel hemorrhage that resolve spontaneously or with simple surgical packing. Despite the absence of uncontrollable hemorrhage, complete rupture of the vessel is certain. Threatened CBS describes exposure of the carotid artery as a result of wound breakdown or neoplastic invasion of the carotid system. Although hemorrhage has not yet occurred, rupture is inevitable if the exposed vessel cannot be promptly covered with healthy vascularized tissue.

Presentation

Patients with cervical hemorrhage can present with an external bleeding, an expanding hematoma, or a hemothorax (Fig. 23.3). Approximately 15–20 % of patients are hypotensive, 15–20 % have external hemorrhage, and 30 % have a cervical hematoma [10]. Overt or potential airway compromise may be present due to a combination of direct compression and laryngeal edema. Neurological status should be determined as associated cerebrovascular injury is common and many patients with traumatic cervical bleeding suffer from polytrauma. "Hard" signs that indicate a likely vascular injury include: expanding hematoma, active external hemorrhage from the wound site, a bruit or thrill over the wound, pulse deficit, or distal ischemia presenting as a neurologic deficit.

Imaging

For traumatic neck injuries, the ATLS algorithm for imaging based on injury location (zones 1, 2, or 3) should be followed [11]. For an immediate postsurgical bleed, no imaging is required. For a delayed bleed, or hemorrhage after tumor resection (a potential carotid blowout), CT angiography (CTA) and/or catheter-directed angiography is recommended.

Treatment

As with all hemorrhage, the ATLS algorithm should be followed initially as a means of stabilizing and evaluating the patient. Temporary hemostasis can often be obtained with

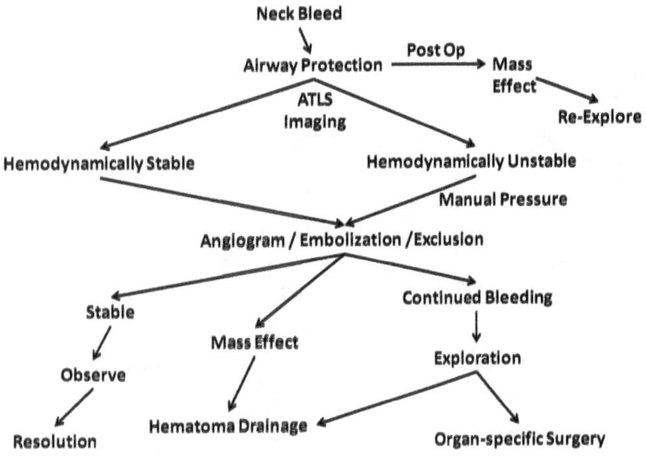

Fig. 23.4 Algorithm for the treatment of a bleed in the neck

direct manual pressure. For traumatic neck injuries, the general consensus is to repair the common and internal carotid arteries. Ligation usually represents a damage control maneuver in patients with hemodynamic compromise or severe neurological deficits. Figure 23.4 depicts a treatment algorithm for patients with cervical hemorrhage.

Immediate Postoperative Hemorrhage

Patients with cervical bleeding in the immediate postoperative period should undergo surgical reexploration. Intubation should be performed by the most experienced practitioner available under controlled conditions in the operating room. Active bleeding should be surgically repaired while quickly correcting any coagulopathy. Drains should be placed in the wound at the time of surgical reexploration, and intubation should be maintained postoperatively to protect the airway.

Endovascular Intervention

Endovascular therapy usually begins with an aortic arch arteriogram followed by selective catheterization of the arch vessels. Active hemorrhage can be initially controlled with proximal balloon occlusion of the bleeding vessel. Definitive therapy can involve intraluminal placement of a stent graft to cover the injury or open exploration and surgical repair under balloon control. Bleeding from an arterial branch can be treated with selective coil embolization. If carotid occlusion is contemplated, contralateral carotid angiography is required to confirm cerebral cross-filling.

Exploration for Penetrating Trauma

As with all exploration for hemorrhage, proximal vascular control prior to violating the hematoma or exploring the actual injury site is recommended if the anatomy and circumstances allow. If a definitive repair requires prolonged clamping of the internal carotid artery, placing an intraluminal shunt can maintain cerebral perfusion. Key surgical principles are aggressive debridement back to viable vessel wall and the use of autologous tissue to achieve a tension-free repair. The most common surgical repairs involve a vein patch angioplasty or vein interposition bypass graft.

Exploration for Carotid Blowout

Surgical intervention for CBS follows the same principles described above for traumatic cervical injuries, namely, proximal vascular control, intraluminal shunting, and vessel debridement with tension-free repair. In a reoperative surgical field, and in the setting of previous neck radiation, endovascular therapy has gained prominence as a definitive treatment or an adjunctive tool to facilitate surgical repair. As previously described, endovascular intervention can involve intraluminal balloon control, stent graft placement, coil embolization of arterial branches, or permanent carotid occlusion.

Outcomes

The current mortality rate in civilians with penetrating neck injuries ranges from 3 to 6 % [12]. Mortality rates for high velocity penetrating neck trauma have decreased from 11 % in World War I to 7 % in World War II to 3.7 % in the current conflicts [13]. Endovascular procedures for cervical traumas are independently associated with a 35 % reduction in mortality risk [14]. Blunt carotid injury continues to carry a poor prognosis.

Groin Hemorrhage

Etiology

Common causes of groin hemorrhage include iatrogenic injury from arterial catheterization, infection with blowout, and penetrating trauma [15].

Presentation

Patients with groin hemorrhage can present with an external bleeding, an expanding hematoma, or a femoral artery pseudoaneurysm. Some patients present with signs and symptoms of acute limb ischemia, while victims of trauma often have other associated injuries. Wound breakdown or a sinus tract with or without purulent drainage suggests an infectious etiology. These patients may describe a minor bleeding episode – "the sentinel bleed" – which heralds impeding major hemorrhage.

Imaging

For immediate postsurgical bleeding, no imaging is required. Likewise, hemodynamically unstable patients with groin hemorrhage do not require imaging before intervention. For hemodynamically stable patients, imaging choices include duplex ultrasound, CTA, and catheter-directed angiography. The ATLS algorithms provide guidance for imaging traumatic injuries.

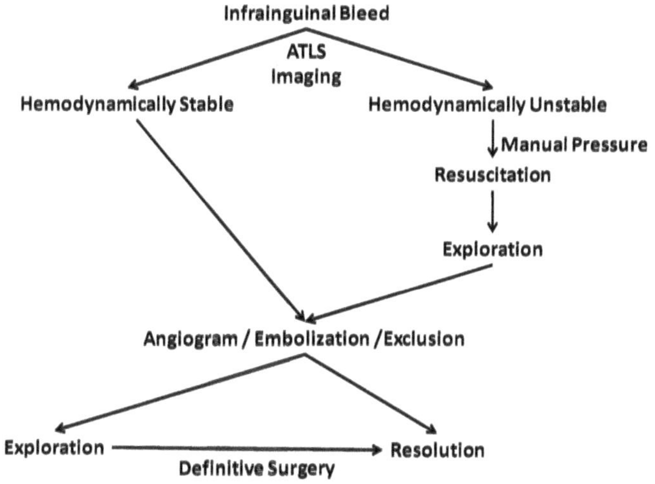

Fig. 23.5 Algorithm for the treatment of a bleed in the groin

Treatment

Active hemorrhage mandates immediate hemostatic maneuvers as delineated in the ATLS algorithm. Direct manual pressure can often provide temporary hemostasis, while arrangements for definitive therapy are made. A treatment algorithm for groin hemorrhage is shown in Fig. 23.5.

Immediate Postoperative Exploration

Postsurgical bleeding should be reexplored under controlled conditions in the operating room. If the case is immediately postoperative, the same proximal site can be used for vascular control. All active bleeding should be addressed and surgically repaired while rapidly correcting coagulopathy. Closed suction wound drainage is recommended postoperatively.

Endovascular Intervention

Angiography of the bleeding groin vessels should be performed via percutaneous access through the contralateral femoral artery. Active hemorrhage can be initially controlled with balloon occlusion of the distal external iliac artery or proximal common femoral artery. Definitive therapy can involve placement of a stent graft or surgical exploration and open repair under balloon control. If arterial branches are bleeding, they can be selectively embolized to achieve hemostasis.

Exploration for Penetrating Trauma

Proximal control for groin hemorrhage may require retroperitoneal exposure of the external iliac artery or isolation of the proximal common femoral artery as it passes deep to the inguinal ligament. If definitive repair requires arterial clamping, shunt placement can be considered but is rarely necessary unless a long delay in reconstituting antegrade flow is anticipated. Concomitant venous injuries may be repaired or ligated depending on the quality of the vessel remaining and the hemodynamic status of the patient. Lower extremity fasciotomies to prevent compartment syndrome should be considered, especially in patients with traumatic injuries. As previously described, surgical principles mandate aggressive debridement of devitalized tissue and the use of autologous tissue for vascular reconstructions. Primary arterial repair can be performed if the defect is less than 2 cm and the edges can be brought together without tension. Vein patch angioplasty or an interposition, reversed vein graft is necessary if primary repair is inadvisable.

Exploration for Femoral Artery/Anastomotic or Pseudoaneurysm Bleeding

Surgical repair of anastomotic or pseudoaneurysm bleeding requires the same techniques previously described for treating penetrating traumatic injuries. The main difference in these clinical scenarios is the possibility of infection which could compromise the long-term integrity of a vascular reconstruction performed within the infected field. If there is evidence or suspicion for infection, an extra-anatomic bypass may be required.

Outcomes

Mortality and morbidity related to groin hemorrhage vary depending on concomitant injuries and preexisting comorbidities. Although a delay in revascularization should be avoided, it is important to note that ischemic time does not correlate precisely with amputation risk nor is it the only factor that determines limb salvage [16].

Arterial Pseudoaneurysm: Diagnosis and Treatment Indications and Options

Etiology

A pseudoaneurysm (PSA) is an arterial rupture in which the bleeding is contained by the surrounding tissues. Blood flow exits through the arterial defect and swirls around within the pseudoaneurysm sac before returning to the artery through the same defect. Unlike a true aneurysm which has all three vessel wall layers, the borders of a PSA do not contain any layers of the arterial wall. PSA is a common complication of percutaneous invasive procedures, occurring in 0.1–0.2 % of diagnostic angiograms and 3.5–5.5 % of interventional procedures [17]. Risk factors for the development of PSA are listed in Table 23.1. Low or high puncture of the common femoral decreases the effectiveness of manual compression resulting in a higher incidence of femoral pseudoaneurysm [18].

Presentation

PSAs commonly present with pain and/or swelling in the groin after catheterization. Swelling from a large PSA or hematoma may lead to compression of nerves and vessels with associated neuropathy, venous thrombosis, claudication, or critical limb ischemia in rare cases. Pressure from the PSA can cause local skin ischemia leading to necrosis and infection. Physical findings associated with PSA include a pulsatile mass, palpable thrill, and audible to-and-fro murmur or systolic bruit. In some cases, none of these physical findings are present, and the patient presents with signs and symptoms of a retroperitoneal hematoma or hemorrhage. These patients have the highest risk for major complications and death.

Table 23.1 Risk Factors for arterial pseudoaneurysm

Antiplatelet agents (aspirin and clopidogrel)
Systemic anticoagulation
Large sheath size (greater than 8 Fr)
Age greater than 65 years
Hypertension
Obesity
Poor postprocedural compression
Simultaneous arterial and venous catheterization
History of peripheral arterial disease
Hemodialysis
Complex interventions with multiple sheath exchanges

Imaging

An arterial duplex ultrasound is the imaging modality of choice for diagnosing a femoral PSA with a sensitivity of 94 % and a specificity of 97 % [19] (Fig. 23.6). A comprehensive duplex ultrasound exam should document the size of the PSA, the degree of thrombus (if any) within the PSA cavity, and the communication with the femoral artery including the blood flow velocity pattern within the artery. The common femoral vein should also be evaluated to detect high velocity flow which would suggest an arteriovenous fistula.

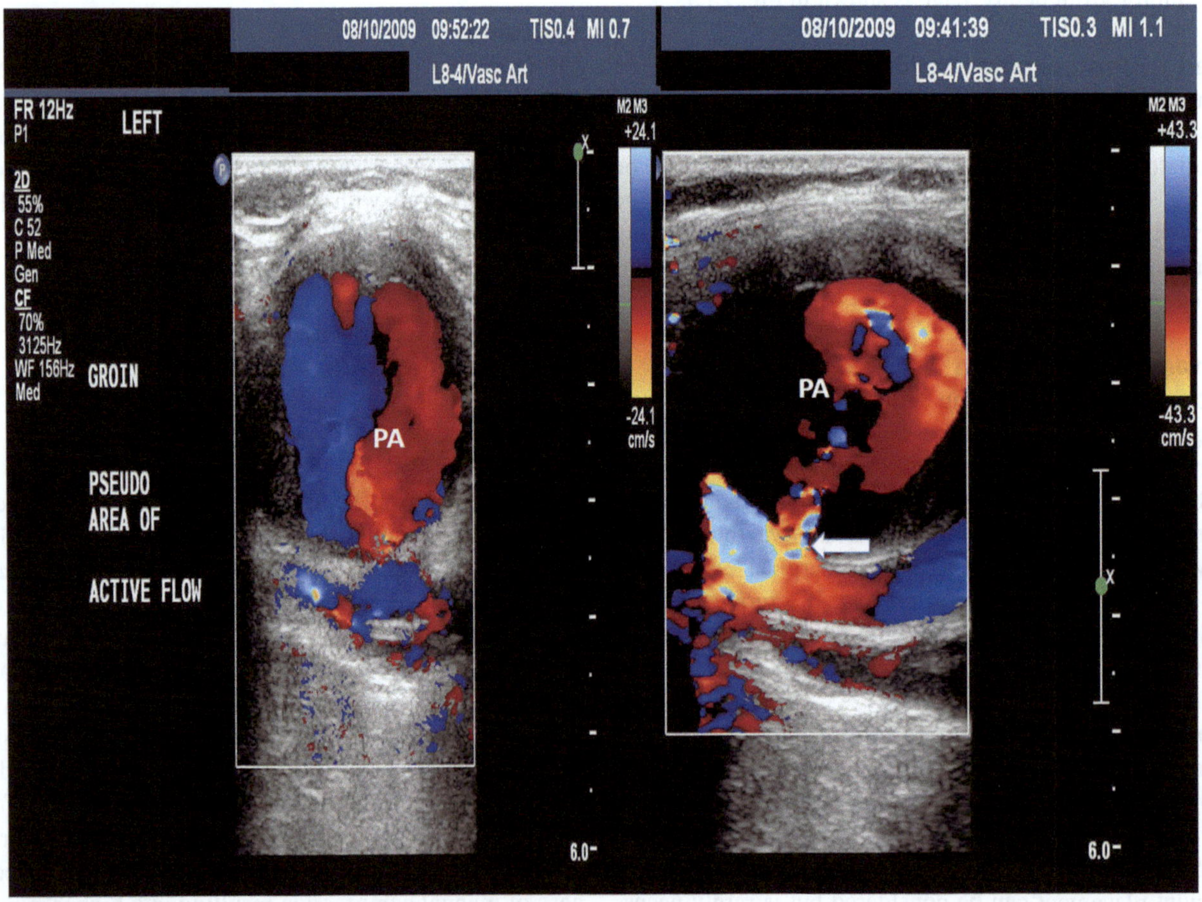

Fig. 23.6 Duplex ultrasound showing a femoral pseudoaneurysm (*PA*) in two views with the right panel demonstrating the defect in the artery (*arrow*)

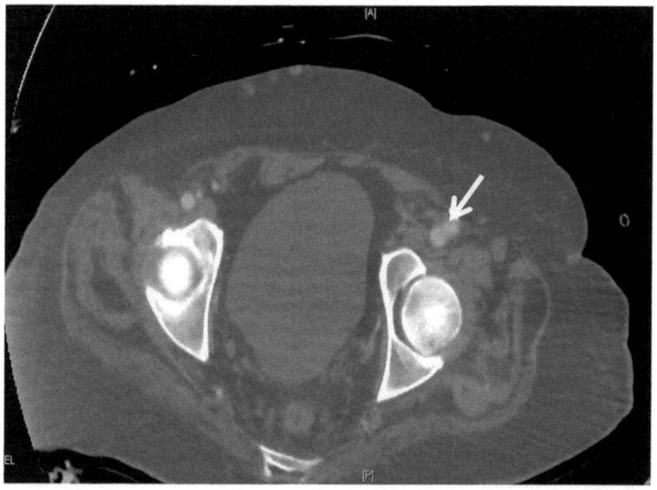

Fig. 23.7 CT scan with contrast showing a common femoral artery pseudoaneurysm (*arrow*)

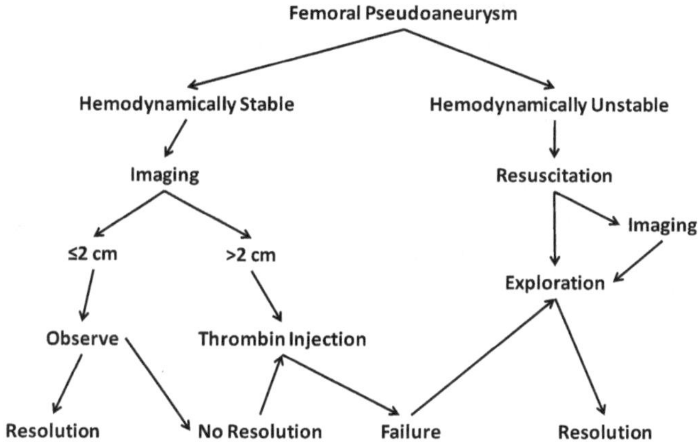

Fig. 23.8 Algorithm for the treatment of an uninfected femoral pseudoaneurysm

In many patients, the imaging quality of ultrasound diminishes above the inguinal ligament. Suspicion of a PSA originating from the external iliac artery should prompt evaluation with a CT scan (Fig. 23.7).

Treatment

Small femoral PSAs less than 2 cm in diameter usually clot spontaneously and do not require treatment. Failure to thrombose spontaneously has been associated with concomitant use of anticoagulation or antiplatelet agents [20]. Larger femoral PSAs usually warrant treatment to prevent subsequent complications including rupture or enlargement with compression of adjacent structures. Compression of the femoral vein can result venous thrombosis, while femoral nerve compression can lead to muscle weakness and dysesthesia. A treatment algorithm for femoral PSA is shown in Fig. 23.8.

Compression

Compression can obliterate flow within the PSA and allow it to thrombose. Ultrasound guidance provides confirmation that the PSA is being compressed while maintaining flow within the parent artery. Successful ultrasound-guided compression can last 30–45 min which often strains the comfort level of the patient and the sonographer.

Ultrasound-Guided Thrombin Injection

Ultrasound-guided thrombin injection (1,000 units) has emerged as the most common treatment for PSA in stable patients. The technique involves percutaneous puncture of the PSA sac to deliver a small volume of thrombin. Thrombosis ensues when the thrombin makes contact with the blood in the PSA. Before pursuing this treatment option, a thorough diagnostic duplex ultrasound should demonstrate a long, small caliber communication to the feeding artery (the so-called neck of the PSA). Injecting thrombin into a PSA with a short, wide neck increases the risk of inducing acute thrombosis of the native artery.

Exploration

Hemodynamic instability warrants prompt resuscitation and surgical exploration. In most cases, proximal vascular control and definitive primary repair can be performed through a groin incision.

Outcomes

While PSA thrombosis occurs within seconds of thrombin injection, the mean time required for ultrasound-guided compression is 30 min. Compression for PSA has fallen out of favor because of its relatively high failure rate and the fact that it is a labor-intensive procedure. A cost analysis shows that thrombin treatment saves vascular laboratory resource use but does not reduce overall hospital expenditures [21].

Aortoenteric Fistula: Diagnosis (Clinical and Imaging Findings), Management Priorities, and Treatment Options

Etiology

An aortoenteric fistula (AEF) is a communication between the aorta and adjacent bowel, which can occur at the level of the esophagus, duodenum, or small bowel. These fistulae can be primary or secondary depending on whether they form spontaneously or after previous surgery, respectively. Primary AEFs have a prevalence of 0.04–0.07 % and most commonly (83 % of cases) occur between the aorta and the third and fourth parts of the duodenum due to an atherosclerotic abdominal aortic aneurysm (AAA) [22] (Fig. 23.9).

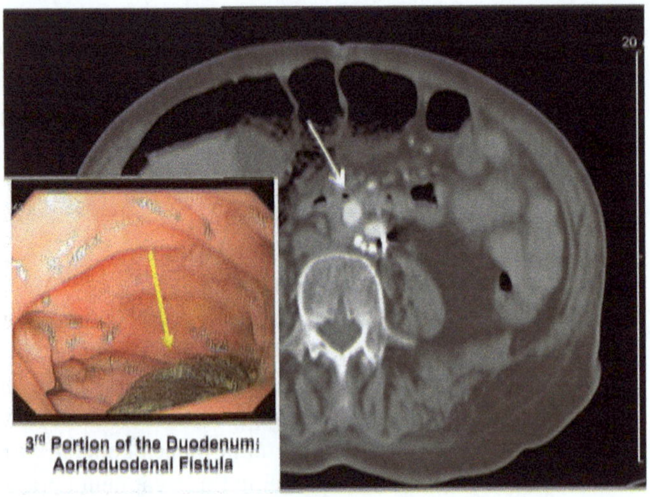

Fig. 23.9 CT scan showing an air pocket on the anterior surface of a limb of an aortobiiliac bypass graft (*white arrow*) at the level of the duodenum. The inset shows exposed Dacron (*yellow arrow*) in the duodenal lumen

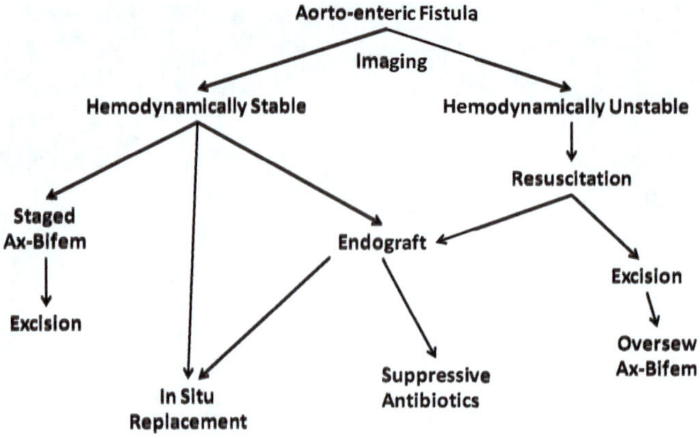

Fig. 23.10 Algorithm for the treatment of an aortoenteric fistula. *Ax-Bifem* axillobifemoral bypass

Other causes of primary AEF include esophageal cancer and mycotic aneurysms due to *Staphylococcus* infections [23]. Secondary AEFs occur after prior aortic surgery and complicate approximately 1.7 % of ruptured AAA repairs and 0.2 % of open elective AAA repairs. Vollmar and Kogel classified AEF as type I for direct aortoenteric communication, type IA and type IB as the absence or presence of a pseudoaneurysm, respectively, and type II as graft enteric erosion [24].

Presentation

The classic clinical triad of AEF consists of gastrointestinal (GI) bleeding, sepsis, and abdominal pain; however, the majority of patients with AEF do not have all three findings. GI bleeding in the form of hematemesis, hematochezia, melena, or chronic anemia is the most common presentation. Most patients present with a sentinel or herald bleed which foreshadows a potentially massive hemorrhage. A large portion of patients rebleed within 24 h of a herald bleed with reported mortality rates ranging from 14 to 46 % [25]. Less common presentations of AEF include sepsis alone, particularly when there are paraprosthetic enteric sinuses, and septic emboli to the legs.

Imaging

Contrast-enhanced CT scan is the imaging modality of choice to diagnose an AEF (Fig. 23.9). Fluid or gas collections around the aortic prosthesis (beyond 2–3 months after implantation) suggest an infection. Other radiographic signs of a vascular infection include false aneurysm formation, loss of normal retroperitoneal tissue planes, and vertebral osteomyelitis in a patient with an aortic graft. CT-guided aspiration is being increasingly used to differentiate a perigraft abscess from a seroma. Technetium (Tc)-99m-labeled white blood cells and indium (In 111) or gallium scintigrams are commonly used along with magnetic resonance imaging (MRI) and CT to define the extent of graft involvement. Positive predictive value of the functional imaging scans ranges from 80 to 90 % in the detection of graft infection [26]. Only 50 % of AEFs can be diagnosed by cross-sectional imaging modalities alone [27].

Treatment

The main treatment goal for AEF is to eradicate the infection while preserving blood flow to the target organs or limbs [28]. Figure 23.10 shows a treatment algorithm for patients with AEF.

Excision and Extra-anatomic Bypass

The most common clinical scenario involves a patient with a prosthetic aortic graft who develops a secondary AEF. If the patient is hemodynamically stable, surgery can be performed in two stages. During the first stage, an axillobifemoral bypass is performed originating from the right axillary artery. The proximal left femoral artery is ligated to prevent competitive flow from the pelvis. The next day, a midline laparotomy or left retroperitoneal approach provides exposure to excise the prosthetic aortic graft and oversew the native aortic stump. Wide debridement of the retroperitoneum and placement of closed suction drains ensures elimination of the infection. An omental flap placed over the native aortic stump provides tissue separation from the overlying small bowel and duodenum. The next step involves repairing the intestinal injuries. Some surgeons perform duodenal exclusion and a loop gastrojejunostomy to bypass the injured duodenum. A feeding jejunostomy tube is usually placed to facilitate postoperative enteral nutrition.

If the patient is hemodynamically unstable, graft excision and extra-anatomic bypass must be performed as part of the same operation. Emergent repair of an AEF uses the same techniques and exposure as an open repair of a ruptured AAA. Proximal and distal vascular control allows for excision of the prosthetic graft. After repairing the small bowel or duodenum, the abdomen is closed, and an axillobifemoral bypass is constructed to restore lower extremity perfusion.

In Situ Interposition Bypass

In situ replacement of the infrarenal aorta can be performed with autologous femoral veins, cryopreserved arterial tissue, or rifampicin-soaked Dacron gel grafts. The neoaortoiliac system (NAIS) technique harvests the femoral vein from both thighs to replace infected aortobiiliac or aortobifemoral bypass grafts. Graft excision and replacement with cryopreserved or rifampicin-soaked Dacron is performed as a single-stage surgery with wide debridement of the retroperitoneum and placement of an omental flap over the new grafts.

Endovascular Exclusion

The rise of endovascular therapy has introduced the technique of endovascular exclusion to treat primary AEFs. Case reports and small series have described thoracic aortic stent graft placement for aortoesophageal fistulae and abdominal aortic stent graft placement for AEFs. The feasibility of endovascular intervention for secondary AEFs depends on the local anatomy and landing sites. Although endovascular exclusion offers a dramatically less invasive treatment option for AEFs, it deviates from the core surgical principle of eliminating the source of infection. Infection can persist after endovascular repair since the prosthetic graft is not removed, the intestinal injury is not repaired, and the surrounding tissue is not debrided or drained. Most vascular surgeons consider endovascular exclusion as a temporizing measure for the hemodynamically unstable patient. Placing the stent graft can stop the bleeding allowing time to resuscitate the patient and plan for removal of the infected graft and definitive revascularization. Foregoing a second stage and leaving the endograft in place may be the only reasonable treatment strategy in severely debilitated patients who would not survive graft removal surgery. In these rare cases, the patient is usually maintained on lifelong suppressive antibiotics.

Outcomes

For in situ Dacron graft replacement, patients have a 30-day operative mortality of 17 % [29]. A 30-day mortality for all cryopreserved arterial grafts is 7.5 % [30].

The NAIS procedure has a 30-day mortality of 10 % and a procedure-related mortality of 14 %. Multivariate analysis of patients undergoing the NAIS procedure identified several independent risk factors for perioperative death including: preoperative sepsis, ASA class 4, and microbial cultures with *Candida* species or gram-negative bacteria. Cumulative primary patency of the reconstructed aortoiliac system was 60–80 % at 72 months; secondary/assisted primary patency was 70–90 %, and limb salvage at 72 was 60–90 %. The overall 5-year survival was less than 50 % [31].

Relatively small case series have reported 30-day mortality rates of 0–10 % after endovascular stent graft placement for secondary AEF involving the thoracic or abdominal aorta [32]. Within 12 months, over half of the patients who survived the initial surgery showed signs of reinfection and required reoperation despite ongoing antibiotic treatment [33]. These results reinforce the principle that endovascular therapy for AEF should be viewed as a temporizing measure to stop exsanguination and allow preparation for definitive graft excision.

Infected Bypass Graft: Pathophysiology, Diagnosis (Clinical and Imaging Findings), and Treatment Principles

Etiology

Vascular prosthetic graft infections occur in approximately 1–5 % of patients, including early and late clinical presentation. The incidence of infection depends on the anatomic site with hemodialysis grafts and infrainguinal grafts having the highest infection rates. Vascular infections occur more commonly in groin incisions (60 % of cases), in subcutaneously tunneled grafts, and in grafts placed under emergency conditions (e.g., acute limb ischemia). Groin wounds can be categorized as superficial infections without exposed vascular graft or suture line (Szilagyi I) or deep infections without (Szilagyi II) or with (Szilagyi III) exposed vascular graft or suture line [34]. Vascular infections can also be classified in terms of appearance time as early (less than 4 weeks after graft implantation) or late (greater than 4 weeks).

Variables that determine the risk of vascular graft infection include: the patient's comorbidities and immune status, the type of procedure, the coexistence of other inflammation sites, the type of perioperative prophylactic antibiotics, and the length of hospital stay. Infection rates increase with reoperative surgery, long operative times, breaks in sterile surgical technique, and postoperative complications (such as hematoma, graft thrombosis). Infections affect autogenous vein bypass grafts and native fistulae at a significantly lower rate than that of prosthetic grafts. Extremely low rates of infection (0.5 %) have also been reported after percutaneous balloon angioplasty and stenting [35].

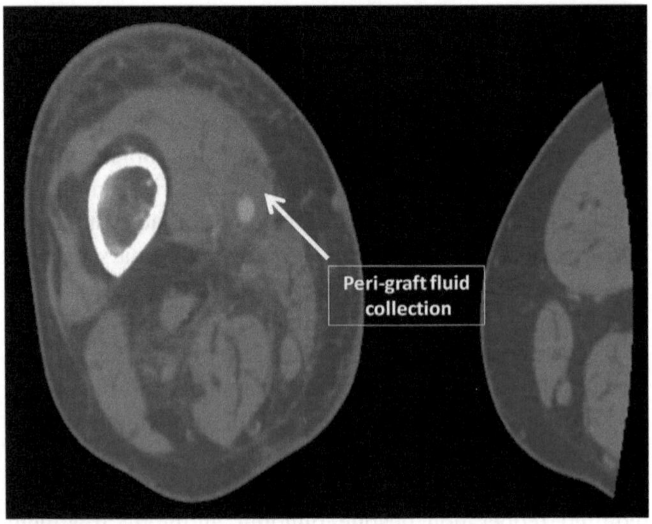

Fig. 23.11 CT scan showing perigraft fluid collection (*arrow*) in a patient with systemic sepsis

Presentation

Infected bypass grafts may present as a fever of unknown origin, purulent drainage from an incision, swelling over a previous anastomotic site, or graft occlusion with resultant ischemia. Some graft infections cause anastomotic dehiscence leading to acute pseudoaneurysm formation and bleeding. In a patient with a vascular graft and a fever, bleeding from an incision can represent a sentinel bleed indicating underlying infection. Although blood cultures are rarely positive (less than 5 %), the presence of bacteremia along with high fever indicates advanced infection and sepsis. Multivariate predictors of infections after bypass surgery include female gender, obesity, chronic obstructive pulmonary disease, hemodialysis, preoperative hyponatremia, and length of operation (greater than 4 h) [36].

Imaging

Duplex ultrasound can evaluate the bypass graft for signs suggesting a vascular infection including the presence of a pseudoaneurysm and perigraft fluid. A contrast CT scan or CT angiography demonstrates the extent of infection and provides images of the inflow and runoff vessels (Fig. 23.11). It is important to note that normal imaging studies do not preclude the presence of vascular graft infection. Purulent drainage in proximity to a vascular graft requires exploration even in the absence of bleeding, pseudoaneurysm formation, and abnormal sonographic or CT findings.

Treatment

Definitive treatment for a vascular graft infection involves complete removal of the bypass graft with debridement and drainage of the perigraft tissue. The morbidity associated with this approach including frequent limb loss spurred interest in techniques aimed at treating the infection without sacrificing the entire graft and risking amputation. Determining which patients are appropriate for graft preservation can be challenging. Selective management of infrainguinal graft infection involves a careful examination of the clinical situation and the application of several important principles:

1. Graft preservation can be attempted when the graft is patent, the anastomosis is intact, and the patient is not septic.
2. Graft excision is mandatory when the patient has a thrombosed infected graft, anastomotic or graft hemorrhage, or significant systemic sepsis.
3. Graft preservation can be attempted in both vein and polytetrafluoroethylene (PTFE) grafts, but is not advised for Dacron grafts.
4. Delayed hemorrhage and continued systemic sepsis represent early failures of graft preservation and mandate graft excision.
5. Although revascularization can be accomplished through the infected bed, an extra-anatomic reconstruction using alternative exposure of the inflow and outflow vessels is generally prudent.

The decision to preserve the bypass graft or proceed with an in situ reconstruction should be tempered by the extent and virulence of the underlying infection, especially when *Pseudomonas aeruginosa* is the pathologic organism [23]. In general, patients, who have gram-negative pathogens or *Staphylococcus aureus* (including methicillin resistant) isolated, require conventional graft excision and extra-anatomic bypass. In contrast, a prosthetic infection secondary to *Staphylococcus epidermidis* can be managed with less extensive procedures which can include segmental resection and in situ replacement with antibiotic-bonded prostheses. A treatment algorithm for vascular graft infection is shown in Fig. 23.12.

Exploration

The wound should be explored with provisions for proximal vascular control and rapid transfusion. If there has been a sentinel bleed or acute hemorrhage, then proximal control should be secured before exploring the primary wound. If the decision to perform extra-anatomic bypass has already been made based on preoperative data, then wound exploration should be performed after completing the new bypass.

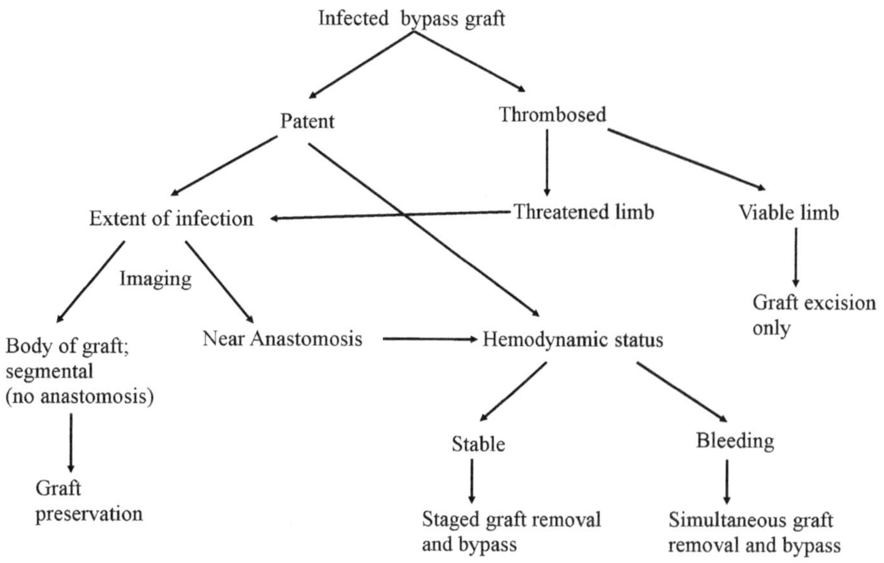

Fig. 23.12 Algorithm for the treatment of an infected bypass graft. *NPWT* negative pressure wound therapy

Debridement

Full and complete debridement of skin, subcutaneous tissue, muscle, and the infected vessels should be performed to eradicate the infection. The extent of purulence and severity of infection should dictate the scope of debridement.

Antibiotic Beads

Antibiotic beads consisting of polymethylmethacrylate cement mixed with two antibiotics can be placed in the wound in an attempt to sterilize it and allow for graft preservation. The beads are then replaced every 2 days until serial deep wound cultures show no growth, and then a muscle flap should be considered. Using this protocol, wound sterilization based on cultures was achieved in over 90 % of cases, and the reinfection rate was 10–20 % [37].

Negative Pressure Wound Therapy (NPWT)

NPWT has been used in a variety of settings to stimulate granulation tissue, decrease edema, and accelerate wound closure. Data suggests that NPWT can also be used in vascular surgical wounds after aggressive debridement and sterilization of the wound. In selected patients, NPWT can help achieve graft preservation rates as high as 70 % [38]. Despite these promising reports, the use of NPWT can trigger life-threatening bleeding from the nearby vascular graft. To reduce this hemorrhagic risk, a tissue layer such as a muscle flap should be interposed between exposed vessels or grafts prior to placing the negative pressure device. NPWT may also not be appropriate for wounds with gross infection, pseudoaneurysm, lack of hemostasis, or weakened or irradiated vessels [39].

Muscle Flaps

The two most common muscle flaps used to cover wounds after treatment of an infected graft are the sartorius and the rectus femoris. After the initial exploration and drainage, wounds with necrotic tissue may require serial surgical debridements, antibiotic beads, NPWT, or wet-to-dry dressing changes. Small wounds can be covered with a turnover sartorius flap, while a muscle or musculocutaneous rectus femoris flap is more appropriate for larger wounds. Most plastic surgeons cite the advantages of a rectus femoris flap over the sartorius muscle for vascular wound coverage. The rectus femoris muscle has an axial blood supply that enters the muscle superiorly and originates from the profunda femoral artery. In contrast, the sartorius muscle has a segmental blood supply originating from the often diseased superficial femoral artery.

Graft Excision

Hemorrhage, pseudoaneurysm, and gross infection usually mandate complete graft excision. Proximal and distal vascular control should be obtained and care taken to preserve the proximal profunda femoral artery. Graft excision is best performed after revascularization unless ongoing bleeding from the graft requires immediate intervention.

Revascularization Options

New Bypass: Graft excision and placement of a new bypass at sites distant from the original bypass has proven to be an effective treatment for vascular infections. Most new bypass conduits are autogenous vein or cryopreserved tissue. Ideally, the procedure can be staged with the new bypass placed before excising the infected bypass graft.

In Situ Replacement: In situ replacement can be performed with autogenous tissue (great saphenous or femoral vein), cryopreserved arterial/venous tissue, or rifampicin-soaked Dacron. This technique is most commonly performed for femoral infections or focal infections involving a vein bypass graft. If the infected bypass originates from the femoral artery but the native artery is intact, a vein patch can be used to repair the vessel.

Extra-anatomic Bypass: Two extra-anatomic bypasses can be used to revascularize the lower extremity after removing an infected bypass graft.

- Transobturator bypass: originates on the external iliac artery and passes through the obturator foramen to the distal femoral vessels.
- Axillofemoral/popliteal bypass: begins on the ipsilateral axillary artery and terminates on the superficial femoral, profunda femoral, or popliteal artery.

Both bypasses route blood flow around the infected groin to restore distal circulation. Choices of conduit include PTFE, rifampicin-soaked Dacron, or cryopreserved arterial/venous tissue.

Endovascular Recanalization: If time permits and the infected graft is a bypass, it may be possible to recanalize the native vessels using an endovascular approach. Restoring some or all circulation can avoid the need for a new bypass. Balloon angioplasty alone is preferred as stents may become infected.

Outcomes

Morbidity and mortality, the likelihood of long-term limb salvage, and the risk of persistent or recurrent infection vary depending on the treatment strategy. In a large historical series, the reported rates for postoperative amputation and mortality were 40 and 18 %, respectively [40].

Conclusion

The aging population and high prevalence of atherosclerosis suggest that the number of patients undergoing vascular procedures will continue to increase. Unfortunately, advances in endovascular technology and minimally invasive surgery will never eliminate the possibility of complications. Hemorrhage or infection following a vascular intervention can have devastating consequences that demand prompt recognition and swift action. This chapter focuses on the most common vascular surgery complications including hemorrhage in the retroperitoneum, neck, and groin; pseudoaneurysms; aortoenteric fistulae; and infected lower extremity bypass grafts. Treatment algorithms provided throughout the chapter outline a rational, stepwise approach to managing each of these potentially life- or limb-threatening conditions.

References

1. Chan YC, Morales JP, Reidy JF, Taylor PR. Management of spontaneous and iatrogenic retroperitoneal haemorrhage: conservative management, endovascular intervention or open surgery? Int J Clin Pract. 2008;62:1604–13.
2. Farouque HM, Tremmel JA, Raissi Shabari F, et al. Risk factors for the development of etroperitoneal hematoma after percutaneous coronary intervention in the era of glycoprotein IIb/IIIa inhibitors and vascular closure devices. J Am Coll Cardiol. 2005;45:363–8.
3. Parmer SS, Carpenter JP, Fairman RM, Velazquez OC, Mitchell ME. Femoral neuropathy following retroperitoneal hemorrhage: case series and review of the literature. Ann Vasc Surg. 2006;20:536–40.
4. Cox N. Managing the femoral artery in coronary angiography. Heart Lung Circ. 2008;17 Suppl 4:S65–9.
5. Farrelly C, Fidelman N, Durack JC, Hagiwara E, Kerlan RK. Transcatheter arterial embolization of spontaneous life-threatening extraperitoneal hemorrhage. J Vasc Interv Radiol. 2011;22:1396–402.
6. Burgess CA, Dale OT, Almeyda R, Corbridge RJ. An evidence based review of the assessment and management of penetrating neck trauma. Clin Otolaryngol. 2012;37:44–52.
7. Biffl WL, Cothren CC, Moore EE, Kozar R, Cocanour C, Davis JW, McIntyre RC. Western Trauma Association critical decisions in trauma: screening for and treatment of blunt cerebrovascular injuries. J Trauma. 2009;67:1150–3.
8. Cohen J, Rad I. Contemporary management of carotid blowout. Curr Opin Otolaryngol Head Neck Surg. 2004;12:110–5.
9. Powitzky R, Vasan N, Krempl G, Medina J. Carotid blowout in patients with head and neck cancer. Ann Otol Rhinol Laryngol. 2010;19:476–84.
10. Kesser BW, Chance E, Kleiner D, et al. Contemporary management of penetrating neck trauma. Am Surg. 2009;75:1–10.
11. American College of Surgeons Committee on Trauma. ATLS student course manual. Chicago: American College of Surgeons; 2008.
12. McConnell DB, Trunkey DD. Management of penetrating trauma to the neck. Adv Surg. 1994;27:97–127.
13. Fox CJ, Gillespie DL, Weber MA, et al. Delayed evaluation of combat-related penetrating neck trauma. J Vasc Surg. 2006;44:86–93.
14. Arthurs ZM, Sohn VY, Starnes BW. Vascular trauma: endovascular management and techniques. Surg Clin North Am. 2007;87:1179–92.
15. Das R, Ahmed K, Athanasiou T, Morgan RA, Belli AM. Arterial closure devices versus manual compression for femoral haemostasis in interventional radiological procedures: a systematic review and meta-analysis. Cardiovasc Intervent Radiol. 2011;34:723–38.
16. Hafez HM, Woolgar J, Robbs JV. Lower extremity arterial injury: results of 550 cases and review of risk factors associated with limb loss. J Vasc Surg. 2001;33:1212–9.
17. Kronzon I. Diagnosis and treatment of iatrogenic femoral artery pseudoaneurysm: a review. J Am Soc Echocardiogr. 1997;10:236–45.
18. Ahmad F, Turner SA, Torrie P, Gibson M. Iatrogenic femoral artery pseudoaneurysms–a review of current methods of diagnosis and treatment. Clin Radiol. 2008;63:1310–6.
19. Tisi PV, Callam MJ. Treatment for femoral pseudoaneurysms. Cochrane Database Syst Rev. 2009;(2):CD004981.
20. Toursarkissian B, Allen BT, Petrinec D, et al. Spontaneous closure of selected iatrogenic pseudoaneurysms and arteriovenous fistulae. J Vasc Surg. 1997;25:803–8.
21. Weinmann EE, Chayen D, Kobzantzev ZV, Zaretsky M, Bass A. Treatment of postcatheterization false aneurysms: ultrasound-guided

compression vs. ultrasound-guided thrombin injection. Eur J Vasc Endovasc Surg. 2002;23:68–72.
22. Ranasinghe W, Loa J, Allaf N, Lewis K, Sebastian MG. Primary aortoenteric fistulae: the challenges in diagnosis and review of treatment. Ann Vasc Surg. 2011;25:386–90.
23. Chiesa R, Astore D, Frigerio S, Garriboli L, Piccolo G, Castellano R, Scalamogna M, Odero A, Pirrelli S, Biasi G, Mingazzini P, Biglioli P, Polvani G, Guarino A, Agrifoglio G, Tori A, Spina G. Vascular prosthetic graft infection: epidemiology, bacteriology, pathogenesis and treatment. Acta Chir Belg. 2002;102:238–47.
24. Vollmar JF, Kogel H. Aorto-enteric fistulas as postoperative complication. J Cardiovasc Surg (Torino). 1987;28:479–84.
25. Armstrong PA, Back MR, Wilson JS, Shames ML, Johnson BL, Bandyk DF. Improved outcomes in the recent management of secondary aortoenteric fistula. J Vasc Surg. 2005;42:660–6.
26. Kashyap VS, O'Hara PJ. Local complications: aortoenteric fistulae. In: Cronenwett JL, Johnston KW, editors. Rutherford's Vascular surgery. 7th ed. Philadelphia: Elsevier; 2010.
27. Saers SJ, Schelting MR. Primary aortoenteric fistula. Br J Surg. 2005;92:143–52.
28. Seeger JM. Management of patients with prosthetic vascular graft infection. Am Surg. 2000;66(2):166–77.
29. Koshiko S, Sasajima T, Muraki S, et al. Limitations in the use of rifampicin-gelatin grafts against virulent organisms. J Vasc Surg. 2002;35:779.
30. Kieffer E, Gomes D, Chiche L, et al. Allograft replacement for infrarenal aortic graft infection: early and late results in 179 patients. J Vasc Surg. 2004;39:1009.
31. Beck AW, Murphy EH, Hocking JA, et al. Aortic reconstruction with femoro-popliteal vein: graft stenosis incidence, risk and reintervention. J Vasc Surg. 2008;47:36.
32. El Sakka K, Halawa M, Kotze C, et al. Complications of open abdominal aortic surgery: the endovascular solution. Interact Cardiovasc Thorac Surg. 2008;7:121.
33. Danneels M, Verhagen H, Teijink J, et al. Endovascular repair for aorto-enteric fistula: a bridge too far or a bridge to surgery. Eur J Vasc Endovasc Surg. 2006;32:27.
34. Szilagyi DE, Smith RF, Elliott JP, Vrandecic MP. Infection in arterial reconstruction with synthetic grafts. Ann Surg. 1972;176: 321–23.
35. Dosluoglu HH, Curl GR, Doerr RJ, et al. Stent-related iliac artery and iliac vein infections: two unreported presentations and review of the literature. J Endovasc Ther. 2001;8:202.
36. Siracuse JJ, Nandivada P, Giles KA, Hamden AD, Wyers MC, Chaikof EL, Pomposelli FB, Schermerhorn ML. Prosthetic graft infections involving the femoral artery. J Vasc Surg. 2013;57: 700–5.
37. Stone PA, Armstrong PA, Bandyk DF, Brumberg RS, Flaherty SK, Back MR, Shames ML. Use of antibiotic-loaded polymethylmethacrylate beads for the treatment of extracavitary prosthetic vascular graft infections. J Vasc Surg. 2006;44:757–61.
38. Dosluoglu H, Schimpf D, Schultz R, Cherr G. Preservation of infected and exposed vascular grafts using vacuum assisted closure without muscle flap coverage. J Vasc Surg. 2005;42:989–92.
39. Sumpio BE, Allie DE, Horvath KA, Marston WA, Meitsell HL, Mills JLR, Orgill DP, Salazar JD, Song DH, Toursarkissian B. Role of negative pressure wound therapy in treating peripheral vascular graft infections. Vascular. 2008;16:194–200.
40. Mertens RA, O'Hara PJ, Hertzer NR, Krajewski LP, Beven EG. Surgical management of infrainguinal arterial prosthetic graft infections: review of a thirty-five year experience. J Vasc Surg. 1995;21:782–91.

Index

V. Gahtan and M.J. Costanza (eds.), *Essentials of Vascular Surgery for the General Surgeon*, DOI 10.1007/978-1-4939-1326-8, © Springer Science+Business Media New York 2015

MIX
Papier aus verantwortungsvollen Quellen
Paper from responsible sources
FSC® C105338

If you have any concerns about our products,
you can contact us on
ProductSafety@springernature.com

In case Publisher is established outside the EU,
the EU authorized representative is:
Springer Nature Customer Service Center GmbH
Europaplatz 3, 69115 Heidelberg, Germany

Printed by Libri Plureos GmbH
in Hamburg, Germany